Advances in Mitochondrial Medicine

Advances in Experimental Medicine and Biology

Editorial Board:

For further volumes:
http://www.springer.com/series/5584

Preface

Mitochondria are far more than the "powerhouse" of the cell as they have classically been described. In fact, mitochondria biological activities have progressively expanded to include not only various bioenergetic processes but also important biosynthetic pathways, calcium homeostasis and thermogenesis, cell death by apoptosis, several different signal transduction pathways mainly related to redox control of gene expression and so on. This functional and structural complexity may undergo important derangements so to justify the definition of 'mitochondrial medicine', which should include all the clinical consequences of congenital or acquired mitochondrial dysfunctions. There are actually a growing number of studies which assign a significant pathogenic role to damaged mitochondria in different diseases: ischemia/reperfusion injury, neurodegenerative diseases, metabolic syndrome, hyperlipidemias, just to mention a few of the most important pathologies.

In this context, a further aspect that should not be disregarded is the interaction of pharmacological agents with mitochondria, not only in regard of the toxicological aspects but, above all, of the potential therapeutic applications. In fact, it is interesting to note that, while the properties of different so-called "mitoxicants" are well-known from a physical, chemical and biochemical point of view, the often subtle linkages between drugs and mitochondria is still in need of a real pharmacological and therapeutic control at the clinical level.

This lack of consideration can often lead to an underestimation of unwanted toxic effects but also of desirable therapeutic activities, both diverging outcomes resulting from drug induced modification of mitochondrial homeostasis.

The aim of this book is to stimulate a re-evaluation of the potential clinical role of mitochondria that could shed new light on some yet debated aspects of human pathophysiology.

Roberto Scatena

Contents

Part I Physiology and Structure of Mitochondria

1 The Oxidative Phosphorylation System in Mammalian Mitochondria 3
Sergio Papa, Pietro Luca Martino, Giuseppe Capitanio, Antonio Gaballo,
Domenico De Rasmo, Anna Signorile, and Vittoria Petruzzella

2 Physiology and Pathophysiology of Mitochondrial DNA 39
Hongzhi Li, Danhui Liu, Jianxin Lu, and Yidong Bai

3 Mitochondrial Ca^{2+} as a Key Regulator of Mitochondrial Activities 53
Tito Calì, Denis Ottolini, and Marisa Brini

4 Mitochondria and Nitric Oxide: Chemistry and Pathophysiology 75
Paolo Sarti, Marzia Arese, Elena Forte, Alessandro Giuffrè,
and Daniela Mastronicola

**5 Mitochondria and Reactive Oxygen Species. Which Role in Physiology
and Pathology?** 93
Giorgio Lenaz

**6 Uncoupling Proteins: Molecular, Functional, Regulatory, Physiological
and Pathological Aspects** 137
Francis E. Sluse

7 The Mitochondrial Pathways of Apoptosis 157
Jérome Estaquier, François Vallette, Jean-Luc Vayssiere, and Bernard Mignotte

Part II Mitochondria and Disease

8 Inherited Mitochondrial Disorders 187
Josef Finsterer

9 Role of Mitochondrial Function in Insulin Resistance 215
Myrte Brands, Arthur J. Verhoeven, and Mireille J. Serlie

10 Mitochondria and Diabetes. An Intriguing Pathogenetic Role 235
Philip Newsholme, Celine Gaudel, and Maurico Krause

11   Mitochondria and Heart Disease 249
Elinor J. Griffiths

12   Mitochondria in Neurodegeneration 269
Lezi E and Russell H. Swerdlow

**13   Mitochondria and Cancer: A Growing Role in Apoptosis, Cancer
Cell Metabolism and Dedifferentiation** 287
Roberto Scatena

Part III   Mitochondria, Aging and Pharmacotoxicological Aspects

14   Mitochondria and Aging 311
Hsin-Chen Lee and Yau-Huei Wei

15   Mitochondria and Drugs 329
Roberto Scatena

**16   Iatrogenic Mitochondriopathies: A Recent Lesson
from Nucleoside/Nucleotide Reverse Transcriptase Inhibitors** 347
George P.H. Leung

**17   Dysfunction of Mitochondrial Respiratory Chain Complex I
in Neurological Disorders: Genetics and Pathogenetic Mechanisms** 371
Vittoria Petruzzella, Anna Maria Sardanelli, Salvatore Scacco,
Damiano Panelli, Francesco Papa, Raffaella Trentadue, and Sergio Papa

18   Anthracyclines and Mitochondria 385
Alvaro Mordente, Elisabetta Meucci, Andrea Silvestrini, Giuseppe Ettore
Martorana, and Bruno Giardina

Part IV   Applications of Mitochondrial Science

**19   Mitochondrial Proteomic Approaches for New Potential Diagnostic
and Prognostic Biomarkers in Cancer** 423
Patrizia Bottoni, Bruno Giardina, Alessandro Pontoglio, Salvatore Scarà,
and Roberto Scatena

20   Mitochondria in Anthropology and Forensic Medicine 441
Tomasz Grzybowski and Urszula Rogalla

Index 455

Contributors

Marzia Arese Department of Biochemical Sciences 'A. Rossi Fanelli', University of Rome "La Sapienza", Rome, Italy

Yidong Bai Zhejiang Provincial Key Laboratory of Medical Genetics, Wenzhou Medical College, Wenzhou, Zhejiang 325035, China

Department of Cellular and Structural Biology, University of Texas Health Sciences Center at San Antonio, San Antonio, TX 78229, USA, baiy@uthscsa.edu

Patrizia Bottoni Institute of Biochemistry and Clinical Biochemistry, School of Medicine, Catholic University, Rome, Italy, patrizia.bottoni@rm.unicatt.it

Myrte Brands Department of Endocrinology and Metabolism, Academic Medical Center, F5-167, Meibergdreef 9, 1105 AZ, Amsterdam, The Netherlands, M.Brands@amc.uva.nl

Marisa Brini Department of Comparative Biomedicine and Food Science, University of Padova, Viale G. Colombo, 3, 35131 Padova, Italy, marisa.brini@unipd.it

Tito Calì Department of Comparative Biomedicine and Food Sciences, University of Padova, Viale G. Colombo, 3, 35131 Padova, Italy

Department of Biomedical Sciences, University of Padova, Padova, Italy

Giuseppe Capitanio Department of Medical Biochemistry, Biology and Physics (DIBIFIM), University of Bari, Bari, Italy

Lezi E Departments of Neurology, Molecular and Integrative Physiology, University of Kansas School of Medicine, MSN 2012, Landon Center on Aging, Kansas City, KS, USA, le2@kumc.edu

Jérome Estaquier Faculté Créteil Henri Mondor, Institut National de la Sante et de la Recherche Médicale, U955, 8 Rue du Général Sarrail, 94010, Créteil, France

Josef Finsterer Danube University Krems, Vienna, Austria, Europe, fifigs1@yahoo.de

Elena Forte Department of Biochemical Sciences 'A. Rossi Fanelli', University of Rome "La Sapienza", Rome, Italy

Antonio Gaballo Institute of Biomembranes and Bioenergetics (IBBE), Italian Research Council, (CNR), Bari, Italy

Celine Gaudel UCD School of Biomolecular and Biomedical Science and UCD Institute of Sport and Health, UCD Dublin, Belfield Dublin 4, Ireland

Bruno Giardina Institute of Biochemistry and Clinical Biochemistry, Catholic University School of Medicine, Rome, Italy, bgiardina@rm.unicatt.it

Alessandro Giuffrè CNR Institute of Molecular Biology and Pathology, University of Rome "La Sapienza", Rome, Italy

Elinor J. Griffiths Department of Biochemistry, School of Medical Sciences, University Walk, Bristol, UK, Elinor.Griffiths@bristol.ac.uk

Bristol Heart Institute and Department of Biochemistry, University of Bristol, Bristol, UK

Tomasz Grzybowski Ludwik Rydygier Collegium Medicum, Department of Molecular and Forensic Genetics, The Nicolaus Copernicus University, M.curie-Sklodowskiej str. 9, 85-094 Bydgoszcz, Poland, tgrzyb@cm.umk.pl

Maurico Krause UCD School of Biomolecular and Biomedical Science and UCD Institute of Sport and Health, UCD Dublin, Belfield Dublin 4, Ireland

Biomedical Research Group (BMRG), Department of Science, Institute of Technology Tallaght, Dublin 24, Ireland

Hsin-Chen Lee Institute of Pharmacology, School of Medicine, National Yang-Ming University, Taipei, Taiwan 112, Republic of China, hclee2@ym.edu.tw

Giorgio Lenaz Dipartimento di Biochimica "G. Moruzzi", Università di Bologna, Via Irnerio 48, 40126 Bologna, Italy, giorgio.lenaz@unibo.it

George P.H. Leung Department of Pharmacology and Pharmacy, The University of Hong Kong, Hong Kong, China, gphleung@hkucc.hku.hk

Hongzhi Li Zhejiang Provincial Key Laboratory of Medical Genetics, Wenzhou Medical College, Wenzhou, Zhejiang 325035, China

Danhui Liu Zhejiang Provincial Key Laboratory of Medical Genetics, Wenzhou Medical College, Wenzhou, Zhejiang 325035, China

Jianxin Lu Zhejiang Provincial Key Laboratory of Medical Genetics, Wenzhou Medical College, Wenzhou, Zhejiang 325035, China

Pietro Luca Martino Department of Medical Biochemistry, Biology and Physics (DIBIFIM), University of Bari, Bari, Italy

Giuseppe Ettore Martorana Institute of Biochemistry and Clinical Biochemistry, Catholic University School of Medicine, Rome, Italy

Daniela Mastronicola Department of Biochemical Sciences 'A. Rossi Fanelli', University of Rome "La Sapienza", Rome, Italy

Elisabetta Meucci Institute of Biochemistry and Clinical Biochemistry, Catholic University School of Medicine, Rome, Italy

Bernard Mignotte Laboratoire de Génétique et Biologie Cellulaire, EA4589, Université Versailles St-Quentin, Ecole Pratique des Hautes Etudes, 45 av des Etats-Units, 78035 Versailles cedex, France, bernard.mignotte@uvsq.fr

Alvaro Mordente Institute of Biochemistry and Clinical Biochemistry, Catholic University School of Medicine, Rome, Italy, alvaro.mordente@rm.unicatt.it

Philip Newsholme UCD School of Biomolecular and Biomedical Science and UCD Institute of Sport and Health, UCD Dublin, Belfield Dublin 4, Ireland

School of Biochemical Sciences, Building 308 Room 122, GPO Box U1987, Curtin University, Perth, Western Australia 6845, philip.newsholme@ucd.ie

Denis Ottolini Department of Biomedical Sciences, University of Padova, Viale G. Colombo 3 35131, Padova, Italy

Department of Experimental Veterinary Sciences, University of Padova, Padova, Italy

Damiano Panelli Department of Medical Biochemistry, Biology and Physics (DIBIFIM), University of Bari, Policlinico, P. zza G. Cesare, 70124 Bari, Italy

Francesco Papa Department of Dental Sciences and Surgery, University of Bari, Bari, Italy

Sergio Papa Department of Medical Biochemistry, Biology and Physics (DIBIFIM), University of Bari, Bari, Italy

Institute of Biomembranes and Bioenergetics (IBBE), Italian Research Council, (CNR), Bari, Italy, s.papa@biochem.uniba.it.

Vittoria Petruzzella Department of Medical Biochemistry, Biology and Physics (DIBIFIM), University of Bari, Policlinico, P. zza G. Cesare, 70124 Bari, Italy

Institute of Biomembranes and Bioenergetics (IBBE), Italian Research Council, (CNR), Bari, Italy

Alessandro Pontoglio Institute of Biochemistry and Clinical Biochemistry, School of Medicine, Catholic University, Rome, Italy, espeedy@libero.it

Domenico De Rasmo Department of Medical Biochemistry, Biology and Physics (DIBIFIM), University of Bari, Bari, Italy

Urszula Rogalla Ludwik Rydygier Collegium Medicum, Department of Molecular and Forensic Genetics, The Nicolaus Copernicus University, M.curie-Sklodowskiej str. 9, 85-094 Bydgoszcz, Poland

Anna Maria Sardanelli Department of Medical Biochemistry, Biology and Physics (DIBIFIM), University of Bari, Bari, Italy

Paolo Sarti Department of Biochemical Sciences 'A. Rossi Fanelli', University of Rome "La Sapienza", Piazzale Aldo Moro 5, I-00185, Rome, Italy, paolo.sarti@uniroma1.it

Salvatore Scacco Department of Medical Biochemistry, Biology and Physics (DIBIFIM), University of Bari, Bari, Italy

Salvatore Scarà Department of Laboratory Medicine, Catholic University, Rome, Italy

Roberto Scatena Institute of Biochemistry and Clinical Biochemistry, School of Medicine, Catholic University, Rome, Italy, r.scatena@rm.unicatt.it

Mireille Serlie Department of Endocrinology and Metabolism, Academic Medical Center, F5-167, Meibergdreef 9, 1105 AZ, Amsterdam, The Netherlands, M.J.Serlie@amc.uva.nl

Anna Signorile Department of Medical Biochemistry, Biology and Physics (DIBIFIM), University of Bari, Bari, Italy

Andrea Silvestrini Institute of Biochemistry and Clinical Biochemistry, Catholic University School of Medicine, Rome, Italy

Francis E. Sluse Laboratory of Bioenergetics and Cellular Physiology, Department of Life Sciences, Faculty of Sciences, University of Liege, Liege, Belgium, F.Sluse@ulg.ac.be

Russel H. Swerdlow Departments of Neurology, Molecular and Integrative Physiology, University of Kansas School of Medicine MSN 2012, Landon Center on Aging, Kansas City, KS, USA, rswerdlow@kumc.edu

Raffaella Trentadue Department of Medical Biochemistry, Biology and Physics (DIBIFIM), University of Bari, Bari, Italy

François Vallette Centre de Recherche en Cancérologie Nantes Angers (UMR 892 INSERM et 6299 CNRS/Université de Nantes), 9 Quai Moncousu, 44007 Nantes, France

Jean-Luc Vayssiere Laboratoire de Génétique et Biologie Cellulaire, EA4589, Université Versailles St-Quentin, Ecole Pratique des Hautes Etudes, 45 av des Etats-Units, 78035 Versailles cedex, France

Yau-Huei Wei Department of Biochemistry and Molecular Biology, National Yang-Ming University, Taipei, Taiwan, Republic of China

Department of Medicine, Mackay Medical College, Danshui, Taipei County, Taiwan, Republic of China

Part I
Physiology and Structure of Mitochondria

Chapter 1
The Oxidative Phosphorylation System in Mammalian Mitochondria

Sergio Papa, Pietro Luca Martino, Giuseppe Capitanio, Antonio Gaballo, Domenico De Rasmo, Anna Signorile, and Vittoria Petruzzella

Abstract The chapter provides a review of the state of art of the oxidative phosphorylation system in mammalian mitochondria. The sections of the paper deal with:

(i) the respiratory chain as a whole: redox centers of the chain and protonic coupling in oxidative phosphorylation
(ii) atomic structure and functional mechanism of protonmotive complexes I, III, IV and V of the oxidative phosphorylation system
(iii) biogenesis of oxidative phosphorylation complexes: mitochondrial import of nuclear encoded subunits, assembly of oxidative phosphorylation complexes, transcriptional factors controlling biogenesis of the complexes.

This advanced knowledge of the structure, functional mechanism and biogenesis of the oxidative phosphorylation system provides a background to understand the pathological impact of genetic and acquired dysfunctions of mitochondrial oxidative phosphorylation.

Keywords F_1F_o ATP synthase • Mitochondrial biogenesis • Mitochondrial protein import • Oxidative phosphorylation • Respiratory chain complexes

S. Papa (✉) • V. Petruzzella • D. De Rasmo
Department of Basic Medical Sciences, Section of Medical Biochemistry, University of Bari, Policlinico, P.zza G. Cesare, 70124 Bari, Italy

Institute of Biomembranes and Bioenergetics (IBBE), Italian Research Council, (CNR), Bari, Italy
e-mail: s.papa@biochem.uniba.it.

P.L. Martino • G. Capitanio • A. Signorile
Department of Basic Medical Sciences, Section of Medical Biochemistry, University of Bari, Policlinico, P.zza G. Cesare, 70124 Bari, Italy

A. Gaballo
Institute of Biomembranes and Bioenergetics (IBBE), Italian Research Council, (CNR), Bari, Italy

R. Scatena et al. (eds.), *Advances in Mitochondrial Medicine*, Advances in Experimental Medicine and Biology 942, DOI 10.1007/978-94-007-2869-1_1,
© Springer Science+Business Media B.V. 2012

1.1   Introduction

House keeping and specialized endoergonic cellular functions of human organs depend on the metabolic cell capacity to extract free energy from nutrients and to convert it to that of the β-γ pyrophosphate bond of adenosintriphosphate. ATP in turn is utilised to drive endoergonic cell functions. In mammalian cells the ATP produced by mitochondrial respiratory chain oxidative phosphorylation (OXPHOS) covers, under normal conditions, more than 80% of the ATP cell need. The remaining is provided by anaerobic cytosolic degradation of nutrients, mainly glycolysis. Mitochondrial respiration accomplishes complete oxidation of substrates, derived from nutrients, to H_2O, CO_2 and NH_3. Mitochondria also perform the initial steps of urea biosynthesis. These final catabolic products are easily excreted from the body, thus preventing, under normal conditions, deleterious accumulation of metabolic scores like oxygen radicals and other radical species, organic acids and NH_3. Under conditions leading to excess of reducing power, in the form of NADH, utilised for biosyntetic reactions after transhydrogenation with $NADP^+$, this results in enhanced production of fatty acids and cholesterol. Elongation of fatty acids and partial reactions of heme biosynthesis and gluconeogenesis also take place in mitochondria.

Mitochondrial production of ATP requires continuous import in mitochondria of respiratory substrates, ADP and P_i and export of ATP. The adenine translocator, P_i carrier, pyruvate carrier, as well as other members of the mitochondrial carrier family work continuously so as to ensure the normal occurrence of cellular energy metabolism and all the other metabolic processes which are partitioned between mitochondria and cytosol (Papa et al. 1971; Palmieri and Klingenberg 2004). A genetic and/or acquired defect in a step of respiratory metabolism, oxidative phosphorylation, mitochondrial biogenesis, biosynthetic pathways or mitochondrial translocators can result in significant metabolic dysfunction. From all this it clearly emerges that primary and secondary dysfunction of mitochondria, in the first place of respiratory chain oxidative phosphorylation, can have profound pathological impact in humans.

1.2   The Respiratory Chain as a Whole

1.2.1   The Redox Centers

The concept of the respiratory chain was developed by Keilin (1966) with the identification of cytochromes a, b, c as redox carriers in aerobic organisms linking in sequence the activating dehydrogenase of Wieland with the oxygen-activating enzyme of Warburg. Figure 1.1 provides the actual picture of the redox centers in the respiratory chain of mammalian mitochondria. Where indicated by a suffix electron transfer by cytochromes and iron-sulphur clusters exhibits pH dependence. This reflects cooperative H^+/e^- linkage at the centers (redox Bohr effect) (Papa et al. 1973; Papa 1976). Dotted boxes circumscribe the inner mitochondrial membrane enzyme complexes I, II, III and IV to which the redox centers are associated (see Sect. 1.3). Specific ubiquinone binding sites are present in complexes I, II and III respectively (Salerno and Ohnishi 1980; Meinhardt and Ohnishi 1992; Ohnishi and Salerno 2005). Reducing equivalents donated by $NADH/NAD^+$ at -320 mV, are accepted by FMN in complex I, passed to a series of Fe-S centers and leave the last Fe-S center (N2) in the complex at an E_m of $-50/-150$ mV (Fig. 1.1). Electrons from complex I, succinate dehydrogenase, acylCoAFp dehydrogenases-ETF-ETF dehydrogenase and glycerolphosphate dehydrogenase converge into the ubiquinone pool (Q_p) at an E_m around zero. Ubiquinone transfers electrons to b cytochromes in complex III. In this complex electrons move down the Fe.S center and cyt c_1, with the involvement of protein bound quinone(s) (Meinhardt and Ohnishi 1992), and are passed to cyt c (E_m +230 mV). Ferrocytochrome c is oxidized in the reduction of molecular oxygen to 2 H_2O by aa_3 cytochrome c oxidase. The free energy made available by electron flow from NADH or flavin nucleotides to O_2 is conserved as a

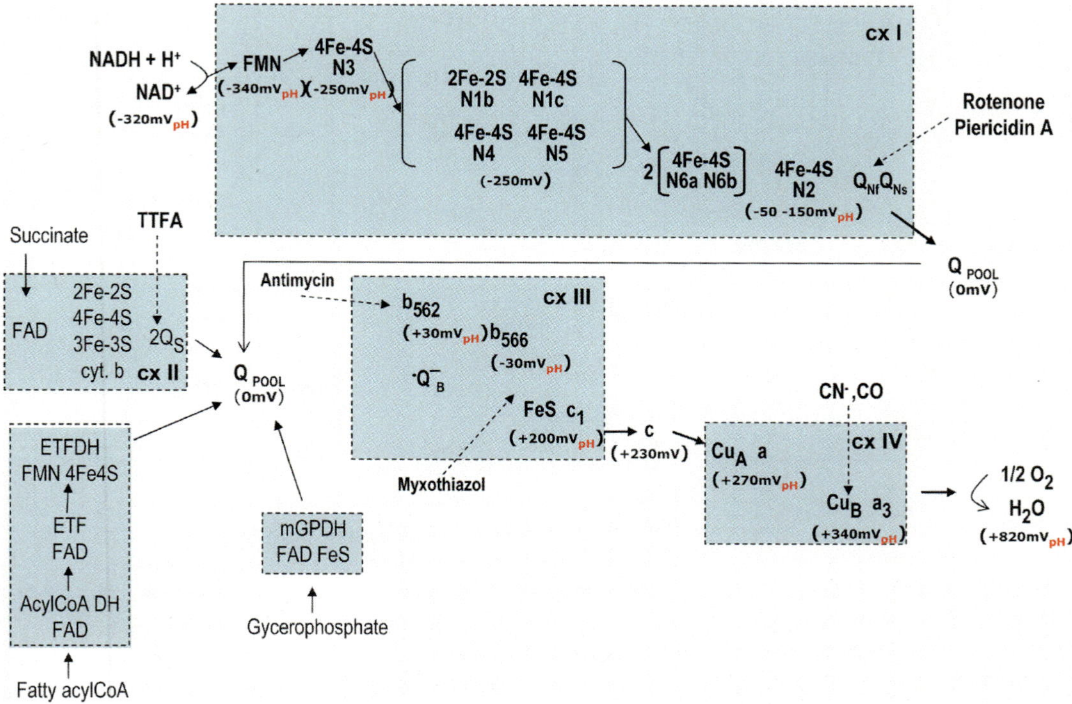

Fig. 1.1 Electron transfer centers of the respiratory chain in mammalian mitochondria. The centers are schematically shown with their midpoint potentials under standard conditions 25°C and pH 7.0. Qpool: ubiquinone of the pool, Q_B: protein bound ubiquinone. Specific inhibitor sites are also shown. Rotenone, antimycin and myxothiazol exert their inhibitory effect by interacting specifically with ubiquinone sites present in complex I (QNs, QNf) and complex III (Qi and Qo). For more details see (Beinert 1986; Brandt 1997; Ohnishi 1998) (Modified from Fig. 2 of Papa et al. 2007)

transmembrane electrochemical proton gradient (protonmotive force, PMF), which is then utilized to make ATP from ADP and P_i (Mitchell 1966; Papa 1976; Wikström et al. 1981a).

Some redox centers in the respiratory chain, like FMN radical and ubisemiquinone in complex I and complex III can be directly oxidized by dioxygen with the transfer of a single electron to O_2 and generation of oxygen superoxide O_2^- (Fig. 1.2) (Chance et al. 1979; Cadenas and Davies 2000). This is an extremely reactive free radical which can directly oxidize proteins, lipids, nucleic acids and/or dismutate to H_2O_2 by the mitochondrial Mn-superoxide dismutase (Mn-SOD). H_2O_2 can be converted to OH· by Fe^{2+}. O_2^- produced at the cytosolic surface of the inner mitochondrial membrane can be oxidized by cytochrome c and cytochrome c oxidase or converted to H_2O_2 by the cytosolic Cu, Zn-SOD. Inactivation of mitochondrial Mn-SOD in transgenic mice has been found to result in lethal dilated cardiomyopathy, with inactivation of mitochondrial enzymes containing iron-sulfur centers (Bironaite et al. 1991). The level of oxygen reactive species (ROS) can be enhanced by defects in respiratory complexes or by inhibitors of complex III and complex I or neurotoxic meperidine analogue derivatives, which cause Parkinsonism-like symptoms (Cortopassi and Wang 1995). A particularly deleterious situation seems to arise in patients with inherited disorders of complex I. Defects in the assembly or activity of the complex result in enhanced O_2^- production. This induces overexpression of the mitochondrial Mn-SOD, which increases production of H_2O_2 (Raha and Robinson 2000). Superoxide can react with NO, produced by the cytosolic nitric oxide synthase or directly by the mitochondrial isozyme (Tatoyan and Giulivi 1998), with formation of the peroxy-nitrite anion ($ONOO^-$). NO can reversibly inhibit cytochrome c oxidase (Brown 1999) and $ONOO^-$ can oxidatively damage respiratory complexes with further production of O_2^-, thus setting in a deleterious cascade of

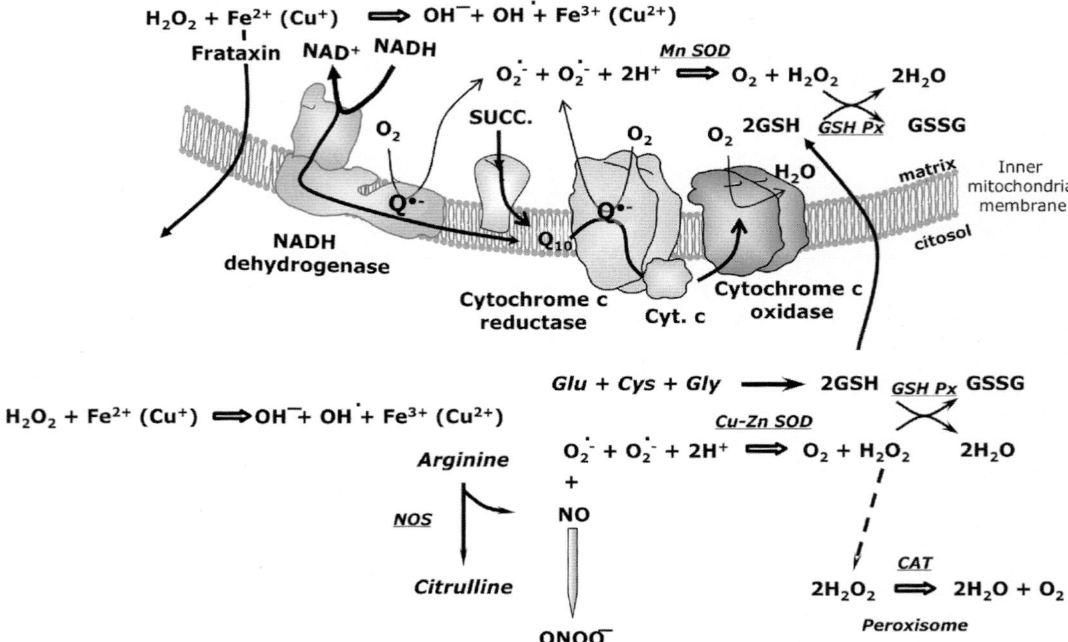

Fig. 1.2 ROS production in complex I and III of the mammalian mitochondrial respiratory chain and ROS scavenger enzymes

events (Papa 1996; Beckman and Koppenol 1996). In both the mitochondrial matrix and cytosol H_2O_2 is reduced to water by glutathione peroxidase. H_2O_2, which diffuses to peroxisomes, is cleaved there by catalase to water and oxygen (Fig. 1.2) (Chance et al. 1979).

1.2.2 Protonic Coupling in Respiratory Chain Oxidative Phosphorylation

The flow of four reducing equivalents down the respiratory chain from NADH to O_2, which is reduced to 2 H_2O, is directly coupled to the translocation of 20 protons from the mitochondrial matrix to the outer mitochondrial space (Fig. 1.3) (Papa 1976; Wikström et al. 1981a; Papa et al. 1999). These protons are utilized by the F_1F_0 ATP synthase (complex V) of the mitochondrial inner membrane to drive the synthesis of 5 ATP molecules from ADP and inorganic phosphate. Fifteen H^+ are directly utilised in the synthesis of ATP, five H^+ for phosphate uptake and charge neutralization of the electrogenic exchange of ATP^{4-} from the matrix with ADP^{3-} from the cytosol (Fig. 1.3). The overall P/O ratio of oxidative phosphorylation is 2.5 and not 3 as previously reported (Hinkle 2005). Of the 20 H^+ expelled from mitochondria, 8 H^+ are released out during electron flow from NADH to ubiquinone of the pool, 8 H^+ in electron flow from ubiquinol to cytochrome c and $4H^+$ for electron flow from reduced cytochrome c to oxygen. H^+ pumping at these three coupling sites is operated by complex I, III and IV respectively (see Sect. 1.3 for the mechanism of proton pumping in these complexes). Electron flow from flavin dehydrogenases to O_2 results in the extrusion of 12 H^+ and the synthesis of ATP with a P/O ratio of 1.5. The flavin dehydrogenases which transfer electrons from the respective substrates to ubiquinone don't pump protons. Controlled dissipation of the PMF by proton back flow mediated by the uncoupling protein of the inner mitochondrial membrane (Ricquier 2005; Sluse et al. 2006) and slips in the proton pump of respiratory chain complexes (Papa et al. 2006a) can contribute under conditions of high reducing power to prevent excessive and harmful metabolic production of fatty acids and cholesterol as well as of oxygen free radicals (Papa and Skulachev 1997).

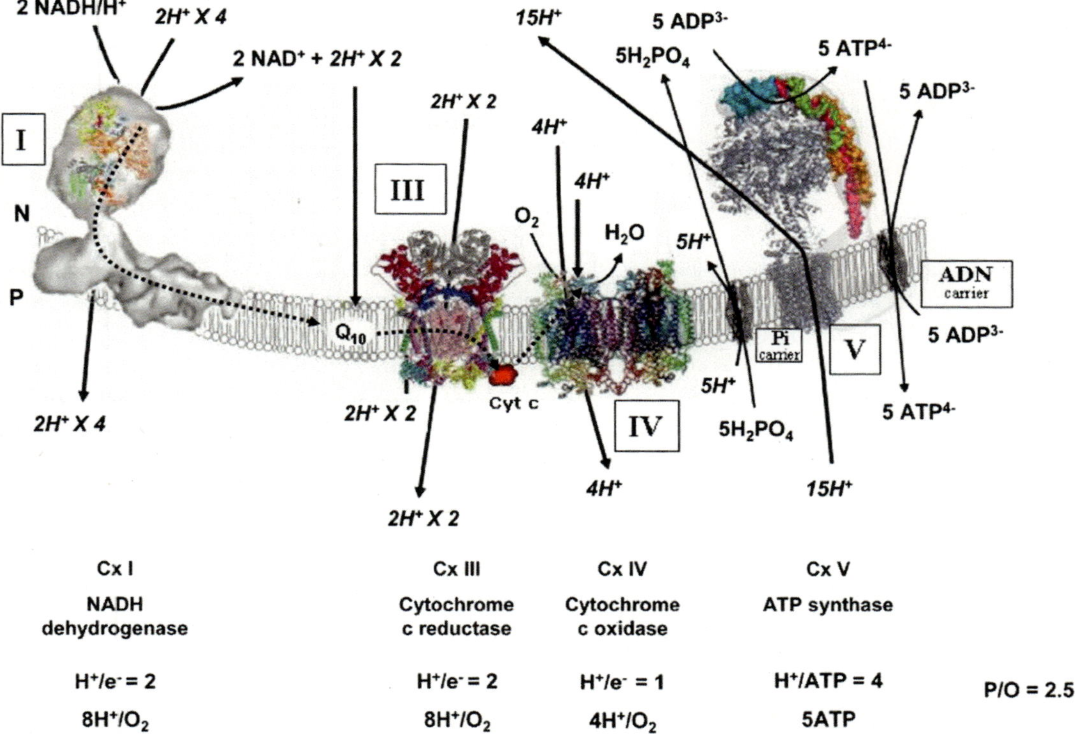

	Cx I		Cx III	Cx IV	Cx V
	NADH dehydrogenase		Cytochrome c reductase	Cytochrome c oxidase	ATP synthase
	$H^+/e^- = 2$		$H^+/e^- = 2$	$H^+/e^- = 1$	$H^+/ATP = 4$
	$8H^+/O_2$		$8H^+/O_2$	$4H^+/O_2$	5ATP

$P/O = 2.5$

Fig. 1.3 Protonic coupling in oxidative phosphorylation in the inner membrane of mammalian mitochondria. The scheme presents the 2D/3D structure of the respiratory complexes I, III and IV, ATP synthase, complex V, the adenine nucleotide translocator (*ADN*) and phosphate carrier inserted in the inner mitochondrial membrane. The shape of complex I results from high resolution electron microscopy image reconstitution (Friedrich and Böttcher 2004; Sazanov and Hinchliffe 2006), those of complex III (Xia et al. 1997; Hunte et al. 2000) and complex IV (Tsukihara et al. 1996) from X-ray crystallographic structures of the bovine heart enzymes. The shape of complex V results from X-ray (Abrahams et al. 1994; Stock et al. 1999) and electron microscopy structure reconstruction (Rubinstein et al. 2003). Complex III, IV and V are shown in the dimeric state as they appear in the structural analysis. The NADH protons are released in the *outer space upon* oxidation of ubiquinone in complex III. The *dotted line* traversing the complexes represents the flow of reducing equivalents from NADH to O_2. The maximal H^+/e^- (proton release per e^- transfer) ratios attainable for the three redox complexes and the H^+/ATP ratio for the ATP synthase are given at the *bottom* of the scheme. Proton and charge translocation for the import of $H_2PO_4^-$ and ADP^{3-} with export of ATP^{4-} is also shown. The overall balance of oxidative phosphorylation results in the production of 5 ATP in the oxidation of two molecules of NADH by one molecule of O_2. The P/O of 2.5 represents the maximal attainable efficiency of oxidative phosphorylation. Under certain physiological conditions the efficiency of oxidative phosphorylation can decrease since of slips in the redox proton pumps (Canton et al. 1995; Papa et al. 1995; Lorusso et al. 1995; Capitanio et al. 1996) and proton *back flow* by leaks, or mediated by the uncoupler protein (Ricquier and Bouillaud 2000). *N* side, matrix space; *P* side, cytosolic side

1.3   Structure and Protonmotive Activity of Oxidative Phosphorylation Complexes

The four redox complexes of the mammalian respiratory chain and F_1F_o ATP synthase can easily be purified in the active enzyme state (Hatefi 1985) and incorporated in phospholipid vesicles (Papa et al. 1996a) or planar phospholipid membranes (Bamberg et al. 1993). In this way it was shown that complex I, III and IV can each, separately, function as a redox-driven proton pump and the ATP synthase (Complex V) as a reversible proton pump. By direct protein analysis and extensive cDNA sequencing the primary structures of all the proteins of the complexes were determined. Nowadays proteomic analysis is providing additional information on these and associated proteins and their post-translational modifications (Taylor et al. 2003a; Palmisano et al. 2007; Pagliarini et al. 2008). The overall subunit pattern of the complexes, and their assembly status in the membrane can easily be obtained by two dimensional non-denaturing blue native electrophoresis/SDS PAGE (Schägger 2001). This procedure is now largely used to screen simultaneously subunit assembly of the five complexes in particular in mitochondrial diseases. It has also provided evidence indicating that the human respiratory complexes can be assembled in the inner mitochondrial membrane as supramolecular structures. Complexes I, III and IV, can apparently associate to form a structure denominated respirasome (Schagger and Pfeiffer 2000, 2001). The loss of complex III prevents respirasome formation and leads to a significant reduction of complex I (Schägger et al. 2004; Acín-Pérez et al. 2004). The possible functional implication of the dimeric form of complexes III, IV and V and of the association of complexes I, III and IV in the respirasome is under investigation in various laboratories. Complex II (succinate-ubiquinone oxidoreductase, SQR, E.C. 1.3.5.1) is an inner mitochondrial membrane intrinsic enzyme which participates in the citric acid cycle. SQR is very similar to the bacterial quinol/fumarate oxidoreductase (QFR) (Cecchini 2003). Succinate ubiquinone oxidoreductases generally contain four subunits, referred to as A, B, C and D. Subunits A and B are hydrophylic, whereas subunits C and D are integral membrane proteins. SQRs contain three iron-sulphur centres which are bound to the B subunit. The larger hydrophylic subunit A carries a covalently-bound flavin adenine dinucleotide (Toogood et al. 2007).

1.3.1 Complex I; NADH – Ubiquinone Oxidoreductase

Complex I (NADH – ubiquinone oxidoreductase, E.C. 1.6.5.3) is the first and the largest enzyme of mammalian and bacterial oxidative phosphorylation systems with a molecular weight ranging from $\approx$1,000 to $\approx$550 kDa respectively. The prokaryotic complex I consists of 14 conserved subunits, the mammalian mitochondrial complex of 45 different subunits (Table 1.1) (Yagi and Matsuno-Yagi 2003; Carroll et al. 2006a), of which seven are encoded by the mitochondrial genome, the others by nuclear genes (Table 1.1) (Hirst et al. 2003; Papa et al. 2007). The 14 conserved subunits constitute the minimal working core of the enzyme harbouring all the redox components (Fig. 1.1) (Guenebaut et al. 1998; Yagi and Matsuno-Yagi 2003): one FMN, eight to nine iron-sulfur clusters and one or two protein bound ubiquinone molecules.

The enzyme catalyzes the oxidation of NADH by ubiquinone conserving the free energy of the reaction as a transmembrane proton gradient (reaction 1.1) (Yagi and Matsuno-Yagi 2003; Papa et al. 2007).

$$\text{NADH} + \text{Q} + 5\text{H}^+_{\text{in}} \rightarrow \text{NAD}^+ + \text{QH}_2 + 4\text{H}^+_{\text{out}} \tag{1.1}$$

Complex I is a regulable pacemaker of the mitochondrial respiratory function (Hüttemann et al. 2007; Papa et al. 2008; Remacle et al. 2008; Yadava et al. 2008), is a major site of cellular oxygen superoxide production (Cadenas and Davies 2000; Grivennikova and Vinogradov 2006; Verkaart et al. 2007; Fato et al. 2008; Murphy 2009) and is involved in apoptosis (Angell et al. 2000; Fearnley et al. 2001; Palmisano et al. 2007) and age-related functional decline (Papa 1996; Ventura et al. 2002).

The first structural model of complex I was derived from two-dimensional crystals of the Neurospora crassa enzyme (Leonard et al. 1987; Hofhaus et al. 1991). Low-resolution structures of Escherichia coli (Guenebaut et al. 1998), Neurospora crassa (Guenebaut et al. 1997, 1998), bovine (Grigorieff 1998), Yarrowia lypolytica (Radermacher et al. 2006) and Aquifex aeolicus (Peng et al. 2003) complex I have also been obtained. A similar L-shaped structure has been determined for these complexes, with the hydrophobic arm embedded in the membrane and the hydrophilic arm protruding into the mitochondrial matrix or the bacterial cytoplasm (Friedrich and Böttcher 2004). The 3-dimensional crystal structure of the hydrophilic domain of complex I from Thermus thermophilus

Table 1.1 Gene nomenclature, protein denomination, molecular weight and functions of subunits of mammalian mitochondrial respiratory complex I (For details see the text)

Gene	Protein denomination	M.W. (kDa)	Redox cofactors	Biochemical features
NDUFA1	MWFE, NIMM	8.1		Phosphorylation
NDUFA2	B8, NI8M	11.0		
NDUFA3	B9, NI9M	9.2		
NDUFA4	MLRQ, NUML	9.3		
NDUFA5	B13, NUFM	13.2		
NDUFA6	B14, NB4M	15.0		
NDUFA7	B14.5a, N4AM	12.6		Ubiquinone binding?, phosphorylation
NDUFA8	PGIV, NUPM	20.0		
NDUFA9/ NDUFSL2	39 kDa, NUEM	39.1		NAD(P)H binding, phosphorylation
NDUFA10	42 kDa, NUDM	36.7		
NDUFAB1	SDAP, ACPM	10.1		Binds phosphopantothenine, ACP
NDUFB1	MNLL, NINM	7.0		
NDUFB2	AGGG, NIGM	8.5		
NDUFB3	B12, NB2M	11.0		
NDUFB4	B15, NB5M	15.1		
NDUFB5	SGDH, NISM	16.7		
NDUFB6	B17, NB7M	15.4		
NDUFB7	B18, NB8M	16.5		
NDUFB8	ASHI, NIAM	18.7		
NDUFB9	B22, NI2M	21.7		
NDUFB10	PDSW, NIDM	20.8		
NDUFC1	KFYI, NIKM	5.8		
NDUFC2	B14.5b, N4BM	14.1		Phosphorylation
NDUFS1	75 kDa, NUAM	77.0	3 (4Fe-4S): N4, N5 (2 Fe-2S): N1b	Electron transfer
NDUFS2	49 kDa, NUCM	49.2		Ubiquinone binding?
NDUFS3	30 kDa, NUGM	26.4		
NDUFS4	18 kDa (AQDQ), NUYM	15.3		Phosphorylation
NDUFS5	15 kDa, NIPM	12.5		
NDUFS6	13 kDa, NUMM	10.5		
NDUFS7	20 kDa (PSST), NUKM	20.1	(4Fe-4S): N2	Electron transfer
NDUFS8	20 kDa (TYKY), NUIM	20.2	2(4Fe-4S): N6a, N6b	Electron transfer, complex assembly-stability
NDUFV1	51 kDa, NUBM	48.4	FMN; (4Fe-4S): N3	NADH binding, electron transfer
NDUFV2	24 kDa, NUHM	23.8	(2Fe-2S): N1a	Antioxidant?
NDUFV3	10 kDa, NUOM	8.4		
–	B17.2	17.2		
NDUFB11	ESSS	13		Phosphorylation, assembly
–	B14.7	14.7		
–	B16.6	16.6		Homologous to GRIM-19, apoptosis?, phosphorylation
ND1 (mt)	NU1M	36.0		
ND2 (mt)	NU2M	39.0		
ND3 (mt)	NU3M	13.0		
ND4 (mt)	NU4M	52.0		
ND5 (mt)	NU5M	67.0		
ND6 (mt)	NU6M	19.0		Assembly
ND4L (mt)	NULM	11.0		

ACP, acyl-carrier protein

has been solved at 3.3 Å resolution (Sazanov and Hinchliffe 2006), establishing the putative electron transfer pathway from the primary electron acceptor flavin mononucleotide (FMN), through seven conserved iron-sulfur clusters, to protein bound semiquinone(s) and ubiquinone of the pool (Sazanov and Hinchliffe 2006). Two additional iron sulfur clusters do not participate to the main electron transfer chain. It has been proposed that they may represent an evolutionary remnant (cluster N7) (Sazanov and Hinchliffe 2006) and a possible anti-oxidant center (cluster N1a) (Yagi and Matsuno-Yagi 2003; Sazanov and Hinchliffe 2006; Kussmaul and Hirst 2006). All EPR detectable clusters, except N2, display a roughly similar midpoint potential (Fig. 1.1) (Dutton et al. 1998) suggesting that cluster N2 is the final electron mediator between the series of Fe-S centers and ubiquinone. The membrane-spanning part of the enzyme which lacks prosthetic groups (Carroll et al. 2006b) contributes to the proton translocation machinery.

Redox proton pumping in mammalian NADH ubiquinone oxidoreductase presents an upper limit stoicheiometry of 2 H^+/e^- (reaction 1.1) (Wikström 1984; Capitanio et al. 1991; Cocco et al. 2009). Various energy coupling mechanism for complex I have been proposed. These can be divided into two main types: (i) direct H^+ coupling mechanism at the redox centers (Vinogradov 1993; Degli Esposti and Ghelli 1994; Dutton et al. 1998); (ii) indirect or conformational H^+ coupling mechanism (Yagi and Matsuno-Yagi 2003; Brandt et al. 2003; Zickermann et al. 2009; Berrisford and Sazanov 2009). Conformational and direct coupling mechanisms are not mutually exclusive. A role of cluster N2 in proton pumping has been suggested (Magnitsky et al. 2002; Flemming et al. 2003). Papa et al. (1994; 1999) have proposed that a protein stabilized UQ^-/UQH_2 couple, transferring $2H^+$ per e^-, can represent the central element of the pump in complex I (see also Ohnishi and Salerno 2005). These authors developed a Q-gated proton pump model (Papa et al. 1999; Ohnishi and Salerno 2005). More recent crystallographic analysis of Esherichia coli (Efremov and Sazanov 2011) and Thermus thermophilus (Efremov et al. 2010) complex I have provided evidence for involvement of membrane-intrinsic subunits in a conformational-mechanical mechanism of proton pumping (see also Brandt et al. 2003; Berrisford and Sazanov 2009; Hunte et al. 2010).

Some of the supernumerary subunits of mammalian complex I participate in the assembly of the complex (Scacco et al. 2003; Antonicka et al. 2003; Scheffler et al. 2004; Papa et al. 2008), others appear to be involved in regulatory function (Papa et al. 2007, 2008; Hüttemann et al. 2007; Remacle et al. 2008; ; Yadava et al. 2008). The GRIM-19 (B16.6) belongs to the group of genes-associated with retinoid-interferon induced mortality (Fearnley et al. 2001). There is evidence showing that subunits NDUFS4 (18 kDa subunit) (Papa et al. 1996b; Technikova-Dobrova et al. 2001), NDUFB11 (ESSS subunit) and NDUFA1 (MWFE subunit) (Chen et al. 2004) are phosphorylated by cAMP dependent protein kinase. Phosphorylation of other subunits by protein kinase(s) has been observed like the NDUFA10 (which presents two isoforms) and NDUFA7 (Palmisano et al. 2007; Pocsfalvi et al. 2007). The phosphorylation state of these subunits "in vivo" and its possible impact on protein stability, import/assembly and functional activity of the complex are under investigation (Papa 2002; Pasdois et al. 2003; Scheffler et al. 2004; Maj et al. 2004; Papa et al. 2008). Additional post translational modifications have also been observed (Taylor et al. 2003a; Burwell et al. 2006). Oxidative damage of complex I subunits may be involved in aging or disease processes.

1.3.2 Complex III; bc$_p$ Ubiquinone-cytochrome c Oxidoreductase

Mitochondrial ubiquinone-cytochrome c oxidoreductase from bovine heart (complex III, bc$_1$ complex, EC. 1.10.2.2) was first isolated in 1961 (Hatefi et al. 1961). It catalyzes reaction (1.2):

$$QH_2 + 2\,ferricyt\,c^{3+} + 2H^+{}_N \rightarrow Q + 2\,ferrocyt\,c^{2+} + 4H^+{}_P \qquad (1.2)$$

Table 1.2 Gene nomenclature, protein denomination, molecular weight and functions of subunits of mammalian mitochondrial respiratory complex III (For details see the text)

Gene	Protein denomination	MW (kDa)	Redox cofactors	Biochemical features
Complex III Sub. I	Core I	53.6		Metal endopeptidase (MPP)
Complex III Sub. II	Core II	46.5		
CYTB (mt)	Cytochrome b	42.6	Heme b (b_{562}); Heme b_1. (b_{566})	Electron transfer
Comples III Sub.IV	Cytochrome C_1	27.3	Heme C_1	Electron donor to cytochrome c
Comples III Sub.V	Reiske ISP	21.6	2Fe.2S	Electron donor to cytochrome c_1
Comples III Sub.VI	Subunit VI	13.3		
Comples III Sub.VII	Subunit VII	9.5		
Comples III Sub.VIII	Subunit VIII	9.2		Interaction with c_1
Comples III Sub.IX	Subunit IX	8.0		
Comples III Sub.X	Subunit X	7.2		
Comples III Sub.XI	Subunit XI	6.4		

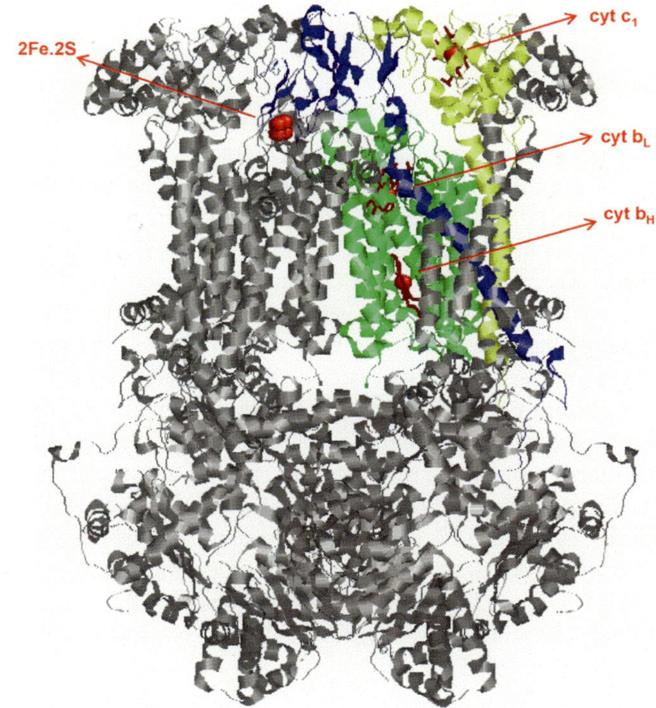

Fig. 1.4 View perpendicular to membrane plane of the complete structure of the 11-subunit bovine mitochondrial cytochrome bc_1 complex in the dimeric form. All the subunits are in *grey* except those, belonginig to right monomer, harbouring the redox active metal center, i.e. cytochrome b (*green*), cytochrome c_1 (*yellow*) and ISP protein (*blue*). The redox centers (cyt b, cyt c_1 and 2Fe.2S cluster) are in *red*. For other details see text (Data from the PDB coordinates (1BGY) of the crystal structure of mitochondrial cytochrome bc_1 complex (Iwata et al. 1998), drawn using RasMol 2.7 program)

The mammalian bc_1 complex ($\approx$240 kDa) is composed of 11 different subunits (Table 1.2) (Hatefi 1985; Schägger et al. 1995). The complex has four prosthetic groups (cyt $b_{L\,(566)}$, cyt $b_{H\,(560)}$, cyt c_1, 2Fe.2S) (Berry et al. 2000). Cytochrome b, cytochrome c_1 and the Rieske iron-sulphur proteins are evolutionary conserved in all the prokaryotic and eukaryotic species analysed and constitute the minimal functional core of the protonmotive complex containing all the prosthetic groups involved in the redox reactions (Berry et al. 2000).

Crystallographic structures of bovine heart (Fig. 1.4) (Xia et al. 1997; Iwata et al. 1998), chicken heart (Berry et al. 1999) and S. Cerevisiae (Hunte et al. 2000) mitochondrial complex III have been

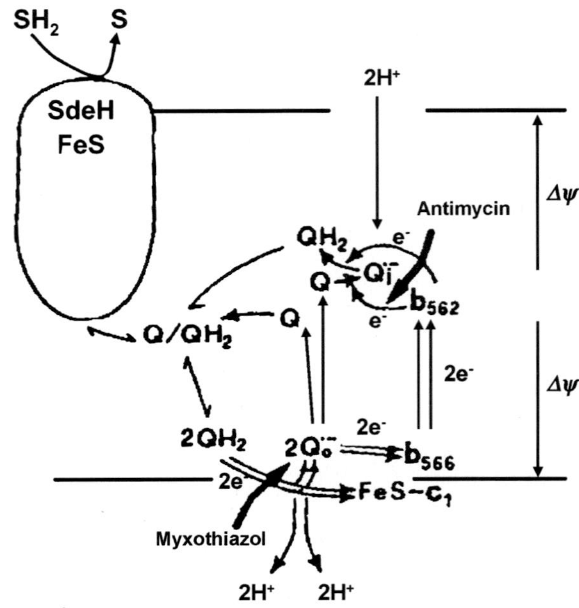

Fig. 1.5 Models of protonmotive activity of complex III (bc_1 complex). The Q-cycle is presented. In bovine complex III, the two b hemes have different midpoint potentials. The low potential heme b_L located near the cytosolic surface of the mitochondrial inner membrane, has an $Em \approx -30$ mV. The high-potential heme b_H, has an $Em \approx 90$ mV and is located near the centre of the membrane (Ohnishi et al. 1989). The iron-sulfur protein (ISP) has an Em of ≈ 280 mV. Cytochrome c_1 has an Em of ≈ 230 mV. All these redox potentials are pH dependent

published and coordinates for bc_1 complexes are available in the Protein Data Banks. The structures of complex III consist of an homodimer of two bc_1 monomers showing a two-fold symmetry about an axis perpendicular to the membrane plane (Berry et al. 2000). The dimer is pear-shaped, with a maximal diameter of 130 Å and a height of 155 Å (Berry et al. 2000). Many contacts between the monomers (especially at the level of subunits core 2 and cytochrome b) suggest that the dimer is the working state of the complex in the native membrane (Berry et al. 2000). Complex III presents three major regions: the transmembrane helix region (42 Å), the matrix region (75 Å) and the intermembrane space region (38 Å). Cytochrome b is largely buried into the membrane (transmembrane helix region), cytochrome c_1 and the Rieske iron-sulphur proteins are almost completely localized in the intermembrane space. In mammalian complex III, eight of the 13 transmembrane helices belong to the cytochrome b protein, the rest, one each, belong to cytochrome c_1, ISP, subunits 7, 10 and 11.

The positions of the heme centers are essentially the same in all the structures examined. The cyt b_L-cyt b_H, cyt b_L-2Fe.2S, 2Fe.2S-cyt c_1 distances are about 21, 27 and 31 Å respectively (Xia et al. 1997). The 2Fe.2S center shows different distances from cyt b_L and cyt c_1 in the various preparations (Xia et al. 1997; Zhang et al. 1998). It has been suggested that the two different positions reflect a movement of the Rieske ISP protein essential for catalysis (Link and Iwata 1996; Zhang et al. 1998; Crofts et al. 1999; Gurung et al. 2005).

Oxidant-induced reduction of *b* cytochromes (Wikström and Berden 1972) and direct measurement of proton pumping associated to electron flow from quinol to cytochrome c, which showed H⁺/e⁻ ratios higher than those predicted by linear redox loops (Lawford and Garland 1972; Papa et al. 1974), brought Mitchell to formulate the ubiquinone cycle to explain proton translocation in complex III (Mitchell 1976) (Fig. 1.5). The non-polar QH_2 diffuses across the membrane and is oxidized at the P side, two H⁺ are released in the P space and the two electrons take two different paths; one electron is transferred to Fe.S cluster $\rightarrow$ cyt c_1 $\rightarrow$ cyt c $\rightarrow$ Complex IV $\rightarrow O_2$, the second electron is transferred back to cyt b_{566}, cyt b_{562} and re-reduces Q to Q⁻ at the inner side. There is no proton uptake in this reduction step. At this point of the Q-cycle, one electron passed from QH_2 to cytochrome c_1 and two protons have been released at the P side of the membrane. The cycle is completed by the oxidation of a second molecule of QH_2 exactly as the first one. Another two H⁺ are released in the P space; one electron is transferred to Fe.S cluster $\rightarrow c_1 \rightarrow c \rightarrow$ Complex IV $\rightarrow O_2$ the second electron cycles back via cyt $b_{566} \rightarrow$ cyt b_{562} and reduces Q^-, transitorily bound at the N side, to QH_2. The reduction of Q^- to QH_2 at the N side takes up two protons from the N side of the membrane completing the cycle. The overall cycle, which involves two turnovers of the bc_1 complex, results in the net oxidation of one QH_2, reduction of 2 molecules of cyt c, release of $4H^+$ in the P space, two of these are substrate protons, two are electrogenically pumped from the N to the P space (Mitchell 1976; Trumpower 1999). The Q-cycle requires two separated ubiquinone-ubiquinol binding sites (Gao et al. 2003; Esser et al. 2004). Antimycin inhibits the one electron reduction of Q by b_H at the N side, myxothiazol blocks the oxidation of QH_2 by ISP (Geier et al. 1993; Link et al. 1993; Miyoshi 2001). Although the Q cycle rationalize different experimental observations and is largely accepted (Trumpower 1999), the proton transfer paths are not clear at the current level of structure resolution and there is not yet unequivocal proof for any one of the steps of the Q-cycle. Alternative mechanisms have been proposed which can equally explain the protonmotive activity of complex III, consistently with the experimental data (Papa et al. 1990; Matsuno-Yagi and Hatefi 2001). In particular Papa et al. (1990) have developed a proton pump model in which redox Bohr effects are conceived to be combined in series with protonmotive redox catalysis by protein bound QH_2/Q^- couple at a catalytic center in the cytochrome b apoprotein (Q-gated proton pump). The protolytic properties of this couple, due to the large difference in the pKs of QH_2 and QH^- results in the translocation of $2H^+$ per e^- transfer in the bc_1 complex. For a detailed discussion of the relative merits of the ubiquinone cycle and alternative mechanisms see (Rieske 1986; Papa et al. 1990; Matsuno-Yagi and Hatefi 2001).

1.3.3   Complex IV; Cytochrome c Oxidase

Mitochondrial and prokaryotic cytochrome c oxidases (CcO) have four redox centers (Wikström et al. 1981b). A binuclear Cu_A center in the extramembrane domain of subunit II, which titrates as one electron redox entity, is the entry point for the electrons delivered by cytochrome c located at the outer (P) side of the membrane. Cu_A transfers electrons to heme a in subunit I. Heme a transfers, in turn, electrons to the heme a_3/Cu_B binuclear center, also bound to subunit I, where dioxygen is reduced to $2 H_2O$ with consumption of 4 protons from the inner (N) aqueous phase. Generation of $\Delta\mu H^+$ by cytochrome c oxidase results also from proton pumping from the N to the P space, coupled to electron flow from ferrocytochrome c to O_2 (Wikström et al. 1981b) with a maximal stoicheiometry of 1 H^+/e^- (reaction 1.3) (Wikström et al. 1981b; Papa et al. 1991; Capitanio et al. 1991, 1996).

$$4\,\text{cytc}^{2+} + 8\,H^+_N + O_2 \rightarrow 4\,\text{cytc}^{3+} + 2\,H_2O + 4\,H^+_P \tag{1.3}$$

X-ray crystallographic structures of cytochrome c oxidase (cytochrome aa_3, complex IV, E.C 1.9.3.1) from bovine heart mitochondria (Tsukihara et al. 1995, 1996), the soil bacterium P. denitrificans (Iwata et al. 1995; Ostermeier et al. 1997), purple bacterium Rhodobacter sphaeroides (Svensson-Ek et al. 2002) are available and coordinates are available in Protein Data Banks. In crystals of purified bovine heart CcO, the enzyme is present as a dimer (Fig. 1.3) (Tsukihara et al. 1996). Prokaryotic CcOs are constituted by four subunits (I, II, III and IV). The mammalian enzyme (M.W. $\approx$ 200 kDa) has, in addition to the conserved subunits I, II and III, which are encoded by the mitochondrial genome, ten additional subunits encoded by nuclear genes (Table 1.3).

Cu_A presents a metal coordination structure similar to the structure of a (2Fe.2S)-type iron sulfur center with a Cu-Cu distance of 2.7 Å (Blackburn et al. 1994; Larsson et al. 1995; Tsukihara et al. 1996). The planes of both hemes lie perpendicular to the membrane plane at approximately one third of depth (Fig. 1.6) (Tsukihara et al. 1996). Heme a and heme a_3 are in close proximity (14 Å). The distances from the center of the two copper atoms of Cu_A to the irons of hemes a and a_3 are 19 and

Table 1.3 Gene nomenclature, protein denomination, molecular weight and functions of subunits of mammalian mitochondrial respiratory complex IV (Kadenbach et al. 1983) (For more details see the text)

Gene	Protein denomination	M.W. (kDa)	Redox cofactors	Biochemical features
Cox1 (mt)	CcO-I	53.6	Heme a, Heme $a_{3,\,CuB}$	Electron transfer, oxygen reduction
Cox2 (mt)	CcO-II	26.0	Cu_A	Cytochrome c binding site, electron transfer
Cox3 (mt)	CcO-III	29.9		
Cox4	CcO-IV	17.1		ATP binding
Cox5a	CcO-Va	12.4		Thyroid hormone (T2) binding
Cox5b	CcO-Vb	10.6		Zn binding
Cox6a	CcO-VIa	9.4		
Cox6b	CcO-VIb	9.4		
Cox6c	Cco-VIc	8.4		
Cox7a	CcO-VIIa	6.2		
Cox7b	CcO-VIIb	6.0		
Cox7c	CcO-VIIc	5.4		
Cox8	CcO-VIII	4.9		

22 Å, respectively. The five-fold coordination of heme a_3 iron leaves one side of the iron available for dioxygen binding. The distance in the crystal structure between the iron of heme a_3 and Cu_B is 4.5 Å. Cu_B^{2+}, in the bovine structure, is coordinated by three histidines. One of them, is covalently bound to one tyrosine forming a conjugated π electron system around Cu_B (Tsukihara et al. 1996). This might lower the pK_a of tyrosine (Yoshikawa et al. 1998) allowing it to participate in the oxygen reduction chemistry (Proshlyakov et al. 2000). The crystal structure of the bovine CcO shows three possible proton translocation networks (Fig. 1.6), named K-, D-, and H-pathway respectively (Tsukihara et al. 1996). The K- and D-pathways connect the binuclear O_2 reduction site with the inner space of the mitochondrial membrane (N space), whereas the H-pathway which extends across the enzyme from the matrix surface to the cytosolic surface involves residues interacting with the porphyrin substituents of heme a (Tsukihara et al. 2003) (Fig. 1.6). This pathway seems to be a specific attribute of the mammalian oxidase (Lee et al. 2000). The D-channel has been proposed to be involved in the translocation of both the pumped protons and two chemical protons (Konstantinov et al. 1997), whereas the K pathway is responsible of the uptake of two chemical protons in the reductive phase of the catalytic cycle (Konstantinov et al. 1997; Brändén et al. 2001). Aminoacid residues (bovine numbering) thought to be involved in the proton translocation pathways are shown in Fig. 1.6.

Various models have been developed in which proton pumping is associated to the oxygen reduction chemistry at the binuclear center (heme a_3/Cu_B) (Wikström 2000; Brzezinski and Larsson 2003; Brzezinski and Gennis 2008). On the other hand, proton pumping models involving coupling at heme a (and Cu_A) have been proposed (Artzatbanov et al. 1978; Babcock and Callahan 1983; Rousseau et al. 1988; Capitanio et al. 1997; Michel 1998; Papa et al. 1998; Tsukihara et al. 2003). Proton pumping models involving coupling at heme a and/or Cu_A require cooperative linkage between oxido-reduction of these centers and proton transfer by acid-base groups in the enzyme. Different functional and structural observations provide evidence for the occurrence of redox-linked allosteric cooperativity in cytochrome c oxidase (Papa et al. 2006b). It has been shown experimentally that heme a and Cu_A share H^+/e^- cooperative coupling with a common acid/base cluster (C_1) (Fig. 1.7), which results in vectorial translocation of around 1 H^+ equivalent per mole of the enzyme undergoing oxido-reduction (Capitanio et al. 2000). While one electron reduction of heme a/Cu_A is sufficient to produce maximal protonation of the cluster, release of the proton bound to the cluster will take place only when both heme a and Cu_A are oxidized. This restriction of one electron at a time might represent one of the causes of slips in the proton pump as observed at high electron pressure imposed on the oxidase (Capitanio et al. 2000).

At steady-state, the catalytic cycle starts with transfer of two electrons from ferrocytochrome c to heme a_3/Cu_B, one at a time, in the fully oxidized enzyme. In this step four protons are taken from the

Fig. 1.6 View perpendicular to the membrane plane of the location in mitochondrial bovine cytochrome c oxidase of the redox centers Cu_A (*green*), Fe_a (*red*), Fe_{a3} (*red*), Cu_B (*green*), and acid/base residues contributing to proton conducting pathways in subunit I. Mg atom (*yellow*) is also shown (Tsukihara et al. 1995). The protolytic residues contributing to the *D channel* (*black solid arrow*), H503, D91, N98, E242, the *K channel* (*green solid arrow*) K265, K319 and the *H channel* (*blue dashed line*) D407, H413, S382, R38, S441, Y440, S205 (subunit II), D51 are also shown. The *blue spheres* show the position of water molecules intercalating protolytic residues along the three channels *above*. R438 and R439, in the proton exit pathway (*black dotted line*) are shown. For other details see text (Data from the PDB (1V54) coordinates of the crystal structure of bovine heart cytochrome c oxidase (Tsukihara et al. 2003), shown using the Ras Mol 2.7 program)

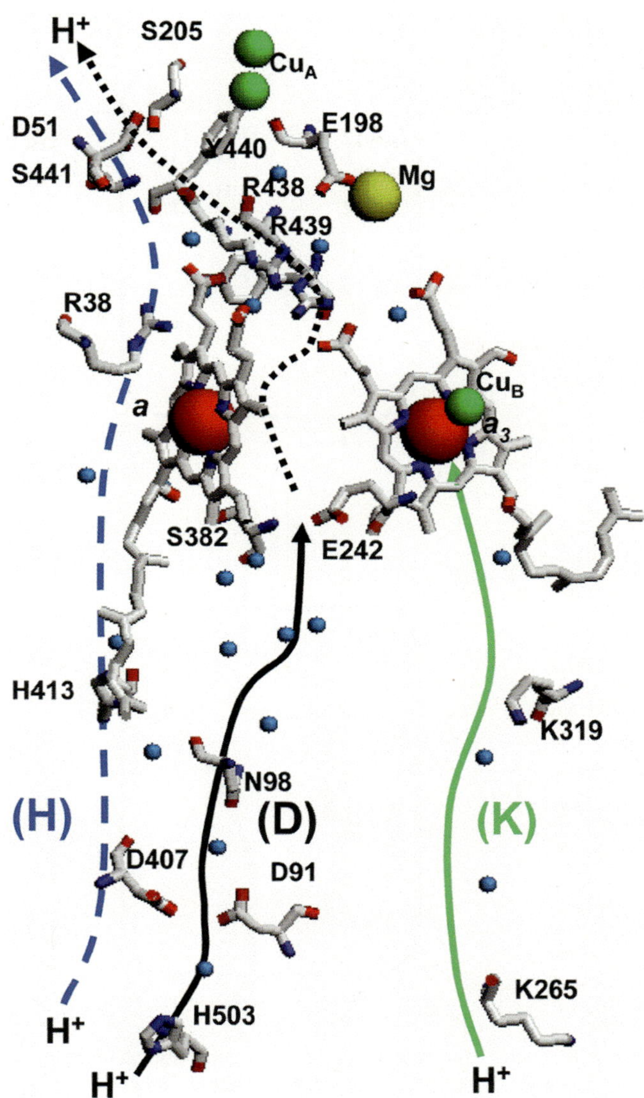

N-side of which two are used for the formation of 2 water molecules, released in the external P space, and 2 are pumped from the N to the P space (Fig. 1.7). O_2, upon binding at the reduced binuclear center, undergoes a four electrons reductive cleavage: two electrons come from the oxidation of Fe_{a3}^{2+} to Fe_{a3}^{4+}, one from Cu_B^{1+} and the fourth, together with a proton, from a Tyr residue (Fig. 1.7), with generation of the P_M intermediate. The transfer of the third electron to the binuclear site, conversion of the P_M to the F intermediate, results in pumping of a third proton. Reduction of the Tyr radical by the third electron is associated with the uptake of the third chemical proton from the N space. The transfer of the fourth electron to the binuclear center (conversion of F to O) is associated with the uptake of $2H^+$ from the N space. One is the fourth chemical proton utilized in the conversion of $Fe_{a3}^{4+}=O$ to $Fe_{a3}^{3+}–OH$, the other is the fourth pumped H^+. In the pump model presented in Fig. 1.7 it is proposed that translocation of each of the four pumped protons is mediated by pK shifts of a residue cluster linked to redox transition of heme a (Papa et al. 1998; Michel 1999; Tsukihara et al. 2003; Belevich et al. 2007). Final release of each pumped proton in the external P side is promoted, upon electrostatic charge neutralization, by arrival of a scalar proton at the binuclear center (Rich 1995). The number of H^+ pumped in the oxidative phase of the catalytic cycle decreases, that in the reductive

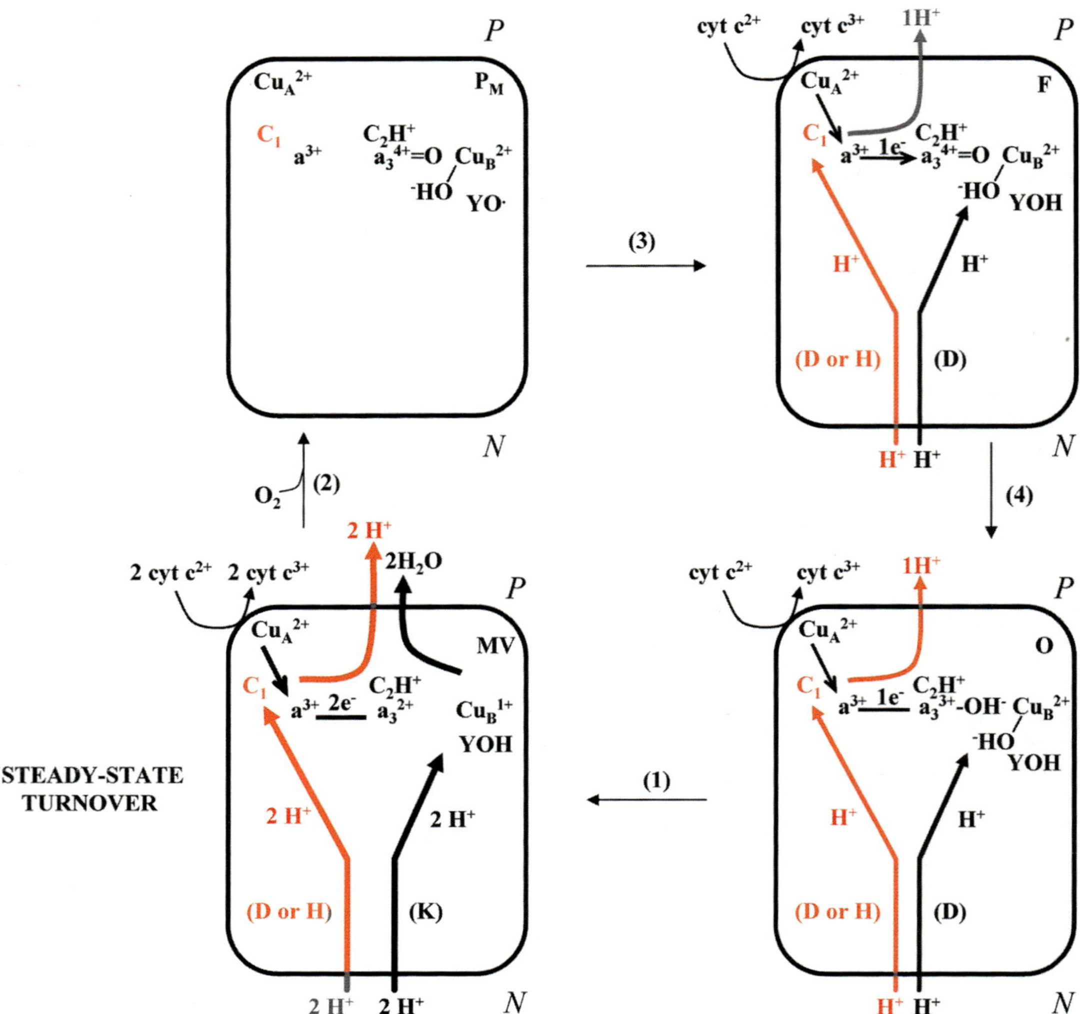

Fig. 1.7 Model of the catalytic cycle and proton pumping in the cytochrome c oxidase in the coupling membrane at the respiratory steady-state. *P*: outer aqueous space, *N*: inner aqueous space. C_1, protolytic cluster cooperatively linked to redox state of heme a; C_2, protolytic cluster apparently linked to heme a_3. The steady-state turnover of the oxidase starts with 2 electrons delivery from ferrocytochrome c to the heme a_3/Cu_B center of the fully oxidized CcO (step 1). The MV (*mixed valence*) state is generated with the uptake of 4H$^+$ from the *N space* of which *2H$^+$* (*black arrow*) are consumed in water formation and release and 2H$^+$ (*red arrow*) are pumped. Molecular oxygen reacting with the MV state is reductively cleaved generating the P_M state (step 2). Transfer of the third electron converts the P_M to the *F state* (step 3) which is finally converted to the *O state* upon delivery of the fourth electron (step 4). In the P_M-F and F-O transition steps, two protons are taken respectively, one chemical in *black*, the other in *red* is pumped from the N to the P space. For more details see text and Papa et al. (2006b)

phase increases, as the pH is raised (Capitanio et al. 2006). This peculiar pH dependence of the two phases of H$^+$ pumping, which is similar to that of the H$^+$ consumption in the formation of H_2O (Capitanio et al. 2003) indicates that the release of the last two protons is associated with protonation of 2 OH$^-$ to 2 H_2O and their release in the external phase. For more details and alternative proposals of proton pumping mechanisms see (Brzezinski and Larsson 2003; Wikström and Verkhovsky 2007; Belevich and Verkhovsky 2008; Brzezinski and Gennis 2008).

Table 1.4 The mitochondrial F1Fo – ATP-synthase subunits

Subunits	n. copies	Location	Mass (Da)	Gene
F_1				
α	3	External hexagon	55,164	Nuclear
β	3	External hexagon	51,595	Nuclear
γ	1	Hexag. cavity and centr. Stalk	30,141	Nuclear
δ	1	Central stalk	15,065	Nuclear
ε	1	Central stalk	5,652	Nuclear
IF_1	1	Surface	9,582	Nuclear
F_0				
F_0I-PVP(b)	1	Lateral stalk	24,670	Nuclear
ATP6(a)	1	Transmembrane	24,815	Mitochondrial
OSCP	1	Surface F_1 and lateral stalk	20,968	Nuclear
d	1	Lateral stalk	18,603	Nuclear
g	1	Transmembrane	11,328	Nuclear
f	1	Transmembrane	10,209	Nuclear
F_6	1	Lateral stalk	8,958	Nuclear
e	1–2	Transmembrane	8,189	Nuclear
c	10–14	Transmembrane	7,608	Nuclear
A6L	1	Transmembrane	7,964	Mitochondrial

Reproduced with kind permission from Springer Science + business media: Gaballo and Papa (2007), chapter 1.6

1.3.4   Complex V; F_1F_0 ATP Synthase

Complex V of the inner mitochondrial membrane utilizes the transmembrane electrochemical proton gradient (PMF) generated by respiration to drive the synthesis of ATP from ADP and inorganic phosphate according to reaction (1.4).

$$ADP + P_i + 3\,H^+_{\,P} \rightarrow ATP + 3\,H^+_{\,N} \tag{1.4}$$

Reaction (1.4) is reversible resulting in H^+ pumping in the reverse direction coupled to ATP hydrolysis. Under conditions of defective generation of respiratory PMF the ATPase activity of complex V, which has high turnover, can result in hydrolytic dissipation of glycolytic ATP. This is a condition, which may acquire pathological significance in respiratory deficiencies like those arising from ischemic tissue conditions or genetic/acquired defects of the respiratory chain. An endogenous inhibitor protein IF_1 is expressed in mammalian cells, which specifically inhibits the ATPase activity of complex V, in particular under conditions of cell acidosis, without any effect on the ATP synthetic activity of the complex (Pullman and Monroy 1963; Papa et al. 1996c; Zanotti et al. 2000).

In mammalian mitochondria, the F_1F_0ATP synthase is composed of 16 subunits (Table 1.4), two ATPase6 and A6L are encoded by the mitochondrial DNA the other by nuclear genes, with an overall molecular weight of about 550 kDa. In mitochondria and chloroplasts, the F_1F_0 complex has been shown to exist as a dimer (Schagger and Pfeiffer 2000; Rexroth et al. 2004; Dudkina et al. 2006) or even as an oligomer (hexamers and/or octamer) (Wittig and Shagger 2009). In yeast, the ATP synthase oligomer is thought to have a role in the formation of mitochondrial cristae (Gavin et al. 2004). In rat liver mitochondria ATP synthase was also shown to be associated with the adenine nucleotide and the Pi carriers to make a supercomplex called the "ATP synthasome" (Chen et al. 2004).

The monomeric ATP synthase complex is made up of two domains, a large globular soluble catalytic portion (the F_1 sector), consisting of 5 subunits with the stoichiometry of $\alpha3\beta3\gamma\delta\varepsilon$, protruding into the mitochondrial matrix, and a membrane embedded portion (the F_0 sector), through which

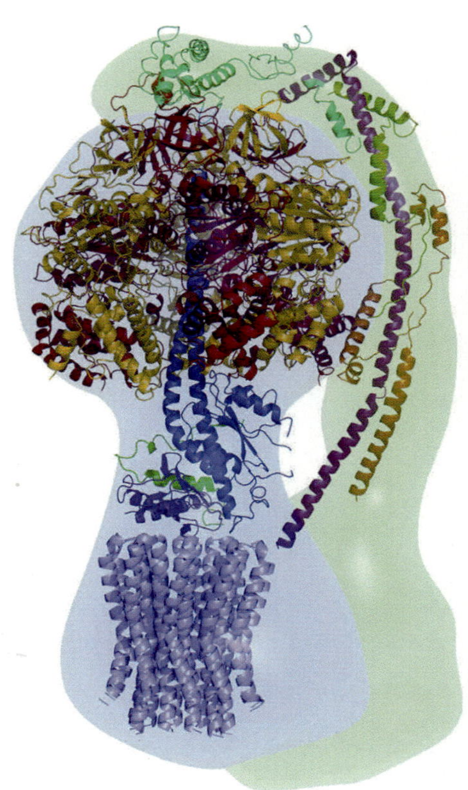

Fig. 1.8 Model of the mitochondrial F_1F_o ATP synthase. Mosaic structure of mitochondrial ATP synthase. The structure is composed by an F_1-stator complex and the c-ring derived from the yeast F_1-c_{10} subcomplex. The mosaic structure was docked into a structure of the intact bovine enzyme determined by electron cryomicroscopy. The region occupied by F_1c_{10} is *blue*, and the peripheral stalk and the membrane subunits *a, e, f, g,* and *A6L* are *green* (Reproduced from Rees et al. (2009). With permission)

transmembrane proton translocation, between the intermembrane P space and the matrix (N space), coupled to enzyme catalysis takes place. The F_o domain has a variable number of different subunits depending on the species. Subunits, *a, b* and the subunit *c* circular oligomer, represent the conserved core of F_o with the stoichiometry in the mitochondrial enzyme of 1:1:10–12 respectively (Fillingame 1997). The F_1 and F_o moieties are structurally and functionally connected by two stalks (Fig. 1.8) (Stock et al. 1999; Gibbons et al. 2000; Lau et al. 2008; Rees et al. 2009).

A breakthrough in understanding the molecular structure/function of complex V has been made in the last 15 years by the results of two lines of investigation: x-ray resolution of the crystallographic structure of the F_1 sector (Abrahams et al. 1994; Menz et al. 2001; Kabaleeswaran et al. 2006; Bowler et al. 2007) and dynamic fluorescence observations showing rotation of the F_1-γ subunit (Sabbert et al. 1996; Noji et al. 1997) and the Fo-subunit *c* (Sambongi et al. 1999; Panke et al. 2000) both driven by ATP hydrolysis. These studies provide definite support to the concept of binding change mechanism of complex V already developed by Boyer in the 1990s (1993, 1997). It should be recalled here that the enzyme kinetics study of Penefsky (1985) had demonstrated that in the synthesis of ATP energy rather than in the formation of β–γ phosphate bond is expended in the removal of ATP from the catalytic site.

The X-ray analysis of the F_1 sector crystallized in the presence of the ATP inhibitory analogue AMP-PNP (Abrahams et al. 1994) shows that the 3α and 3β subunits are alternatively arranged to form a spherical hexamer with six nucleotide binding sites, 3 of these catalytically competent, 3 non catalytic sites each binding AMP-PNP. The catalytic sites in the 3β subunits present different structural binding sites; the first β binds Mg-AMP-PNP, the second Mg-ADP, and the third is empty (no bound nucleotide). These subunits are termed β_{TP}, β_{DP} and β_E and correspond to "tight", "loose" and "open" conformations respectively (Fig. 1.9a). The empty conformation of β_E appears to be induced by the γ subunit which pushes the β lower C-terminal part towards the central axis of F_1 (Fig. 1.9a) (Abrahams et al. 1994).

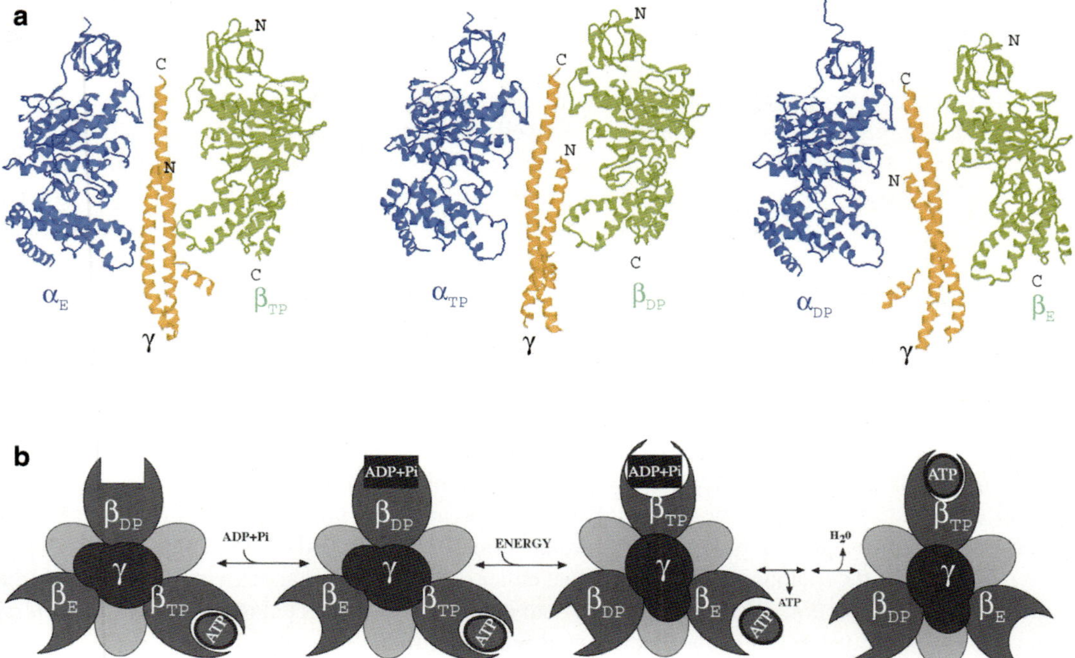

Fig. 1.9 (**a**) Different structural conformations of F_1 α, β and γ subunits as observed in the AMP-PNP inhibited F_1 crystal structure. Longitudinal sections of the F_1 moiety each showing partially resolved subunit γ facing α and β subunits. The three different conformations $β_{TP}$; $β_{DP}$ and $β_E$ are visible (Structural data are from the bovine heart mitochondrial F_1 crystal structure (Abrahams et al. 1994) (PDB ID = 1bmf). Molecular graphic by RasMol 2.6), (**b**) The binding change mechanism. Catalysis scheme in which only two catalytic sites in the β subunits are occupied by adenine nucleotides (ATP and ADP + P_i) during steady state catalysis. Looking at the scheme from *left* to *right* (ATP synthesis) it can be seen an ATP molecule bound at the high affinity site ($β_{TP}$); the binding of ADP and Pi at the loose site ($β_{DP}$) and the catalytic sites interconversion in association with rotation of the γ subunit. In the last step ATP is released from the open site ($β_E$) (Reproduced with kind permission from Springer Science + business media: Gaballo and Papa (2007), chapter 1.6,, fig. 1.6–2)

Subunit γ protrudes out of the α3β3 hexamer (Abrahams et al. 1994; Stock et al. 1999), and contacts the polar inner loop of Fo membrane-embedded c subunits (Fillingame 1997). During catalysis, the three catalytic sites in β subunits undergo cyclically through three different nucleotide conformations and cooperative interconversion of the states is due to γ subunit rotation (F_1motor) (Fig. 1.9b) (Boyer 1993, 1997; Noji et al. 1997). A crystallographic analysis at 2.4 Å resolution of bovine F_1 (Gibbons et al. 2000) revealed that the γ subunit, together with subunits δ and ε, constitutes the central stalk which is in contact with the F_o subunit c oligomer which, in turn, constitutes the Fo part of the rotary motor (Sambongi et al. 1999; Panke et al. 2000; Tsunoda et al. 2001).

Conversion of PMF into mechanochemical energy is assured by proton flow, through the Fo moiety, that drives rotation of the c subunit ring (Sambongi et al. 1999; Panke et al. 2000; Tsunoda et al. 2001). Rotation of the *c* ring induces rotation of the γ subunit, which finally, causes conformational changes in the β subunits catalytic sites causing a decrease of the affinity of F_1 for ATP (and probably increase in the affinity for ADP and Pi) with ATP release in the medium (Fig. 1.9b).

In addition to the γδε central stalk, the F_1 moiety is also connected to the Fo membrane domain by a non rotating peripheral stalk which has the function of a stator in the ATP synthase rotary motor (Fig.1.8). This lateral stalk is made up of part of subunits *b* and *d*, plus the whole F6 and the oligomycin sensitive conferring protein (OSCP) subunit (Dickson et al. 2006; Lau et al. 2008; Rees et al. 2009). The N-terminal domain of OSCP contacts the N terminal region of an α subunit at the top of the F_1 sector. The C-terminal of OSCP interacts, on the opposite part of F_1 with the C-terminus of subunit *b*. Subunits d and F6 lie alongside subunit b and appear to stiffen it. The Fo sector of mammalian mt ATP synthase includes in addition to the conserved subunits *a*, *b* and *c* other subunits, namely *e, f, g*, and *A6L* whose function is not yet well characterized (Devenish et al. 2008).

Subunit *c* (sub 9) is a highly hydrophobic subunit that folds in the membrane as a hairpin with two membrane spanning α-helices connected by a polar loop region in contact with the F_1 sector (Girvin et al. 1998; Dmitriev et al. 1999). There are several copies (10–12) of the *c* subunit organized in an oligomer with a ring-like structure. In the middle of the C-terminal helix of subunit c there is a highly conserved residue (D61 in E. coli; E65 in mitochondria) essential for proton translocation through Fo (Miller et al. 1990).

Subunit *a* (sub 6) of F_o is located at one side of the *c* subunit ring. It consists of five membrane spanning helices (Wada et al. 1999). Arg 210 in helix 4 of subunit *a* interacts with D61 in subunit *c*. The passage of protons through Fo occurs at this interface between subunits *a* and *c* where these two residues, are in close proximity and causes a rotation of the $\gamma\delta\epsilon\text{-}c_{10\text{-}12}$ central rotor (Fillingame et al. 2002; Fillingame and Dmitriev 2002). According to Vik and Antonio (1994) two half proton channels within subunit *a*, provide a gate for protons towards or from subunit *c* carboxylate (D61 in E. coli; E65 in mitochondria). The sequential protonation/deprotonation of subunit *c* carboxylate is coupled to a stepwise movement of the *c* subunit ring. It can rotate either clockwise or anticlockwise depending on the direction of the proton flow. This rotation is in both cases strictly connected to rotation of the central stalk, this allowing the transfer of mechanical energy from or to the catalytic sites.

Various human mitochondrial diseases are caused by mutations in the mitochondrial gene encoding the ATP synthase subunit *a*, such Leber's hereditary optic neuropathy (LHON), the maternally inherited Leigh syndrome (MILS) and the neurogenic ataxia and retinitis pigmentosa (NARP) (reviewed in Kucharczyk et al. 2009 and references therein).

1.4 Biogenesis of Oxidative Phosphorylation Complexes

Biogenesis of mitochondria involves the formation of the organelle during the cell life cycle (Attardi and Schatz 1988; Leaver and Lonsdale 1989). Pre-existing mitochondria grow and divide during mitosis, providing daughter cells with a normal complement of mitochondria. Although the mass of mitochondria increases from the onset of S-phase through M-phase (Sanger et al. 2000) there are instances in which mitochondrial divisions are not tied to the cell cycle. Division of mitochondria is controlled by a framework of cellular signalling that culminates in the coordinated expression of the two cellular genomes: nuclear DNA and mitochondrial DNA. The mitochondrial genome encodes protein components of the respiratory chain and ATP synthase complexes but hundreds of nuclear-encoded proteins involved in respiration and in different functions must be synthesized in the rough endoplasmic reticulum and imported into mitochondria (Neupert 1997; Pfanner et al. 1997; Neupert and Herrmann 2007). The study of the machinery of mitochondrial protein expression, import, biogenesis, assembly of the oxidative phosphorylation complexes, as well as of metal transport, fusion and segregation of mitochondria, has been greatly facilitated by using model organisms, such as *Saccharomyces cerevisiae* and *Neurospora crassa*. These allowed the isolation of several human genes based on their sequence homology. In humans, the search for the nuclearly encoded mitochondrial proteins has been further boosted by studies on mitochondrial disorders. More recently, the identification of mitochondrial proteins has benefited of global approaches in the fields of comparative genomics and proteomics for human mitochondria (Taylor et al. 2003b; Cotter et al. 2004), and for other model organisms (Mootha et al. 2003; Premsler et al. 2009). For description of mtDNA structure, expression and genetics see the following chapter by Ian Holt.

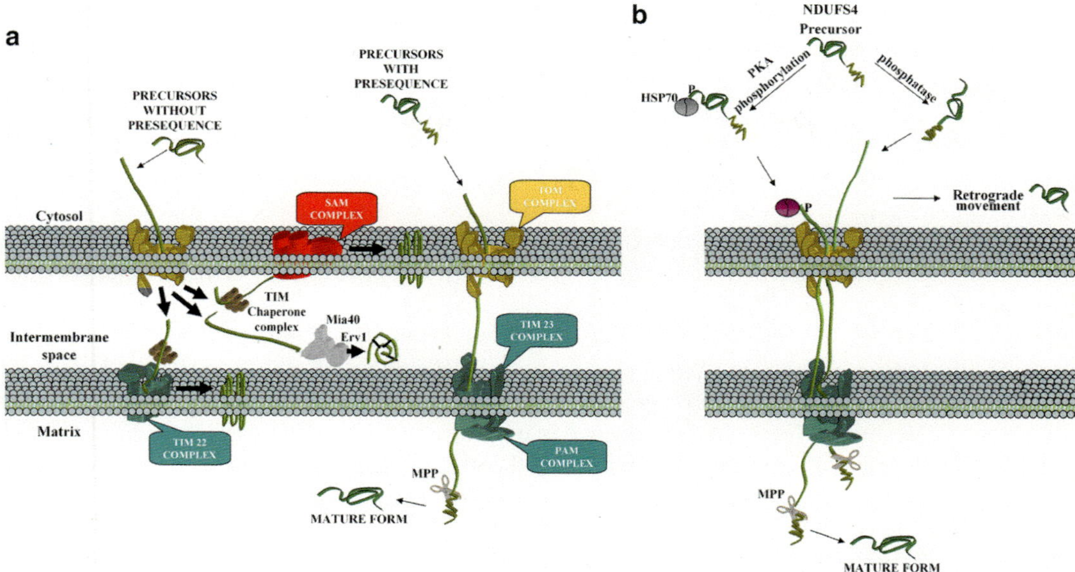

Fig. 1.10 (**a**) Protein import pathways in mitochondria, (**b**) Scheme describing the impact on mitochondrial import of serine phosphorylation in the C-terminus of the *NDUFS4* subunit of complex I. Phosphorylation of NDUFS4 C-terminus mediates binding of the NDUFS4 protein to the cytosolic Hsp70. Binding of the NDUFS4/Hsp70 complex to *TOM* contributes to maintain the NDUFS4 precursor protein in unfolded translocation competent configuration and prevents retrograde release from mitochondria of the mature protein from which the positively charged leader sequence has been removed

1.4.1   Mitochondrial Import of Nuclear Encoded Proteins

Newly synthesized mitochondrial proteins have four destinations including the outer membrane (OM), the intermembrane space (IMS), the inner membrane (IM) and the matrix (Fig. 1.10a). Protein import into mitochondria is mediated by translocator complexes crossing the membranes and chaperones acting in the proximity of intermembrane space and within the matrix. Nuclear-encoded mitochondrial proteins can be distinguished into two main classes. The first includes precursor proteins with N-terminal cleavable presequences. The positively charged presequences function as targeting signals that interact with the mitochondrial import receptors thus directing the pre-proteins across both outer and inner membranes (Koehler et al. 1999; Pfanner and Geissler 2001; Neupert and Herrmann 2007). The second class of proteins, without cleavable presequences, carry various internal targeting signals (Brix et al. 1999; Endres et al. 1999). There is also evidence of presence of target sequence in the C-terminal region of the proteins (Robin et al. 2002). The mitochondrial import of mitochondrial inner membrane and matrix space proteins is dependent on ATP and mitochondrial $\Delta\psi$.

The TOM40 (Translocase of the Outer mitochondrial Membrane) complex represents the main entry for almost all nuclear-encoded mitochondrial proteins and consists of several preprotein receptors and a general import pore. Most of the mitochondrial precursor proteins are imported after cytosolic translation (*post-translational import*), likely guided to mitochondria by cytosolic chaperones, which include the heat shock proteins (Young et al. 2003) and additional cytosolic factors (Komiya et al. 1998; Yano et al. 2003). In some instances, the presequence is inserted into the TOM machinery while a C-terminal portion is still undergoing synthesis on the ribosome (*co-translational import*) (Knox et al. 1998). After crossing the TOM complex, the imported proteins are sorted to one of the four sub-compartments following one of the four main pathways. (i) the precursors of the mitochondrial outer membrane, without the target presequence, like porin, are sorted from the TOM complex to the SAM complex (Sorting and Assembly Machinery) by the small Tim proteins which behave as chaperones of the mitochondrial intermembrane space. The SAM complex assembles the newly imported proteins in the outer membrane (Paschen et al. 2005; Becker et al. 2008). (ii) Proteins directed to the intermembrane space, characterized by the presence of cystein motifs, follow the MIA40/ERV1 pathway (Chacinska et al. 2004). Mia40 (Mitocondrial Import and Assembly machinery) introduces disulfide bonds into proteins within the intermembrane space to facilitate their import and folding (Mesecke et al. 2005; Dabir et al. 2007; Banci et al. 2009). (iii) Hydrophobic precursors of the inner membrane, from TOM complex are bound to Tim9–Tim10 or Tim8–Tim13 complex in the intermembrane space which, acting as a chaperone, prevents protein aggregation (Webb et al. 2006; Gebert et al. 2008). The chaperon complexes drive the proteins to the TIM22 (Translocase of Inner Membrane 22) complex; this releases the transported protein in the inner membrane in a $\Delta\psi$-dependent manner (Rehling et al. 2003). (iv) The precursors of the matrix space carrying a cleavable presequence, are transferred to TIM23 (Translocase of Inner Membrane 23) complex. Once the presequence is transferred to the matrix side, through the Tim23 import channel using ATP and $\Delta\psi$, it is bound by the mitochondrial Hsp70 (mtHsp70) to complete translocation of the entire precursor protein into the matrix. The mtHsp70 is the import motor of the PAM complex (Presequence translocase-Associated Motor). It interacts with the TIM23 complex in order to trap and pull the precursors into the matrix space (Neupert and Brunner 2002).

Once the precursor proteins arrive into the matrix, the Mitochondrial Processing Protease, MPP, cleaves the targeting sequence. A second intermediate processing protease, MIP, can be utilized in Fe-S assembly. For a few intermembrane space proteins, the inner membrane processing protease complex (IMP) cleaves the sorting sequence after the initial cleavage by the MPP.

TIM23 complex, without PAM complex, can also physically associate with complexes III and IV of mitochondrial respiratory chain (Chacinska et al. 2005). It has been proposed that this interaction allows mitochondrial import in condition of low electrochemical gradient using the local gradient generated by complex III and IV of the respiratory chain (van der Laan et al. 2006, 2010).

cAMP signalling (via PKA) is able to enhance the level of some proteins in mitochondria by PKA dependent phosphorylation of precursor proteins. This is the case of the NDUFS4 protein (De Rasmo et al. 2008), a subunit of complex I (Fig. 1.10b), cytochrome P4502B1 (Anandatheerthavarada et al. 1999), CY2E1 (Robin et al. 2002) and glutathione S-transferase (GSTA4-4) (Robin et al. 2003). PKA-dependent phosphorylation promotes the level of proteins in mitochondria also through post-transcriptional regulation in which phosphorylation of AKAP protein, in outer mitochondrial membrane enhances its affinity for mRNAs coding for mitochondrial SOD and Fo-f subunit of ATP synthase complex (Ginsberg et al. 2003). It is proposed that this binding promotes the stability of mRNA or the cotranslational import mechanism (Ginsberg et al. 2003). More detailed aspects of the import machinery are reviewed in (Wiedemann et al. 2004; Neupert and Herrmann 2007).

1.4.2 Assembly of Oxidative Phosphorylation Complexes

The elucidation of the protein factors and assembly steps involved in the biosynthesis of oxidative phosphorylation complexes is mostly based on yeast studies (Fontanesi et al. 2008; Zara et al. 2009; Rak et al. 2009). In humans information is becoming available mainly for complex I and IV assembly mechanisms and only partially for complex III and V from studies in patients with OXPHOS deficiency. Much of what is known about the assembly of complex I comes from studies in the fungus *Neurospora crassa*, which contains only 35 subunits (Videira and Duarte 2001). It has been shown that there is an independent formation of the membrane part with respect to the protruding arm of the complex (see Fig. 1.11) since the peripheral arm can still be formed in the absence of mitochondrially encoded subunits (Tuschen et al. 1990; Duarte et al. 1995). To date, it is, however, unclear whether

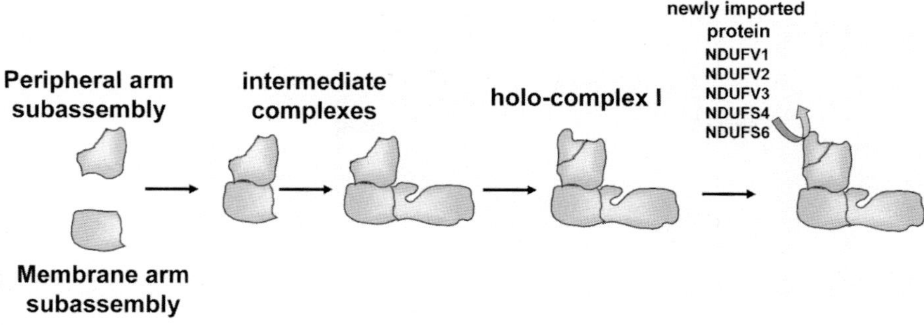

Fig. 1.11 Assembly scheme of complex I. De novo assembly of complex I occurs via the preassembly of intermediate complexes. A pre-assembled peripheral arm is formed, which associates with a pre-assembled membrane arm to form an intermediate complex, to which other subunits are attached to form holo-complex I (Ugalde et al. 2004). Dynamic assembly occurs by exchanging of peripheral subunits which, once oxidized, are displaced and replaced by newly imported subunits (Lazarou et al. 2007)

complex I assembly in mammalian cells is comparable to the *N. crassa* model. Studies on the pattern of partially assembled complexes I in patients, either with mtDNA or nDNA mutations, has allowed to propose two different models for complex I assembly. A first model suggests no separate formation of the peripheral and membrane arms (Antonicka et al. 2003). In an alternative model complex I assembly is proposed to be a semi-sequential process in which pre-assembled subcomplexes are joined to form holo-complex I (Ugalde et al. 2004) (Fig. 1.11). In addition to the "de novo" assembly of complex I, another process, named dynamic assembly, proposes that complex I is able to "rejuvenate" by exchanging the peripheral subunits which, once damaged, are displaced and replaced by subunits newly imported into mitochondria (Fig. 1.11) (Lazarou et al. 2007).

In *Neurospora*, two proteins, the complex I intermediate associated proteins, CIA30 and CIA84, have been shown to associate with intermediates of the assembly process but not with the mature complex (Kuffner et al. 1998). A human homologue has been found for CIA30 (Janssen et al. 2002) and shown to be a chaperone for complex I assembly (Vogel et al. 2005). Another chaperone protein, called the B17.2-like, for its homology with the B17.2 subunit of complex I, has been found to be associated with intermediates of the assembly process of about 850 kDa in human fibroblasts (Ogilvie et al. 2005; Lazarou et al. 2007). In addition other proteins, ECSITE (Evolutionary Conserved Signaling Intermediate in Toll pathways) (Vogel et al. 2007), mainly localized in the cytosol, but also present in small amounts in mitochondria, and the C6orf66 protein (Saada et al. 2008), have been found to be involved in the assembly of complex I. More recently, a phylogenetic profiling approach identified 19 complex I associated proteins (Pagliarini et al. 2008) and, among these, the C8orf38 protein was found to be mutated in an inherited CI deficiency disease (Pagliarini et al. 2008).

For Complex II assembly the group of Lemire (Lemire and Oyedotun 2002) has reported that in the course of assembly, three [Fe-S] clusters must be incorporated into the IP subunit. A heme (bL) group is coordinated with two integral membrane subunits, and a FAD cofactor becomes covalently linked to the largest FP subunit. It seems that in the absence of the integral membrane subunit there is no assembly of a functional SDH activity (Oostveen et al. 1995).

Of the 11 subunits of complex III only one, cytochrome *b*, is encoded by the mitochondrial genome, the other subunits by nuclear genes. These latter are synthesized in the cytosol, imported into mitochondria and assembled in the inner membrane as a homo-dimer complex. The similarities between the yeast and mammalian bc_1 complex, despite the fact that mammalian complex contains 9 additional subunits, has made possible to use the yeast enzyme as a model to understand how it is assembled. The assembly is a dynamic, stepwise process in which there is formation of three different subcomplexes. These subcomplexes assemble together to form a cytochrome bc1 precomplex to which other two subunits, Rieske Fe–S (RISP) and Qcr10p, are added (Cruciat et al. 1999; Zara et al. 2004). The complete assembly in the homo-dimer takes place before full assembly of the complex III monomer is completed. In yeast, several genes have been demonstrated to be involved in assembly of the complex III such as cbp3 (Wu and Tzagoloff 1989), cbp4 (Crivellone 1994), bcs1 (Nobrega et al. 1992), and abc1 (Bousquet et al. 1991). So far only one such gene, bcs1l, has been identified in humans (Petruzzella et al. 1998). The BCS1L protein is a chaperon like protein that promotes the incorporation of RISP into the precomplex (Fernandez-Vizarra et al. 2007).

The precursor proteins of the nuclear encoded subunits of cytochrome c oxidase are imported into the mitochondrial inner membrane and assembled, along with two haem a groups, three copper, one zinc and one magnesium ion, into a functional complex (Stiburek et al. 2006; Fernández-Vizarra et al. 2009). The assembly of CcO is believed to be a sequential process in which pools of unassembled subunits exist and at least two assembly intermediates have been detected (Wielburski and Nelson 1983; Nijtmans et al. 1998). In a first step a subcomplex S1 containing COXI, possibly with associated haem groups is formed and then COXIV is incorporated and subcomplex S2 is formed. COXII and COXIII are added to this subcomplex together with COXVa,b, COXVIb,c, COXVII a or b, VII c and COXVIII to obtain the subcomplex S3. Finally, COXVIa, COXVIIa or VIIb are added which gives S4 (holo-CcO) and subsequently the dimer is formed (Nijtmans et al. 1998; Taanman and Williams 2001). In humans, mutations have been found that affect the stability and incorporation of CcO subunits into the assembled complex, associated with different phenotypical presentations of CcO deficiency (see later). At least 25 factors have been identified for complex IV assembly largely based on analysis of CcO yeast deficient mutants. SURF1/Shy1 was identified as responsible for Leigh disease associated to CcO deficiency (Tiranti et al. 1998). In yeast there are the Cox10, CoX11, CoX14-20, and Cox23, the Pet100, Pet117, and Pet191 genes, the Shy1 gene (SURF-1 in mammals), Sco1 and Sco2 genes, Mba1 and MSS51 genes, the Oxa1gene and more. An up-to date discussion of each of these can be found in the review by (Herrmann and Funes 2005). Some of these genes are required for the translation of CcO mRNAs in the matrix and the insertion of the peptides into the membrane; others are involved in heme synthesis. The Sco gene products together with other chaperones are needed for insertion of copper ions into the two centers (Papadopoulou et al. 1999; Valnot et al. 2000).

Most of the study on the biogenesis of ATP synthase have been performed in yeast and a detailed discussion of the results can be found in Ackerman and Tzagoloff 2005. The core subunits of the F1 subcomplexes (α, β, γ) and the core subunits of the Fo subcomplex (c, a, b) assemble separately, to combine then with other subunits to form the functional complex. Assembly factors or molecular chaperones are involved in the process. Molecular chaperone proteins called Atp11p and Atp12p, have been described for the assembly of the mitochondrial alpha and beta subunits into the F(1) oligomer of F(1)F(0) ATP synthase and the human counterparts of these two proteins have been described (Wang et al. 2001). F_1Fo-ATP synthase together with the respiratory chain supercomplexes accumulate in the cristae membrane domains which are believed to generate a microenvironment for energy-transduction reactions (Bornhövd et al. 2006; Strauss et al. 2008; Zick et al. 2009).

Two subunits, e and g, were first described to be required for dimerization of complex V. Dimerization and oligomerization can have an essential role in establishing the mitochondrial cristae morphology (Paumard et al. 2002; Arselin et al. 2004; Bornhövd et al. 2006). Su k and Su i play an important role in the stepwise assembly and stabilization of mature ATP synthase dimers.

1.4.3 Transcriptional Factors Controlling the Biogenesis of Respiratory Chain Complexes

Mitochondrial biogenesis requires pre-protein translocation, assembly of the mitochondrial respiratory chain complexes, division, fusion, fission of mitochondria, all processes requiring careful coordinate expression of the nuclear and mitochondrial genomes (Nisoli et al. 2004) and depend upon trans-acting nuclear encoded factors (for more details Scarpulla 2008). Mitochondrial biogenesis responds to a variety of stimuli. In mammalian cells promotion of mitochondrial biogenesis by various agents involves cAMP and Ca^{2+} mediated signal transduction pathways. Recruitment of these pathways results in phosphorylation by cAMP and Ca^{2+} dependent protein kinases of CREB protein that controls the expression of some 100 genes (Shaywitz and Greenberg 1999; Mayr and Montminy 2001). The role of CREB in mitochondrial biogenesis was highlighted by the discovery that the CREB translational complex controls the expression of the transcriptional coactivator PPARγ coactivator 1α (PGC-1α) (Herzig et al. 2001). In certain cell types activation of cAMP and/or Ca^{2+} dependent protein kinases results in phosphorylation of members of the transducer of regulated CREB binding protein family (TORCs) (Screaton et al. 2004), causing translocation of these proteins from the cytoplasm to the nucleus where they bind to the CREB complex and exert their transcriptional coactivator action (Screaton et al. 2004; Bittinger et al. 2004). The CREB-TORC complex stimulates the transcriptional level of the PGC-1α gene (Wu et al. 2006). The PGC-1α transcription coactivator is a central node in the control of mitochondrial biogenesis. Its activity and/or expression responds to a variety positive and negative signal pathways (Fig. 1.12). PGC-1α is also activated by post-translational modifications, like deacetylation by SIRT1, and phosphorylation by other kinases, like AMPK and P38MAPK.

Induced expression of PGC-1α a member of the PGC-1 family of coactivators, in turn activates a transcriptional regulatory cascade which amplifies the impact of CREB mediated signal transduction on mitochondrial biogenesis (López-Lluch et al. 2008). PGC-1α promotes the expression and activity of the nuclear respiratory transcription factors NRF1 and NRF2 (Wu et al. 1999; Scarpulla 2008; Wenz 2009). NRF1 and NRF2 control the expression of many nuclear genes coding for structural proteins of the mitochondrial respiratory chain and the F_1F_o-ATP synthase, enzymes of heme biosynthesis, proteins involved in mitochondrial import of nuclear encoded subunits of OXPHOS complexes and complex assembly (Scarpulla 1997; Takahashi et al. 2002; Blesa et al. 2004; Kelly and Scarpulla 2004) as well as proteins involved in the transcription of the mitochondrial genome like the transcription factor A (TFAM). TFAM, once imported in mitochondria, interacts with one of two additional transcription factors, TFB1 or TFB2, and with the mitochondrial RNA polymerase (Blesa et al. 2004; Kelly and Scarpulla 2004; Wenz 2009). In this way a transcriptional cascade, which involves, in a downstream sequence, CREB (and TORCs), PGC-1α, NRF1, NRF2, TFAM, TFB1, TFB2, confers to mammalian cells the capacity to upregulate in a concerted process the expression of nuclear and mitochondrial genes encoding subunits of OXPHOS complexes.

More recently a second process has been discovered which contributes to coordinate the expression of nuclear and mitochondrial genes. This consists in the translocation of CREB from the cytoplasm to mitochondria by a membrane potential and TOM complex dependent mechanism. In mitochondria, CREB binds to the mtDNA D-loop and activates the biosynthesis of mitochondrial encoded subunits (Cammarota et al. 1999; Lee et al. 2005; Ryu et al. 2005; De Rasmo et al. 2009).

1.5 Remarks and Perspectives

What reported has marked important progress in the elucidation of the atomic structure and functional mechanisms, molecular genetics and transcriptional regulation of the expression of the respiratory chain oxidative phosphorylation system in mammalian cells. Mitochondria in all eukaryotic organisms are adapted to a variety of niches with the mitochondrial proteomes reflecting large diversity of functions (Gabaldon and Huynen 2004). Mitochondria number per cell can substantially vary from tissue to tissue. In mammalian cells the number of mtDNA copies, encoding subunits of

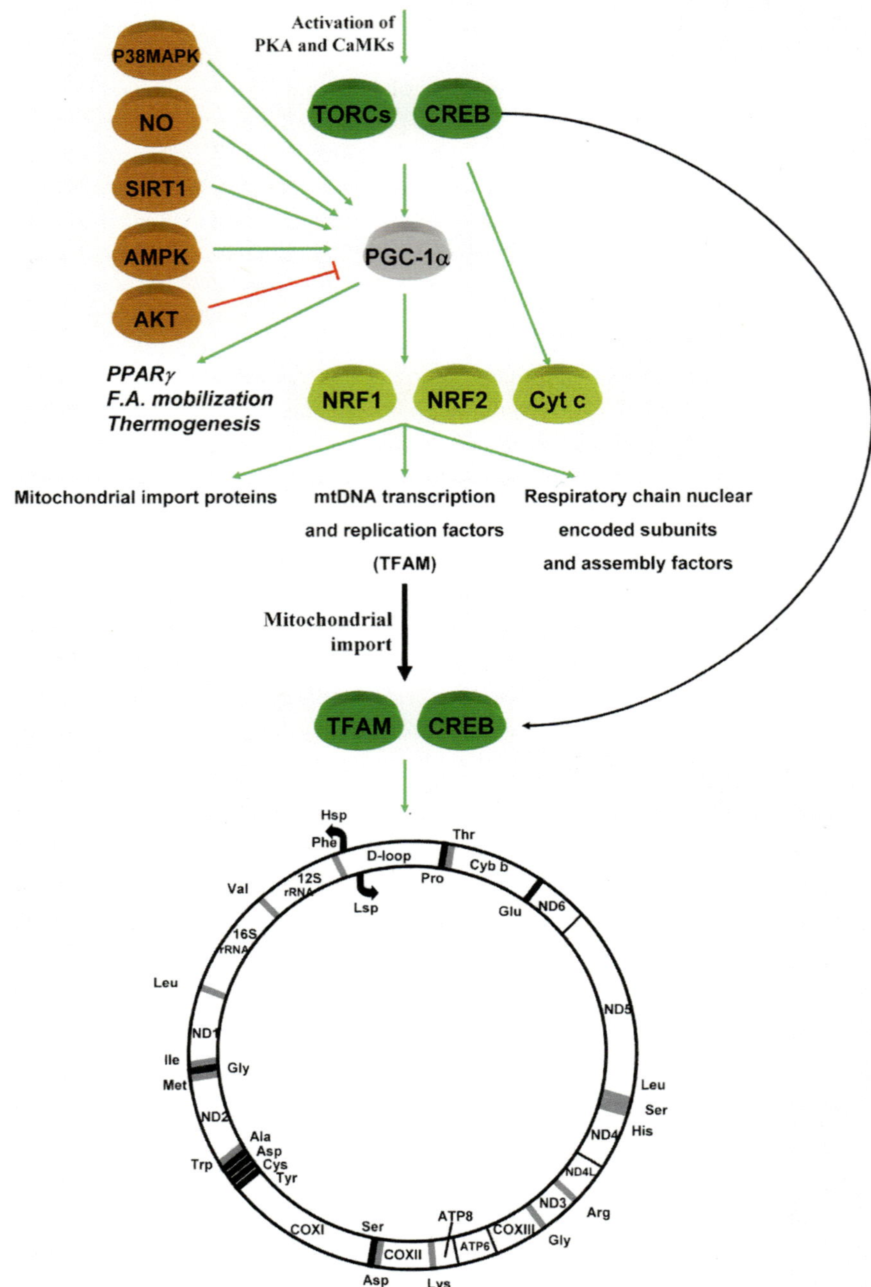

Fig. 1.12 Schematic representation of transcription factors which control mitochondrial biogenesis. Activation of protein kinases by cAMP and/or Ca²⁺ results in phosphorylation of *CREB* and members of the transducer of regulated CREB binding protein family (*TORCs*) (Screaton et al. 2004; Bittinger et al. 2004). CREB and TORC together promote the transcription of *PGC-1α* and cytochrome c genes. The activity and/or expression of PGC-1α responds to a variety positive and negative signal pathways (López-Lluch et al. 2008). The transcriptional level of PGC-1α is also increased by *NO*. PGC-1α is also activated by post-translational modifications, like deacetylation by *SIRT1*, phosphorylation by *AMPK* and *P38MAPK* and inhibited by phosphorylation by *AKT* which is activated by insulin pathway. PGC-1α in combination with other factors, activates the expression of enzymes of fatty acid oxidation and of the nuclear respiratory transcription factors, *NRF1* and *NRF2*. NRF1 and NRF2 activate, in turn, the expression of the mitochondrial transcription and replication factors, like *TFAM*, nuclear genes coding for structural proteins and assembly factors of OXPHOS complexes, mitochondrial import proteins, ion channel and shuttle proteins. The *mTFA* and CREB proteins, after mitochondrial import, promote the expression of *mtDNA*

the oxidative phosphorylation complexes, is thought to be regulated by the energy requirement (Hecht et al. 1984; Hecht and Liem 1984; Satoh and Kuroiwa 1991; Moyes et al. 1998). This contributes to confer to the OXPHOS system the functional capacity to respond to the specific ATP requirement of the various tissues, which, in addition, varies continuously depending on the phases of the cell cycle and the energy demand for specialized cell functions. This knowledge is useful to decipher the impact and pathogenetic mechanisms of hereditary and acquired defects in structural and ancillary genes of oxidative phosphorylation complexes. Further progress along these lines can substantially contribute to devise rational therapeutical measures for prevention and treatment of diseases in which dysfunction of mitochondrial oxidative phosphorylation plays a primary or a contributing role.

Acknowledgements This work was supported by: National Project, "Progetto FIRB Rete Nazionale per lo Studio della Proteomica Umana (Italian Human ProteomeNet)", 2009, Ministero dell' Istruzione, dell'Università e della Ricerca (MIUR) and University of Bari Research grant, 2009.

References

Abrahams JP, Leslie AG, Lutter R, Walker JE (1994) Structure at 2.8 Å resolution of F1-ATPase from bovine heart mitochondria. Nature 370:621–628

Acín-Pérez R, Bayona-Bafaluy MP, Fernández-Silva P, Moreno-Loshuertos R, Pérez-Martos A, Bruno C, Moraes CT, Enríquez JA (2004) Respiratory complex III is required to maintain complex I in mammalian mitochondria. Mol Cell 13(6):805–815

Ackerman SH, Tzagoloff A (2005) Function, structure, and biogenesis of mitochondrial ATP synthase. Prog Nucleic Acid Res Mol Biol 80:95–133

Anandatheerthavarada H, Biswas G, Mullick J, Sepuris N, Pain D, Avadhani G (1999) Dual targeting of cytochrome P4502B1 to endoplasmic reticulum and mitochondria involves a novel signal activation by cyclic AMP-dependent phosphorylation at ser128. EMBO J 18:5494–5504

Angell JE, Lindner DJ, Shapiro PS, Hofmann ER, Kalvakolanu DV (2000) Identification of GRIM-19, a novel cell death-regulatory gene induced by the interferon and retinoic acid combination, using a genetic approach. J Biol Chem 275:33416–33426

Antonicka H, Ogilvie I, Taivassalo T, Anitori RP, Haller RG, Vissing J, Kennaway NG, Shoubridge EA (2003) Identification and characterization of a common set of complex I assembly intermediates in mitochondria from patients with complex I deficiency. J Biol Chem 278:43081–43088

Arselin G, Vaillier J, Salin B, Schaeffer J, Giraud MF, Dautant A, Brèthes D, Velours J (2004) The modulation in subunits e and g amounts of yeast ATP synthase modifies mitochondrial cristae morphology. J Biol Chem 279: 40392–40399

Artzatbanov VY, Konstantinov AA, Skulachev VP (1978) Involvement of intramitochondrial protons in redox reactions of cytochrome *a*. FEBS Lett 87:180–185

Attardi G, Schatz G (1988) Biogenesis of mitochondria. Annu Rev Cell Biol 4:289–333

Babcock GT, Callahan PM (1983) Redox-linked hydrogen bond strength changes in cytochrome *a*: implications for a cytochrome oxidase proton pump. Biochemistry 22(10):2314–2319

Bamberg E, Butt HJ, Eisenraunch A, Fendler K (1993) Charge transport of ion pumps on lipid bilayer membranes. Q Rev Biophys 26:1–25

Banci L, Bertini I, Cefaro C, Ciofi-Baffoni S, Gallo A, Martinelli M, Sideris DP, Karakili N, Tokatlidis K (2009) MIA40 is an oxidoreductase that catalyzes oxidative protein folding in mitochondria. Nat Struct Mol Biol 16:198–206

Becker T, Vogtle FN, Stojanovski D, Meisinger C (2008) Sorting and assembly of mitochondrial outer membrane proteins. Biochim Biophys Acta 1777:557–563

Beckman JS, Koppenol WH (1996) Nitric oxide, superoxide, and peroxynitrite: the good, the bad, and ugly. Am J Physiol 271(5 Pt 1):C1424–C1437

Beinert H (1986) Iron-sulphur clusters: agents of electron transfer and storage, and direct participants in enzymic reactions. Tenth Keilin memorial lecture. Biochem Soc Trans 14:527–533

Belevich I, Verkhovsky MI (2008) Molecular mechanism of proton translocation by cytochrome c oxidase. Antioxid Redox Signal 10(1):1–29

Belevich I, Bloch DA, Belevich N, Wikstrom M, Verkhovsky MI (2007) Exploring the proton pump mechanism of cytochrome c oxidase in real time. Proc Natl Acad Sci USA 104(8):2685–90

Berrisford JM, Sazanov LA (2009) Structural basis for the mechanism of respiratory complex I. J Biol Chem 284(43):29773–29783

Berry EA, Huang LS, Zhang Z, Kim SH (1999) Structure of the avian mitochondrial cytochrome bc1 complex. J Bioenerg Biomembr 31(3):177–190

Berry EA, Guergova-Kuras M, Huang LS, Crofts AR (2000) Structure and function of cytochrome *bc* complexes. Annu Rev Biochem 69:1005–1075

Bironaite DA, Cenas NK, Kulys JJ (1991) The rotenone-insensitive reduction of quinones and nitrocompounds by mitochondrial NADH:ubiquinone reductase. Biochim Biophys Acta 1060(2):203–209

Bittinger MA, McWhinnie E, Meltzer J, Iourgenko V, Latario B, Liu X, Chen CH, Song C, Garza D, Labow M (2004) Activation of cAMP response element-mediated gene expression by regulated nuclear transport of TORC proteins. Curr Biol 14:2156–2161

Blackburn NJ, Barr ME, Woodruff WH, van der Oost J, de Vries S (1994) Metal-metal bonding in biology: EXAFS evidence for a 2.5 A copper-copper bond in the CuA center of cytochrome oxidase. Biochemistry 33(34): 10401–10407

Blesa JR, Hernandez JM, Hernandez-Yago J (2004) NRF-2 transcription factor is essential in promoting human Tomm70 gene expression. Mitochondrion 3:251–259

Bornhövd C, Vogel F, Neupert W, Reichert AS (2006) Mitochondrial membrane potential is dependent on the oligomeric state of F_1F_o-ATP synthase supracomplexes. J Biol Chem 281:13990–13998

Bousquet I, Dujardin G, Slonimski PP (1991) ABC1, a novel yeast nuclear gene has a dual function in mitochondria: it suppresses a cytochrome b mRNA translation defect and is essential for the electron transfer in the bc_1 complex. EMBO J 10:2023–2031

Bowler MW, Montgomery MG, Leslie AG, Walker JE (2007) Ground state structure of F1-ATPase from bovine heart mitochondria at 1.9 A resolution. J Biol Chem 282:14238–14242

Boyer PD (1993) The binding change mechanism for ATP synthase–some probabilities and possibilities. Biochim Biophys Acta 1140:215–250

Boyer PD (1997) The ATP synthase-a splendid molecular machine. Annu Rev Biochem 66:717–749

Brändén M, Sigurdson H, Namslauer A, Gennis RB, Adelroth P, Brzezinski P (2001) On the role of the K-proton transfer pathway in cytochrome c oxidase. Proc Natl Acad Sci USA 98(9):5013–5018

Brandt U (1997) Proton-translocation by membrane-bound NADH: ubiquinoneoxidoreductase (complex I) through redox-gated ligand conduction. Biochim Biophys Acta 1318:79–91

Brandt U, Kerscher S, Dröse S, Zwicker K, Zickermann V (2003) Proton pumping by NADH:ubiquinone oxidoreductase. A redox driven conformational change mechanism? FEBS Lett 545(1):9–17

Brix J, Rudiger S, Bukau B, Schneider-Mergener J, Pfanner N (1999) Distribution of binding sequences for the mitochondrial import receptors Tom20, Tom22, and Tom70 in a presequence-carrying preprotein and a non-cleavable preprotein. J Biol Chem 274:16522–16530

Brown GC (1999) Nitric oxide and mitochondrial respiration. Biochim Biophys Acta 1411(2–3):351–369

Brzezinski P, Gennis RB (2008) Cytochrome c oxidase: exciting progress and remaining mysteries. J Bioenerg Biomembr 40:521–531

Brzezinski P, Larsson G (2003) Redox-driven proton pumping by heme-copper oxidases. Biochim Biophys Acta 1605:1–13

Burwell LS, Nadtochiy SM, Tompkins AJ, Young S, Brookes PS (2006) Direct evidence for S-nitrosation of mitochondrial complex I. Biochem J 394(3):627–634

Cadenas E, Davies KJ (2000) Mitochondrial free radical generation, oxidative stress, and aging. Free Radic Biol Med 29:222–230

Cammarota M, Paratcha G, Bevilaqua LR, Levi de Stein M, Lopez M, Pellegrino de Iraldi A, Izquierdo I, Medina JH (1999) Cyclic AMP-responsive element binding protein in brain mitochondria. J Neurochem 72:2272–2277

Canton M, Luvisetto S, Schmehl I, Azzone GF (1995) The nature of mitochondrial respiration and discrimination between membrane and pump properties. Biochem J 310:477–481

Capitanio N, Capitanio G, De Nitto E, Villani G, Minuto M, Papa S (1991) Variable H^+/e^- stoichiometry of mitochondrial respiratory chain. In: 36th congress Italian biochemical society, Ferrara, Italy IBST, vol 2, p 98 and 15th international congress of biochemistry, Jerusalem, Israel, Abstract volume p 195

Capitanio N, Capitanio G, Demarinis DA, De Nitto E, Massari S, Papa S (1996) Factors affecting the H^+/e^- stoichiometry in mitochondrial cytochrome c oxidase: influence of the rate of electron flow and transmembrane delta pH. Biochemistry 35(33):10800–10806

Capitanio N, Vygodina TV, Capitanio G, Konstantinov AA, Nicholls P, Papa S (1997) Redox-linked protolytic reactions in soluble cytochrome-c oxidase from beef-heart mitochondria: redox Bohr effects. Biochim Biophys Acta 1318(1–2):255–265

Capitanio N, Capitanio G, Boffoli D, Papa S (2000) The proton/electron coupling ratio at heme a and Cu(A) in bovine heart cytochrome c oxidase. Biochemistry 39(50):15454–15461

Capitanio N, Capitanio G, De Nitto E, Boffoli D, Papa S (2003) Proton transfer reactions associated with the reaction of the fully reduced, purified cytochrome c oxidase with molecular oxygen and ferricyanide. Biochemistry 42(16):4607–4612

Capitanio G, Martino PL, Capitanio N, De Nitto E, Papa S (2006) pH dependence of proton translocation in the oxidative and reductive phases of the catalytic cycle of cytochrome c oxidase. The role of H_2O produced at the oxygen-reduction site. Biochemistry 45(6):1930–1937

Carroll J, Fearnley IM, Skehel JM, Shannon RJ, Hirst J, Walker JE (2006a) Bovine complex I is a complex of 45 different subunits. J Biol Chem 281(43):32724–32727

Carroll J, Fearnley IM, Walker JE (2006b) Definition of the mitochondrial proteome by measurement of molecular masses of membrane proteins. Proc Natl Acad Sci USA 103:16170–16175

Cecchini G (2003) Function and structure of complex II of the respiratory chain. Annu Rev Biochem 72:77–109

Chacinska A, Pfannschmidt S, Wiedemann N, Kozjak V, Sanjuan-Szklarz LK, Schulze-Specking A, Truscott KN, Guiard B, Meisinger C, Pfanner N (2004) Essential role of Mia40 in import and assembly of mitochondrial inter-membrane space proteins. EMBO J 23:3735–3746

Chacinska A, Lind M, Frazier AE, Dudek J, Meisinger C, Geissler A, Sickmann A, Meyer HE, Truscott KN, Guiard B, Pfanner N, Rehling P (2005) Mitochondrial presequence translocase: switching between TOM tethering and motor recruitment involves Tim21 and Tim17. Cell 120:817–829

Chance B, Sies H, Boveris A (1979) Hydroperoxide metabolism in mammalian organs. Physiol Rev 59(3):527–605

Chen C, Ko Y, Delannoy M, Ludtke SJ, Chiu W, Pedersen PL (2004) Mitochondrial ATP synthasome: three-dimensional structure by electron microscopy of the ATP synthase in complex formation with carriers for Pi and ADP/ATP. J Biol Chem 279:31761–31768

Cocco T, Pacelli C, Sgobbo P, Villani G (2009) Control of OXPHOS efficiency by complex I in brain mitochondria. Neurobiol Aging 30(4):622–629

Cortopassi G, Wang E (1995) Modelling the effects of age-related mtDNA mutation accumulation; complex I deficiency, superoxide and cell death. Biochim Biophys Acta 1271(1):171–176

Cotter D, Guda P, Fahy E, Subramaniam S (2004) MitoProteome: mitochondrial protein sequence database and annotation system. Nucleic Acids Res 32:D463–D467

Crivellone MD (1994) Characterization of CBP4, a new gene essential for the expression of ubiquinol-cytochrome c reductase in Saccharomyces cerevisiae. J Biol Chem 269:21284–21292

Crofts AR, Guergova-Kuras M, Huang LS, Kuras R, Zhang Z, Berry EA (1999) The mechanism of ubiquinol oxidation by the bc_1 complex: the role of the iron sulfur protein, and its mobility. Biochemistry 38:15791–15806

Cruciat CM, Hell K, Folsch H, Neupert W, Stuart RA (1999) Bcs1p, an AAA-family member, is a chaperone for the assembly of the cytochrome bc(1) complex. EMBO J 18:5226–5233

Dabir DV, Leverich EP, Kim SK, Tsai FD, Hirasawa M, Knaff DB, Koehler CM (2007) A role for cytochrome c and cytochrome c peroxidase in electron shuttling from Erv1. EMBO J 26:4801–4811

De Rasmo D, Panelli D, Sardanelli AM, Papa S (2008) cAMP-dependent protein kinase regulates the mitochondrial import of the nuclear encoded NDUFS4 subunit of complex I. Cell Signal 20:989–997

De Rasmo D, Signorile A, Roca E, Papa S (2009) cAMP response element-binding protein (CREB) is imported into mitochondria and promotes protein synthesis. FEBS J 276:4325–4333

Degli Esposti M, Ghelli A (1994) The mechanism of proton and electron transport in mitochondrial complex I. Biochim Biophys Acta 1187:116–120

Devenish RJ, Prescott M, Rodgers AJ (2008) The structure and function of mitochondrial F_1F_0-ATP synthases. Int Rev Cell Mol Biol 267:1–58

Dickson VK, Silvester JA, Fearnley IM, Leslie AG, Walker JE (2006) On the structure of the stator of the mitochondrial ATP synthase. EMBO J 25:2911–2918

Dmitriev OY, Jones PC, Fillingame RH (1999) Structure of the subunit c oligomer in the F_1F_0 ATP synthase: model derived from solution structure of the monomer and cross-linking in the native enzyme. Proc Natl Acad Sci USA 96:7785–7790

Duarte M, Sousa R, Videira A (1995) Inactivation of genes encoding subunits of the peripheral and membrane arms of Neurospora mitochondrial complex I and effects on enzyme assembly. Genetics 139:1211–1221

Dudkina NV, Sunderhaus S, Braun HP, Boekema EJ (2006) Characterization of dimeric ATP synthase and cristae membrane ultrastructure from Saccharomyces and Polytomella mitochondria. FEBS Lett 580:3427–3432

Dutton PL, Moser CC, Sled VD, Daldal F, Ohnishi T (1998) A reductant-induced oxidation mechanism for complex I. Biochim Biophys Acta 1364(2):245–257

Efremov RG, Baradaran R, Sazanov LA (2010) The architecture of respiratory complex I. Nature. 465:441–445

Efremov RG, Sazanov LA (2011) Structure of the membrane domain of respiratory complex I. Nature. 476:414–420

Endres M, Neupert W, Brunner M (1999) Transport of the ADP/ATP carrier of mitochondria from the TOM complex to the TIM22.54 complex. EMBO J 18:3214–3221

Esser L, Quinn B, Li YF, Zhang M, Elberry M, Yu L, Yu CA, Xia D (2004) Crystallographic studies of quinol oxidation site inhibitors: a modified classification of inhibitors for the cytochrome bc(1) complex. J Mol Biol 341(1):281–302

Fato R, Bergamini C, Leoni S, Strocchi P, Lenaz G (2008) Generation of reactive oxygen species by mitochondrial complex I: implications in neurodegeneration. Neurochem Res 33:2487–2501

Fearnley IM, Carroll J, Shannon RJ, Runswick MJ, Walker JE, Hirst J (2001) GRIM-19, a cell death regulatory gene product, is a subunit of bovine mitochondrial NADH:ubiquinone oxidoreductase (complex I). J Biol Chem 276:38345–38348

Fernandez-Vizarra E, Bugiani M, Goffrini P, Carrara F, Farina L, Procopio E, Donati A, Uziel G, Ferrero I, Zeviani M (2007) Impaired complex III assembly associated with BCS1L gene mutations in isolated mitochondrial encephalopathy. Hum Mol Genet 16:1241–1252

Fernández-Vizarra E, Tiranti V, Zeviani M (2009) Assembly of the oxidative phosphorylation system in humans: what we have learned by studying its defects. Biochim Biophys Acta 1793:200–211

Fillingame RH (1997) Coupling H+ transport and ATP synthesis in F_1F_0-ATP synthases: glimpses of interacting parts in a dynamic molecular machine. J Exp Biol 200:217–224

Fillingame RH, Dmitriev OY (2002) Structural model of the transmembrane F_0 rotary sector of H^+-transporting ATP synthase derived by solution NMR and intersubunit cross-linking in situ. Biochim Biophys Acta 1565:232–245

Fillingame RH, Angevine CM, Dmitriev OY (2002) Coupling proton movements to c-ring rotation in F(1)F(o) ATP synthase: aqueous access channels and helix rotations at the a-c interface. Biochim Biophys Acta 1555:29–36

Flemming D, Hellwig P, Friedrich T (2003) Involvement of tyrosines 114 and 139 of subunit NuoB in the proton pathway around cluster N2 in Escherichia coli NADH:ubiquinone oxidoreductase. J Biol Chem 278(5):3055–3062

Fontanesi F, Soto IC, Barrientos A (2008) Cytochrome c oxidase biogenesis: new levels of regulation. IUBMB Life 60:557–568

Friedrich T, Böttcher B (2004) The gross structure of the respiratory complex I: a Lego System, Review. Biochim Biophys Acta 1657:71–83

Gabaldon T, Huynen MA (2004) Shaping the mitochondrial proteome. Biochim Biophys Acta 1659:212–220

Gaballo A, Papa S (2007) The mitochondrial F_1F_0 ATP synthase. In: Lajtha A, Dienel G, Gibson G (eds) Handbook of neurochemistry and molecular neurobiology. Springer, Berlin/Heidelberg, pp 120–134

Gao X, Wen X, Esser L, Quinn B, Yu L, Yu CA, Xia D (2003) Structural basis for the quinone reduction in the bc1 complex: a comparative analysis of crystal structures of mitochondrial cytochrome bc1 with bound substrate and inhibitors at the Qi site. Biochemistry 42(30):9067–9080

Gavin PD, Prescott M, Luff SE, Devenish RJ (2004) Cross-linking ATP synthase complexes in vivo eliminates mitochondrial cristae. J Cell Sci 117:2333–2343

Gebert N, Chacinska A, Wagner K, Guiard B, Koehler CM, Rehling P, Pfanner N, Wiedemann N (2008) Assembly of the three small Tim proteins precedes docking to the mitochondrial carrier translocase. EMBO Rep 9:548–554

Geier BM, Haase U, von Jagow G (1993) Inhibitor binding to the Qp-site of bc1 complex: comparative studies of yeast mutants and natural inhibitor resistant fungi. Biochem Soc Trans 22:203–209

Gibbons C, Montgomery MG, Leslie AGW, Walker JE (2000) The structure of the central stalk in bovine F(1)-ATPase at 2.4 A resolution. Nat Struct Biol 7:1055–1061

Ginsberg MD, Feliciello A, Jones JK, Avvedimento EV, Gottesman ME (2003) PKA-dependent binding of mRNA to the mitochondrial AKAP121 protein. J Mol Biol 327:885–897

Girvin ME, Rastogi VK, Abildgaard F, Markley JL, Fillingame RH (1998) Solution structure of the transmembrane H+-transporting subunit c of the F_1F_0 ATP synthase. Biochemistry 37:8817–8824

Grigorieff N (1998) Three-dimensional structure of bovine NADH:ubiquinone oxidoreductase (complex I) at 22 Å in ice. J Mol Biol 277:1033–1046

Grivennikova VG, Vinogradov AD (2006) Generation of superoxide by the mitochondrial complex I. Biochim Biophys Acta 1757:553–561

Guenebaut V, Vincentelli R, Mills D, Weiss H, Leonard KR (1997) Three-dimensional structure of NADH-dehydrogenase from Neurospora crassa by electron microscopy and conical tilt reconstruction. J Mol Biol 265:409–418

Guenebaut V, Schlitt A, Weiss H, Leonard K, Friedrich T (1998) Consistent structure between bacterial and mitochondrial NADH: ubiquinone oxidoreductase (complex I). J Mol Biol 276:105–112

Gurung B, Yu L, Xia D, Yu CA (2005) The iron-sulfur cluster of the Rieske iron-sulfur protein functions as a proton-exiting gate in the cytochrome bc(1) complex. J Biol Chem 280(26):24895–24902

Hatefi Y (1985) The mitochondrial electron transport and oxidative phosphorylation system. Annu Rev Biochem 54:1015–1069

Hatefi Y, Haavik AG, Griffiths DE (1961) Reconstitution of the electron transport system II. Reconstitution of DPNH-cytochrome c reductase. succinic-cytochrome c reductase and DPNH, succinic-cytochrome c reductase. Biochem Biophys Res Commun 4:447–453

Hecht NB, Liem H (1984) Mitochondrial DNA is synthesized during meiosis and spermiogenesis in the mouse. Exp Cell Res 154:293–298

Hecht NB, Liem H, Kleene KC, Distel RJ, Ho SM (1984) Maternal inheritance of the mouse mitochondrial genome is not mediated by a loss or gross alteration of the paternal mitochondrial DNA or by methylation of the oocyte mitochondrial DNA. Dev Biol 102:452–461

Herrmann JM, Funes S (2005) Biogenesis of cytochrome oxidase-sophisticated assembly lines in the mitochondrial inner membrane. Gene 354:43–52

Herzig S, Long F, Jhala US, Hedrick S, Quinn R, Bauer A, Rudolph D, Schutz G, Yoon C, Puigserver P, Spiegelman B, Montminy M (2001) CREB regulates hepatic gluconeogenesis through the coactivator PGC-1. Nature 413:179–183

Hinkle PC (2005) P/O ratios of mitochondrial oxidative phosphorylation. Biochim Biophys Acta 1706(1–2):1–11

Hirst J, Carrol J, Fearnley IM, Shannnon RJ, Walker JE (2003) The nuclear encoder subunits of complex I from bovine heart mitochondria. Biochim Biophys Acta 1604:135–150

Hofhaus G, Weiss H, Leonard K (1991) Electron microscopic analysis of the peripheral and membrane parts of mitochondrial NADH dehydrogenase (complex I). J Mol Biol 221:1027–1043

Hunte C, Koepke J, Lange C, Rossmanith T, Michel H (2000) Structure at 2.3 A resolution of the cytochrome bc(1) complex from the yeast Saccharomyces cerevisiae cocrystallized with an antibody Fv fragment. Struct Fold Des 8:669–684

Hunte C, Zickermann V, Brandt U (2010) Functional modules and structural basis of on formational coupling in mitochondrial complex I. Science 329:448–451

Hüttemann M, Lee I, Samavati L, Yu H, Doan JW (2007) Regulation of mitochondrial oxidative phosphorylation through cell signalling. Biochim Biophys Acta 1773:1701–1720

Iwata S, Ostermeier C, Ludwig B, Michel H (1995) Structure at 2.8 Å resolution of cytochrome c oxidase from Paracoccus denitrificans. Nature 376:660–669

Iwata S, Lee JW, Okada K, Lee JK, Iwata M, Rasmussen B, Link TA, Ramaswamy S, Jap BK (1998) Complete structure of the 11-subunit bovine mitochondrial cytochrome bc1 complex. Science 281:64–71

Janssen R, Smeitink J, Smeets R, van den Heuvel L (2002) CIA30 complex I assembly factor: a candidate for human complex I deficiency? Hum Genet 110:264–270

Kabaleeswaran V, Puri N, Walker JE, Leslie AG, Mueller DM (2006) Novel features of the rotary catalytic mechanism revealed in the structure of yeast F1 ATPase. EMBO J 25(22):5433–5442

Kadenbach B, Jarausch J, Hartmann R, Merle P (1983) Separation of mammalian cytochrome c oxidase into 13 polypeptides by a sodium dodecyl sulfate-gel electrophoretic procedure. Anal Biochem 129(2):517–521

Keilin D (1966) The history of cell respiration and cytochrome. Cambridge University Press, Cambridge

Kelly DP, Scarpulla RC (2004) Transcriptional regulatory circuits controlling mitochondrial biogenesis and function. Genes Dev 18:357–368

Knox C, Sass E, Neupert W, Pines O (1998) Import into mitochondria, folding and retrograde movement of fumarase in yeast. J Biol Chem 273:25587–25593

Koehler CM, Merchant S, Schatz G (1999) How membrane proteins travel across the mitochondrial intermembrane space. Trends Biochem Sci 24:428–432

Komiya T, Rospert S, Koehler C, Looser R, Schatz G, Mihara K (1998) Interaction of mitochondrial targeting signals with acidic receptor domains along the protein import pathway: evidence for the 'acid chain' hypothesis. EMBO J 17:3886–3898

Konstantinov AA, Siletsky S, Mitchell D, Kaulen A, Gennis RB (1997) The roles of the two proton input channels in cytochrome c oxidase from Rhodobacter sphaeroides probed by the effects of site-directed mutations on time-resolved electrogenic intraprotein proton transfer. Proc Natl Acad Sci USA 94(17):9085–9090

Kucharczyk R, Zick M, Bietenhader M, Rak M, Couplan E, Blondel M, Caubet SD, di Rago JP (2009) Mitochondrial ATP synthase disorders: molecular mechanisms and the quest for curative therapeutic approaches. Biochim Biophys Acta 1793:186–199

Kuffner R, Rohr A, Schmiede A, Krull C, Schulte U (1998) Involvement of two novel chaperones in the assembly of mitochondrial NADH: ubiquinone oxidoreductase (complex I). J Mol Biol 283:409–417

Kussmaul L, Hirst J (2006) The mechanism of superoxide production by NADH: ubiquinone oxidoreductase (complex I) from bovine heart mitochondria. Proc Natl Acad Sci USA 103:7607–7612

Larsson S, Kullebring B, Wittung P, Malmstrom BG (1995) The Cu_A center of cytochrome-c oxidase: electronic structure and spectra of models compared to the properties of Cu_A domains. Proc Natl Acad Sci USA 92:7167–7171

Lau WC, Baker LA, Rubinstein JL (2008) Cryo-EM structure of the yeast ATP synthase. J Mol Biol 382(5):1256–1264

Lawford HG, Garland PB (1972) Proton translocation coupled to quinone reduction by reduced nicotinamide-adenine dinucleotide in rat liver and ox heart mitochondria. Biochem J 130(4):1029–1044

Lazarou M, McKenzie M, Ohtake A, Thorburn DR, Ryan MT (2007) Analysis of the assembly profiles for mitochondrial and nuclear-DNA-encoded subunits into Complex I. Mol Cell Biol 27:4228–4237

Leaver CJ, Lonsdale DM (1989) Mitochondrial biogenesis. Cambridge University Press, London

Lee HM, Das TK, Rousseau DL, Mills D, Ferguson-Miller S, Gennis RB (2000) Mutations in the putative H-channel in the cytochrome c oxidase from Rhodobacter sphaeroides show that this channel is not important for proton conduction but reveal modulation of the properties of heme a. Biochemistry 39(11):2989–2996

Lee J, Kim CH, Simon DK, Aminova LR, Andreyev AY, Kushnareva YE, Murphy AN, Lonze BE, Kim KS, Ginty DD, Ferrante RJ, Ryu H, Ratan RR (2005) Mitochondrial cyclic AMP response element-binding protein (CREB) mediates mitochondrial gene expression and neuronal survival. J Biol Chem 280:40398–40401

Lemire BD, Oyedotun KS (2002) The Saccharomyces cerevisiae mitochondrial succinate:ubiquinone oxidoreductase. Biochim Biophys Acta 1553:102–116

Leonard K, Haiker H, Weiss H (1987) Three dimensional structure of NADH: ubiquinone reductase (complex I) from Neurospora mitochondria determined by electron microscopy of membrane crystals. J Mol Biol 194:277–286

Link TA, Iwata S (1996) Functional implications of the structure of the 'Rieske' iron-sulfur protein of bovine heart mitochondrial cytochrome bc1 complex. Biochim Biophys Acta 1275(1–2):54–60

Link TA, Haase U, Brandt U, von Jagow G (1993) What information do inhibitors provide about the structure of the hydroquinone oxidation site of ubihydroquinone: cytochrome c oxidoreductase? J Bioenerg Biomembr 25:221–232

López-Lluch G, Irusta PM, Navas P, de Cabo R (2008) Mitochondrial biogenesis and healthy aging. Exp Gerontol 43:813–819

Lorusso M, Cocco T, Minuto M, Capitanio N, Papa S (1995) Proton/electron stoichiometry of mitochondrial bc1 complex. Influence of pH and transmembrane delta pH. J Bioenerg Biomembr 27:101–118

Magnitsky S, Toulokhonova L, Yano T, Sled VD, Hägerhäll C, Grivennikova VG, Burbaev DS, Vinogradov AD, Ohnishi T (2002) EPR characterization of ubisemiquinones and iron-sulfur cluster N2, central components of the energy coupling in the NADH-ubiquinone oxidoreductase (complex I) in situ. J Bioenerg Biomembr 34(3):193–208

Maj MC, Raha S, Myint T, Robinson BH (2004) Regulation of NADH/CoQ oxidoreductase: do phosphorylation events affect activity? Protein J 23:25–32

Matsuno-Yagi A, Hatefi Y (2001) Ubiquinol: cytochrome c oxidoreductase (complex III). Effect of inhibitors on cytochrome b reduction in submitochondrial particles and the role of ubiquinone in complex III. J Biol Chem 276:19006–19011

Mayr B, Montminy M (2001) Transcriptional regulation by the phosphorylation- dependent factor CREB. Nat Rev Mol Cell Biol 2:599–609

Meinhardt SW, Ohnishi T (1992) Determination of the position of the Qi.-quinone binding site from the protein surface of the cytochrome bc1 complex in Rhodobacter capsulates chromatofores. Biochim Biophys Acta 1100(1):67–74

Menz RI, Walker JE, Leslie AG (2001) Structure of bovine mitochondrial F(1)-ATPase with nucleotide bound to all three catalytic sites: implications for the mechanism of rotary catalysis. Cell 106:331–341

Mesecke N, Terziyska N, Kozany C, Baumann F, Neupert W, Hell K, Herrmann JM (2005) A disulfide relay system in the intermembrane space of mitochondria that mediates protein import. Cell 121:1059–1069

Michel H (1998) The mechanism of proton pumping by cytochrome c oxidase. Proc Natl Acad Sci USA 95(22): 12819–12824

Michel H (1999) Cytochrome c oxidase: catalytic cycle and mechanisms of proton pumping – a discussion. Biochemistry 38(46):15129–15140

Miller MJ, Oldenburg M, Fillingame RH (1990) The essential carboxyl group in subunit c of the F_1F_0 ATP synthase can be moved and H(+)-translocating function retained. Proc Natl Acad Sci USA 87:4900–4904

Mitchell P (1966) Chemiosmotic coupling in oxidative and photosynthetic phosphorylation. Biol Rev Camb Philos Soc 41(3):445–502

Mitchell P (1976) Possible molecular mechanisms of the protonmotive function of cytochrome systems. J Theor Biol 62:327–367

Miyoshi H (2001) Probing the ubiquinone reduction site in bovine mitochondrial complex I using a series of synthetic ubiquinones and inhibitors. J Bioenerg Biomembr 33(3):223–231

Mootha VK, Bunkenborg J, Olsen JV, Hjerrild M, Wisniewski JR, Stahl E, Bolouri MS, Ray HN, Sihag S, Kamal M, Patterson N, Lander ES, Mann M (2003) Integrated analysis of protein composition, tissue diversity, and gene regulation in mouse mitochondria. Cell 115:629–640

Moyes CD, Battersby BJ, Leary SC (1998) Regulation of muscle mitochondrial design. J Exp Biol 201:299–307

Murphy MP (2009) How mitochondria produce reactive oxygen species. Biochem J 417:1–13

Neupert W (1997) Protein import into mitochondria. Annu Rev Biochem 66:863–917

Neupert W, Brunner M (2002) The protein import motor of mitochondria. Nat Rev Mol Cell Biol 3:555–565

Neupert W, Herrmann JM (2007) Translocation of proteins into mitochondria. Annu Rev Biochem 76:723–749

Nijtmans LG, Taanman JW, Muijsers AO, Speijer D, Van den Bogert C (1998) Assembly of cytochrome-c oxidase in cultured human cells. Eur J Biochem 254:389–394

Nisoli E, Clementi E, Moncada S, Carruba MO (2004) Mitochondrial biogenesis as a cellular signaling framework. Biochem Pharmacol 67:1–15

Nobrega FG, Nobrega MP, Tzagoloff A (1992) BCS1, a novel gene required for the expression of functional Rieske iron-sulfur protein in Saccharomyces cerevisiae. EMBO J 11:3821–3829

Noji H, Yasuda R, Yoshida M, Kinosita K (1997) Direct observation of the rotation of F1-ATPase. Nature 386:299–302

Ogilvie I, Kennaway NG, Shoubridge EA (2005) A molecular chaperone for mitochondrial complex I assembly is mutated in a progressive encephalopathy. J Clin Invest 115:2784–2792

Ohnishi T (1998) Iron–sulfur clusters/semiquinones in complex I. Biochim Biophys Acta 1364:186–206

Ohnishi T, Salerno JC (2005) Conformation-driven and semiquinone-gated protonpump mechanism in the NADH-ubiquinone oxidoreductase (complex I). FEBS Lett 579:4555–4561

Ohnishi T, Schägger H, Meinhardt SW, LoBrutto R, Link TA, von Jagow G (1989) Spatial organization of redox active centers in the bovine heart ubiquinol-cytochrome c oxidoreductase. J Biol Chem 264:735–744

Oostveen FG, Au HC, Meijer PJ, Scheffler IE (1995) A Chinese hamster mutant cell line with a defect in the integral membrane protein CII-3 of complex II of the mitochondrial electron transport chain. J Biol Chem 270:26104–26108

Ostermeier C, Harrenga A, Ermler U, Michel H (1997) Structure at 2.7 Å resolution of the Paracoccus denitrificans two-subunit cytochrome c oxidase complexed with an antibody Fv fragment. Proc Natl Acad Sci USA 94:10547–10553

Pagliarini DJ, Calvo SE, Chang B, Sheth SA, Vafai SB, Ong SE, Walford GA, Sugiana C, Boneh A, Chen WK, Hill DE, Vidal M, Evans JG, Thorburn DR, Carr SA, Mootha VK (2008) A mitochondrial protein compendium elucidates complex I disease biology. Cell 134:112–123

Palmieri F, Klingenberg M (2004) Mitochondrial metabolite transporter family. In: Lennarz WJ, Lane MD (eds) Encyclopedia of biological chemistry, vol 2. Elsevier, Oxford, pp 725–732

Palmisano G, Sardanelli AM, Signorile A, Papa S, Larsen MR (2007) The phosphorylation pattern of bovine heart complex I subunits. Proteomics 7(10):1575–1583

Panke O, Gumbiowski K, Junge W, Engelbrecht S (2000) F-ATPase: specific observation of the rotating c subunit oligomer of EF(O) EF(1). FEBS Lett 472:34–38

Papa S (1976) Proton translocation reactions in respiratory chains. Biochim Biophys Acta 456:39–84

Papa S (1996) Mitochondrial oxidative phosphorylation changes in the life span. Molecular aspects and physiopathological implications. Biochim Biophys Acta 1276:87–105

Papa S (2002) The NDUFS4 nuclear gene of complex I of mitochondria and the cAMP cascade. Biochim Biophys Acta 1555:147–153

Papa S, Skulachev VP (1997) Reactive oxygen species, mitochondria, apoptosis and aging. Mol Cell Biochem 174:305–319

Papa S, Lofrumento NE, Quagliariello E, Meijer AJ, Tager JM (1971) Coupling mechanisms in anionic substrate transport across the inner membrane of rat-liver mitochondria. J Bioenerg 1:287–307

Papa S, Guerrieri F, Lorusso M, Simone S (1973) Proton translocation and energy transduction in mitochondria. Biochimie 55(6):703–716

Papa S, Guerrieri F, Lorusso M (1974) Mechanism of respiration-driven proton translocation in the inner mitochondrial membrane. Analysis of proton translocation associated to oxido-reductions of the oxygen-terminal respiratory carriers. Biochim Biophys Acta 357(2):181–192

Papa S, Lorusso M, Cocco T, Boffoli D, Lombardo M (1990) Protonmotive ubiquinolcytochrome c oxidoreductase of mitochondria. A possible example of co-operative anisotropy of protolytic redox catalysis. In: Lenaz G, Barnabei O, Rabbi A, Battino M (eds) Highlights in ubiquinone research. Taylor & Francis, London/New York/Philadelphia, pp 122–135

Papa S, Capitanio N, Capitanio G, De Nitto E, Minuto M (1991) The cytochrome chain of mitochondria exhibits variable H^+/e^- stoichiometry. FEBS Lett 288(1–2):183–186

Papa S, Lorusso M, Capitanio N (1994) Mechanistic and phenomenological features of proton pumps in the respiratory chain of mitochondria. J Bioenerg Biomembr 26:609–618

Papa S, Lorusso M, Capitanio N (1995) On the mechanism of proton pumps in respiratory chains. In: Papa S, Tager JM (eds) Biochemistry of cell membranes. Birkhäuser Verlag, Basel, pp 151–166

Papa S, Lorusso M, Capitanio N, Zanotti F (1996a) Liposomes in reconstitution of protonmotive proteins. In: Barenholtz Y, Lasic DD (eds) Handbook of nonmedical applications of liposomes, vol II. CRC Press, Boca Raton, pp 245–259

Papa S, Sardanelli AM, Cocco T, Speranza F, Scacco S, Technikova-Dobrova Z (1996b) The nuclear-encoded 18 kDa (IP) AQDQ subunit of bovine heart complex I is phosphorylated by the mitochondrial cAMP-dependent protein kinase. FEBS Lett 379:299–301

Papa S, Zanotti F, Cocco T, Perrucci C, Candita C, Minuto M (1996c) Identification of functional domains and critical residues in the adenosinetriphosphatase inhibitor protein of mitochondrial F_oF_1 ATP synthase. Eur J Biochem 240:461–467

Papa S, Capitanio N, Villani G (1998) A cooperative model for protonmotive heme-copper oxidases. The role of heme a in the proton pump of cytochrome c oxidase. FEBS Lett 439:1–8

Papa S, Capitanio N, Villani G (1999) Proton pumps of respiratory chain enzymes. In: Papa S, Guerrieri F, Tager JM (eds) Frontiers of cellular bioenergetics: molecular biology, biochemistry and physiopathology. Plenum Press, London, pp 49–88

Papa S, Lorusso M, Di Paola M (2006a) Cooperativity and flexibility of the protonmotive activity of mitochondrial respiratory chain. Biochim Biophys Acta 1757:428–436

Papa S, Capitanio G, Martino PL (2006b) Concerted involvement of cooperative proton-electron linkage and water production in the proton pump of cytochrome c oxidase. Biochim Biophys Acta 1757(9–10):1133–1143

Papa S, Petruzzella V, Scacco S (2007) Electron transport, Structure, redox-coupled protonmotive activity and pathological disorders of respiratory chain complexes. In: Lajtha A, Dienel G, Gibson G (eds) Handbook of neurochemistry and molecular neurobiology. Springer, Berlin/Heidelberg, pp 93–118

Papa S, De Rasmo D, Scacco S, Signorile A, Technikova-Dobrova Z, Palmisano G, Sardanelli AM, Papa F, Panelli D, Scaringi R, Santeramo A (2008) Mammalian complex I: a regulable and vulnerable pacemaker in mitochondrial respiratory function. Biochim Biophys Acta 1777:719–728

Papadopoulou LC, Sue CM, Davidson MM, Tanji K, Nishino I, Sadlock JE, Krishna S, Walker W, Selby J, Glerum DM, Coster RV, Lyon G, Scalais E, Lebel R, Kaplan P, Shanske S, De Vivo DC, Bonilla E, Hirano M, DiMauro S, Schon EA (1999) Fatal infantile cardioencephalomyopathy with COX deficiency and mutations in SCO2, a COX assembly gene. Nat Genet 23:333–337

Paschen SA, Neupert W, Rapaport D (2005) Biogenesis of b-barrel membrane proteins of mitochondria. Trends Biochem Sci 30:575–582

Pasdois P, Deveaud C, Voisin P, Bouchaud V, Rigoulet M, Beauvoit B (2003) Contribution of the phosphorylable complex I in the growth phase-dependent respiration of C6 glioma cells in vitro. J Bioenerg Biomembr 35:439–450

Paumard P, Vaillier J, Coulary B, Schaeffer J, Soubannier V, Mueller DM, Brèthes D, di Rago JP, Velours J (2002) The ATP synthase is involved in generating mitochondrial cristae morphology. EMBO J 21:221–230

Penefsky HS (1985) Energy-dependent dissociation of ATP from high affinity catalytic sites of beef heart mitochondrial adenosine triphosphatase. J Biol Chem 260:13735–13741

Peng G, Fritzsch G, Zickermann V, Schagger H, Mentele R, Lottspeich F et al (2003) Isolation, characterization and electron microscopic single particle analysis of the NADH:ubiquinone oxidoreductase (complex I) from the hyperthermophilic eubacterium Aquifex aeolicus. Biochemistry 42:3032–3039

Petruzzella V, Tiranti V, Fernandez P, Ianna P, Carrozzo R, Zeviani M (1998) Identification and characterization of human cDNAs specific to BCS1, PET112, SCO1, COX15, and COX11, five genes involved in the formation and function of the mitochondrial respiratory chain. Genomics 54:494–504

Pfanner N, Geissler A (2001) Versatility of the mitochondrial protein import machinery. Nat Rev Mol Cell Biol 2(5):339–349

Pfanner N, Craig EA, Honlinger A (1997) Mitochondrial preprotein translocase. Annu Rev Cell Dev Biol 13:25–51

Pocsfalvi G, Cuccurullo M, Schlosser G, Scacco S, Papa S, Malorni A (2007) Phosphorylation of B14.5a subunit from bovine heart complex I identified by titanium dioxide selective enrichment and shotgun proteomics. Mol Cell Proteomics 6(2):231–237

Premsler T, Zahedi RP, Lewandrowski U, Sickmann A (2009) Recent advances in yeast organelle and membrane proteomics. Proteomics 9:4731–4743

Proshlyakov DA, Pressler MA, DeMaso C, Leykam JF, DeWitt DL, Babcock GT (2000) Oxygen activation and reduction in respiration: involvement of redox-active tyrosine 244. Science 290(5496):1588–1591

Pullman ME, Monroy GC (1963) A naturally occurring inhibitor of mitochondrial adenosine triphosphatase. J Biol Chem 238:3762–3769

Radermacher M, Ruiz T, Clason T, Benjamin S, Brandt U, Zickermann V (2006) The three dimensional structure of complex I from Yarrowia lipolytica: a highly dynamic enzyme. J Struct Biol 154:269–279

Raha S, Robinson BH (2000) Mitochondria, oxygen free radicals, disease and ageing. Trends Biochem Sci 25(10):502–508

Rak M, Zeng X, Brière JJ, Tzagoloff A (2009) Assembly of F_O in Saccharomyces cerevisiae. Biochim Biophys Acta 1793:108–116

Rees DM, Leslie AG, Walker JE (2009) The structure of the membrane extrinsic region of bovine ATP synthase. Proc Natl Acad Sci USA 106:21597–21601

Rehling P, Model K, Brandner K, Kovermann P, Sickmann A, Meyer HE, Kühlbrandt W, Wagner R, Truscott KN, Pfanner N (2003) Protein insertion into the mitochondrial inner membrane by a twin-pore translocase. Science 299:1747–1751

Remacle C, Barbieri MR, Cardol P, Hamel PP (2008) Eukaryotic complex I: functional diversity and experimental systems to unravel the assembly process. Mol Genet Genomics 280:93–110

Rexroth S, Meyer Zu Tittingdorf JM, Schwassmann HJ, Krause F, Seelert H, Dencher NA (2004) Dimeric H^+-ATP synthase in the chloroplast of Chlamydomonas reinhardtii. Biochim Biophys Acta 1658(3):202–211

Rich PR (1995) Towards an understanding of the chemistry of oxygen reduction and proton translocation in the iron-copper respiratory oxidases. Aust J Plant Physiol 22:479–486

Ricquier D (2005) Respiration uncoupling and metabolism in the control of energy expenditure. Proc Nutr Soc 64:47–52

Ricquier D, Bouillaud F (2000) The uncoupling protein homologues: UCP1, UCP2, UCP3, StUCP and AtUCP. Biochem J 345:161–179

Rieske JS (1986) Experimental observations on the structure and function of mitochondrial complex III that are unresolved by the protonmotive ubiquinone-cycle hypothesis. J Bioenerg Biomembr 18:235–257

Robin M, Anandatheerthavarada H, Biswas G, Sepuris N, Gordon D, Pain D, Avadhani G (2002) Bimodal targeting of microsomal CYP2E1 to mitochondria through activation of an N-terminal chimeric signal by cAMP-mediated phosphorylation. J Biol Chem 277:40583–40593

Robin M, Prabu S, Raza H, Anandatheerthavarada H, Avadhani G (2003) Phosphorylation enhances mitochondrial targeting of GSTA4-4 through increased affinity for binding to cytoplasmic Hsp70. J Biol Chem 278:18960–18970

Rousseau DL, Sassaroli M, Ching YC, Dasgupta S (1988) The role of water near cytochrome a in cytochrome c oxidase. Ann N Y Acad Sci 550:223–237

Rubinstein JL, Walker JE, Henderson R (2003) Structure of the mitochondrial ATP synthase by electron cryomicroscopy. EMBO J 22:6182–6192

Ryu H, Lee J, Impey S, Ratan RR, Ferrante RJ (2005) Antioxidants modulate mitochondrial PKA and increase CREB binding to D-loop DNA of the mitochondrial genome in neurons. Proc Natl Acad Sci USA 102:13915–13920

Saada A, Edvardson S, Rapoport M, Shaag A, Amry K, Miller C, Lorberboum-Galski H, Elpeleg O (2008) C6ORF66 is an assembly factor of mitochondrial complex I. Am J Hum Genet 82:32–38

Sabbert D, Engelbrecht S, Junge W (1996) Intersubunit rotation in active F-ATPase. Nature 381:623–625

Salerno JC, Ohnishi T (1980) Studies on the stabilized ubisemiquinone species in the succinate cytochrome c reductase segment of the intact mitochondrial membrane system. Biochem J 192:769–781

Sambongi Y, Iko Y, Tanabe M, Omote H, Iwamoto-Kihara A, Ueda I, Yanagida T, Wada Y, Futai M (1999) Mechanical rotation of the c subunit oligomer in ATP synthase (F_0F_1): direct observation. Science 286:1722–1724

Sanger N, Strohmeier R, Kaufmann M, Kuhl H (2000) Cell cycle-related expression and ligand binding of peripheral benzodiazepine receptor in human breast cancer cell lines. Eur J Cancer 36:2157–2163

Satoh M, Kuroiwa T (1991) Organization of multiple nucleoids and DNA molecules in mitochondria of a human cell. Exp Cell Res 196:137–140

Sazanov LA, Hinchliffe P (2006) Structure of the hydrophilic domain of respiratory complex I from Thermus thermophilus. Science 311:1430–1436

Scacco S, Petruzzella V, Budde S, Vergari R, Tamborra R, Panelli D, van den Heuvel LP, Smeitink JA, Papa S (2003) Pathological mutations of the human NDUFS4 gene of the 18-kDa (AQDQ) subunit of complex I affect the expression of the protein and the assembly and function of the complex. J Biol Chem 278:44161–44167

Scarpulla RC (1997) Nuclear control of respiratory chain expression in mammalian cells. J Bioenerg Biomembr 29:109–119

Scarpulla RC (2008) Nuclear control of respiratory chain expression by nuclear respiratory factors and PGC-1-related coactivator. Ann N Y Acad Sci 1147:321–334

Schägger H (2001) Blue-native gels to isolate protein complexes from mitochondria. Methods Cell Biol 65:231–244

Schagger H, Pfeiffer K (2000) Supercomplexes in the respiratory chains of yeast and mammalian mitochondria. EMBO J 19:1777–17783

Schägger H, Pfeiffer K (2001) The ratio of oxidative phosphorylation complexes I-V in bovine heart mitochondria and the composition of respiratory chain supercomplexes. J Biol Chem 276(41):37861–37867

Schägger H, Brandt U, Gencic S, von Jagow G (1995) Ubiquinol-cytochrome-c reductase from human and bovine mitochondria. Methods Enzymol 260:82–96

Schägger H, de Coo R, Bauer MF, Hofmann S, Godinot C, Brandt U (2004) Significance of respirasomes for the assembly/stability of human respiratory chain complex I. J Biol Chem 279(35):36349–36353

Scheffler IE, Yadava N, Potluri P (2004) Molecular genetics of complex I-deficient Chinese hamster cell lines. Biochim Biophys Acta 1659:160–171

Screaton RA, Conkright MD, Katoh Y, Best JL, Canettieri G, Jeffries S, Guzman E, Niessen S, Yates JR III, Takemori H, Okamoto M, Montminy M (2004) The CREB coactivator TORC2 functions as a calcium- and cAMP-sensitive coincidence detector. Cell 119:61–74

Shaywitz AJ, Greenberg ME (1999) CREB: a stimulus-induced transcription factor activated by a diverse array of extracellular signals. Annu Rev Biochem 68:821–861

Sluse FE, Jarmuszkiewicz W, Navet R, Douette P, Mathy G, Sluse-Goffart CM (2006) Mitochondrial UCPs: new insights into regulation and impact. Biochim Biophys Acta 1757:480–485

Stiburek L, Hansikova H, Tesarova M, Cerna L, Zeman J (2006) Biogenesis of eukaryotic cytochrome c oxidase. Physiol Res 55:S27–S41

Stock D, Leslie AG, Walker JE (1999) Molecular architecture of the rotary motor in ATP synthase. Science 286:1700–1705

Strauss M, Hofhaus G, Schröder RR, Kühlbrandt W (2008) Dimer ribbons of ATP synthase shape the inner mitochondrial membrane. EMBO J 27:1154–1160

Svensson-Ek M, Abramson J, Larsson G, Tornroth S, Brezezinski P, Iwata S (2002) The X-ray crystal structures of wild-type and Eq(I-286) mutant cytochrome c oxidases from Rhodobacter sphaeroides. J Mol Biol 321:329–339

Taanman JW, Williams SL (2001) Assembly of cytochrome c oxidase: what can we learn from patients with cytochrome c oxidase deficiency? Biochem Soc Trans 29:446–451

Takahashi Y, Kako K, Arai H, Ohishi T, Inada Y, Takehara A, Fukamizu A, Munekata E (2002) Characterization and identification of promoter elements in the mouse COX17 gene. Biochim Biophys Acta 1574:359–364

Tatoyan A, Giulivi C (1998) Purification and characterization of a nitric-oxide synthase from rat liver mitochondria. J Biol Chem 273(18):11044–11048

Taylor ER, Hurrell F, Shannon RJ, Lin TK, Hirst J, Murphy MP (2003a) Reversible glutathionylation of complex I increases mitochondrial superoxide formation. J Biol Chem 278(22):19603–19610

Taylor RW, McDonnell MT, Blakely EL, Chinnery PF, Taylor GA, Howell N, Zeviani M, Briem E, Carrara F, Turnbull DM (2003b) Genotypes from patients indicate no paternal mitochondrial contribution. Ann Neurol 54:521–524

Technikova-Dobrova Z, Sardanelli AM, Speranza F, Scacco S, Signorile A, Lorusso V, Papa S (2001) Cyclic adenosine monophosphate-dependent phosphorylation of mammalian mitochondrial proteins: enzyme and substrate characterization and functional role. Biochemistry 40:13941–13947

Tiranti V, Hoertnagel K, Carrozzo R, Galimberti C, Munaro M, Granatiero M, Zelante L, Gasparini P, Marzella R, Rocchi M, Bayona-Bafaluy MP, Enriquez JA, Uziel G, Bertini E, Dionisi-Vici C, Franco B, Meitinger T, Zeviani M (1998) Mutations of SURF-1 in Leigh disease associated with cytochrome c oxidase deficiency. Am J Hum Genet 63:1609–1621

Toogood HS, Leys D, Scrutton NS (2007) Dynamics driving function: new insights from electron transferring flavoproteins and partner complexes. FEBS J 274(21):5481–5504

Trumpower BL (1999) Energy transduction in mitochondrial respiration by the protonmotive Q-cycle mechanism of the cytochrome bc1 complex. In: Tager JM (ed) Frontiers of cellular bioenergetics: molecular biology, biochemistry, and physiopathology. Kluwer Academic/Plenum Publishers, New York, pp 233–261

Tsukihara T, Aoyama H, Yamashita E, Tomizaki T, Yamaguchi H, Shinzawa-Itoh K, Nakashima R, Yaono R, Yoshikawa S (1995) Structures of metal sites of oxidized bovine heart cytochrome c oxidase at 2.8 Å. Science 269:1069–1074

Tsukihara T, Aoyama H, Yamashita E, Tomizaki T, Yamaguchi H, Shinzawa-Itoh K, Nakashima R, Yaono R, Yoshikawa S (1996) The whole structure of the 13-subunit oxidized cytochrome c oxidase at 2.8 A. Science 272:1136–1144

Tsukihara T, Shimokata K, Katayama Y, Shimada H, Muramoto K, Aoyama H, Mochizuki M, Shinzawa-Itoh K, Yamashita E, Yao M, Ishimura Y, Yoshikawa S (2003) The low-spin heme of cytochrome c oxidase as the driving element of the proton-pumping process. Proc Natl Acad Sci USA 100:15304–15309

Tsunoda SP, Aggeler R, Yoshida M, Capaldi RA (2001) Rotation of the c subunit oligomer in fully functional F_1F_o ATP synthase. Proc Natl Acad Sci USA 98:898–902

Tuschen G, Sackmann U, Nehls U, Haiker H, Buse G, Weiss H (1990) Assembly of NADH: ubiquinone reductase (complex I) in Neurospora mitochondria. Independent pathways of nuclear-encoded and mitochondrially encoded subunits. J Mol Biol 213:845–857

Ugalde C, Vogel R, Huijbens R, Van Den Heuvel B, Smeitink J, Nijtmans L (2004) Human mitochondrial complex I assembles through the combination of evolutionary conserved modules: a framework to interpret complex I deficiencies. Hum Mol Genet 13:2461–2472

Valnot I, Osmond S, Gigarel N, Mehaye B, Amiel J, Cormier-Daire V, Munnich A, Bonnefont JP, Rustin P, Rötig A (2000) Mutations of the SCO1 gene in mitochondrial cytochrome c oxidase deficiency with neonatal-onset hepatic failure and encephalopathy. Am J Hum Genet 67:1104–1109

van der Laan M, Wiedemann N, Mick DU, Guiard B, Rehling P, Pfanner N (2006) A role for Tim21 in membrane-potential-dependent preprotein sorting in mitochondria. Curr Biol 16:2271–2276

van der Laan M, Hutu DP, Rehling P (2010) On the mechanism of preprotein import by the mitochondrial presequence translocase. Biochim Biophys Acta 1803:732–739

Ventura B, Genova ML, Bovina C, Formiggini G, Lenaz G (2002) Control of oxidative phosphorylation by Complex I in rat liver mitochondria: implications for aging. Biochim Biophys Acta 1553:249–260

Verkaart S, Koopman WJ, Cheek J, van Emst-de Vries SE, van den Heuvel LW, Smeitink JA, Willems PH (2007) Mitochondrial and cytosolic thiol redox state are not detectably altered in isolated human NADH:ubiquinone oxidoreductase deficiency. Biochim Biophys Acta 1772:1041–1051

Videira A, Duarte M (2001) On complex I and other NADH: ubiquinone reductases of Neurospora crassa mitochondria. J Bioenerg Biomembr 33:197–203

Vik SB, Antonio BJ (1994) A mechanism of proton translocation by F_1F_o ATP synthases suggested by double mutant of the a subunit. J Biol Chem 269:30364–30369

Vinogradov AD (1993) Kinetics, control, and mechanism of ubiquinone reduction by the mammalian respiratory chain-linked NADH-ubiquinone reductase. J Bioenerg Biomembr 25(4):367–375

Vogel RO, Janssen RJ, Ugalde C, Grovenstein M, Huijbens RJ, Visch HJ, van den Heuvel LP, Willems PH, Zeviani M, Smeitink JA, Nijtmans LG (2005) Human mitochondrial complex I assembly is mediated by NDUFAF1. FEBS J 272:5317–5326

Vogel RO, Janssen RJ, van den Brand MA, Dieteren CE, Verkaart S, Koopman WJ, Willems PH, Pluk W, van den Heuvel LP, Smeitink JA, Nijtmans LG (2007) Cytosolic signaling protein Ecsit also localizes to mitochondria where it interacts with chaperone NDUFAF1 and functions in complex I assembly. Genes Dev 21:615–624

Wada T, Long JC, Zhang D, Vik SB (1999) A novel labeling approach supports the five-transmembrane model of subunit a of the Escherichia coli ATP synthase. J Biol Chem 274:17353–17357

Wang ZG, White PS, Ackerman SH (2001) Atp11p and Atp12p are assembly factors for the F(1)-ATPase in human mitochondria. J Biol Chem 276:30773–30778

Webb CT, Gorman MA, Lazarou M, Ryan MT, Gulbis JM (2006) Crystal structure of the mitochondrial chaperone TIM9.10 reveals a six-bladed alpha-propeller. Mol Cell 21:123–133

Wenz T (2009) PGC-1alpha activation as a therapeutic approach in mitochondrial disease. IUBMB Life 61: 1051–1062

Wiedemann N, Frazier AE, Pfanner N (2004) The protein import machinery of mitochondria. J Biol Chem 279: 14473–14476

Wielburski A, Nelson BD (1983) Evidence for the sequential assembly of cytochrome oxidase subunits in rat liver mitochondria. Biochem J 212:829–834

Wikström M (1984) Two protons are pumped from the mitochondrial matrix per electron transferred between NADH and ubiquinone. FEBS Lett 169:300–304

Wikström M (2000) Mechanism of proton translocation by cytochrome c oxidase: a new four-stroke histidine cycle. Biochim Biophys Acta 1458(1):188–198

Wikström MK, Berden JA (1972) Oxidoreduction of cytochrome b in the presence of antimycin. Biochim Biophys Acta 283(3):403–420

Wikström M, Verkhovsky MI (2007) Mechanism and energetics of proton translocation by the respiratory heme-copper oxidases. Biochim Biophys Acta 1767:1200–1214

Wikström M, Krab K, Saraste M (1981a) Proton-translocating cytochrome complexes. Annu Rev Biochem 50:623–655

Wikström M, Krab K, Saraste M (1981b) Cytochrome c oxidase. A synthesis. Academic Press INC. (London) LTD, London/New York

Wittig I, Shagger H (2009) Supramolecular organization of ATP synthase and respiratory chain in mitochondrial membranes. Biochim Biophys Acta 1787:672–680

Wu M, Tzagoloff A (1989) Identification and characterization of a new gene (CBP3) required for the expression of yeast coenzyme QH2-cytochrome c reductase. J Biol Chem 264:11122–11130

Wu Z, Puigserver P, Andersson U, Zhang C, Adelmant G, Mootha V, Troy A, Cinti S, Lowell B, Scarpulla RC, Spiegelman BM (1999) Mechanisms controlling mitochondrial biogenesis and respiration through the thermogenic coactivator PGC-1. Cell 98:115–124

Wu Z, Huang X, Feng Y, Handschin C, Feng Y, Gullicksen PS, Bare O, Labow M, Spiegelman B, Stevenson SC (2006) Transducer of regulated CREB-binding proteins (TORCs) induce PGC-1alpha transcription and mitochondrial biogenesis in muscle cells. Proc Natl Acad Sci USA 103:14379–14384

Xia D, Yu CA, Kim H, Xia JZ, Kachurin AM, Zhang L, Yu L, Deisenhofer J (1997) Crystal structure of the cytochrome bc_1 complex from bovine heart mitochondria. Science 277:60–66

Yadava N, Potluri P, Scheffler IE (2008) Investigations of the potential effects of phosphorylation of the MWFE and ESSS subunits on complex I activity and assembly. Int J Biochem Cell Biol 40:447–460

Yagi T, Matsuno-Yagi A (2003) The proton-translocating NADH-quinone oxidoreductase in the respiratory chain: the secret unlocked. Biochemistry 42:2266–2274

Yano M, Terada K, Mori M (2003) AIP is a mitochondrial import mediator that binds to both import receptor Tom20 and preproteins. J Cell Biol 163:45–56

Yoshikawa S, Shinzawa-Itoh K, Nakashima R, Yaono R, Yamashita E, Inoue N, Yao M, Fei MJ, Libeu CP, Mizushima T, Yamaguchi H, Tomizaki T, Tsukihara T (1998) Redox-coupled crystal structural changes in bovine heart cytochrome c oxidase. Science 280(5370):1723–1729

Young JC, Hoogenraad NJ, Hartl FU (2003) Molecular chaperones Hsp90 and Hsp70 deliver preproteins to the mitochondrial import receptor Tom70. Cell 112:41–50

Zanotti F, Raho G, Vuolo R, Gaballo A, Papa F, Papa S (2000) Functional domains of the ATPase inhibitor protein from bovine heart mitochondria. FEBS Lett 482:163–166

Zara V, Palmisano I, Conte L, Trumpower BL (2004) Further insights into the assembly of the yeast cytochrome bc1 complex based on analysis of single and double deletion mutants lacking supernumerary subunits and cytochrome b. Eur J Biochem 271:1209–1218

Zara V, Conte L, Trumpower BL (2009) Biogenesis of the yeast cytochrome bc1 complex. Biochim Biophys Acta 1793:89–96

Zhang Z, Huang L, Shulmeister VM, Chi YI, Kim KK, Hung LW, Crofts AR, Berry EA, Kim SH (1998) Electron transfer by domain movement in cytochrome bc_1. Nature 392:677–684

Zick M, Rabl R, Reichert AS (2009) Cristae formation-linking ultrastructure and function of mitochondria. Biochim Biophys Acta 1793:5–19

Zickermann V, Kerscher S, Zwicker K, Tocilescu MA, Radermacher M, Brandt U (2009) Architecture of complex I and its implications for electron transfer and proton pumping. Biochim Biophys Acta 1787(6):574–583

Chapter 2
Physiology and Pathophysiology of Mitochondrial DNA

Hongzhi Li, Danhui Liu, Jianxin Lu, and Yidong Bai

Abstract Mitochondria are the only organelles in animal cells which possess their own genomes. Mitochondrial DNA (mtDNA) alterations have been associated with various human conditions. Yet, their role in pathogenesis remains largely unclear. This review focuses on several major features of mtDNA: (1) mtDNA haplogroup, (2) mtDNA common deletion, (3) mtDNA mutations in the control region or D-loop, (4) mtDNA copy number alterations, (5) mtDNA mutations in translational machinery, (6) mtDNA mutations in protein coding genes (7) mtDNA heteroplasmy. We will also discuss their implications in various human diseases.

Keywords Mitochondrial DNA mutation • Mitochondrial haplogroup • D-loop region • Common deletion • Heteroplasmy

2.1 Mitochondrial DNA

The mammalian mitochondrial genome is a double-stranded circular DNA of about 16,500 nucleotides. It encodes 13 peptides for the oxidative phosphorylation apparatus, 7 for subunits of complex I (ND1, 2, 3, 4L, 4, 5, 6), 1 for subunit of complex III (cytb), 3 for subunits of complex IV (COI, II, III) and 2 for subunits of complex V (ATP 6 & 8), as well as 22 tRNAs and 2 rRNAs (12S, 16S) which are essential for protein synthesis within mitochondria (Fig. 2.1). Besides these coding regions, there is a main control region, or D-loop which contains the mtDNA replication origin (O_H) and promoters (P_H and P_L) for mtRNA transcription (Fig. 2.1).

H. Li • D. Liu • J. Lu
Zhejiang Provincial Key Laboratory of Medical Genetics, Wenzhou Medical College,
Wenzhou, Zhejiang 325035, China

Y. Bai, Ph.D. (✉)
Zhejiang Provincial Key Laboratory of Medical Genetics, Wenzhou Medical College,
Wenzhou, Zhejiang 325035, China

Department of Cellular and Structural Biology, University of Texas Health Science Center at San Antonio,
San Antonio, TX 78229, USA
e-mail: baiy@uthscsa.edu

R. Scatena et al. (eds.), *Advances in Mitochondrial Medicine*, Advances in Experimental
Medicine and Biology 942, DOI 10.1007/978-94-007-2869-1_2,
© Springer Science+Business Media B.V. 2012

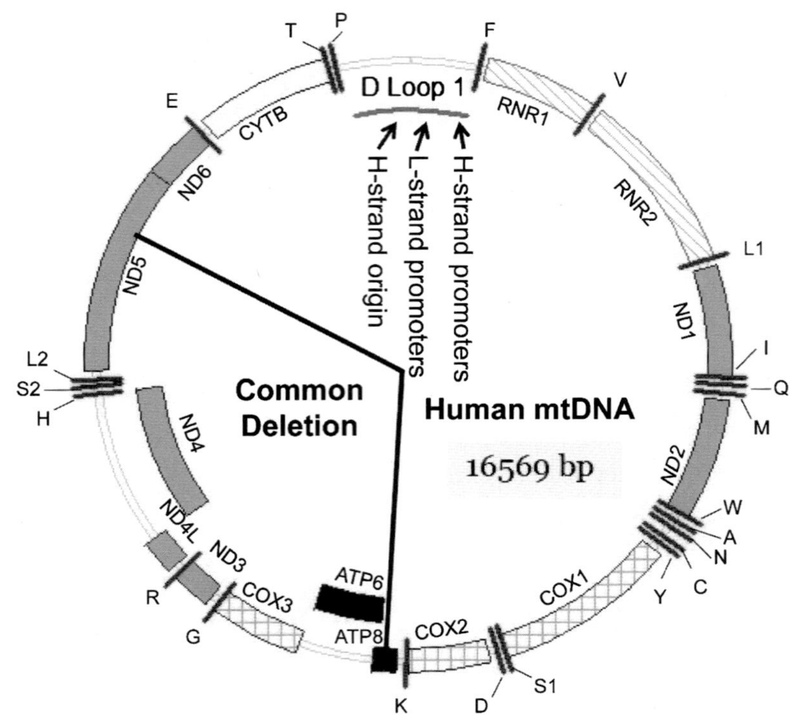

Fig. 2.1 Human mitochondrial genome. It encodes 13 peptides, 22 tRNA and 2 rRNA. The D-loop contains mtDNA replication origin and transcription promoters. The 4,977-bp common deletion is indicated

mtDNA is predominantly maternal transmission. Most mammalian cells contain many copies of mitochondrial genomes. mtDNA within a cell could be a mixture of both wild-type and mutant species, a condition called "heteroplasmy", while "homoplasmy" refers the situation when all mtDNAs are identical. The pathogenic mutations are usually heteroplasmic in nature. It is expected that, due to the multiplicity of mitochondrial genomes in each cell, a threshold of mutant mtDNA must be reached before cellular dysfunction caused by defective mitochondria becomes apparent. Thus mtDNA heteroplasmy is very important in regulating mitochondrial function.

2.2   mtDNA Alterations in Human Diseases

As discussed in previous chapters, mitochondria play important roles in regulating energy production, metabolism, signal transduction and apoptosis, it is not surprising that more and more mtDNA alterations and mitochondrial dysfunctions have been reported in various human diseases. Clinical manifestations that have been related to mtDNA mutations affect the brain, heart, skeletal muscle, kidney, endocrine system and other organs. Specific symptoms include forms of blindness, deafness, dementia, cardiovascular disease, muscle weakness, movement disorders, renal dysfunction, and endocrine disorders. Recently, mutations in both the non-coding and coding regions of the mtDNA have also been identified in almost all types of human cancer (Lu et al. 2009).

2.3 mtDNA Haplogroup

A human mtDNA haplogroup refers to a unique set of mtDNA polymorphisms, reflecting mutations accumulated by a discrete maternal lineage. The haplogroups are associated with region-specific mtDNA sequence variation as a result of genetic drift and/or adaptive selection for an environment-favored mitochondrial function. Difference in redox signaling as a consequence of haplogroup-associated oxidative phosphorylation capacity has been reported (Tanaka et al. 2004; Wallace 2005). Some typical haplogroups and their determination sites in Wenzhou population which we have studied were described as in Fig. 2.2.

The implications of mtDNA haplogroups in various conditions including aging, neurodegenerative diseases, metabolic diseases, infectious diseases and cancer have been explored. For example, haplogroups D4a and D5 were reported to be enriched in centenarians in Japanese population (Bilal et al. 2008), while D4 was found to be increased in female and N9 to be decreased in a Chinese population in Rugao area (Cai et al. 2009). mtSNP at 10398, which is a major diagnostic site of macro-haplogroups M and N, has been implicated not only in longevity, but also in Parkinson's disease and breast cancer, in various populations. The population-specific haplogroup implication was also reported on D4a as it was observed to increase susceptibility in a Chinese population to esophageal carcinoma (Li et al. 2007).

In addition, haplogroup T was associated with coronary artery disease and diabetic retinopathy in Middle European Caucasian populations (Kofler et al. 2009). H5 was reported as a risk factor for late onset Alzheimer's disease for females without APOE genotype (Santoro et al. 2010). The haplogroup cluster IWX was associated with front temporal lobar degeneration (Kruger et al. 2010). Haplogroup K was suggested as an independent determinant of risk of cerebral, but not coronary ischemic vascular events, which provided a new means for the identification of individuals with a high susceptibility of developing ischemic stroke (Chinnery et al. 2010). The LHON patients with the primary mtDNA mutation at 14484T>C had significantly higher frequency of haplogroups C, G, M10 and Y, but a lower frequency of haplogroup F (Yu et al. 2010). Our own study indicated that mitochondrial haplogroups could have a tissue-specific, population-specific and stage-specific role in modulating cancer development (Shen et al. 2010).

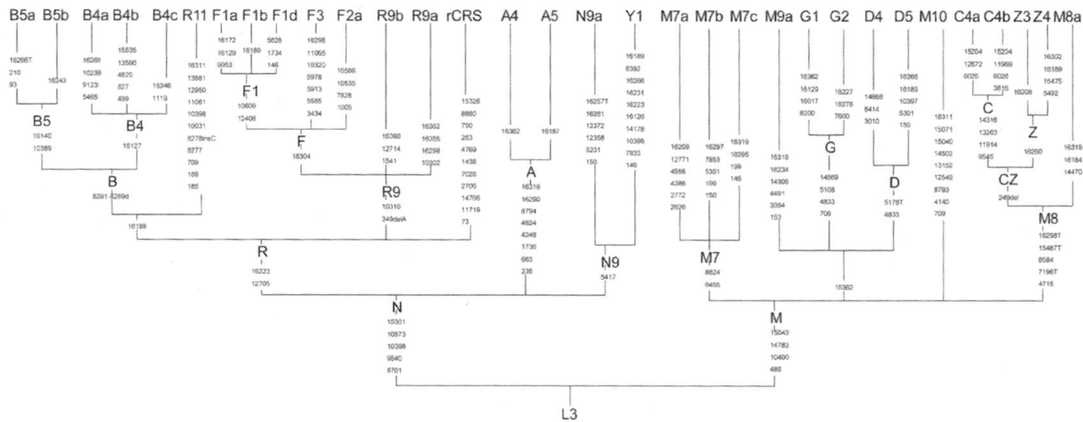

Fig. 2.2 Classification of mtDNA haplogroups in Wenzhou population. The defining sites utilized in this study are listed in the branches. "d" indicates a deletion; "9bpd" indicates a 9bp deletion in the intergenic mtDNA region between nucleotides 8,195–8,316

2.4 mtDNA Common Deletion

It has been shown that oxidative damaged DNA is especially prone to mispairing of repetitive elements and is correlated with DNA deletions. The uncharacterized DNA repairing machineries may mediate the formation of deleted species, by homologous recombination and non-homologous end-joining (Fukui and Moraes 2009; Vermulst et al. 2008). mtDNA deletions are most likely to occur during repair of damaged mtDNA (Krishnan et al. 2008). More than 100 mtDNA deletions have been reported to be associated with various diseases (http://www.mitomap.org/). In fact, large scale deletions were among the first mtDNA mutations identified to cause human diseases. In particular, large scale deletions in individual neurons from the substantial nigra of patients with Parkinson's disease were detected, with various sizes ranging from 1,763bp to 9,445bp within the major arc (Reeve et al. 2008).

Among these deletions, a 4,977-bp deletion (Fig. 2.1) occurring between two 13-bp direct repeats at positions 13,447–13,459 and 8,470–8,482 has attracted tremendous interests since it is the common cause of several sporadic diseases including Pearson's disease(PD), Kearns-Sayre syndrome (KSS), mitochondrial myopathies (MM) and progressive external ophthalmoplegia (PEO) (Sadikovic et al. 2010), and is therefore called the "common" deletion. This deletion also accumulates in many tissues during aging (Schroeder et al. 2008), and has been used as an mtDNA damage biomarker (Meissner et al. 2008). As shown in Fig. 2.1, the common deletion removes all or part of the genes encoding four complex I subunits, one complex IV subunit, two complex V subunits and five tRNA genes, which are indispensable for maintaining normal mitochondrial function. Consequently, the common deletion could lead to energy production catastrophes (Peng et al. 2006). We found that the mtDNA 4,977 bp deletion may play a role in the early stage of colorectal cancer, and it is also implicated in alteration of mtDNA content in cancer cells (Chen et al. 2011).

2.5 mtDNA Mutations in D-Loop

The mtDNA D-loop, is a DNA structure where the two strands of a double-stranded mtDNA molecule are separated and held apart by a third strand of DNA. The third strand has a sequence which is complementary to one of the main strands and pairs with it, thus displacing the other main strand in the region. The D-loop locates in the main non-coding area, a segment also called the main control region (Fig. 2.1). D-loop is the most variable region in mtDNA. The mutation rate at two hypervariable regions (HV-I, HV-II) in D-loop was estimated 100- to 200-fold that of nuclear DNA (Sharawat et al. 2010). It was suggested that in the D-loop region, a poly-C stretch (poly-C tract) termed the D310 region is more susceptible to oxidative damage and electrophilic attack compared with other regions of mtDNA (Mambo et al. 2003).

mtDNA alterations in D-loop region have been reported as a frequent event in cervical cancer, breast cancer, gastric carcinoma, colorectal cancer, hepatocellular cancer, lung cancer and renal cell carcinoma in the forms of point mutations, insertions, deletions, and mitochondrial microsatellite instability (mtMSI) (Lu et al. 2009). Our own results indicate that mtDNA alterations in D-loop region could happen before tumorigenesis in thyroid, and they might also accumulate during tumorigenesis (Ding et al. 2010). Cancer patients with D-loop mutations (Lievre et al. 2005), or in particular with heteroplasmy of the mtDNA D-loop (CA) (n) polymorphism (Ye et al. 2008) were reported to have significantly poorer prognosis. One large investigation showed three variations in HV-I, namely m.16126T>C, m.16224T>C and m.16311T>C, could serve as a potential prognostic marker in paediatric acute myeloid leukemia (AML) (Sharawat et al. 2010).

D-loop mutations have also been associated with other diseases. For example, T16189C was reported in patients with coronary artery disease (CAD) in a Middle European population (Mueller et al. 2011). The same mutation was also found in European type 2 diabetes patients (Mueller et al. 2011).

2.6   mtDNA Mutations in Translational Machinery

Point mutations in mitochondrial protein synthesis genes (including 2 rRNA and 22 tRNA genes) can result in multisystem disorders with a wide range of symptoms, including deafness, diabetes, mitochondrial myopathy, movement disorders, cardiomyopathy, intestinal dysmotility, dementia, etc (Wallace 2005) (Fig. 2.3).

The tRNA (Lys) A8344G mutation is a classical one which was associated with myoclonic epilepsy and ragged red fiber (MERRF) disease (Fan et al. 2006). Perhaps the most common mtDNA protein synthesis mutation is the A3243G in the tRNA (Leu) gene. The A3243G mutation in the tRNA (Leu) was first associated with mitochondrial encephalomyopathy, lactic acid and stroke-like episodes, mitochondrial encephalomyopathy lactic acidosis and stroke-like syndrome (MELAS). This mutation is remarkable in the variability of its clinical manifestations. When the A3243G mutation is present at relatively low levels (10–30%) in the blood, the patient may manifest only type II diabetes with or without deafness, accounting for 0.5–1% of all type II diabetes worldwide. Interestingly, when

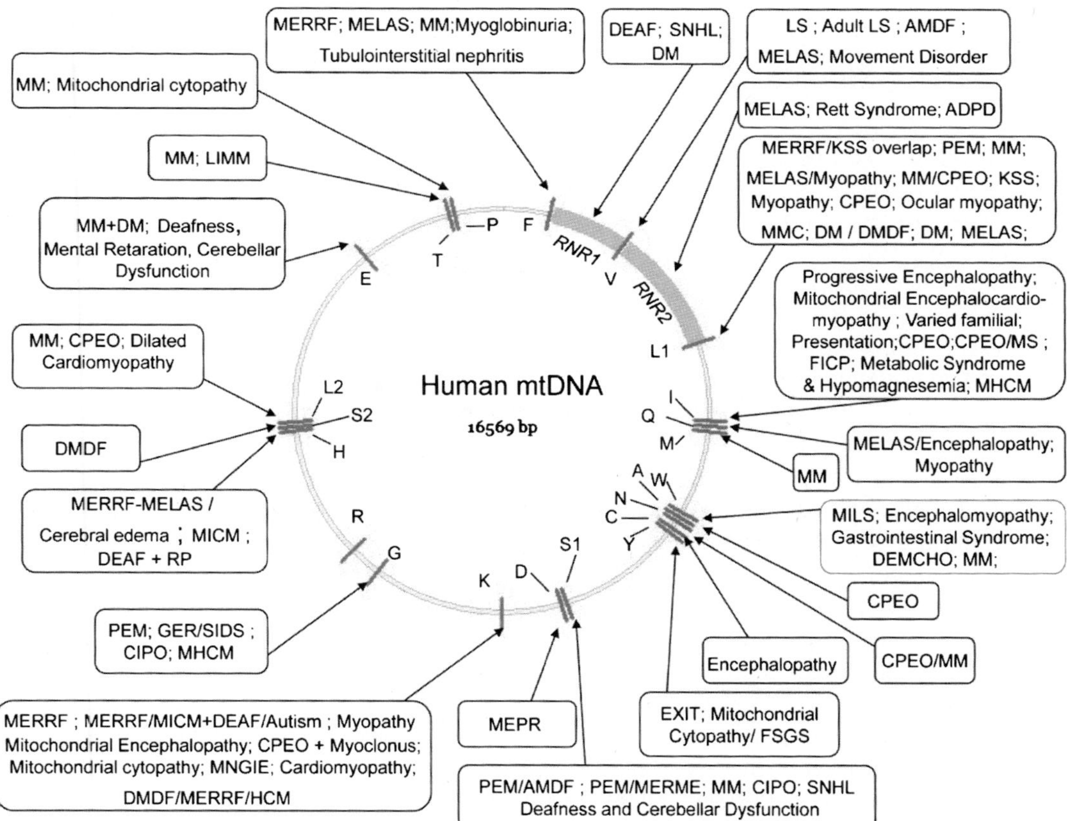

Fig. 2.3 mtDNA tRNA/rRNA mutation map. *ADPD* Alzheimer's Disease and Parkinsons's Disease, *CIPO* Chronic Intestinal Pseudoobstruction with myopathy and Ophthalmoplegia, *CPEO* Chronic Progressive External Ophthalmoplegia, *DEMCHO* Dementia and Chorea, *DM* Diabetes Mellitus, *DMDF* Diabetes Mellitus & Deafness, *EXIT* exercise intolerance, *FICP* Fatal Infantile Cardiomyopathy Plus, a MELAS-associated cardiomyopathy, *HCM* Hypertrophic Cardio Myopathy, *LS* Leigh Tyndrome, *MELAS* Mitochondrial Encephalomyopathy, Lactic Acidosis, and Stroke-like episodes, *MERRF* Myoclonic Epilepsy and Ragged Red Muscle Fibers, *MHCM* Maternally Inherited Hypertrophic Cardiomyopathy, *MICM* Maternally Inherited Cardiomyopathy, *MM* Mitochondrial Myopathy, *SNHL* Sensorineural Hearing Loss

the A3243G mutation is present at relatively high levels (>70% of the mtDNAs), it causes more severe symptoms including short stature, cardiomyopathy, chronic progressive external ophthalmoplegia (CPEO), mitochondrial encephalomyopathy, lactic acid and stroke-like episodes (Wallace 2005). Deleterious mutations in the mitochondrial tRNA (Phe) gene may solely manifest with epilepsy when segregating to homoplasmy (Zsurka et al. 2010). In benign cytochrome c oxidase deficiency myopathy patients, a homoplasmic T14674C or T14674G tRNA (Glu) mutation within tRNA (Glu) gene was identified (Mimaki et al. 2010).

mtDNA mutations, those in the 12S rRNA gene and tRNA genes in particular have been associated with hearing loss (Xing et al. 2007). The A1555G mutation of 12S rRNA gene was a primary contributing factor underlying the development of deafness but not sufficient to produce a clinical phenotype. The T1095C mutation of 12S rRNA gene was suggested to play a role in the phenotypic expression of A1555G mutation, as it disrupted an evolutionarily conserved base pair at a stem-loop structure, resulting in impaired translation in mitochondrial protein synthesis and a significant reduction of cytochrome c oxidase activity (Dai et al. 2008). The alteration of the tertiary or quaternary structure of 12S rRNA by an A827G mutation may play a role in the pathogenesis of hearing loss and aminoglycoside hypersensitivity (Chaig et al. 2008).

2.7 mtDNA Mutations in Protein Coding Genes

All mtDNA-encoded 13 polypeptide are subunits of mitochondrial oxidative phosphorylation complexes, and mutations in these genes can result in an array of clinical manifestations (Wallace 2005) (Fig. 2.4).

The T8993G mutation in ATP6 gene is associated with neurogenic muscle weakness, ataxia, retinitis pigmentosa (NARP) when presents at lower percentages of mutant, and lethal childhood Leigh syndrome when present at higher percentages of mutant (Wallace 2005). Missense and nonsense mutations in the cytb gene have been linked to progressive muscle weakness (Wallace 2005). Rare nonsense or frameshift mutations in COI have been associated with encephalomyopathies (Wallace 2005). Missense mutations in mtDNA encoded complex I subunit genes have been linked to Leigh syndrome, generalized dystonia and deafness, and Leber hereditary optic neuropathy (LHON) (Wallace 2005). Three primary mutations at G3460A of ND1, G11778A of ND4, and T14484C of ND6 account for over 90% of LHON cases in European population (Yu-Wai-Man et al. 2011).

Among mitochondrial genes, ND5 encoded the largest peptide. Mutations in the ND5 gene are also a frequent cause of oxidative phosphorylation disease, especially for those with MELAS- and Leigh-like syndrome with a complex I deficiency (Blok et al. 2007). The sequence variant A13511T occurred in a patient with a Leigh-like syndrome. Mutation G13513A, associated with MELAS and MELAS/Leigh/LHON overlap syndrome, was found in two patients from two different families, one with a MELAS/Leigh phenotype and the other with a MELAS/CPEO phenotype. Mutation G13042A which was detected previously in a patient with a MELAS/MERRF phenotype and in a family with a prevalent ocular phenotype, was also found in a patient with a Leigh-like phenotype. The sequence variant G12622A which was reported once in a control database as a polymorphism, was reported to have a fatal effect in three brothers, all with infantile encephalopathy (Leigh syndrome).

2.8 mtDNA Heteroplasmy

The mtDNA has a relatively high mutation rate, presumably due to its chronic exposure to mitochondrial ROS. When a new mtDNA mutation arises in a cell, a mixed population of mtDNAs is generated, a state known as heteroplasmy. As mtDNA replicates and segregates, the mutant and normal molecules

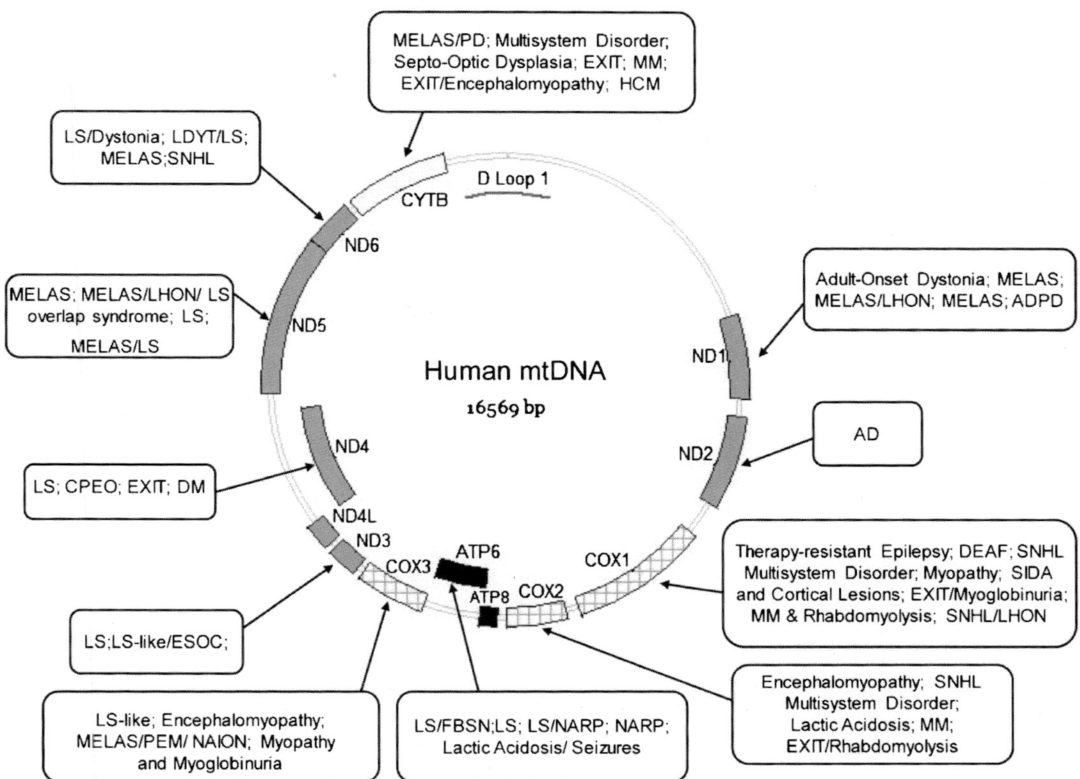

Fig. 2.4 mtDNA coding region mutation map. *AD* Alzheimer's Disease, *ADPD* Alzheimer's Disease and Parkinsons's Disease, *CPEO* Chronic Progressive External Ophthalmoplegia, *DM* Diabetes Mellitus, *EXIT* exercise intolerance, *FBSN* Familial Bilateral Striatal Necrosis, *HCM* Hypertrophic Cardio Myopathy, *LHON* Leber Hereditary Optic Neuropathy, *LS* Leigh Syndrome, *MELAS* Mitochondrial Encephalomyopathy, Lactic Acidosis, and Stroke-like episodes, *MM* Mitochondrial Myopathy, *NAION* Nonarteritic Anterior Ischemic Optic Neuropathy, *NARP* Neurogenic muscle weakness, Ataxia, and Retinitis Pigmentosa, *SIDA* Sideroblastic Anemia, *SNHL* Sensorineural Hearing Loss

are randomly distributed into the daughter cells. As a consequence, the proportion of mutant and normal mtDNAs can drift toward homoplasmic mutant type or homoplasmic wild type. A threshold is reached when the mutant mtDNA accumulates to a certain level that the normal mitochondrial function can not be sustained.

The regulation of mtDNA heteroplamy could happen at the replication level. A replicative advantage of the mutant mtDNA molecules was described for mtDNA carrying the mutation associated with the mitochondrial encephalomyopathy (Yoneda et al. 1992). As a result, mutant mtDNA enriched. The regulation could also be achieved by specific turnover of mitochondria. It was reported that longterm overexpression of cytosolic E3 ligase Parkin may signal the selective removal of defective mitochondria within cells. Parkin can eliminate mitochondria with deleterious COXI mutations in heteroplasmic cybrid cells, thereby enriching cells for wild-type mtDNA and restoring cytochrome c oxidase activity (Suen et al. 2010).

Although it had been considered to be homogeneous, one recent study found widespread heteroplasmy in the mtDNA of normal human cells. Moreover, the frequency of heteroplasmic variants varied considerably between different tissues in the same individual. Cancer cells have been reported to harbor both homoplasmic and heteroplasmic mtDNA mutations. These results provide insights into the nature and variability of mtDNA sequences. In particular, they demonstrate that individual humans are characterized by a complex mixture of mitochondrial genotypes rather than a single genotype (He et al. 2010).

mtDNA heteroplasmy has been related to severe inherited syndromes, such as myopathy, encephalopathy, MELAS, neuropathy, ataxia, NARP-MILS, and LHON (Suen et al. 2010).

We recently examined the contribution of heteroplasmic and homoplasmic ND5 mutations in tumorigenesis, the same mutation was previously identified in a human colorectal cancer cell line (Park et al. 2009). With increasing mutant ND5 mtDNA content, respiratory function, including oxygen consumption and ATP generation through oxidative phosphorylation, declined progressively, whereas lactate production and dependence on glucose increased. Both heteroplasmic and homoplasmic mtDNA mutation caused an increased production of mitochondrial ROS. However in cells with heteroplasmic ND5 mutation, the cytosolic ROS level was somewhat reduced, probably due to the upregulation of antioxidant enzymes. As a result, only cells with homoplasmic ND5 mutation exhibited enhanced apoptotic potency. Furthermore, anchorage dependence and tumor-forming capacity of cells carrying wild type and mutant mtDNA were tested by a growth assay in soft agar and subcutaneous implantation of the cells in nude mice. Surprisingly, the cell line carrying the heteroplasmic ND5 mtDNA mutation showed significantly enhanced tumor growth, whereas tumor formation was inhibited for cells with the homoplasmic form of the same mutation.

2.9 mtDNA Copy Number Alterations

Regulation of mitochondrial biogenesis is essential for proper cellular functioning. mtDNA depletion and the resulting mitochondrial malfunction have been implicated in cancer, neurodegeneration, diabetes, aging, and many other human diseases (Clay Montier et al. 2009). The mtDNA control region is believed to play an important role in mtDNA replication. The mutation T16189C at mtDNA D-loop cit was suggested to interfere with the replication process of mtDNA, which in turn decreased the mtDNA copy number and caused mitochondrial dysfunction (Liou et al. 2010). Large deletions in mtDNA control region are rarely found, as they are expected to interfere with the replication of mtDNA. However, a recent report showed a 50-bp deletion and a 154-bp deletion in the human mtDNA control region do not affect the mtDNA copy number, suggesting that the control of mtDNA replication may be more complex than we had thought (Bi et al. 2010).

Alterations in mtDNA content have been reported in increasing numbers of cancer types (Lee and Wei 2009). Low mtDNA content has been reported to be associated with increased risk of renal cancer carcinoma, and a decrease in mtDNA copy number was also found in gastric cancer, breast cancer and hepatocellular carcinoma. On the other hand, an increase in mtDNA copy number was reported in the majority of head and neck cancer, endometrial cancer, ovarian cancer and colorectal cancer (Lee and Wei 2009). Recent reports suggested that mtDNA copy number may be positively associated with subsequent risk of lung cancer (Hosgood et al. 2010) and non-Hodgkin lymphoma (Lan et al. 2008).

The age-related decrease in mtDNA copy number observed in human pancreatic islet preparations may explain the age-dependent decline in pancreatic beta cell insulin secretory capacity (Cree et al. 2008). The mtDNA copy number was reported decreased in Friedreich's ataxia (FRDA) patients. Adriamycin (ADR) is a commonly used chemotherapeutic agent that also produces significant tissue damage. mtDNA mutations and reductions in mtDNA copy number have been identified as contributors to ADR-induced injury (Papeta et al. 2010).

2.10 Pitfalls in mtDNA Studies

As described in previous sections, mtDNA alterations in human diseases have drawn more and more attentions and more and more mtDNA mutations have been associated expanding numbers of human diseases. To avoid flaws in the experimental procedures and interpretation of the data, some cautions are required. Following are some guidelines we have followed in our own research.

The DNA source for sequencing analysis is critical. In cancer study, it's very important to extract DNA from the very samples that used for pathological diagnosis. The percentages of cancer cells are different in different fractions of the cancer tissue. We suggest that one should extract DNA for sequencing analysis from the material on slides used for pathological diagnosis with microdissection technology (Eltoum et al. 2002).

Both positive and negative controls should be included in PCR, especially in cases where nested PCR strategy is utilized. Cautions have been taken according to Kraytsberg's suggestions to avoiding contamination in PCR (Kraytsberg and Khrapko 2005). It is important to include a mtDNA-less rho zero cell as a control to avoid amplification of mitochondrial pseudogenes in nuclear genome (Yao et al. 2008).

Artificially generated phantom mutations through the sequencing and editing process have been found in some reports (Bandelt et al. 2007). One should be very careful about phantom mutations when only one strand of mtDNA is analyzed.

Another important issue is that one should be very careful when they conclude that mtDNA mutations they found are novel and/or pathogenic. In fact, many reported 'novel' mtDNA mutations turned out to be having been reported previously, and some previously reported 'pathogenic' mutations are generally considered to be polymorphic variants now. MITOMAP is widely used for deciding if the mtDNA alteration is novel for it is a convenient source for the information required. But it may be misleading if the user was not aware of its limitations and did not perform multiple searches throughout the published record. We suggest other databases such as mtDB (http://www.genpat.uu.se/mtDB), mtDNA (http://www.ianlogan.co.uk/mtdna.htm), FBI mtDNA population database (http://www.fbi. gov/hq/lab/fsc/backissu/april2002/miller1.htm) or GenBank (http://www.ncbi.nlm.nih.gov/Genbank/ index.html) should be included in data analysis. A straightforward Google or Yahoo search can help to define the "novelty" of mtDNA polymorphisms. The other useful advice is to identify potential pathogenic mutations with phylogenetic methods (Fang et al. 2009).

2.11   Experimental Approaches to Study mtDNA

Over the years, a set of unique experimental approaches to study of mitochondrial function has been established, and these tools are very useful in investigating physiology and pathology of mtDNA.

(1) **Labeling mitochondrial proteins**

Based on the difference in sensitivity to certain antibiotics, we can selectively label the mtDNA encoded proteins (Bai et al. 2004). In particular, mitochondrial proteins are labeled with [^{35}S] methionine in the presence of emetine, to inhibit cytoplasmic protein synthesis. The labeled products are then electrophoresed through SDS-polyacrylamide gradient gel. The electrophoretic patterns between wild-type and mutant cell lines could indicate the possible mutation site on mtDNA as shown in our studies in identification of mouse ND5 and ND6 mutation (Bai and Attardi 1998; Bai et al. 2000).

(2) **Generation of cytoplasmic hybrid (cybrid)**

Because mitochondria are under dual genetic control, nuclear and mitochondrial, mutations in either genome could potentially cause mitochondrial dysfunctions. To verify that a mutation in mtDNA is solely responsible for the respiration deficiency observed, an mtDNA-less (ρ^0) cell repopulation approach has been established (King and Attardi 1988). For example, mtDNAs carrying a mutation in the ND5 or ND6 gene were transferred to mouse ρ^0 cells by cytoplast-cell fusion, thus placing those mutant genomes in a new nuclear background. The co-segregation of mtDNA with the mitochondrial dysfunction usually indicates a pathogenic role of mutation residing on these mtDNA (Bai et al. 2004).

(3) **Generation of trans-mitochondrial mice**

Up to now, two procedures have been successful established in introducing exogenous mtDNA mutations into the mouse female germline: (a) to fuse cytoplasts from mutant cells directly to mouse single-cell embryos and then to implant the embryos into the oviduct of pseudo-pregnant females, and (b) to fuse enucleated cell cytoplasts bearing mutant mtDNA to undifferentiated female mouse embryonic stem (ES) cells, and then to inject the stem cell cybrids into mouse blastocysts, and to implant the chimeric embryos into a foster mother (Wallace and Fan 2009). The former method was used to create mice harboring a heteroplasmic mtDNA deletion (Nakada et al. 2008), while the latter has permitted the creation of variety of mouse strains bearing heteroplasmic or homoplasmic mtDNA point mutations (Fan et al. 2008).

2.12 Perspectives

So far forward genetics has made important contributions in our understanding of the putative role of mtDNA mutations in various human diseases. It is well-established that accumulation of mtDNA mutations is associated with a wide variety of diseases. However, there is still no convincing evidence to explain whether accumulation of these pathogenic mutant mtDNAs in tissues is responsible for the expressions of various clinical phenotypes.

To complement, reverse genetic study is required to provide model systems for studying exactly how pathogenic mutant mtDNAs are transmitted and distributed in tissues and result in the pathogenesis of mitochondrial diseases with various clinical phenotypes. However, so far we are still facing serious technical challenges to perform such experiments. First there are no procedures are available for introducing mutagenized mammalian whole mtDNA genome into mitochondria in living cells or even into isolated mitochondria (Nakada et al. 2008). The investigation of the effects of mtDNA mutations have lagged behind due to lack of effective technologies to modify the mammalian mtDNA.

We also need a better system to investigate the role of nuclear modifiers in manifestation of tissue-specific pathogenesis of various mtDNA mutations. The recent developed iPS systems might provide some hopes in this regard.

Finally animal models carrying the corresponding mtDNA mutations identified in human diseases would be great assets in understanding the molecular pathways mediating the clinical phenotypes, and the generation of such animals will open new ways to develop therapeutic approaches.

Acknowledgements The work in the laboratory of the authors has been supported by NIH (R01 AG025223) and Chinese National Science Foundation (31070765/C050605, and 810004611/H1409).

References

Bai Y, Attardi G (1998) The mtDNA-encoded ND6 subunit of mitochondrial NADH dehydrogenase is essential for the assembly of the membrane arm and the respiratory function of the enzyme. EMBO J 17:4848–4858

Bai Y, Shakeley RM, Attardi G (2000) Tight control of respiration by NADH dehydrogenase ND5 subunit gene expression in mouse mitochondria. Mol Cell Biol 20:805–815

Bai Y, Hu P, Park JS, Deng JH, Song X, Chomyn A, Yagi T, Attardi G (2004) Genetic and functional analysis of mitochondrial DNA-encoded complex I genes. Ann N Y Acad Sci 1011:272–283

Bandelt HJ, Yao YG, Salas A, Kivisild T, Bravi CM (2007) High penetrance of sequencing errors and interpretative shortcomings in mtDNA sequence analysis of LHON patients. Biochem Biophys Res Commun 352:283–291

Bi R, Zhang AM, Zhang W, Kong QP, Wu BL, Yang XH, Wang D, Zou Y, Zhang YP, Yao YG (2010) The acquisition of an inheritable 50-bp deletion in the human mtDNA control region does not affect the mtDNA copy number in peripheral blood cells. Hum Mutat 31:538–543

Bilal E, Rabadan R, Alexe G, Fuku N, Ueno H, Nishigaki Y, Fujita Y, Ito M, Arai Y, Hirose N, Ruckenstein A, Bhanot G, Tanaka M (2008) Mitochondrial DNA haplogroup D4a is a marker for extreme longevity in Japan. PLoS One 3:e2421

Blok MJ, Spruijt L, de Coo IF, Schoonderwoerd K, Hendrickx A, Smeets HJ (2007) Mutations in the ND5 subunit of complex I of the mitochondrial DNA are a frequent cause of oxidative phosphorylation disease. J Med Genet 44:e74

Cai XY, Wang XF, Li SL, Qian J, Qian DG, Chen F, Yang YJ, Yuan ZY, Xu J, Bai Y, Yu SZ, Jin L (2009) Association of mitochondrial DNA haplogroups with exceptional longevity in a Chinese population. PLoS One 4:e6423

Chaig MR, Zernotti ME, Soria NW, Romero OF, Romero MF, Gerez NM (2008) A mutation in mitochondrial 12S rRNA, A827G, in Argentinean family with hearing loss after aminoglycoside treatment. Biochem Biophys Res Commun 368:631–636

Chen T, He J, Shen L, Fang H, Nie H, Jin T, Wei X, Xin Y, Jiang Y, Li H, Chen G, Lu J, Bai Y (2011) The mitochondrial DNA 4,977-bp deletion and its implication in copy number alteration in colorectal cancer. BMC Med Genet 12:8

Chinnery PF, Elliott HR, Syed A, Rothwell PM (2010) Mitochondrial DNA haplogroups and risk of transient ischaemic attack and ischaemic stroke: a genetic association study. Lancet Neurol 9:498–503

Clay Montier LL, Deng JJ, Bai Y (2009) Number matters: control of mammalian mitochondrial DNA copy number. J Genet Genomics 36:125–131

Cree LM, Patel SK, Pyle A, Lynn S, Turnbull DM, Chinnery PF, Walker M (2008) Age-related decline in mitochondrial DNA copy number in isolated human pancreatic islets. Diabetologia 51:1440–1443

Dai D, Lu Y, Chen Z, Wei Q, Cao X, Xing G (2008) Co-segregation of the T1095C with the A1555G mutation of the mitochondrial 12S rRNA gene in a patient with non-syndromic hearing loss. Biochem Biophys Res Commun 377:1152–1155

Ding Z, Ji J, Chen G, Fang H, Yan S, Shen L, Wei J, Yang K, Lu J, Bai Y (2010) Analysis of mitochondrial DNA mutations in D-loop region in thyroid lesions. Biochim Biophys Acta 1800:271–274

Eltoum IA, Siegal GP, Frost AR (2002) Microdissection of histologic sections: past, present, and future. Adv Anat Pathol 9:316–322

Fan H, Civalier C, Booker JK, Gulley ML, Prior TW, Farber RA (2006) Detection of common disease-causing mutations in mitochondrial DNA (mitochondrial encephalomyopathy, lactic acidosis with stroke-like episodes MTTL1 3243 A>G and myoclonic epilepsy associated with ragged-red fibers MTTK 8344A>G) by real-time polymerase chain reaction. J Mol Diagn 8:277–281

Fan W, Waymire KG, Narula N, Li P, Rocher C, Coskun PE, Vannan MA, Narula J, Macgregor GR, Wallace DC (2008) A mouse model of mitochondrial disease reveals germline selection against severe mtDNA mutations. Science 319:958–962

Fang H, Lu J, Wei J, Shen LJ, Ding Z, Li H, Bai Y (2009) Mitochondrial DNA mutations in the D-loop region may not be frequent in cervical cancer: a discussion on pitfalls in mitochondrial DNA studies. J Cancer Res Clin Oncol 135:649–651

Fukui H, Moraes CT (2009) Mechanisms of formation and accumulation of mitochondrial DNA deletions in aging neurons. Hum Mol Genet 18:1028–1036

He Y, Wu J, Dressman DC, Iacobuzio-Donahue C, Markowitz SD, Velculescu VE, Diaz LA JR, Kinzler KW, Vogelstein B, Papadopoulos N (2010) Heteroplasmic mitochondrial DNA mutations in normal and tumour cells. Nature 464:610–614

Hosgood HD, 3rd Liu CS, Rothman N, Weinstein SJ, Bonner MR, Shen M, Lim U, Virtamo J, Cheng WL, Albanes D, Lan Q (2010) Mitochondrial DNA copy number and lung cancer risk in a prospective cohort study. Carcinogenesis 31:847–849

King MP, Attardi G (1988) Injection of mitochondria into human cells leads to a rapid replacement of the endogenous mitochondrial DNA. Cell 52:811–819

Kofler B, Mueller EE, Eder W, Stanger O, Maier R, Weger M, Haas A, Winker R, Schmut O, Paulweber B, Iglseder B, Renner W, Wiesbauer M, Aigner I, Santic D, Zimmermann FA, Mayr JA, Sperl W (2009) Mitochondrial DNA haplogroup T is associated with coronary artery disease and diabetic retinopathy: a case control study. BMC Med Genet 10:35

Kraytsberg Y, Khrapko K (2005) Single-molecule PCR: an artifact-free PCR approach for the analysis of somatic mutations. Expert Rev Mol Diagn 5:809–815

Krishnan KJ, Reeve AK, Samuels DC, Chinnery PF, Blackwood JK, Taylor RW, Wanrooij S, Spelbrink JN, Lightowlers RN, Turnbull DM (2008) What causes mitochondrial DNA deletions in human cells? Nat Genet 40:275–279

Kruger J, Hinttala R, Majamaa K, Remes AM (2010) Mitochondrial DNA haplogroups in early-onset Alzheimer's disease and frontotemporal lobar degeneration. Mol Neurodegen 5:8

Lan Q, Lim U, Liu CS, Weinstein SJ, Chanock S, Bonner MR, Virtamo J, Albanes D, Rothman N (2008) A prospective study of mitochondrial DNA copy number and risk of non-Hodgkin lymphoma. Blood 112:4247–4249

Lee HC, Wei YH (2009) Mitochondrial DNA instability and metabolic shift in human cancers. Int J Mol Sci 10:674–701

Li XY, Su M, Huang HH, Li H, Tian DP, Gao YX (2007) mtDNA evidence: genetic background associated with related populations at high risk for esophageal cancer between Chaoshan and Taihang Mountain areas in China. Genomics 90:474–481

Lievre A, Chapusot C, Bouvier AM, Zinzindohoue F, Piard F, Roignot P, Arnould L, Beaune P, Faivre J, Laurent-Puig P (2005) Clinical value of mitochondrial mutations in colorectal cancer. J Clin Oncol 23:3517–3525

Liou CW, Lin TK, Chen JB, Tiao MM, Weng SW, Chen SD, Chuang YC, Chuang JH, Wang PW (2010) Association between a common mitochondrial DNA D-loop polycytosine variant and alteration of mitochondrial copy number in human peripheral blood cells. J Med Genet 47:723–728

Lu J, Sharma LK, Bai Y (2009) Implications of mitochondrial DNA mutations and mitochondrial dysfunction in tumorigenesis. Cell Res 19:802–815

Mambo E, Gao X, Cohen Y, Guo Z, Talalay P, Sidransky D (2003) Electrophile and oxidant damage of mitochondrial DNA leading to rapid evolution of homoplasmic mutations. Proc Natl Acad Sci USA 100:1838–1843

Meissner C, Bruse P, Mohamed SA, Schulz A, Warnk H, Storm T, Oehmichen M (2008) The 4977 bp deletion of mitochondrial DNA in human skeletal muscle, heart and different areas of the brain: a useful biomarker or more? Exp Gerontol 43:645–652

Mimaki M, Hatakeyama H, Komaki H, Yokoyama M, Arai H, Kirino Y, Suzuki T, Nishino I, Nonaka I, Goto Y (2010) Reversible infantile respiratory chain deficiency: a clinical and molecular study. Ann Neurol 68:845–854

Mueller EE, Eder W, Ebner S, Schwaiger E, Santic D, Kreindl T, Stanger O, Paulweber B, Iglseder B, Oberkofler H, Maier R, Mayr JA, Krempler F, Weitgasser R, Patsch W, Sperl W, Kofler B (2011) The Mitochondrial T16189C Polymorphism Is Associated with Coronary Artery Disease in Middle European Populations. PLoS One 6:e16455

Nakada K, Sato A, Hayashi J (2008) Reverse genetic studies of mitochondrial DNA-based diseases using a mouse model. Proc Jpn Acad Ser B Phys Biol Sci 84:155–165

Papeta N, Zheng Z, Schon EA, Brosel S, Altintas MM, Nasr SH, Reiser J, D'Agati VD, Gharavi AG (2010) Prkdc participates in mitochondrial genome maintenance and prevents Adriamycin-induced nephropathy in mice. J Clin Invest 120:4055–4064

Park JS, Sharma LK, Li H, Xiang R, Holstein D, Wu J, Lechleiter J, Naylor SL, Deng JJ, Lu J, Bai Y (2009) A heteroplasmic, not homoplasmic, mitochondrial DNA mutation promotes tumorigenesis via alteration in reactive oxygen species generation and apoptosis. Hum Mol Genet 18:1578–1589

Peng TI, Yu PR, Chen JY, Wang HL, Wu HY, Wei YH, Jou MJ (2006) Visualizing common deletion of mitochondrial DNA-augmented mitochondrial reactive oxygen species generation and apoptosis upon oxidative stress. Biochim Biophys Acta 1762:241–255

Reeve AK, Krishnan KJ, Elson JL, Morris CM, Bender A, Lightowlers RN, Turnbull DM (2008) Nature of mitochondrial DNA deletions in substantia nigra neurons. Am J Hum Genet 82:228–235

Sadikovic B, Wang J, El-Hattab A, Landsverk M, Douglas G, Brundage EK, Craigen WJ, Schmitt ES, Wong LJ (2010) Sequence homology at the breakpoint and clinical phenotype of mitochondrial DNA deletion syndromes. PLoS One 5:e15687

Santoro A, Balbi V, Balducci E, Pirazzini C, Rosini F, Tavano F, Achilli A, Siviero P, Minicuci N, Bellavista E, Mishto M, Salvioli S, Marchegiani F, Cardelli M, Olivieri F, Nacmias B, Chiamenti AM, Benussi L, Ghidoni R, Rose G, Gabelli C, Binetti G, Sorbi S, Crepaldi G, Passarino G, Torroni A, Franceschi C (2010) Evidence for sub-haplogroup h5 of mitochondrial DNA as a risk factor for late onset Alzheimer's disease. PLoS One 5:e12037

Schroeder P, Gremmel T, Berneburg M, Krutmann J (2008) Partial depletion of mitochondrial DNA from human skin fibroblasts induces a gene expression profile reminiscent of photoaged skin. J Invest Dermatol 128:2297–2303

Sharawat SK, Bakhshi R, Vishnubhatla S, Bakhshi S (2010) Mitochondrial D-loop variations in paediatric acute myeloid leukaemia: a potential prognostic marker. Br J Haematol 149:391–398

Shen L, Wei J, Chen T, He J, Qu J, He X, Jiang L, Qu Y, Fang H, Chen G, Lu J, Bai Y (2010) Evaluating mitochondrial DNA in patients with breast cancer and benign breast disease. J Cancer Res Clin Oncol 137:669–675

Suen DF, Narendra DP, Tanaka A, Manfredi G, Youle RJ (2010) Parkin overexpression selects against a deleterious mtDNA mutation in heteroplasmic cybrid cells. Proc Natl Acad Sci USA 107:11835–11840

Tanaka M, Takeyasu T, Fuku N, Li-Jun G, Kurata M (2004) Mitochondrial genome single nucleotide polymorphisms and their phenotypes in the Japanese. Ann N Y Acad Sci 1011:7–20

Vermulst M, Wanagat J, Kujoth GC, Bielas JH, Rabinovitch PS, Prolla TA, Loeb LA (2008) DNA deletions and clonal mutations drive premature aging in mitochondrial mutator mice. Nat Genet 40:392–394

Wallace DC (2005) A mitochondrial paradigm of metabolic and degenerative diseases, aging, and cancer: a dawn for evolutionary medicine. Annu Rev Genet 39:359–407

Wallace DC, Fan W (2009) The pathophysiology of mitochondrial disease as modeled in the mouse. Genes Dev 23:1714–1736

Xing G, Chen Z, Cao X (2007) Mitochondrial rRNA and tRNA and hearing function. Cell Res 17:227–239

Yao YG, Kong QP, Salas A, Bandelt HJ (2008) Pseudomitochondrial genome haunts disease studies. J Med Genet 45:769–772

Ye C, Gao YT, Wen W, Breyer JP, Shu XO, Smith JR, Zheng W, Cai Q (2008) Association of mitochondrial DNA displacement loop (CA)n dinucleotide repeat polymorphism with breast cancer risk and survival among Chinese women. Cancer Epidemiol Biomarkers Prev 17:2117–2122

Yoneda M, Chomyn A, Martinuzzi A, Hurko O, Attardi G (1992) Marked replicative advantage of human mtDNA carrying a point mutation that causes the MELAS encephalomyopathy. Proc Natl Acad Sci USA 89:11164–11168

Yu D, Jia X, Zhang AM, Li S, Zou Y, Zhang Q, Yao YG (2010) Mitochondrial DNA sequence variation and haplogroup distribution in Chinese patients with LHON and m.14484 T>C. PLoS One 5:e13426

Yu-Wai-man P, Griffiths PG, Chinnery PF (2011) Mitochondrial optic neuropathies – disease mechanisms and therapeutic strategies. Prog Retin Eye Res 30:81–114

Zsurka G, Hampel KG, Nelson I, Jardel C, Mirandola SR, Sassen R, Kornblum C, Marcorelles P, Lavoue S, Lombes A, Kunz WS (2010) Severe epilepsy as the major symptom of new mutations in the mitochondrial tRNA(Phe) gene. Neurology 74:507–512

Chapter 3
Mitochondrial Ca²⁺ as a Key Regulator of Mitochondrial Activities

Tito Calì, Denis Ottolini, and Marisa Brini

Abstract Mitochondria play a central role in cell biology, not only as producers of ATP but also as regulators of the Ca^{2+} signal. The translocation by respiratory chain protein complexes of H^+ across the ion-impermeable inner membrane generates a very large H^+ electrochemical gradient that can be employed not only by the H^+ ATPase to run the endoergonic reaction of ADP phosphorylation, but also to accumulate cations into the matrix. Mitochondria can rapidly take up Ca^{2+} through an electrogenic pathway, the uniporter, that acts to equilibrate Ca^{2+} with its electrochemical gradient, and thus accumulates the cation into the matrix, and they can release it through two exchangers (with H^+ and Na^+, mostly expressed in non-excitable and excitable cells, respectively), that utilize the electrochemical gradient of the monovalent cations to prevent the attainment of electrical equilibrium.

The uniporter, due to its low Ca^{2+} affinity, demands high local Ca^{2+} concentrations to work. In different cell systems these high Ca^{2+} concentration microdomains are generated, upon cell stimulation, in proximity of the plasma membrane and the sarco/endoplasmic reticulum Ca^{2+} channels.

Recent work has revealed the central role of mitochondria in signal transduction pathways: evidence is accumulating that, by taking up Ca^{2+}, they not only modulate mitochondrial activities but also tune the cytosolic Ca^{2+} signals and their related functions. This review analyses recent developments in the area of mitochondrial Ca^{2+} signalling and attempts to summarize cell physiology aspects of the mitochondrial Ca^{2+} transport machinery.

Keywords Mitochondria • Ca^{2+} transport • ER/mitochondria connection • Mitochondrial Ca^{2+} regulated processes • Mitochondrial dynamics

T. Calì
Department of Comparative Biomedicine and Food Science, University of Padova,
Viale G. Colombo, 3, 35131 Padova, Italy

D. Ottolini
Department of Biomedical Sciences, University of Padova, Padova, Italy

M. Brini (✉)
Department of Comparative Biomedicine and Food Science, University of Padova,
Viale G. Colombo, 3, 35131 Padova, Italy
e-mail: marisa.brini@unipd.it

R. Scatena et al. (eds.), *Advances in Mitochondrial Medicine*, Advances in Experimental
Medicine and Biology 942, DOI 10.1007/978-94-007-2869-1_3,
© Springer Science+Business Media B.V. 2012

3.1 Introduction

3.1.1 General Concepts on Calcium Signalling

Calcium ions (Ca^{2+}) control many cellular processes such as secretion, muscle contraction, gene expression, energy metabolism, proliferation and cell death. Cells evolved several mechanisms to maintain Ca^{2+} homeostasis and to specifically support the different Ca^{2+}-regulated cellular functions. Unfortunately, the high Ca^{2+} concentration of the extracellular medium (in the mM range) does not allow a fine regulation of the cellular processes. To cope with this, two energy-dependent Ca^{2+} extrusion mechanisms, the plasma membrane Ca^{2+} ATPase (PMCA) and the Na^+/Ca^{2+} exchanger (NCX), work against a large unfavourable Ca^{2+} concentration gradient to maintain a low basal cytosolic free Ca^{2+} concentration (in the nM range). By converse, the Ca^{2+} entry from the extracellular ambient is mediated by the opening of plasma membrane Ca^{2+} channels that can be generally classified on the basis of their gating mechanisms as voltage-operated channels (VOCs), receptor-operated channels (ROCs), second-messenger-operated channels (SMOCs) and store-operated channels (SOCs) (Berridge et al. 2003).

Eukaryotic cells can also store Ca^{2+} into intracellular deposits, in particular in the lumen of the sarco/endoplasmic reticulum (SR/ER) and of the Golgi apparatus. The organellar Ca^{2+} sequestration requires ATP hydrolysis and is mediated by the SR/ER ATPase (SERCA) and the Secretory Pathway Ca^{2+} ATPase (SPCA) that accumulate Ca^{2+} at values ranging from hundreds of μM to mM, thereby creating a new "internal" electrochemical gradient (Brini and Carafoli 2009). Once it is stored, organellar Ca^{2+} represents a tunable potential energy to be rapidly released on demand. The SR/ER Ca^{2+} release occurs through the non-specific cations channels inositol 1,4,5 trisphosphate receptor (InsP$_3$R, (Mikoshiba 2007)) and ryanodine receptor (RyR, especially in skeletal and cardiac muscle and cells) which opening is induced by the soluble second messenger InsP$_3$ (or cyclic ADP ribose, cADPR, in the case of RyR) or through the coupling with voltage-gated plasma membrane Ca^{2+} channels in muscle cells (Zalk et al. 2007). The other intracellular organelles, i.e. mitochondria, peroxisomes, secretory vesicles, nucleus, together with the cytosolic Ca^{2+} binding proteins cooperate in shaping the changes in intracellular Ca^{2+} concentration to achieve the fine control the Ca^{2+} regulated processes (Brini and Carafoli 2000).

In particular, mitochondria display an exquisite flexibility that allows them to adapt Ca^{2+} signals to the cell demand in a strongly regulated manner thus contributing to the handling and the decoding of cellular Ca^{2+} signals. This aim is achieved by sensing the cytosolic Ca^{2+} fluctuations and by balancing the rates of Ca^{2+} uptake and release according to them.

Ca^{2+} itself is necessary for the mitochondrial functions: three dehydrogenases of the Krebs cycle (pyruvate dehydrogenase, the α-ketoglutarate dehydrogenase and the isocytrate dehydrohgenase) are activated by Ca^{2+}. Other sites such as the electron transport chain, the F_1F_0 ATPase and the ATP translocator have been proposed to be regulated by Ca^{2+} (McCormack et al. 1990). A fine regulation is necessary to make opposite decisions such as energy production or apoptotic cell death. The maintenance of a correct architecture of the mitochondrial network within the cell is also a Ca^{2+} regulated-process. Mitochondria are not restricted to serve as passive Ca^{2+} sinks rather they communicate with cells in a "mutual crosstalk", Ca^{2+} being the key to decipher their language.

Here we will discuss the role of Ca^{2+} as a modulator of mitochondrial activities and the role of mitochondria as Ca^{2+}-dependent modulators of cellular activities.

3.1.2 Main Players in Mitochondrial Ca^{2+} Handling

Mitochondrial Ca^{2+} homeostasis is regulated by transporters that concertedly accomplish the organelle's demand by handling Ca^{2+} in a tunable fashion (Fig. 3.1). In early 1960s, the discovery that isolated respiring mitochondria were capable to sustain Ca^{2+} accumulation (Vasington and Murphy 1962),

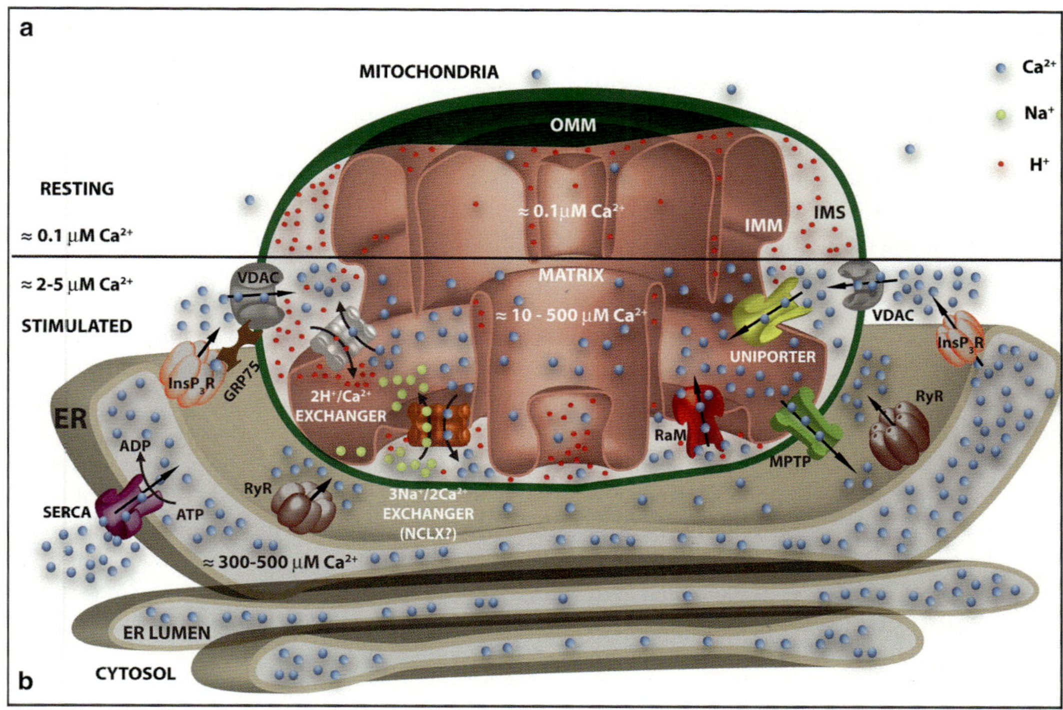

Fig. 3.1 Mitochondrial Ca²⁺ homeostasis at resting conditions (**a**) and following stimulation that induces the opening of the InsP₃R or the RyR (**b**). The players involved in mitochondrial Ca²⁺ transport are indicated. *VDAC* voltage-dependent anion channel, *RaM* rapid mode of uptake, *GRP75* glucose-regulated protein 75, *InsP₃R* and *RyR* inositol 1,4,5 trisphosphate and Ryanodine receptors, *MPTP* mitochondrial permeability transition pore, *OMM* outer mitochondrial membrane, *IMS* intermembrane space, *IMM* inner mitochondrial membrane

already raised the question on how the low sensitivity of the mitochondrial Ca²⁺ uptake machinery could fit with the extremely low cytosolic Ca²⁺ concentration: thus for a long time it was assumed that Ca²⁺ sequestration by mitochondria in living cells was physiologically irrelevant. At the beginning of 1990s the specific targeting to mitochondrial matrix of recombinant Ca²⁺ sensors clearly demonstrated that in intact cells mitochondria promptly sequester Ca²⁺ upon cell stimulation under physiological conditions (Rizzuto et al. 1992) and solved the question of the low affinity of the mitochondrial uptake system proposing that mitochondria could sense localized microdomains at high Ca²⁺ concentration generated close to the mouth of the Ca²⁺ channels (Rizzuto et al. 1993). Such microdomains are achieved by a close proximity of mitochondrial Ca²⁺ uptake sites with those of Ca²⁺ release at the endoplasmic reticulum (ER) (Rizzuto et al. 1998) and/or presumably also by functional coupling with Ca²⁺ entry channels at the plasma membrane (Hoth et al. 1997; Malli et al. 2003). This finding re-opened new possibility on the meaning of mitochondrial Ca²⁺ uptake.

The renewed interest in mitochondrial Ca²⁺ not only encouraged the studies on its physiological role but also increased the interest in identifying the unknown mitochondrial Ca²⁺ transporters.

Starting from the 1960s, during 50 years of intense research, many aspects of the mitochondrial Ca²⁺ uptake and extrusion mechanisms have been clarified but the molecular identity of the players involved remained elusive for a long time despite different actors were proposed. The Na⁺/Ca²⁺ exchanger (one of the two Ca²⁺ extrusion system) and the uniporter have been molecularly identified only very recently (Baughman et al. 2011; De Stefani et al. 2011; Palty et al. 2010). During the trip in/out the mitochondrial matrix, Ca²⁺ must overcome two barriers with decreasing ions permeability properties: the outer (OMM) and the inner (IMM) mitochondrial membranes. The OMM contains many porines and it was traditionally considered freely permeable to Ca^{2+}, but recent evidence suggested that its permeability could be regulated by the voltage dependent anion-selective channels (VDAC) (Szabadkai et al. 2006 and see below).

The IMM represents the impermeable barrier to the free diffusion of ions and metabolites. It is the location where the oxidative phosphorylation occurs since it contains the respiratory chain complexes, but it also contains the proteins deputed to the Ca^{2+} influx and efflux from the matrix.

Mitochondrial Ca^{2+} uptake is an electrogenic process and is countered by Ca^{2+} egress so that electrochemical gradient equilibrium does not occur (Nicholls and Crompton 1980). The translocation of H^+ from the matrix into the intermembrane space coupled to electron fluxes between the complexes of the respiratory chain generates a -180 mV membrane potential at the IMM (Mitchell 1961). This potential represents the driving force for Ca^{2+} entry thus, the dissipation of the proton gradient across the IMM abolishes mitochondrial Ca^{2+} uptake. Given that the cytosolic free Ca^{2+} concentration in most cell types is about 100 nM, equilibrium should be reached at 0.1 M Ca^{2+} values inside the mitochondria. However the equilibrium is not reached since Ca^{2+} uptake is matched by Ca^{2+} efflux via distinct pathways.

The Ca^{2+} uniporter (MCU), which has been proposed to be a gated and highly selective ion channel (Kirichok et al. 2004; Saris and Allshire 1989) and the so-called "rapid mode" (RaM) of uptake (Sparagna et al. 1995) are responsible for mitochondrial Ca^{2+} uptake; while a Na^+-dependent and a Na^+-independent Ca^{2+} efflux mechanisms are associated with the activity of the $3Na^+/Ca^{2+}$ and $2H^+/Ca^{2+}$ antiporters, which action is coupled to the proton motive force developed by the respiratory chain (Carafoli et al. 1974).

3.1.2.1 Mitochondrial Ca^{2+} Uptake

Patch clamp experiments on mitoblasts (swollen mitochondria without the OMM) showed that MCU is a highly selective hardly saturable Ca^{2+} channel (half-activation constant, $K_{0.5}$ of 19 mM Ca^{2+}) with an activation domain as well as a transport site (Kirichok et al. 2004). The selectivity series of the uniporter is: $Ca^{2+} > Sr^{2+} > Mn^{2+} > Ba^{2+} > Fe^{2+} > La^{3+}$ and many pharmacological studies led to the identification of compounds able to either inhibit or activate it. While Ca^{2+} itself is thought to activate MCU, other ions like the lanthanides, Mg^{2+}, ruthenium red (RR) and its derivate Ru360 (reviewed in Carafoli 2010; Rizzuto et al. 2000) and the plasma membrane Na^+/Ca^{2+} exchange inhibitor KB-R7943 (Santo-Domingo et al. 2007) inhibit it. Physiological concentrations of polyamines, such as spermine and related compounds (Rustenbeck et al. 1998), have instead been shown to activate mitochondrial Ca^{2+} uptake at low Ca^{2+} concentrations, suggesting that polyamines may have important physiological roles in intracellular Ca^{2+} handling. The uniporter can also be activated by physiological (mM) amounts of taurine (Palmi et al. 1999), while nucleotides were shown to either inhibit or stimulate the MCU (Litsky and Pfeiffer 1997). Interestingly, the p38 MAPK inhibitor SB202190 has been shown to increase mitochondrial Ca^{2+} sequestration in intact as well as permeabilized cells, suggesting that in physiological conditions the MCU activity could be modulated through a protein kinase dependent mechanism (Montero et al. 2002). The molecular identity of the MCU remained elusive for a long time. Some proteins (with already known function) have been proposed to be involved in the MCU-mediated Ca^{2+} influx, among them the RyR (Beutner et al. 2001) and the Uncoupling Proteins, a family of inner membrane anion transporters that increase protons conductance by transporting free fatty acid anions from mitochondrial matrix to the intermembrane space (Trenker et al. 2007). However, a general consensus was missing and none of them have been further confirmed to be involved in mitochondrial Ca^{2+} transport. Recently, an uniporter regulator (named MICU1), was identified *in silico* in the MitoCarta database (Perocchi et al. 2010). MICU1 is associated with the mitochondrial inner membrane and has two canonical EF hands indicating a role in Ca^{2+} sensing.

Looking at the same database, few months later, two independent groups have identified an integral inner membrane protein satisfying the criteria for being MCU (Baughman et al. 2011; De Stefani et al. 2011). MCU is ubiquitously expressed in mammals, it has two predicted transmembrane regions connected through a loop enriched in acidic residues and forms oligomers in the inner mitochondrial membrane. The channel activity of purified MCU reconstituted in a planar lipid bilayer revealed the properties previously reported for the uniporter, thus definitively demonstrating that MCU per se represents the pore-forming channel (De Stefani et al. 2011).

Mitochondrial Ca^{2+} uptake via Rapid Mode (RaM) has been described in heart and liver as an alternative/additional pathway to the uniporter (Gunter et al. 2000; Sparagna et al. 1995). It is characterized by the very rapidly Ca^{2+} transfer into mitochondria during brief Ca^{2+} pulses. It differs from uniporter since it has a high rate of uptake at the beginning of the Ca^{2+} pulse and it is inhibited very rapidly possibly by Ca^{2+} itself. Ca^{2+} uptake via the RaM is also inhibited by uncouplers, RR (although at higher concentration than that required for the inhibition of the uniporter) and strongly activated by physiological concentrations of spermine, and millimolar levels of ATP and GTP (Sparagna et al. 1995). The sensitivity of the RaM to the same modulators of the uniporter, although with different affinity, suggests a relationship between the two inward transport mechanisms. To date, the physiological function of RaM is unknown, and it is difficult to say whether the RaM is an alternative conformation of the uniporter complex or a really different transport mechanism.

At the end of this section covering mitochondrial Ca^{2+} uptake it is necessary to mention a paper by Clapham and coworkers that has recently appeared on a genome-wide *Drosophila* RNA interference (RNAi) screen study searching the genes that regulate mitochondrial Ca^{2+} and H^+ concentrations. The paper reported the finding of a mammalian homolog of *Drosophila* gene Letm1 (leucine zipper EF-hand–containing transmembrane protein 1), responsible for mediating the coupled Ca^{2+}/H^+ exchange. RNAi knockdown, overexpression, and liposome reconstitution of the purified Letm1 protein suggested that it acts as $Ca^{2+}/2H^+$ antiporter which mediates the Ca^{2+} entry in the matrix (Jiang et al. 2009). However, other studies on Letm1 homologous in yeast and *Drosophila* did not support a role for it in mitochondrial Ca^{2+} homeostasis rather they indicated that Letm1 is responsible for mitochondrial K^+/H^+ exchange (Frazier et al. 2006; McQuibban et al. 2010; Nowikovsky et al. 2007).

3.1.2.2 Mitochondrial Ca²⁺ Efflux

The efflux mechanisms displace Ca^{2+} concentrations to reach the thermodynamic equilibrium inside the mitochondrial matrix, therefore the free Ca^{2+} concentration depends on the concentrations of phosphate and of adenine nucleotides (Nicholls and Scott 1980) that control it through the formation of reversible Ca^{2+}-phosphate complexes (Zoccarato and Nicholls 1982). The balance between free and buffered Ca^{2+} is also strongly related to pH values: matrix acidification induced by protonophores neutralizes the formation of Ca^{2+}-phosphate complexes thus reducing mitochondrial Ca^{2+} buffer capacity and enhancing mitochondrial Ca^{2+} release (Nicholls 2005). This buffering helps to maintain nanomolar free Ca^{2+} levels in the matrix, but an active role is certainly played by the two efflux pathways: the $Ca^{2+}/3Na^+$ exchanger (mNCX) and the $Ca^{2+}/2H^+$ exchanger (mHCX).

The existence of a Na^+-dependent Ca^{2+} flux was initially based on the observation that, in isolated mitochondria, after the addition of RR, the rate of Ca^{2+} efflux can be substantially stimulated by the addition of Na^+ (Carafoli et al. 1974). Later, the pharmacological characterization of this pathway further supported its existence. The transport was electrogenic and thus the transport stoichiometry was probably 3 to 1 as in the case of the plasma membrane NCX (Baysal et al. 1994). The mNCX is inhibited by Sr^{2+}, Ba^{2+}, Mg^{2+} or Mn^{2+}, and by many compounds of pharmacological interest including diltiazem, clonazepam, verapamil, tetraphenyl-phosphonium, trifluoperazine amiloride and its derivatives. In particular, the chloro-5-(2-chlorophenyl)-1,5-dihydro-4,1-benzothiazepin-2(3H)-one (CGP 37157) was shown to inhibit with high specificity the Na^+ dependent Ca^{2+} efflux and it is now widely used (Cox and Matlib 1993). A very recent study proposed that NCLX, a mammalian member of the phylogenetically ancestral Ca^{2+}/anion exchangers family initially characterized as a novel plasma membrane Na^+/Ca^{2+} exchanger that catalyzes Na^+ or Li^+ dependent Ca^{2+} transport, is enriched in mitochondrial cristae. Strong evidence suggests that NCLX may represent the long elusive mNCX, since its overexpression or silencing enhances or reduces mitochondrial Na^+-dependent Ca^{2+} efflux, respectively, and its activity is selectively inhibited by CGP-37157 (Palty et al. 2010).

As the Na^+-independent Ca^{2+} extrusion mechanism, it has been firstly described in liver mitochondria (Fiskum et al. 1979). It transports Ca^{2+}, but also Sr^{2+}, or Mn^{2+} from the matrix to the intermembrane space against the Ca^{2+} electrochemical gradient. The observation that the rate of efflux via this mechanism decreases with increasing ΔpH (internally alkaline) (Gunter et al. 1983) suggests that the mechanism is an active Ca^{2+}/H^+ exchanger. The transport is electroneutral and it has been characterized as a 1 Ca^{2+} for 2H^+ exchanger (Gunter et al. 2000). Cyanide, low levels of uncouplers and very high levels of RR have been described to inhibit it (Wingrove and Gunter 1986).

In addition to the antiporters, another mechanism of Ca^{2+} transport can be considered to play an important role in the mitochondrial Ca^{2+} efflux, especially in condition in which mitochondrial Ca^{2+} concentration reaches threshold levels. This pathway is represented by a non-specific pore, the mitochondrial permeability transition pore (MPTP), a multi-protein complex which properties are well defined, but, still molecularly unknown. In conditions that expose mitochondria to the risk of Ca^{2+} overload the MPTP opening through transient spontaneous flickering could be responsible for the modulation of mitochondrial Ca^{2+} homeostasis in a physiological way (Rasola et al. 2010). Ca^{2+} entering the mitochondrial matrix enhances MPTP opening because of the presence of a Ca^{2+}-binding site, which is competitively inhibited by other ions such as Mg^{2+}, Sr^{2+} and Mn^{2+} (Nicolli et al. 1996). Together with a Ca^{2+} rise in the mitochondrial matrix, many factors such as pH, adenine nucleotides, free radicals and mitochondrial membrane potential ($\Delta\Psi_m$) modulate the opening of the MPTP. Mitochondrial Ca^{2+} overload and increases in Reactive Oxygen Species (ROS) in the matrix are the "point of no return" that cause permeabilization of the inner mitochondrial membrane, proton electrochemical gradient dissipation, ATP depletion, further ROS production and organelle swelling. These events are collectively termed "mitochondrial permeability transition" (MPT), a process that, in turn, causes the release of cytochrome c and culminates in apoptotic cell death.

The voltage-dependent anion channel VDAC, the adenine nucleotide translocase (ANT) and cyclophilin D (CypD) (Baines 2009; Bernardi and Forte 2007) modify the MPTP sensitivity to Ca^{2+}, irrespective of whether they take directly part in PTP formation. Reconstitution of a VDAC-ANT-CypD complex in phosphatidylcholine liposomes indicated that the complex was able to form a Ca^{2+}-dependent CsA-sensitive channel similar to the MPTP (Crompton et al. 1998). Recent evidence suggests that VDAC is indeed not a component of the MPTP, rather it mediates the formation of contact sites between the mitochondrial membranes and that of the ER, thus facilitating the transfer of ER Ca^{2+} to the mitochondrial matrix (Szabadkai et al. 2006), thus implying that also the OMM may play an important role in controlling mitochondrial fluxes.

Inhibition of ANT and CypD by pharmacological drugs, e.g., bongkrekic acid and cyclosporine-A (CsA) respectively, or their knocking out, reduced the Ca^{2+} sensitivity of the MPTP with an inhibitory effect that can be overcome by increasing Ca^{2+} and P_i (Baines et al. 2005; Haworth and Hunter 2000); indicating they are fundamental regulators. Recent studies also shed light on the possible contribution of these components in the molecular composition of the MPTP (see (Baines 2009) for an extensive review on the topic).

3.2 Ca^{2+}-Mediated Mitochondrial Functions

3.2.1   *ER-Mitochondria: Let's Keep in Touch*

The re-evaluation of the mitochondrial Ca^{2+} transport has permitted to establish that mitochondria Ca^{2+} uptake can modulate cellular events as diverse as aerobic metabolism, cytoplasmic diffusion of Ca^{2+} signals and induction of apoptotic cell death (Fig. 3.2). The work by Denton, McCormack and

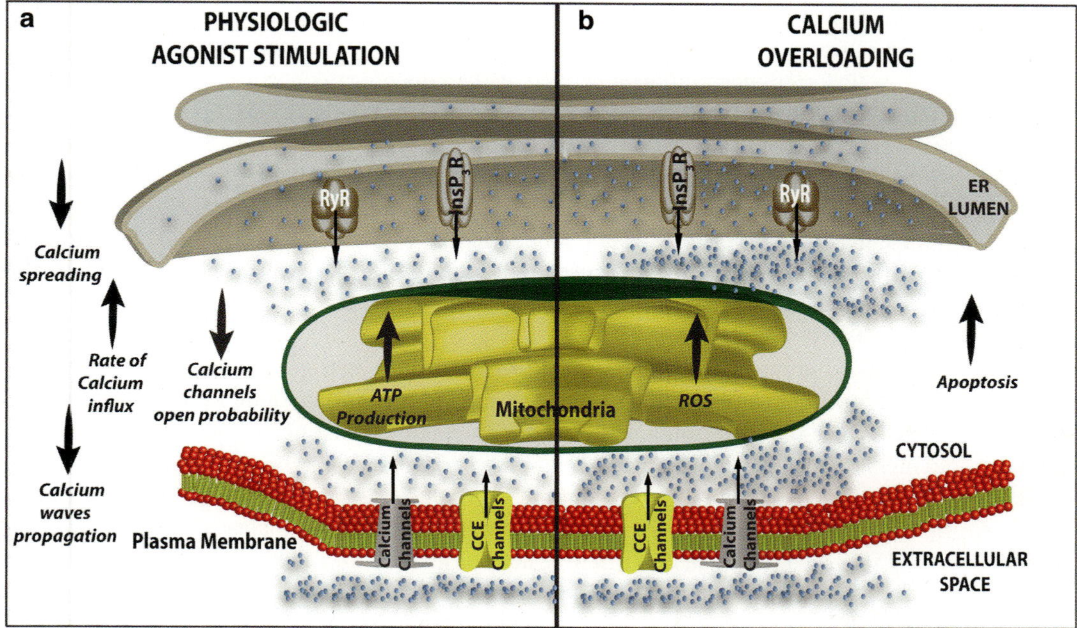

Fig. 3.2 Ca²⁺ as a key regulator of mitochondrial activities. (**a**) Mitochondrial calcium handling influences mitochondrial activities (i.e., ATP production) and the cytosolic Ca²⁺ signaling by buffering and shaping the cytoslic Ca²⁺ spreading. (**b**) Prolonged and sustained cytosolic Ca²⁺ increases lead to mitochondrial Ca²⁺ overload, enhanced ROS production and apoptosis mediated cell death

Hansford in the 1960s demonstrated that three key metabolic enzymes (the pyruvate, α-ketoglutarate and isocitrate dehydrogenases) are activated by Ca²⁺ by different mechanisms (Denton 2009): in the case of pyruvate dehydrogenase through a Ca²⁺-dependent dephosphorylation step, in the latter two cases through the direct binding of Ca²⁺ to the enzyme complex. How the Ca²⁺ signal originated in the cytoplasm could be extended to the mitochondria and could serve the purpose of transmitting an activatory signal to the energy powerhouse of the cell was still unclear until the 1990s, when novel experimental tools allowed to specifically measure the Ca²⁺ concentration in the mitochondrial matrix. Using molecularly engineered chimeras of the Ca²⁺-sensitive photoprotein aequorin, that include mitochondrial targeting sequences and are thus exclusively localized in the mitochondrial matrix (Rizzuto et al. 1992), and, later on, positively charged fluorescent indicators that are largely accumulated in the mitochondria it was possible to demonstrate that, in a variety of cell systems (ranging from epithelial cells to skeletal and cardiac myocytes, from hepatocytes to neurons (Rizzuto et al. 1999), the cytosolic Ca²⁺ rises evoked by physiological stimulations are always paralleled by rapid mitochondrial Ca²⁺ increases, that reach values well above those of the bulk cytosol, even up to ~500 μM in chromaffin cells (Montero et al. 2000). The obvious discrepancy between this prompt response and the low affinity of the Ca²⁺ uniporter was reconciled by the demonstration that mitochondria are exposed to microdomains of high Ca²⁺ that largely exceed the values reported in the bulk cytosol and meet the low affinity of the uniporter. This is achieved through a close interaction between the mitochondria and the ER, the intracellular Ca²⁺ store, that could be directly demonstrated using targeted chimeras of a fluorescent recombinant protein (GFP) and a high resolution imaging system (Rizzuto et al. 1998). These experiments revealed the presence of overlapping regions of the two organelles (thus establishing an upper limit of 100 nm for their distance) and allowed to estimate the area of the contact sites as 5–20% of total mitochondrial surface. More recently, electron tomography techniques allowed to estimate an even smaller distance (10–25 nm) as well as the presence of trypsin-sensitive (hence proteinaceous) tethers between the two membranes. A consequence of this morphological arrangement is the capacity of mitochondria to "sense" the microenvironment at the mouth of the $InsP_3$-sensitive channel, and thus the high cytosolic Ca^{2+} concentration generated by their opening upon cell stimulation. Following this seminal observation the ER/mitochondria connection became a paradigm (Csordas et al., 2006) and the same concept could be extended to the plasma membrane Ca^{2+} channels. However, it must be extended with caution since it was recently shown that activation of voltage-operated Ca^{2+} channels results in substantially larger rises of Ca^{2+} concentration at the OMM of organelles close to the plasma membrane than in more deeply located mitochondria, whereas upon activation of capacitative Ca^{2+} entry no difference between the two organelle populations was observed, suggesting that mitochondria are excluded from the regions where store-operated Ca^{2+} channels are activated (Giacomello et al. 2010).

Despite of these differences, the general idea of Ca^{2+} microheterogeneity as a way to transmit specific signal has now large consensus and the work has evolved in searching how different partner molecules could further modulate mitochondrial Ca^{2+} uptake optimizing it. On this line the outer mitochondrial membrane channel VDAC has been shown to enhance Ca^{2+} signal propagation into the mitochondria increasing the extent of mitochondrial Ca^{2+} uptake, acting at the ER/mitochondria contact sites forming a physical link with the $InsP_3R$, through the molecular chaperone glucoe-regulated protein 75 (GRP75) (Szabadkai et al. 2006). These notions have a direct impact on mitochondrial Ca^{2+} transport, as variations in OMM permeability to Ca^{2+} can represent a bottleneck for the efficient ion transfer from the high Ca^{2+} concentration microdomains generated by the opening of the $InsP_3R$ to the intermembrane space.

Other intriguing examples are that of sigma-1 and mitofusin-2. Sigma-1 is a novel ER chaperone serendipitously identified in cellular distribution studies and shown to be involved in the Ca^{2+}-mediated stabilization of $InsP_3Rs$ (Hayashi and Su 2007). Sigma-1 is normally localized in the so-called "mitochondria-associated membrane" (MAM), bound to another ER chaperone (BiP). When the luminal Ca^{2+} concentration of the ER drops, following the opening of $InsP_3Rs$, sigma-1 dissociates from BiP and binds to $InsP_3R$, thus preventing degradation by the proteasome. Thus, sigma-1 appears to be involved in maintaining, from the ER luminal side, the integrity of the ER/mitochondrial Ca^{2+} crosstalk in conditions (e.g. ER stress) that could impair signal transmission. Mitofusin-2 is a mitochondrial dynamin-related protein enriched at the ER-mitochondria interface. Silencing of mitofusin 2 disrupts ER morphology and loosens ER-mitochondria interactions, thereby reducing the efficiency of mitochondrial Ca^{2+} uptake in response to stimuli that generate $InsP_3$. Several evidences support a model in which ER-mitofusin 2 engages complexes with mitofusin 1 or 2 on the surface of mitochondria thus tethering the two organelles to allow an efficient mitochondrial Ca^{2+} uptake (de Brito and Scorrano 2008).

3.2.2 ATP Production and Mitochondrial Ca²⁺ Increase: a close relationship

As mentioned above, the role of Ca^{2+} in the regulation of energetic metabolism was already established by Denton and MacCormack at the beginning of the 1980s, but the improvement of molecular tools to directly measure intraorganellar Ca^{2+} concentration and also mitochondrial ATP production contributed to deeply explore the Ca^{2+} regulation of metabolic processes (Griffiths and Rutter 2009).

Cytosolic Ca^{2+} increases in conjunction to the triggering of energy-consuming processes in the cytosol (contraction, secretion, etc.) induce, through mitochondrial Ca^{2+} transients generation, the stimulation of mitochondrial dehydrogenases, thus adapting aerobic metabolism to the increased needs of an active cell (Fig. 3.3). Using the luciferase based probe for ATP, it was possible to demonstrate that a rise in mitochondrial ATP levels strictly depends on the mitochondrial Ca^{2+} increase

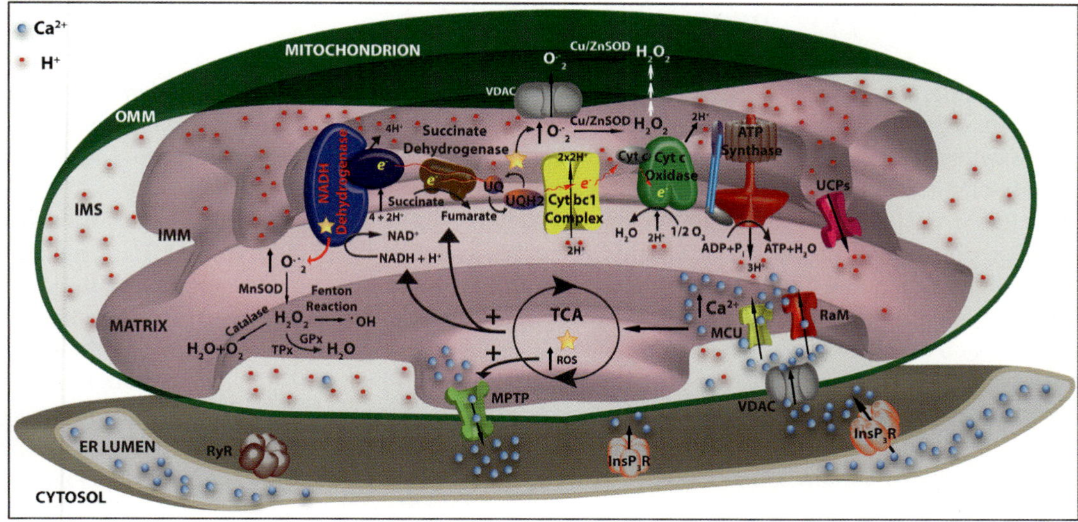

Fig. 3.3 Ca²⁺ stimulation of oxidative-phosphorylation and ROS production. Increases in mitochondrial Ca²⁺ stimulate the TCA (Tricarbossilic acids) cycle enzymes and ROS production. Superoxide (O2·⁻) is generated by the respiratory chain complexes (especially complex I and III as indicated by the *stars*) and is dismuted to H₂O₂ by matrix manganese superoxide dismutase (MnSOD) or cytosolic copper/zinc superoxide dismutase (Cu/ZnSOD). H₂O₂ is detoxified in the matrix by catalase and thioredoxin (TPx) or glutathione (GPx) peroxidase. H₂O₂ can also react with metal ions to generate the highly reactive hydroxyl radical (•OH) via Fenton reaction or pass freely through membranes (*dashed arrows*). The respiratory chain complexes are represented. e⁻, electrons. *OMM* outer mitochondrial membrane, *IMS* intermembrane mitochondrial space, *IMM* inner mitochondrial membrane, *VDAC* voltage-dependent anion channel, *RaM* rapid mode of uptake, *MCU* mitochondrial calcium uniporter, *MPTP* mitochondrial permeability transition pore, *UCPs* uncoupling proteins (see text), *InsP₃R* and *RyR* InsP₃ and Ryanodine receptors

evoked by cell stimulation: if the latter is prevented by the use of Ca²⁺ chelators, such as BAPTA, also the ATP concentration rise does not occur. Interestingly, it was also shown that increases in NADH levels and ATP production directly paralleled with the entity of mitochondrial Ca²⁺ increases (Jouaville et al. 1999; Rizzuto et al. 1994), and that if an impairment in mitochondrial Ca²⁺ uptake is corrected by blocking the mitochondrial Ca²⁺ efflux, as was the case in cellular model of mitochondrial myopathies, also the impairment in energy production can be recovered (Brini et al. 1999). The correlation is even more complex as suggested by observations made on hepatocytes where it has been shown that mitochondrial Ca²⁺ oscillations induced by InsP₃-dependent cytosolic Ca²⁺ oscillations result in a sustained increase in NADH production. It is no necessary to keep high mitochondrial Ca²⁺ levels for long time (that could result in cell damage) to maximally stimulate mitochondria Krebs cycle: Ca²⁺ oscillations are decoded by mitochondria to optimize ATP production according the specific cell demands (Hajnoczky et al. 1995).

In addition to the intramitochondrial Ca²⁺ regulation of the energy metabolism, it has been postulated the existence of an additional mechanism causing a stimulation of mitochondria by extramitochondrial Ca²⁺ which acts together with the Ca²⁺ activation of the mitochondrial deydrogenases. As shown by the extensive work of Satrustegui (del Arco and Satrustegui 1998) and Palmieri' s groups (Lasorsa et al. 2003), the aspartate/glutamate carrier (AGC1 or aralar) – as a central enzyme of the malate–aspartate shuttle (MAS) – transports reducing hydrogen equivalents (of cytosolic NADH) into the mitochondria. This reaction is strongly regulated by extra-mitochondrial Ca²⁺ through the AGC1/aralar regulatory EF-hand Ca²⁺ binding sites that face the IMS (Satrustegui et al. 2007). Thus, extramitochondrial Ca²⁺ increases could be responsible for enhanced glutamate inside the mitochondria, implying a regulation also of the oxidative phosphorylation (Gellerich et al. 2010).

3.2.3   Shaping a Ca²⁺ Wave

Work by different groups has clarified that the role of mitochondrial Ca²⁺ uptake is not limited to the control of organelle function, but has a direct impact on the Ca²⁺ signals evoked by agonist stimulation in the cytosol. Moreover, being the mitochondria extremely dynamic in terms of movement (see below) their role in the control of Ca²⁺ signals can be very versatile.

In this respect, mitochondria act essentially through two different mechanisms. The first occurs at the microdomains where mitochondria and Ca²⁺ release channels get in close contact. Here, the efficiency of mitochondrial Ca²⁺ accumulation accounts for the rapid clearing of the high Ca²⁺ concentration at the mouth of the release channel, and thus reduces the (positive or negative) feedback effect of the cation on the channel itself. Such a mechanism has been shown in a variety of experimental systems ranging from *Xenopus oocytes* ((Jouaville et al. 1995) in which the diffusion properties of Ca²⁺ waves correlates with the energization state of mitochondria) to mammalian cells such as hepatocytes (Hajnoczky et al. 1999), lymphocytes (Hoth et al. 1997) and glial cells (Boitier et al. 1999), where it was demonstrated that the kinetics of Ca²⁺ release from the ER (through the InsP$_3$ receptor) and of Ca²⁺ entry from the extracellular medium (through the VOCCS or the CCE channels) are influenced by the process of mitochondrial Ca²⁺ uptake that in turn also influences the spatio-temporal properties of the cytosolic Ca²⁺ rise. The consequences can be extended to the different Ca²⁺-regulated processes including gene expression as initially proposed by Lewis and co-workers: the inhibition of mitochondrial Ca²⁺ uptake in lymphocytes inactivated CRAC-channel activity and, as a consequence, the nuclear translocation of the transcription factor NFAT (Hoth et al. 2000).

The second mechanism by which mitochondrial Ca²⁺ uptake affects cytosolic Ca²⁺ signals has been initially demonstrated in pancreatic acinar cells, where the Ca²⁺ uptake by mitochondria clustered below the apical region act as a "firewall" preventing the spreading of the cytosolic Ca²⁺ rise. When the mitochondrial "belt" is overwhelmed (e.g. upon intense stimulation, or when the Ca²⁺ uptake capacity of mitochondria is experimentally impaired), then the Ca²⁺ signal can freely diffuse to the rest of the cell (Tinel et al. 1999). This concept has been extended to several different cell models, and it was also proposed that in some cell types, i.e. chromaffin cells, the Ca²⁺ accumulation was remarkably large and exceeded the clearance by the plasma membrane Ca²⁺ extrusion systems and the SERCA pumps (Babcock et al. 1997).

Recent work in sensory neurons has shown that mitochondria following cell stimulation accumulate Ca²⁺ very rapidly but release it slowly thus contributing to maintain a long plateau in cytosolic Ca²⁺ concentration (Medvedeva et al. 2008). It has also been proposed that the release of Ca²⁺ accumulated by mitochondria located close to the SOC channels could efficiently contribute to ER Ca²⁺ re-load (Jousset et al. 2007).

Finally, in the past years a more "dangerous" role for mitochondrial Ca²⁺ uptake has emerged. Work from various laboratories has revealed that the alteration of the Ca²⁺ signal reaching the mitochondria and/or the combined action of apoptotic agents or pathological conditions (e.g. oxidative stress) can induce a profound alteration of organelle structure and function. As a consequence, proteins normally retained in the organelle (such as an important component of the respiratory chain, cytochrome c, as well as other proteins, such as AIF and Smac/Diablo) are released into the cytoplasm, where they activate effector caspases and drive cells to apoptotic cell death. These aspects will be treated in a specific section of this chapter (see Sect. 3.2.5).

3.2.4   The Ca²⁺/ROS Crosstalk: How to Keep the Balance

Mitochondria are the primary sources of reactive oxygen species (ROS) production inside the cells (Csordas and Hajnoczky 2009). During the electron transport, O_2 is converted to H_2O and, particularly at complexes I and III the free radical superoxide is generated (Fig. 3.3). Coenzyme Q at complex III and cytochrome c at complex IV are also important in modulating free radicals production. In addition to the respiratory chain complexes, matrix dehydrogenases like α-ketoglutarate dehydrogenase complex (KGDHC), succinate dehydrogenase (SDH), aconitase and mitochondrial monoamine oxidases (MAOA and MAOB), the enzymes involved in the metabolism of serotonin, norepinphrine and dopamine, are involved in ROS production. Mitochondria also harbour numerous ROS defence systems that guarantee the correct balance between ROS production and detoxification. In the last years, emerging consensus suggested that endogenously generated ROS may not necessarily represent dangerous products, rather, they could act as modulators of different signalling cascades. The main ROS species produced inside cells are superoxide anions (O_2^-) that rapidly react with different molecules (among them with nitric oxide to generate peroxynitrite $ONOO^-$, which induces nitration of proteins on tyrosine residues impairing their function) unless promptly dismuted by the superoxide dismutase (SOD) enzymes, being MnSOD particularly active in mitochondria (Okado-Matsumoto and Fridovich 2001). O_2^- can also spontaneously dismute into O_2 and hydrogen peroxide (H_2O_2). Usually, H_2O_2 is efficiently converted to water by catalase or by GSH-peroxidase, and directly scavenged by GSH, a cysteine containing tripeptide, or by thioredoxin (TR), a disulfide containing protein. NADPH-dependent GSH- and TR-reductase then re-establish the non-oxidized form of GSH and TR. However, H_2O_2 can react with metal ions (Fe^{2+} and Cu^+) to form hydroxyl radicals (•OH) via Fenton reaction.

In normal conditions, electrons transport from NAD-linked substrates through the respiratory chain complexes causes a very low production of O_2^-, but when the electron transport chain is inhibited electrons accumulate at complex I and coenzyme Q level, where they can be donated directly to molecular oxygen. High mitochondrial membrane potential ($\Delta\Psi_m$) favours ROS production from complex I, thus Ca^{2+} uptake inside mitochondria that causes a mild depolarization of the organelle and stimulates metabolic pathways could theoretically increase ROS production. On the other hand, it must be also mentioned that a slight increase in ROS contributes to sensitize Ca^{2+} signaling pathways being the RyR and InsP$_3$R mediated ER Ca^{2+} release stimulated by ROS (Anzai et al. 1998; Kourie 1998; Suzuki and Ford 1992) .Whether ROS could modulate also mitochondrial Ca^{2+} transport is presently unclear, but numerous evidences suggest that the Ca^{2+}/ROS crosstalk at the mitochondrial level is essential to maintain the cell function. As soon as mitochondrial dysfunctions are emerging the cells take the way to degeneration and death (Feissner et al. 2009).

The sarco/endoplasmic reticulum Ca^{2+} ATPase (SERCA) and plasma membsurane Ca^{2+} ATPase (PMCA) are instead inhibited by ROS increases (Kaplan et al. 2003; Zaidi and Michaelis 1999), thus contributing to augment Ca^{2+} level inside cells and mitochondria. The mitochondria can cope with this situation balancing the Ca^{2+} efflux pathway through the transient opening of the MPTP, until Ca^{2+} overload becomes massive and induces its irreversible opening, that further increases ROS production by altering conformation and activity of complex I (Bernardi and Rasola 2007).

3.2.5 A Wave of Death: Ca²⁺-Mediated Apoptosis

Apoptosis is a process of programmed cell death that occurs in all multicellular organisms as different as nematodes, insects and mammals (Twomey and McCarthy 2005). It is essential for normal tissue development and its dysregulation has very deleterious effects: a lot of pathological conditions like neurodegeneration or cancer find their genesis in a defective apoptosis (Thompson 1995). The final outcome of the apoptotic process are macroscopic morphological changes, as formation of membrane blebs, chromatin condensation, chromosomal DNA fragmentation, that bring the cell to collapse (Saraste and Pulkki 2000). The process can be induced through different pathways that selectively involve specific proteins and intracellular compartments. Activation of apoptosis starts principally in two way: the extrinsic pathway, through the engagement of plasma membrane receptors belonging to a subgroup of the TNF-receptor superfamily known as death receptors and the activation of the death-inducing caspase cascade (Ashkenazi 2002), and the intrinsic pathway, through the engagement of

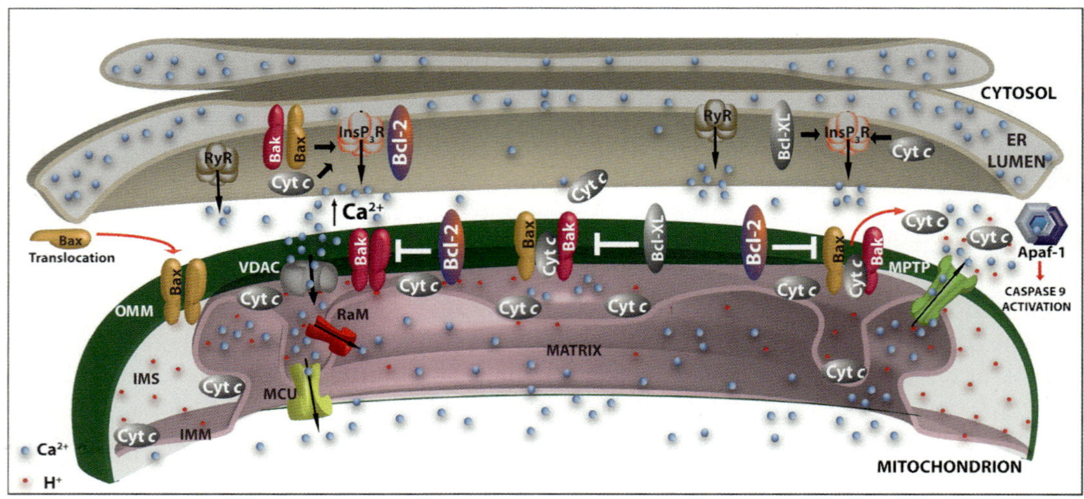

Fig. 3.4 Ca^{2+}-mediated apoptosis. In resting conditions, the anti-apoptotic protein Bcl-2 directly interacts with the InsP$_3$R by modulating its activity and promotes ER Ca^{2+} leak. In response to cell damage and persistent stimulation, the pro-apoptotic proteins Bax/Bak enhance the InsP$_3$R-mediated Ca^{2+}-release and mitochondria are more sensitive to Ca^{2+}-overload. Opening of the mitochondrial permeability transition pore (*MPTP*) and specific channels formed by Bax/Bak oligomers allows the release of Cytochrome c (*Cyt c*) and other proapoptotic factors (e.g., Apaf-1). Cyt c release further increases InsP$_3$R Ca^{2+} release thus promoting mitochondrial Ca^{2+}-overload. The anti-apoptotic proteins Bcl-2 and Bcl-xL can protect the cell by forming heteropolymers with Bax and Bak and thus reducing their proapoptotic function (see text)

Bcl-2-related proteins upon cellular insults (Youle and Strasser 2008). The Ca^{2+} link with the apoptotic pathways has been established very clearly when it was shown that the anti-apoptotic Bcl-2 protein can control the Ca^{2+} signal and that Ca^{2+} can sensitize cells to apoptotic challenges, acting on the mitochondrial checkpoint (Fig. 3.4). The idea was reinforced by the finding that Bcl-2, in addition to be localized in the cytoplasm and at the nuclear envelope, is also associated to the ER and mitochondrial membranes, two organelles strictly involved in the control of Ca^{2+} homeostasis, for a review see (Pinton and Rizzuto 2006). The first evidence that Bcl-2 overexpression could directly affect Ca^{2+} homeostasis was given in hematopoietic cells, where its overexpression was suggested to prevent the cytosolic free Ca^{2+} level reduction induced by withdrawal of interleukin-3 and to protect from apoptosis (Baffy et al. 1993). Successive studies, performed using targeted probes, showed that HeLa cells overexpressing Bcl-2 have reduced Ca^{2+} levels in ER and in the Golgi apparatus lumen, and, as a consequence, also displayed a reduction in Ca^{2+} release following InsP$_3$-stimulation and thus in cytosolic and mitochondrial Ca^{2+} transients (Pinton et al. 2000). Bcl-2 overexpression also promoted survival of HeLa cells upon ceramide treatment (Pinton et al. 2001) and Bax/Bak MEF double knockout are resistant to several apoptotic stimuli (Scorrano et al. 2003). Accordingly, when the pro-apoptotic Bcl-2 family member proteins Bax and Bak are knocked down, the Ca^{2+} content of ER decrease; instead Bax overexpression increased ER Ca^{2+} concentration (Chami et al. 2004; Danial and Korsmeyer 2004). Bcl-2, and similarly Bcl-XL, another antiapoptotic member of Bcl-2 family, directly interacted with InsP$_3$R on the ER membrane, and sensitizes it to low agonist doses, promoting the leakage of Ca^{2+} from ER. All these effects are reverted by overexpression of Bax (White et al. 2005).

Considering that the ER/mitochondria connection is strictly linked to the coupling of the InsP$_3$R to mitochondrial outer membrane proteins such as VDAC and that the amount of Ca^{2+} released is critical to the transduction of the signal in mitochondria, it is evident that the modulation of InsP$_3$R opening by pro or antiapoptotic proteins is a key element to determine mitochondrial changes in morphology but also in physio/pathological responses. Mitochondria are the depositaries of several proapoptotic proteins like Smac/DIABLO, Omi/HtrA2, AIF and EndoG which are in equilibrium with other antiapoptotic proteins as XIAP, cIAP-1 and cIAP-2 to finely regulate the balance between cell death and life: thus the role of mitochondria and Ca^{2+} appears evidently essential in concurring the key determinant events leading to cell death. Ca^{2+} loads were shown to sensitize the MPTP to apoptotic stimuli, inducing its opening, mitochondrial changes in morphology and the release of cytochrome c (Pacher and Hajnoczky 2001). Cytochrome c release promotes the oligomerization of Apaf-1 and the activation of caspases (Kroemer and Reed 2000; Pinton et al. 2008). Interestingly, it has been shown that cytochrome c binds to $InsP_3R$ and increases its conductance, causing a larger release of Ca^{2+} that in turn promotes mitochondrial Ca^{2+} overload (Boehning et al. 2003).

3.3 Mitochondria on the Move: Trafficking, Fission and Fusion

The ER–mitochondrial network is strictly dependent on the fact that these organelles are intrinsically highly dynamic structures continuously moving and remodelling in their shape (Pacher et al. 2008). The molecular determinants of this dynamism are the so-called "mitochondria-shaping proteins" (essentially the dynamin–related protein Drp1, the mitofusins Mfns and the optic atrophy 1 Opa1) that regulate the process of mitochondrial fission and fusion (Jahani-Asl et al. 2010; Jeyaraju et al. 2009) and the Miro/Milton machinery that controls mitochondrial trafficking (Liu and Hajnoczky 2009; MacAskill and Kittler 2010) (Fig. 3.5).

The process of fission/fusion is strictly connected with mitochondrial trafficking and both of them concur to the maintenance of the mitochondrial network according to the cell demand. Emerging evidence has shown that the distribution of mitochondria reflects the state of the cell and may influence the cell response to physiological and pathological conditions by modulating functions such as energy supply, programmed cell death, and Ca^{2+} signalling. Interestingly, in both these processes Ca^{2+} plays an emerging role: it acts as transducer to modulate the intracellular distribution of the organelles at sites of high energy demand (mitochondrial trafficking) and as molecular switch for the mitochondrial membrane remodelling proteins during the mitochondrial fission-fusion events.

3.3.1 Mitochondrial Trafficking

Mitochondria are transported along cytoskeletal tracks to sites in the cell where the energy demands are high and/or where Ca^{2+} buffering is required. This movement is especially important in neurons because of their peculiar morphological characteristics. Rapid, long distance, movement of mitochondria is accomplished via the microtubule network, whereas actin plays a role in anchoring mitochondria and in tracking their short range transport (Ligon and Steward 2000; Rube and van der Bliek 2004). In polarized cells, like budding yeast and neurons, the organelle movements along the major axis of the cell are prominent, and occur both away from the nucleus (anterograde transport) and toward the centre of the cell and nucleus (retrograde transport) (Frederick et al. 2004), being the two transport machineries functionally coupled.

The anterograde (plus end-directed) transport of mitochondria along microtubules is mediated by kinesins (KIFs). KIFs act as molecular motors also in other transport processes such as that of lysosomes and tubulin oligomers (Nakata and Hirokawa 2007) but their specific binding to mitochondria is mediated by the kinesin binding protein Milton and the atypical GTPase Miro (Mitochondrial rho) that have been originally identified in *Drosophila* to act as adaptor proteins (Glater et al. 2006; Guo et al. 2005). Other possible specific adaptor proteins linking mitochondria to kinesin motors have been described, they include syntabulin, KBP and the scaffold protein RanBP2 (Cai et al. 2005;

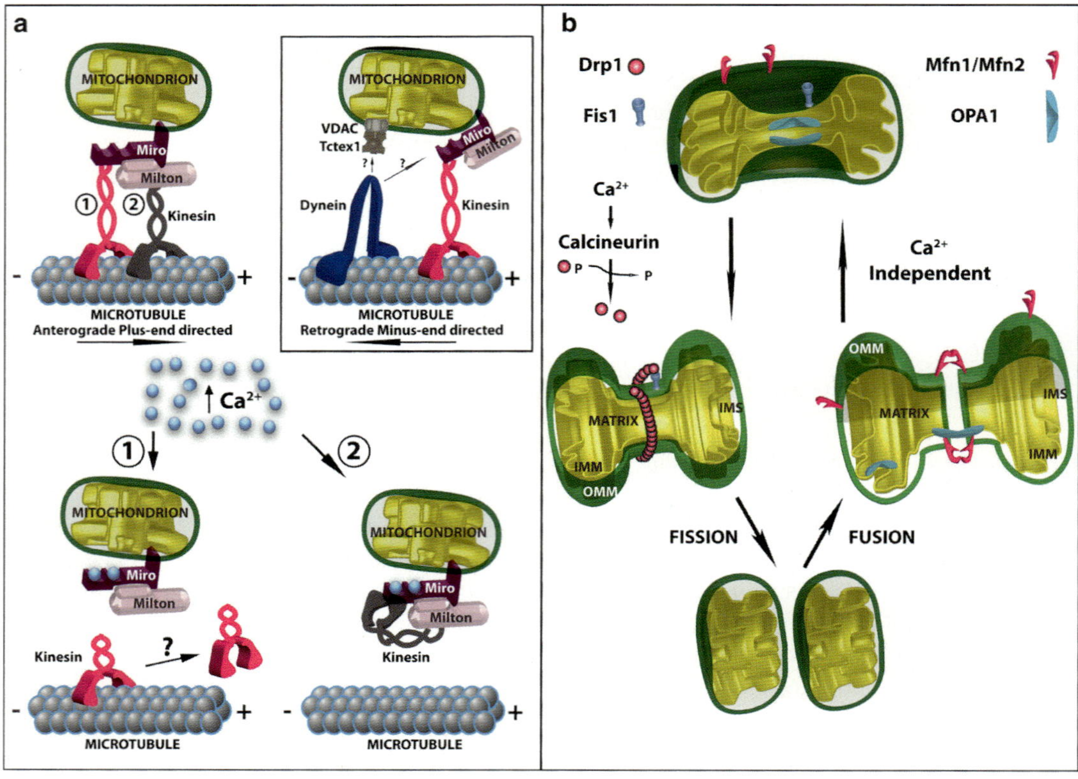

Fig. 3.5 Mitochondrial trafficking (**a**) and fission-fusion (**b**) machineries. (**a**) At resting intracellular Ca^{2+} levels (<0.1 μM) microtubule-based anterograde transport is supported by Kinesins (KIFs) and Kinesin adaptors (Miro/Milton). High levels of Ca^{2+} inhibit mitochondrial movement via Ca^{2+}-binding to the EF-hands Ca^{2+} binding sites of Miro. The two proposed mechanisms are represented: in (1) Ca^{2+} binding to Miro inhibits the Miro/Kinesin interaction and thus the coupling between mitochondria and the transport machinery (Macaskill et al. 2009), and in (2) Ca^{2+} binding to Miro promotes the direct Miro/Kinesin interaction liberating Milton form the interaction, thus resulting in the uncoupling of mitochondria from the microtubule pathway (Wang and Schwarz 2009). Inset: Retrograde minus-end directed transport is supported by dynein motors. (**b**) Ca^{2+}-induced Drp1 de-phosphorylation promotes Drp1 oligomerization into 8–12 subunit spiral chains recruited around the mitochondria via the adaptor Fis1. Drp1 GTPase activity is required for mitochondrial fission. Mitochondrial fusion of the outer and inner membranes involves trans-dimerization of Mfn1 (or its homologue Mfn2) and OPA1. GTPase activity is then responsible for fusion of the two membranes

Cho et al. 2007; Wozniak et al. 2005), but whether these proteins are recruited by Miro to the mitochondria or may themselves regulate the Miro/KIFs trafficking is presently unclear.

Miro proteins belong to the Ras GTPases mitochondrial subfamily and are well conserved from yeast to humans, being Miro1 and Miro2 the two members present in mammals. Miro1 and Miro2 have two GTPase domains at the N and C terminus, a C terminus transmembrane domain which confers targeting to the OMM and two Ca^{2+}-binding EF-hand motifs responsible for their Ca^{2+} sensitivity (Fransson et al. 2006). Milton proteins are cytosolic and are proposed to support mitochondrial traffic by directly binding both Miros and kinesin heavy chain (KHC). However, it has been also proposed that Milton acts as an essential bridging molecule necessary to link Miro to kinesin motors and thus to confer Ca^{2+} sensitivity to the mitochondria trafficking process (Glater et al. 2006).

Ca^{2+} regulation has a double way of action: at resting Ca^{2+} concentrations mitochondrial movement is maximal, whereas increases in Ca^{2+} concentrations within a physiological range result in mitochondria trafficking arrest and in keeping mitochondria at the sites of cytosolic Ca^{2+} elevation

(Liu and Hajnoczky 2009). Two distinct models have been proposed for the molecular mechanism of the Ca²⁺ regulation: in one model Ca²⁺ binding to Miro inhibits the Miro/KHC interaction and thus the coupling between mitochondria and the transport machinery (Macaskill et al. 2009), in the other, Ca²⁺ concentration rises switch the Miro binding to KIF through the adaptor Milton to the direct Miro/KIF interaction thus resulting in the uncoupling of mitochondria from the motor/microtubule pathway (Wang and Schwarz 2009) (Fig. 3.5a).

The retrograde (minus end-directed) axonal transport is mediated by dynein motors (Hirokawa and Takemura 2005), but it also requires kinesin function to transport dynein to the periphery of cells. Since the anterograde transport of mitochondria has an essential role in supporting the bioenergetic demands of the cells, it has been widely investigated. Instead, the mechanisms of mitochondria trafficking to the cell body are less known, despite this movement is probably essential to remove damaged mitochondria and thus to maintain the correct equilibrium between functional and unfunctional mitochondria. As in the kinesins-mediated transport, a large number of accessory proteins allows selective coupling between dynein motors and the different cargoes (Susalka et al. 2000), however it is still unclear whether dynein is directly involved in mitochondria transport. Interestingly, among the different adaptor proteins, Tctex1 has been shown to interact with VDAC suggesting a possible link with mitochondria and dynein, but also with Ca²⁺ in the regulation of this process (Schwarzer et al. 2002) (Fig. 3.5a inset). Recently the mitochondria/Ca²⁺ link to dynein has became even more probable since the kinesin adaptator Miro has also been proposed as adaptor recruiting dynein to mitochondria (Russo et al. 2009).

3.3.2 Mitochondria Fission and Fusion

As well as undergoing regulated movement throughout the cell, mitochondria undergo cycles of fission and fusion events to create multiple small or single large tubular mitochondrial networks, and regulating their morphology (Fig. 3.5b). In mammals, mitochondrial fission is dependent on Drp1, a soluble, cytosolic GTPase that is recruited to the outer mitochondrial membrane. In yeast, in addition to the DRp1 homologous Dnm1, the assembly of the fission machinery, requires the outer mitochondrial membrane protein Fis1. Also in mammals Fis1 acts as Drp1 receptor, but Drp1 recruitment to mitochondria is also mediated by actin filaments and microtubules. Activity of additional proteins, such as Endophilin B1 and MTP18, have also been reported to play a role, being their downregulation responsible for the formation of highly interconnected mitochondrial reticulum suggesting an impairment of physiological mitochondrial fission events (Jeyaraju et al. 2009).

Drp1 inhibition or down-regulation result in an overall dominant effect of membrane fusion activities, causing mitochondria to be fused and interconnected. Recent evidence suggests that Ca²⁺ controls Drp1-dependent mitochondrial fission through calcineurin and CaM kinase activities: Drp1 calcineurin dependent dephosphorylation drives its translocation to mitochondria where it causes their fission; however it has also been shown that Drp1 phosphorylation by CaM kinase (but also by PKA) recruits Drp1 to mitochondria, probably increasing Drp1 affinity for its mitochondrial receptor Fis1 (Cereghetti et al. 2008; Cribbs and Strack 2007; Han et al. 2008), thus suggesting that multiple Ca²⁺ and cAMP dependent pathways may interact to regulate mitochondrial dynamics. Drp1 is also regulated by a Miro-dependent Ca²⁺-induced mechanism: in addition to governing mitochondria trafficking, Miro has been shown to modulate the mitochondrial morphology. It enhances the fusion state of the mitochondria at resting Ca²⁺ levels but promotes mitochondrial fragmentation at high Ca²⁺ concentrations, probably acting through Drp1 suppression and activation, respectively. Thus, Miro proteins serve as a Ca²⁺-sensitive bifunctional regulator for both the motility and fusion-fission dynamics of the mitochondria (Saotome et al. 2008).

As mitochondrial fusion in mammals, the main players are mitofusin-1 (Mfn1), mitofusin-2 (Mfn2), optic atrophy 1 (Opa1), and presenilin-associated rhomboid-like protein (Parl) (Hoppins and

Nunnari 2009; Soubannier and McBride 2009). Mfn1 and 2 are integral outer membrane proteins and mediate the OMM fusion, whereas Opa1, which is localized at the intermembrane space, is probably involved in the fusion of the IMM and in the regulation of cristae structure. Loss of Mfn1, Mfn2 and Opa1 leads to mitochondrial fragmentation and increases sensitivity to cell death stimuli (Jahani-Asl et al. 2007), while their overexpression increases survival in several cell types including neurons (Barsoum et al. 2006).

Mitofusins possess GTPase activity, and Mfn1 has higher GTPase activity than Mfn2 and induces fusion more efficiently (Ishihara et al. 2004). Unlike Drp1, their regulation seems to be Ca^{2+}-independent, even if, as mentioned above, they play a crucial role in tethering ER and mitochondria membranes and thus in the generation of ER/mitochondria contact sites that have a big relevance in the regulation of mitochondrial Ca^{2+} (de Brito and Scorrano 2008). Genetic ablation of Mfn2 causes an increase in the distance between the two organelles with a consequent impairment of mitochondrial Ca^{2+} uptake. The ER–mitochondrial apposition performed by Mfn2 predisposes mitochondria to high Ca^{2+} microdomains and to the consequent overloading, leading eventually to apoptosis by excessive Ca^{2+} transfer. Opa1 has also GTPase activity, requires Mfn1 but not Mfn2 to mediate fusion (Cipolat et al. 2004) and it is proteolitically regulated by Parl. No evidences are present to support this pathways as a Ca^{2+}-related process.

3.4 Concluding Remarks

Mitochondria have been recently recognized as multifunctional organelles: they play a crucial role in energy metabolism, cell survival and death but also, thanks to their dynamic behaviour they are now considered essential in the process of Ca^{2+} buffering and thus in the regulation of signal transduction pathways. Mitochondria and their Ca^{2+} handling have been extensively investigated for 50 years but they are still extremely intriguing. The big improvement of the methodology, essentially based on the development of genetically encoded Ca^{2+} indicators, has opened the possibility to deeply investigate mitochondrial Ca^{2+} fluxes. Recombinant probes now represent a wonderful tool to dissect physiological from pathological situations: mitochondrial Ca^{2+} dysregulation appears to be a common hallmark of numerous pathological conditions ranging from cardiovascular, neuromuscular to neurodegenerative diseases. It has still to be defined whether the mitochondrial dysfunctions are the consequences or the causes of the pathological situations, but emerging consensus suggests that mitochondrial impairments can be a cause of selective vulnerability of specific cell populations rather than simply a late stage consequence. The very recent identification of molecular actors in mitochondrial transport, i.e. the uniporter and the Na^+/Ca^{2+} exchanger, opens the possibility to generate animal models and to develop new targeted drugs to manipulate processes regulated by mitochondrial Ca^{2+} signals, such as aerobic metabolism and cell death.

Acknowledgements The original work described in this review by the authors has been supported over the years by grants to M.B from the Italian National Research Council (CNR), the Italian Ministry of University and Research (PRIN 2003, 2005 and 2008), the Telethon Foundation (Project GGP04169) and the local fundings of the University of Padova (Progetto di Ateneo 2008).

References

Anzai K, Ogawa K, Kuniyasu A, Ozawa T, Yamamoto H, Nakayama H (1998) Effects of hydroxyl radical and sulfhydryl reagents on the open probability of the purified cardiac ryanodine receptor channel incorporated into planar lipid bilayers. Biochem Biophys Res Commun 249:938–942

Ashkenazi A (2002) Targeting death and decoy receptors of the tumour-necrosis factor superfamily. Nat Rev Cancer 2:420–430

Babcock DF, Herrington J, Goodwin PC, Park YB, Hille B (1997) Mitochondrial participation in the intracellular Ca^{2+} network. J Cell Biol 136:833–844

Baffy G, Miyashita T, Williamson JR, Reed JC (1993) Apoptosis induced by withdrawal of interleukin-3 (IL-3) from an IL-3-dependent hematopoietic cell line is associated with repartitioning of intracellular calcium and is blocked by enforced Bcl-2 oncoprotein production. J Biol Chem 268:6511–6519

Baines CP (2009) The molecular composition of the mitochondrial permeability transition pore. J Mol Cell Cardiol 46:850–857

Baines CP, Kaiser RA, Purcell NH, Blair NS, Osinska H, Hambleton MA, Brunskill EW, Sayen MR, Gottlieb RA, Dorn GW et al (2005) Loss of cyclophilin D reveals a critical role for mitochondrial permeability transition in cell death. Nature 434:658–662

Barsoum MJ, Yuan H, Gerencser AA, Liot G, Kushnareva Y, Graber S, Kovacs I, Lee WD, Waggoner J, Cui J et al (2006) Nitric oxide-induced mitochondrial fission is regulated by dynamin-related GTPases in neurons. EMBO J 25:3900–3911

Baughman JM, Perocchi F, Girgis HS, Plovanich M, Belcher-Timme CA, Sancak Y, Bao XR, Strittmatter L, Goldberger O, Bogorad RL et al (2011) Integrative genomics identifies MCU as an essential component of the mitochondrial calcium uniporter. Nature 476:341–345

Baysal K, Jung DW, Gunter KK, Gunter TE, Brierley GP (1994) Na(+)-dependent Ca^{2+} efflux mechanism of heart mitochondria is not a passive Ca^{2+}/2Na+ exchanger. Am J Physiol 266:C800–C808

Bernardi P, Forte M (2007) The mitochondrial permeability transition pore. Novartis Found Symp 287:157–164, discussion 164–159

Bernardi P, Rasola A (2007) Calcium and cell death: the mitochondrial connection. Subcell Biochem 45:481–506

Berridge MJ, Bootman MD, Roderick HL (2003) Calcium signalling: dynamics, homeostasis and remodelling. Nat Rev Mol Cell Biol 4:517–529

Beutner G, Sharma VK, Giovannucci DR, Yule DI, Sheu SS (2001) Identification of a ryanodine receptor in rat heart mitochondria. J Biol Chem 276:21482–21488

Boehning D, Patterson RL, Sedaghat L, Glebova NO, Kurosaki T, Snyder SH (2003) Cytochrome c binds to inositol (1,4,5) trisphosphate receptors, amplifying calcium-dependent apoptosis. Nat Cell Biol 5:1051–1061

Boitier E, Rea R, Duchen MR (1999) Mitochondria exert a negative feedback on the propagation of intracellular Ca^{2+} waves in rat cortical astrocytes. J Cell Biol 145:795–808

Brini M, Carafoli E (2000) Calcium signalling: a historical account, recent developments and future perspectives. Cell Mol Life Sci 57:354–370

Brini M, Carafoli E (2009) Calcium pumps in health and disease. Physiol Rev 89:1341–1378

Brini M, Pinton P, King MP, Davidson M, Schon EA, Rizzuto R (1999) A calcium signaling defect in the pathogenesis of a mitochondrial DNA inherited oxidative phosphorylation deficiency. Nat Med 5:951–954

Cai Q, Gerwin C, Sheng ZH (2005) Syntabulin-mediated anterograde transport of mitochondria along neuronal processes. J Cell Biol 170:959–969

Carafoli E (2010) The fateful encounter of mitochondria with calcium: how did it happen? Biochim Biophys Acta 1797:595–606

Carafoli E, Tiozzo R, Lugli G, Crovetti F, Kratzing C (1974) The release of calcium from heart mitochondria by sodium. J Mol Cell Cardiol 6:361–371

Cereghetti GM, Stangherlin A, Martins de Brito O, Chang CR, Blackstone C, Bernardi P, Scorrano L (2008) Dephosphorylation by calcineurin regulates translocation of Drp1 to mitochondria. Proc Natl Acad Sci USA 105: 15803–15808

Chami M, Prandini A, Campanella M, Pinton P, Szabadkai G, Reed JC, Rizzuto R (2004) Bcl-2 and Bax exert opposing effects on Ca^{2+} signaling, which do not depend on their putative pore-forming region. J Biol Chem 279: 54581–54589

Cho KI, Cai Y, Yi H, Yeh A, Aslanukov A, Ferreira PA (2007) Association of the kinesin-binding domain of RanBP2 to KIF5B and KIF5C determines mitochondria localization and function. Traffic 8:1722–1735

Cipolat S, Martins de Brito O, Dal Zilio B, Scorrano L (2004) OPA1 requires mitofusin 1 to promote mitochondrial fusion. Proc Natl Acad Sci USA 101:15927–15932

Cox DA, Matlib MA (1993) Modulation of intramitochondrial free Ca^{2+} concentration by antagonists of Na(+)-Ca^{2+} exchange. Trends Pharmacol Sci 14:408–413

Cribbs JT, Strack S (2007) Reversible phosphorylation of Drp1 by cyclic AMP-dependent protein kinase and calcineurin regulates mitochondrial fission and cell death. EMBO Rep 8:939–944

Crompton M, Virji S, Ward JM (1998) Cyclophilin-D binds strongly to complexes of the voltage-dependent anion channel and the adenine nucleotide translocase to form the permeability transition pore. Eur J Biochem 258:729–735

Csordas G, Hajnoczky G (2009) SR/ER-mitochondrial local communication: calcium and ROS. Biochim Biophys Acta 1787:1352–1362

Csordas G, Renken C, Varnai P, Walter L, Weaver D, Buttle KF, Balla T, Mannella CA, Hajnoczky G (2006) Structural and functional features and significance of the physical linkage between ER and mitochondria. J Cell Biol 174:915–921

Danial NN, Korsmeyer SJ (2004) Cell death: critical control points. Cell 116:205–219

de Brito OM, Scorrano L (2008) Mitofusin 2 tethers endoplasmic reticulum to mitochondria. Nature 456:605–610

De Stefani D, Raffaello A, Teardo E, Szabo I, Rizzuto R (2011) A forty-kilodalton protein of the inner membrane is the mitochondrial calcium uniporter. Nature 476(7360):336–340

del Arco A, Satrustegui J (1998) Molecular cloning of Aralar, a new member of the mitochondrial carrier superfamily that binds calcium and is present in human muscle and brain. J Biol Chem 273:23327–23334

Denton RM (2009) Regulation of mitochondrial dehydrogenases by calcium ions. Biochim Biophys Acta 1787: 1309–1316

Feissner RF, Skalska J, Gaum WE, Sheu SS (2009) Crosstalk signaling between mitochondrial Ca^{2+} and ROS. Front Biosci 14:1197–1218

Fiskum G, Lehninger AL (1979) Regulated release of Ca2+ from respiring mitochondria by $Ca^{2+}/2H+$ antiport. J Biol Chem. Jul 25;254(14):6236–9. PubMed PMID:36390

Fransson S, Ruusala A, Aspenstrom P (2006) The atypical Rho GTPases Miro-1 and Miro-2 have essential roles in mitochondrial trafficking. Biochem Biophys Res Commun 344:500–510

Frazier AE, Taylor RD, Mick DU, Warscheid B, Stoepel N, Meyer HE, Ryan MT, Guiard B, Rehling P (2006) Mdm38 interacts with ribosomes and is a component of the mitochondrial protein export machinery. J Cell Biol 172:553–564

Frederick RL, McCaffery JM, Cunningham KW, Okamoto K, Shaw JM (2004) Yeast Miro GTPase, Gem1p, regulates mitochondrial morphology via a novel pathway. J Cell Biol 167:87–98

Gellerich FN, Gizatullina Z, Trumbeckaite S, Nguyen HP, Pallas T, Arandarcikaite O, Vielhaber S, Seppet E, Striggow F (2010) The regulation of OXPHOS by extramitochondrial calcium. Biochim Biophys Acta 1797:1018–1027

Giacomello M, Drago I, Bortolozzi M, Scorzeto M, Gianelle A, Pizzo P, Pozzan T (2010) Ca^{2+} hot spots on the mitochondrial surface are generated by Ca^{2+} mobilization from stores, but not by activation of store-operated Ca^{2+} channels. Mol Cell 38:280–290

Glater EE, Megeath LJ, Stowers RS, Schwarz TL (2006) Axonal transport of mitochondria requires milton to recruit kinesin heavy chain and is light chain independent. J Cell Biol 173:545–557

Griffiths EJ, Rutter GA (2009) Mitochondrial calcium as a key regulator of mitochondrial ATP production in mammalian cells. Biochim Biophys Acta 1787:1324–1333

Gunter TE, Chace JH, Puskin JS, Gunter KK (1983) Mechanism of sodium independent calcium efflux from rat liver mitochondria. Biochemistry 22:6341–6351

Gunter TE, Buntinas L, Sparagna G, Eliseev R, Gunter K (2000) Mitochondrial calcium transport: mechanisms and functions. Cell Calcium 28:285–296

Guo X, Macleod GT, Wellington A, Hu F, Panchumarthi S, Schoenfield M, Marin L, Charlton MP, Atwood HL, Zinsmaier KE (2005) The GTPase dMiro is required for axonal transport of mitochondria to Drosophila synapses. Neuron 47:379–393

Hajnoczky G, Robb-Gaspers LD, Seitz MB, Thomas AP (1995) Decoding of cytosolic calcium oscillations in the mitochondria. Cell 82:415–424

Hajnoczky G, Hager R, Thomas AP (1999) Mitochondria suppress local feedback activation of inositol 1,4, 5-trisphosphate receptors by Ca^{2+}. J Biol Chem 274:14157–14162

Han XJ, Lu YF, Li SA, Kaitsuka T, Sato Y, Tomizawa K, Nairn AC, Takei K, Matsui H, Matsushita M (2008) CaM kinase I alpha-induced phosphorylation of Drp1 regulates mitochondrial morphology. J Cell Biol 182:573–585

Haworth RA, Hunter DR (2000) Control of the mitochondrial permeability transition pore by high-affinity ADP binding at the ADP/ATP translocase in permeabilized mitochondria. J Bioenerg Biomembr 32:91–96

Hayashi T, Su TP (2007) Sigma-1 receptor chaperones at the ER-mitochondrion interface regulate Ca(2+) signaling and cell survival. Cell 131:596–610

Hirokawa N, Takemura R (2005) Molecular motors and mechanisms of directional transport in neurons. Nat Rev Neurosci 6:201–214

Hoppins S, Nunnari J (2009) The molecular mechanism of mitochondrial fusion. Biochim Biophys Acta 1793:20–26

Hoth M, Fanger CM, Lewis RS (1997) Mitochondrial regulation of store-operated calcium signaling in T lymphocytes. J Cell Biol 137:633–648

Hoth M, Button DC, Lewis RS (2000) Mitochondrial control of calcium-channel gating: a mechanism for sustained signaling and transcriptional activation in T lymphocytes. Proc Natl Acad Sci USA 97:10607–10612

Ishihara N, Eura Y, Mihara K (2004) Mitofusin 1 and 2 play distinct roles in mitochondrial fusion reactions via GTPase activity. J Cell Sci 117:6535–6546

Jahani-Asl A, Cheung EC, Neuspiel M, MacLaurin JG, Fortin A, Park DS, McBride HM, Slack RS (2007) Mitofusin 2 protects cerebellar granule neurons against injury-induced cell death. J Biol Chem 282:23788–23798

Jahani-Asl A, Germain M, Slack RS (2010) Mitochondria: joining forces to thwart cell death. Biochim Biophys Acta 1802:162–166

Jeyaraju DV, Cisbani G, Pellegrini L (2009) Calcium regulation of mitochondria motility and morphology. Biochim Biophys Acta 1787:1363–1373

Jiang D, Zhao L, Clapham DE (2009) Genome-wide RNAi screen identifies Letm1 as a mitochondrial Ca²⁺/H+ antiporter. Science 326:144–147

Jouaville LS, Ichas F, Holmuhamedov EL, Camacho P, Lechleiter JD (1995) Synchronization of calcium waves by mitochondrial substrates in Xenopus laevis oocytes. Nature 377:438–441

Jouaville LS, Pinton P, Bastianutto C, Rutter GA, Rizzuto R (1999) Regulation of mitochondrial ATP synthesis by calcium: evidence for a long-term metabolic priming. Proc Natl Acad Sci USA 96:13807–13812

Jousset H, Frieden M, Demaurex N (2007) STIM1 knockdown reveals that store-operated Ca²⁺ channels located close to sarco/endoplasmic Ca²⁺ ATPases (SERCA) pumps silently refill the endoplasmic reticulum. J Biol Chem 282: 11456–11464

Kaplan P, Babusikova E, Lehotsky J, Dobrota D (2003) Free radical-induced protein modification and inhibition of Ca²⁺-ATPase of cardiac sarcoplasmic reticulum. Mol Cell Biochem 248:41–47

Kirichok Y, Krapivinsky G, Clapham DE (2004) The mitochondrial calcium uniporter is a highly selective ion channel. Nature 427:360–364

Kourie JI (1998) Interaction of reactive oxygen species with ion transport mechanisms. Am J Physiol 275:C1–C24

Kroemer G, Reed JC (2000) Mitochondrial control of cell death. Nat Med 6:513–519

Lasorsa FM, Pinton P, Palmieri L, Fiermonte G, Rizzuto R, Palmieri F (2003) Recombinant expression of the Ca(²⁺)-sensitive aspartate/glutamate carrier increases mitochondrial ATP production in agonist-stimulated Chinese hamster ovary cells. J Biol Chem 278:38686–38692

Ligon LA, Steward O (2000) Role of microtubules and actin filaments in the movement of mitochondria in the axons and dendrites of cultured hippocampal neurons. J Comp Neurol 427:351–361

Litsky ML, Pfeiffer DR (1997) Regulation of the mitochondrial Ca²⁺ uniporter by external adenine nucleotides: the uniporter behaves like a gated channel which is regulated by nucleotides and divalent cations. Biochemistry 36:7071–7080

Liu X, Hajnoczky G (2009) Ca²⁺-dependent regulation of mitochondrial dynamics by the Miro-Milton complex. Int J Biochem Cell Biol 41:1972–1976

Loew LM, Carrington W, Tuft RA, Fay FS (1994) Physiological cytosolic Ca²⁺ transients evoke concurrent mitochondrial depolarizations. Proc Natl Acad Sci USA 91:12579–12583

MacAskill AF, Kittler JT (2010) Control of mitochondrial transport and localization in neurons. Trends Cell Biol 20:102–112

Macaskill AF, Rinholm JE, Twelvetrees AE, Arancibia-Carcamo IL, Muir J, Fransson A, Aspenstrom P, Attwell D, Kittler JT (2009) Miro1 is a calcium sensor for glutamate receptor-dependent localization of mitochondria at synapses. Neuron 61:541–555

Malli R, Frieden M, Osibow K, Graier WF (2003) Mitochondria efficiently buffer subplasmalemmal Ca²⁺ elevation during agonist stimulation. J Biol Chem 278:10807–10815

McCormack JG, Halestrap AP, Denton RM (1990) Role of calcium ions in regulation of mammalian intramitochondrial metabolism. Physiol Rev 70:391–425

McQuibban AG, Joza N, Megighian A, Scorzeto M, Zanini D, Reipert S, Richter C, Schweyen RJ, Nowikovsky K (2010) A Drosophila mutant of LETM1, a candidate gene for seizures in Wolf-Hirschhorn syndrome. Hum Mol Genet 19:987–1000

Medvedeva YV, Kim MS, Usachev YM (2008) Mechanisms of prolonged presynaptic Ca²⁺ signaling and glutamate release induced by TRPV1 activation in rat sensory neurons. J Neurosci 28:5295–5311

Mikoshiba K (2007) IP3 receptor/Ca²⁺ channel: from discovery to new signaling concepts. J Neurochem 102: 1426–1446

Mitchell P (1961) Coupling of phosphorylation to electron and hydrogen transfer by a chemi-osmotic type of mechanism. Nature 191:144–148

Montero M, Alonso MT, Carnicero E, Cuchillo-Ibanez I, Albillos A, Garcia AG, Garcia-Sancho J, Alvarez J (2000) Chromaffin-cell stimulation triggers fast millimolar mitochondrial Ca²⁺ transients that modulate secretion. Nat Cell Biol 2:57–61

Montero M, Lobaton CD, Moreno A, Alvarez J (2002) A novel regulatory mechanism of the mitochondrial Ca²⁺ uniporter revealed by the p38 mitogen-activated protein kinase inhibitor SB202190. FASEB J 16:1955–1957

Nakata T, Hirokawa N (2007) Neuronal polarity and the kinesin superfamily proteins. Sci STKE 2007:pe6

Nicholls DG (2005) Mitochondria and calcium signaling. Cell Calcium 38:311–317

Nicholls DG, Crompton M (1980) Mitochondrial calcium transport. FEBS Lett 111:261–268

Nicholls DG, Scott ID (1980) The regulation of brain mitochondrial calcium-ion transport. The role of ATP in the discrimination between kinetic and membrane-potential-dependent calcium-ion efflux mechanisms. Biochem J 186:833–839

Nicolli A, Basso E, Petronilli V, Wenger RM, Bernardi P (1996) Interactions of cyclophilin with the mitochondrial inner membrane and regulation of the permeability transition pore, and cyclosporin A-sensitive channel. J Biol Chem 271:2185–2192

Nowikovsky K, Reipert S, Devenish RJ, Schweyen RJ (2007) Mdm38 protein depletion causes loss of mitochondrial K+/H+ exchange activity, osmotic swelling and mitophagy. Cell Death Differ 14:1647–1656

Okado-Matsumoto A, Fridovich I (2001) Subcellular distribution of superoxide dismutases (SOD) in rat liver: Cu, Zn-SOD in mitochondria. J Biol Chem 276:38388–38393

Pacher P, Hajnoczky G (2001) Propagation of the apoptotic signal by mitochondrial waves. EMBO J 20:4107–4121

Pacher P, Sharma K, Csordas G, Zhu Y, Hajnoczky G (2008) Uncoupling of ER-mitochondrial calcium communication by transforming growth factor-beta. Am J Physiol Renal Physiol 295:F1303–F1312

Palmi M, Youmbi GT, Fusi F, Sgaragli GP, Dixon HB, Frosini M, Tipton KF (1999) Potentiation of mitochondrial Ca^{2+} sequestration by taurine. Biochem Pharmacol 58:1123–1131

Palty R, Silverman WF, Hershfinkel M, Caporale T, Sensi SL, Parnis J, Nolte C, Fishman D, Shoshan-Barmatz V, Herrmann S et al (2010) NCLX is an essential component of mitochondrial $Na+/Ca^{2+}$ exchange. Proc Natl Acad Sci USA 107:436–441

Perocchi F, Gohil VM, Girgis HS, Bao XR, McCombs JE, Palmer AE, Mootha VK (2010) MICU1 encodes a mitochondrial EF hand protein required for $Ca^{(2+)}$ uptake. Nature 467:291–296

Pinton P, Rizzuto R (2006) Bcl-2 and Ca^{2+} homeostasis in the endoplasmic reticulum. Cell Death Differ 13:1409–1418

Pinton P, Ferrari D, Magalhaes P, Schulze-Osthoff K, Di Virgilio F, Pozzan T, Rizzuto R (2000) Reduced loading of intracellular $Ca^{(2+)}$ stores and downregulation of capacitative Ca^{2+} influx in Bcl-2-overexpressing cells. J Cell Biol 148:857–862

Pinton P, Ferrari D, Rapizzi E, Di Virgilio F, Pozzan T, Rizzuto R (2001) The Ca^{2+} concentration of the endoplasmic reticulum is a key determinant of ceramide-induced apoptosis: significance for the molecular mechanism of Bcl-2 action. EMBO J 20:2690–2701

Pinton P, Giorgi C, Siviero R, Zecchini E, Rizzuto R (2008) Calcium and apoptosis: ER-mitochondria Ca^{2+} transfer in the control of apoptosis. Oncogene 27:6407–6418

Rasola A, Sciacovelli M, Pantic B, Bernardi P (2010) Signal transduction to the permeability transition pore. FEBS Lett 584:1989–1996

Rizzuto R, Simpson AW, Brini M, Pozzan T (1992) Rapid changes of mitochondrial Ca^{2+} revealed by specifically targeted recombinant aequorin. Nature 358:325–327

Rizzuto R, Brini M, Murgia M, Pozzan T (1993) Microdomains with high Ca^{2+} close to IP3-sensitive channels that are sensed by neighboring mitochondria. Science 262:744–747

Rizzuto R, Bastianutto C, Brini M, Murgia M, Pozzan T (1994) Mitochondrial Ca^{2+} homeostasis in intact cells. J Cell Biol 126:1183–1194

Rizzuto R, Pinton P, Carrington W, Fay FS, Fogarty KE, Lifshitz LM, Tuft RA, Pozzan T (1998) Close contacts with the endoplasmic reticulum as determinants of mitochondrial Ca^{2+} responses. Science 280:1763–1766

Rizzuto R, Pinton P, Brini M, Chiesa A, Filippin L, Pozzan T (1999) Mitochondria as biosensors of calcium microdomains. Cell Calcium 26:193–199

Rizzuto R, Bernardi P, Pozzan T (2000) Mitochondria as all-round players of the calcium game. J Physiol 529(Pt 1):37–47

Rube DA, van der Bliek AM (2004) Mitochondrial morphology is dynamic and varied. Mol Cell Biochem 256–257:331–339

Russo GJ, Louie K, Wellington A, Macleod GT, Hu F, Panchumarthi S, Zinsmaier KE (2009) Drosophila Miro is required for both anterograde and retrograde axonal mitochondrial transport. J Neurosci 29:5443–5455

Rustenbeck I, Eggers G, Reiter H, Munster W, Lenzen S (1998) Polyamine modulation of mitochondrial calcium transport. I. Stimulatory and inhibitory effects of aliphatic polyamines, aminoglucosides and other polyamine analogues on mitochondrial calcium uptake. Biochem Pharmacol 56:977–985

Santo-Domingo J, Vay L, Hernandez-Sanmiguel E, Lobaton CD, Moreno A, Montero M, Alvarez J (2007) The plasma membrane Na^+/Ca^{2+} exchange inhibitor KB-R7943 is also a potent inhibitor of the mitochondrial Ca^{2+} uniporter. Br J Pharmacol 151:647–654

Saotome M, Safiulina D, Szabadkai G, Das S, Fransson A, Aspenstrom P, Rizzuto R, Hajnoczky G (2008) Bidirectional Ca^{2+}-dependent control of mitochondrial dynamics by the Miro GTPase. Proc Natl Acad Sci USA 105:20728–20733

Saraste A, Pulkki K (2000) Morphologic and biochemical hallmarks of apoptosis. Cardiovasc Res 45:528–537

Saris NE, Allshire A (1989) Calcium ion transport in mitochondria. Methods Enzymol 174:68–85

Satrustegui J, Pardo B, Del Arco A (2007) Mitochondrial transporters as novel targets for intracellular calcium signaling. Physiol Rev 87:29–67

Schwarzer C, Barnikol-Watanabe S, Thinnes FP, Hilschmann N (2002) Voltage-dependent anion-selective channel (VDAC) interacts with the dynein light chain Tctex1 and the heat-shock protein PBP74. Int J Biochem Cell Biol 34:1059–1070

Scorrano L, Oakes SA, Opferman JT, Cheng EH, Sorcinelli MD, Pozzan T, Korsmeyer SJ (2003) BAX and BAK regulation of endoplasmic reticulum Ca^{2+}: a control point for apoptosis. Science 300:135–139

Soubannier V, McBride HM (2009) Positioning mitochondrial plasticity within cellular signaling cascades. Biochim Biophys Acta 1793:154–170

Sparagna GC, Gunter KK, Sheu SS, Gunter TE (1995) Mitochondrial calcium uptake from physiological-type pulses of calcium. A description of the rapid uptake mode. J Biol Chem 270:27510–27515

Susalka SJ, Hancock WO, Pfister KK (2000) Distinct cytoplasmic dynein complexes are transported by different mechanisms in axons. Biochim Biophys Acta 1496:76–88

Suzuki YJ, Ford GD (1992) Superoxide stimulates IP3-induced Ca²⁺ release from vascular smooth muscle sarcoplasmic reticulum. Am J Physiol 262:H114–H116

Szabadkai G, Bianchi K, Varnai P, De Stefani D, Wieckowski MR, Cavagna D, Nagy AI, Balla T, Rizzuto R (2006) Chaperone-mediated coupling of endoplasmic reticulum and mitochondrial Ca²⁺ channels. J Cell Biol 175:901–911

Thompson CB (1995) Apoptosis in the pathogenesis and treatment of disease. Science 267:1456–1462

Tinel H, Cancela JM, Mogami H, Gerasimenko JV, Gerasimenko OV, Tepikin AV, Petersen OH (1999) Active mitochondria surrounding the pancreatic acinar granule region prevent spreading of inositol trisphosphate-evoked local cytosolic Ca²⁺ signals. EMBO J 18:4999–5008

Trenker M, Malli R, Fertschai I, Levak-Frank S, Graier WF (2007) Uncoupling proteins 2 and 3 are fundamental for mitochondrial Ca²⁺ uniport. Nat Cell Biol 9:445–452

Twomey C, McCarthy JV (2005) Pathways of apoptosis and importance in development. J Cell Mol Med 9:345–359

Vasington FD, Murphy JV (1962) Ca ion uptake by rat kidney mitochondria and its dependence on respiration and phosphorylation. J Biol Chem 237:2670–2677

Wang X, Schwarz TL (2009) The mechanism of Ca²⁺ -dependent regulation of kinesin-mediated mitochondrial motility. Cell 136:163–174

White C, Li C, Yang J, Petrenko NB, Madesh M, Thompson CB, Foskett JK (2005) The endoplasmic reticulum gateway to apoptosis by Bcl-X(L) modulation of the InsP₃R. Nat Cell Biol 7:1021–1028

Wingrove DE, Gunter TE (1986) Kinetics of mitochondrial calcium transport. I. Characteristics of the sodium-independent calcium efflux mechanism of liver mitochondria. J Biol Chem 261:15159–15165

Wozniak MJ, Melzer M, Dorner C, Haring HU, Lammers R (2005) The novel protein KBP regulates mitochondria localization by interaction with a kinesin-like protein. BMC Cell Biol 6:35

Youle RJ, Strasser A (2008) The BCL-2 protein family: opposing activities that mediate cell death. Nat Rev Mol Cell Biol 9:47–59

Zaidi A, Michaelis ML (1999) Effects of reactive oxygen species on brain synaptic plasma membrane Ca²⁺-ATPase. Free Radic Biol Med 27:810–821

Zalk R, Lehnart SE, Marks AR (2007) Modulation of the ryanodine receptor and intracellular calcium. Annu Rev Biochem 76:367–385

Zoccarato F, Nicholls D (1982) The role of phosphate in the regulation of the independent calcium-efflux pathway of liver mitochondria. Eur J Biochem 127:333–338

Chapter 4
Mitochondria and Nitric Oxide: Chemistry and Pathophysiology

Paolo Sarti, Marzia Arese, Elena Forte, Alessandro Giuffrè, and Daniela Mastronicola

Abstract Cell respiration is controlled by nitric oxide (NO) reacting with respiratory chain complexes, particularly with Complex I and IV. The functional implication of these reactions is different owing to involvement of different mechanisms. Inhibition of complex IV is rapid (milliseconds) and reversible, and occurs at nanomolar NO concentrations, whereas inhibition of complex I occurs after a prolonged exposure to higher NO concentrations. The inhibition of Complex I involves the reversible S-nitrosation of a key cysteine residue on the ND3 subunit. The reaction of NO with cytochrome c oxidase (CcOX) directly involves the active site of the enzyme: two mechanisms have been described leading to formation of either a relatively stable nitrosyl-derivative (CcOX-NO) or a more labile nitrite-derivative (CcOX-NO_2^-). Both adducts are inhibited, though with different K_i; one mechanism prevails on the other depending on the turnover conditions and availability of substrates, cytochrome c and O_2. SH-SY5Y neuroblastoma cells or lymphoid cells, cultured under standard O_2 tension, proved to follow the mechanism leading to degradation of NO to nitrite. Formation of CcOX-NO occurred upon rising the electron flux level at this site, artificially or in the presence of higher amounts of endogenous reduced cytochrome c. Taken together, the observations suggest that the expression level of mitochondrial cytochrome c may be crucial to determine the respiratory chain NO inhibition pathway prevailing *in vivo* under nitrosative stress conditions. The putative patho-physiological relevance of the interaction between NO and the respiratory complexes is addressed.

Keywords Nitrosative stress • Cell respiration • Cytochromes • ROS • Mitochondria • Bioenergetics

P. Sarti (✉) • M. Arese • E. Forte • D. Mastronicola
Department of Biochemical Sciences 'A. Rossi Fanelli', University of Rome "La Sapienza",
Piazzale Aldo Moro 5, I-00185 Rome, Italy
e-mail: paolo.sarti@uniroma1.it

A. Giuffrè
CNR Institute of Molecular Biology and Pathology, University of Rome "La Sapienza",
I-00185 Rome, Italy

R. Scatena et al. (eds.), *Advances in Mitochondrial Medicine*, Advances in Experimental
Medicine and Biology 942, DOI 10.1007/978-94-007-2869-1_4,
© Springer Science+Business Media B.V. 2012

Abbreviations

CcOX	cytochrome *c* oxidase
I/R	ischemia and reperfusion
Mb	myoglobin
NO	nitric oxide
NOS	nitric oxide synthase
ONOO⁻	peroxynitrite
OXPHOS	oxidative phosphorylation
ROS	reactive oxygen species
SNO-MPG	S-nitroso-2-mercaptopropionyl-glicine.
TMPD	tetramethyl-p-phenylendiamine

4.1   Introduction

About 20 years ago nitric oxide (NO) was discovered to act as an efficient, to a large extent reversible inhibitor of cellular respiration (Bolanos et al. 1994; Brown and Cooper 1994; Carr and Ferguson 1990; Cleeter et al. 1994; Schweizer and Richter 1994). No wonder, therefore, if over the past few years the bioenergetic relevance of the NO chemistry has gained attention in several basic and applied biomedical areas (Bryan et al. 2007; Cooper and Giulivi 2007; Hendgen-Cotta et al. 2008; Lundberg et al. 2008). To account for NO bioavailability, a number of mechanisms, enzymatic *via* specific NO-synthases (NOSs) or involving direct bulk chemistry and redox recycling of higher NO oxides (NO_x), have been proposed as responsible for generation of NO able to react, among other targets, with many metalloproteins. In this contribution, we will focus our attention on the reactions involving NO and mitochondria, thus responsible for the control of the oxidative phosphorylation (OXPHOS). This control occurs primarily but not solely at the level of Complex I and IV (Fig. 4.1). Depending on a variety of parameters, at cellular and tissue level these reactions cause physiologic or pathologic effects, particularly under ischemic/hypoxic and reperfusion conditions favouring nitrosative reactions.

Before entering into the specific chemistry, it is worth mentioning that these studies started in the 1980s mostly highlighting, over the years, the *negative* effects of the NO inhibition on both Complex I and IV. Later on, as the reaction mechanisms became better understood and detailed, also signalling-like *positive* effects have been discovered and assigned to the reaction of NO with mitochondrial respiratory complexes.

The predominance of *positive* or *negative* effects of NO on mitochondrial respiration is, indeed, linked to the actual concentration and persistence in the mitochondrial environment of NO and related species. To understand this peculiar duality, it may help considering the paradigmatic sequence of events characteristic of the ischemia-reperfusion (I/R) injury. This is a pathological condition in which cells first have to face an hypoxic environment, followed by sudden reoxygenation. In a view oversimplified for the sake of the argument, under I/R conditions, much of the cellular damage observed is the result of mitochondrial events such as Ca^{2+} overload, leading to overproduction of reactive oxygen species (ROS) (Brookes et al. 2004), and eventually opening of the mitochondrial permeability transition pore with cytochrome *c* release, apoptosis or necrosis (Di Lisa and Bernardi 2006). Interestingly, in the presence of NO, produced enzymatically or directly *via* the reduction of bulk nitrite, as during hypoxia (Zweier et al. 1999), the inhibition of Complex I and Complex IV may become cytoprotective (Moncada and Erusalimsky 2002; Keynes and Garthwaite 2004). Under transient ischemic conditions, in fact, the controlled inhibition of Complex I by decreasing ROS generation decreases the mitochondrial reperfusion damage and cell oxidative injury (Dezfulian et al. 2009). On the other hand, if the OXPHOS inhibition by NO persists, then the lowered ATP synthesis will become predominant, leading to cell damage.

Fig. 4.1 *Scheme illustrating the interaction of mitochondrial respiratory chain complexes with nitric oxide.* Unequivocal evidence has been collected showing that NO reacts with Complex I and IV with important patho-physiological consequences. The reaction with Complex III has been also demonstrated, but its relevance needs to be further substantiated. NO is produced *in situ* by the cell NOS isoforms or, particularly under hypoxic conditions, by the direct or the enzymatic reduction of nitrite

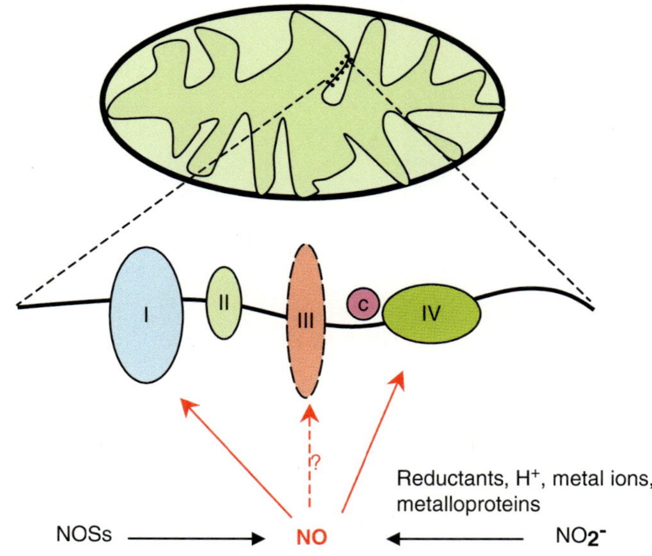

4.2 The Reactions of Nitric Oxide with Complex I and Complex IV

Complex I and IV react with NO according to different mechanisms, the former being targeted at the level of crucial thiol residues exposed during turnover and the latter at the catalytic (heme a_3-Cu_B) binuclear site.

4.2.1 *Nitric Oxide and Complex I*

Mitochondrial Complex I (NADH-ubiquinone oxidoreductase) is a 46 subunit enzyme, responsible for the NADH oxidation and reduction of the ubiquinone at the electron entry site of the respiratory chain (Vinogradov 1998). Likewise Complex IV (see below), Complex I is inhibited by NO (Stuehr and Nathan 1989; Clementi et al. 1998; Brown and Cooper 1994, Fig. 4.1). The functional implication of the reaction is different for these two respiratory complexes, owing to involvement of different reaction mechanisms. Inhibition of complex IV occurs at nanomolar NO concentrations, is rapid and reversible, whereas inhibition of complex I is more persistent and occurs after a prolonged exposure to higher NO concentration (Clementi et al. 1998). In the presence of NO, artificially produced by the donor mole-cule   (Z)-1-[N-(2-aminoethyl)-N-(2-ammonioethyl)amino]diazen-1-ium-1,2-diolate   (DETA-NO), Complex I in mitochondria or cells is inhibited *via* S-nitrosation of critical thiol residues, the inhibition being reverted by the thiol-reducing agent dithiothreitol (DTT) or by exposing the inhibited enzyme to the light (Borutaite et al. 2000); both treatments lead to destabilization of S-nitrosothiols.

The S-nitrosation of Complex I crucially depends on the structural conformation of the complex (Fig. 4.2), which in turn depends on the availability of O_2 and mitochondrial NADH (Galkin and Moncada 2007). Under hypoxic conditions and temperature above 30°C (Galkin and Moncada 2007; Galkin et al. 2009), Complex I undergoes a transition from the active (A) form to the so-called *dormant* (D) or de-activated form, also favoured by the duration of hypoxia (Vinogradov 1998). Relevant to the S-nitrosation of the complex, the cysteine residues exposed at the surface of the enzyme are different in the A and D conformation (Gavrikova and Vinogradov 1999). The A-form exposes several

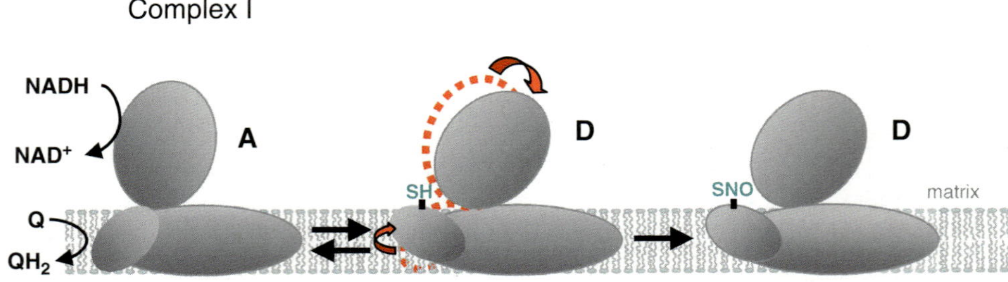

Fig. 4.2 *Schematic representation of the S-nitrosation of Complex I.* Depending on the metabolic conditions, including NADH availability and temperature, Complex I undergoes a conformational transition from the active (*A*) form to the dormant (*D*) inactive form. Number and type of cysteine residues exposed, thus accessible to S-nitrosation, depend on the A to D transition. The D form exposes Cys-39 on ND3 subunit, whose S-nitrosation causes the enzymatic reversible inhibition

(up to 10–15) cysteine residues, whose S-nitrosation or derivatization with thiol-blocking agents, such as N-ethyl maleimide (NEM), is almost ineffective (Galkin et al. 2009). Once in the D-state, the enzyme exposes on the surface of the mitochondrially-encoded ND3 subunit the residue cys 39 whose blockage fully inhibits the enzyme (Gavrikova and Vinogradov 1999, Fig. 4.2). Thus the A to D conformational change of Complex I, provides a feasible mechanistic interpretation of its inactivation by NO observed in turnover and under conditions favouring nitrosative stress, such as during hypoxia.

This attracting hypothesis has been tested recently by experiments designed to measure the rate of respiration in human epithelial kidney cells (HEK293), where the A to D transition of Complex I was induced by exposing the cells to hypoxia for different periods of time (Galkin et al. 2009). In the presence of NO endogenously released, and consistent with the accumulation of the D conformer able to react with NO, the rate of oxygen consumption after ischemia and re-oxygenation of the cells was found to be lower than that measured before anaerobiosis; moreover the extent of Complex I inhibition was proportional to the duration of the anaerobic phase as expected based on the accumulation of the D form under these conditions (Galkin et al. 2009).

It is important to notice that, under circumstances such as tissue re-oxygenation following hypoxia, the severe inhibition of the S-nitrosated Complex I, rather than detrimental, may be protective for the cells. Stabilization of the nitroso-derivative of the D form during hypoxia indeed contributes to prevent the accumulation of reducing equivalents in the respiratory chain and consequent downhill ROS production following re-oxygenation (Zweier et al. 1999).

Thus, similarly to complex IV (see below), also Complex I upon reacting with NO may trigger cell physiological or pathological events (Brown and Cooper 1994; Cleeter et al. 1994; Clementi et al. 1998; Hess et al. 2005).

4.2.2 *Nitric Oxide and Complex IV*

In 1990 Carr and Ferguson (1990) showed that NO, catalytically produced by the *Paracoccus denitrificans* nitrite reductase, was able to inhibit O_2 consumption of beef heart mitochondrial particles. The same Authors proposed that the target of NO inhibition was cytochrome *c* oxidase (CcOX), a suggestion which was confirmed a few years later by several groups (Bolanos et al. 1994; Brown and Cooper 1994; Cleeter et al. 1994; Schweizer and Richter 1994). NO was shown to inhibit the enzyme potently (low K_i), rapidly, in competition with O_2 and, importantly, in a reversible manner. Inhibition of CcOX by NO is very efficient, with an apparent inhibition constant whose value increases with $[O_2]$ and is in favour of NO over O_2 by a factor of at least 50 (Brown and Cooper 1994; Torres et al. 1995): as an example, 60 nM NO reportedly causes half inhibition of synaptosomal respiration at 30 μM O_2 (Brown and Cooper 1994). As proved by stopped-flow spectroscopy, the onset of CcOX inhibition by NO is fast, occurring within milliseconds even in the presence of a large excess of O_2 (Giuffrè et al. 1996): a result quite unexpected given that O_2 and NO bind to the fully reduced active site of CcOX with similar rate constants. Another important feature of the inhibition of CcOX by NO is that it is reversible. NO-inhibited CcOX recovers its activity spontaneously under aerobic conditions, as NO is slowly but progressively degraded by the excess of O_2 in solution. Reversal of inhibition is enhanced if NO in solution is rapidly scavenged, for example by addition of oxyhemoglobin, or by specifically inhibiting the cell NOSs (Brown et al. 1995; Sarti et al. 2000).

Given the involvement of NO as a signalling molecule in many patho-physiological processes, a large number of investigations on the reactions of NO with CcOX were carried out (reviewed in Cooper and Giulivi 2007; Cooper 2002; Sarti et al. 2003; Brunori et al. 2004, 2006) showing that the NO inhibition of the enzyme can occur at all integration levels ranging from the isolated enzyme, to mitochondria, cells and tissues (Bolanos et al. 1994; Brown and Cooper 1994; Cleeter et al. 1994; Schweizer and Richter 1994; Brown et al. 1995; Borutaite and Brown 1996; Clementi et al. 1999; Sarti et al. 1999; Shen et al. 1995; Hare et al. 1995; Xie et al. 1996; Zhao et al. 1999; Shiva et al. 2001).

Over the last two decades, several studies have been designed aimed at unravelling the mechanism for CcOX inhibition by NO.

4.2.2.1 The 'Nitrosyl' Pathway

As mentioned above the reaction of NO with CcOX involves the catalytic metals in the active site of the enzyme. Cytochrome oxidase contains four redox centers, Cu_A, heme a, heme a_3 and Cu_B. The bimetallic Cu_A site accepts one electron from reduced cytochrome c and in turn rapidly reduces intramolecularly heme a, a bis-histidine low-spin heme buried within the membrane-embedded part of the enzyme. From heme a electrons are transferred intramolecularly to the active site, the binuclear heme a_3-Cu_B center, where O_2 and other gaseous ligands (CO and NO) bind. The heme a_3-Cu_B center can accept up to two electrons; thereby it can exist in a fully oxidized (**O**), in a single-electron reduced (**E**) and in a two-electron reduced (**R**) state (Fig. 4.3).

NO binds to R at a rate ($k = 0.4-1 \times 10^8$ $M^{-1}s^{-1}$, Gibson and Greenwood 1963; Blackmore et al. 1991) similar to that of O_2, yielding a high affinity Fe^{2+} nitrosyl adduct (Fig. 4.3) with a characteristic UV/vis absorption spectrum. A first important consequence of these features is that all conditions favoring the electron donation to the catalytic site of CcOX also favor CcOX nitrosylation, indeed in the presence of NO. Mitochondrial CcOX cannot reduce the NO bound at reduced heme a_3 to N_2O (Stubauer et al. 1998), whereas a few bacterial cytochrome c oxidases were shown to be endowed with a slow, but measurable NO-reductase activity (Giuffrè et al. 1999; Forte et al. 2001), whose existence was interpreted in view of the common phylogenesis between heme-copper oxidases and bacterial heme b_3-containing NO reductases.

The dissociation of NO from the reduced heme a_3 of CcOX, as measured by Sarti et al. (2000), is relatively slow ($k_{off} = 3.9 \times 10^{-3}$ s^{-1} at 20°C), but unexpectedly high compared, for example, to haemoglobin ($k_{off} \approx 10^{-4}$ to 10^{-5} s^{-1} at 20°C). The nitrosyl adduct is photosensitive and the apparent k_{off} for NO increases therefore substantially under illumination (Fig. 4.3): this property has been widely used by Sarti and co-workers in studies where the light-induced NO displacement from CcOX and the recovery rate of respiration was explored under different experimental conditions to gain insight into the mechanism of NO inhibition of CcOX (see below Sect. 4.2.2.3). R can also react with O_2, thus CcOX

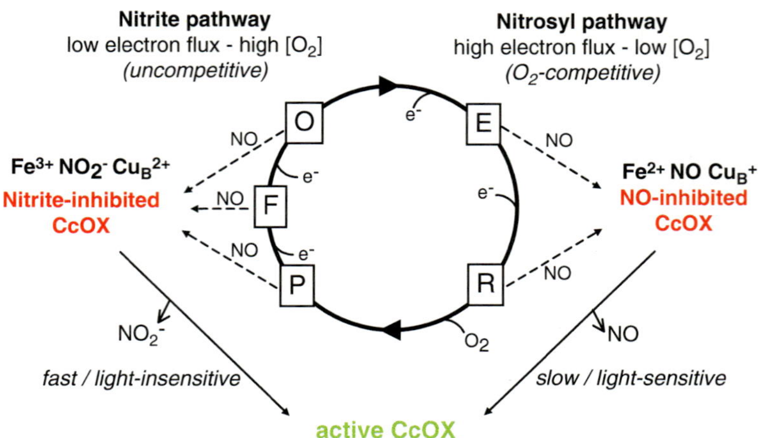

Fig. 4.3 *The catalytic cycle of cytochrome oxidase and the double mechanism of inhibition by NO.* For simplicity, the scheme highlights only the redox (e^-) and NO-ligation state of the heme a_3-Cu_B active site of CcOX. In a catalytic cycle*, the fully oxidised species **O** is fully reduced to **R**, by two single-electron donations, thus *via* formation of the so called (half-reduced) intermediate **E**. The **R** species reacts with O_2, forming in sequence **P** (peroxy) and **F** (ferryl), regenerating eventually **O**. Evidence has been collected suggesting that the partially or fully reduced intermediates bind NO to give a ferrous nitrosyl derivative, the so-called nitrosyl-adduct, whereas **O**, **P** and **F** yield a nitrite-adduct of the oxidized heme a_3
* For the definition of the redox state of the intermediate species **O**, **E**, **R**, **P** and **F** see Sects. 4.2.2.1 and 4.2.2.2

inhibition by NO is expected to be competitive with respect to O_2 when it proceeds *via* formation of a nitrosyl adduct of the enzyme. Under these conditions, the inhibition reverts upon exposing the enzyme to O_2 and the rate of activity recovery matches that one of NO dissociation from reduced heme a_3. The reversal of inhibition has been proposed (Pearce et al. 2002) to involve formation of superoxide (O_2^-) produced by reaction of O_2 with reduced Cu_B reacting, in turn, with the NO molecule bound to heme a_3, to yield peroxynitrite ($ONOO^-$). According to this hypothesis, the peroxynitrite formed at the active site would be rapidly reduced to nitrite, and eventually released as such in the bulk. Although intriguing, a more recent study disproved this mechanism, showing that recovery of CcOX activity simply results from O_2-mediated displacement of NO bound to reduced heme a_3 (Giuffrè et al. 2005, Fig. 4.3). The NO dissociation from the nitrosyl adduct is a fairly slow process for mitochondrial CcOX (minutes at 37°C in the dark, as *in vivo*); interestingly, the same process is much faster in the Cu-lacking cytochrome *bd* oxidase from *E. coli* (Borisov et al. 2004; Borisov et al. 2007) pointing to a role of Cu_B in this reaction. It is worth mentioning that the remarkably higher dissociation rate measured for this bacterial enzyme possibly represents a defense mechanism that ensures a higher resistance of bacterial respiration to nitrosative stress (Borisov et al. 2007; Mason et al. 2009a).

While O_2 and CO binding requires the complete reduction of the binuclear active site, NO has been suggested (Torres et al. 1995; Giuffrè et al. 1996) to combine also with the single-electron reduced (**E**) site, in which the electron resides either on heme a_3 or on Cu_B (Fig. 4.3). If this was the case, then the kinetic efficiency of NO in competing with O_2 may be more easily accounted for, as shown previously by performing kinetic model simulations (Giuffrè et al. 1996). Giuffrè et al. (2002) reported an experiment on a mutant (K354M) of the *Paracoccus denitrificans* cytochrome oxidase which indeed supports the contention that NO can bind rapidly to Fe^{2+} in the single-electron reduced binuclear site. However the issue is debated since others proposed that (i) the reaction of NO with **E** occurs at Cu_B^+, and not at ferrous heme a_3 (Torres et al. 1995) and (ii) the reaction with **E** is unnecessary to account for steady-state data (Mason et al. 2006; Cooper et al. 2008).

4.2.2.2 The 'Nitrite' Pathway

Beyond binding to reduced heme a_3, NO can also be oxidized by reacting with the fully oxidized **O** binuclear site of CcOX (Cooper et al. 1997; Giuffrè et al. 1998) or with the same site in catalytic intermediates (**P** and **F**) generated during reaction of the enzyme with O_2 (Torres et al. 1998; Giuffrè et al. 2000, Fig. 4.3). In all cases, by reacting with CcOX, NO is oxidized to nitrite (NO_2^-). O_2 rapidly combines with reduced heme a_3 of species **R** yielding the so-called compound **A**, in which O_2 is complexed to Fe^{2+}. Compound **A** is short-lived, due to very fast delivery of electrons to bound O_2. The resulting intermediate (**P**) was initially assigned to a peroxy-complex with oxidized heme a_3 and Cu_B, though now-a-days there is consensus on the idea that **P** is a ferryl-oxo adduct of heme a_3 ($Fe^{4+}=O$) (Weng and Baker 1991; Babcock 1999; Fabian et al. 1999), with the O-O bond already cleaved off. **P** in turn converts to the **F** intermediate, that is also a ferryl-oxo adduct of heme a_3, which eventually converts to the fully oxidized state **O** upon arrival of one more electron from Cu_A/heme a.

In the early 1980s, NO was reported to bind Cu_B in the fully oxidized (**O**) CcOX very slowly (Brudvig et al. 1980). Those experiments were performed on the so-called *resting* form of the enzyme that displays markedly different redox and ligand binding properties compared to the so-called *pulsed* enzyme discovered by Antonini et al. (1977). The *pulsed* state of CcOX is generated immediately after exposing the fully reduced *resting* enzyme to O_2, thus representing the CcOX species populated during turnover. The reactivity of the fully oxidized enzyme with NO was clarified by Cooper et al. (1997). Using a *pulsed* (*fast*) preparation of CcOX, these authors found that NO reacts much more rapidly than with the *resting* enzyme. With the *pulsed* enzyme NO reacts at Cu_B injecting one electron at the level of this redox site that rapidly equilibrates intramolecularly, and by reverse electron transfer, with heme a (Cooper et al. 1997). As a result, NO is oxidized to nitrosonium ion (NO^+) that in turn is subsequently hydroxylated (or hydrated) to nitrite (or nitrous acid). The enzyme displays eventually nitrite bound to ferric heme a_3, which accounts for inhibition. Later on, Giuffrè et al. (1998) confirmed those findings and showed that the rapid reaction of oxidized Cu_B with NO follows second-order kinetics ($k = 2 \times 10^5$ $M^{-1} s^{-1}$ at 20°C) and does not occur with the enzyme as prepared, due to chloride bound at the oxidized binuclear site. The pulsing process of oxidase, as performed in the experiments reported by Cooper et al. (1997), removes chloride from the enzyme, thereby allowing fast reaction with NO. In agreement with the proposal that NO has a peculiar reactivity towards oxidized Cu_B, recent evidence was provided that the **O** species of *E. coli* cytochrome *bd*, which lacks Cu_B, reacts with NO much more slowly ($k = 1.5 \times 10^2$ $M^{-1} s^{-1}$ at 20°C) than mitochondrial CcOX and does not lead to nitrite formation (Borisov et al. 2009).

An interesting point emerging from these findings is that the reaction of NO with Cu_B in the **O** species of CcOX leads to *in situ* formation of NO_2^- that eventually binds to the (nearby) oxidized heme a_3 with formation of a nitrite-complex. This species is optically undistinguishable from the one obtained by addition of a large excess (>mM) of nitrite to the oxidized enzyme. The NO_2^- adduct of CcOX is inhibited in standard cytochrome *c* oxidation assays. However, the affinity of nitrite for oxidized heme a_3 is much greater than for the reduced heme a_3. Accordingly, nitrite dissociation from the oxidized enzyme is very slow ($t_{1/2} \sim 80$ min at room temperature) but, upon reduction of the active site, nitrite dissociation and consequent activity restoration occur promptly (Giuffrè et al. 2000; Torres et al. 2000). Relevant for the discussion about the pathways of CcOX inhibition by NO, nitrite dissociation upon reduction of heme a_3 ($k \sim 6 \times 10^{-2}$ s^{-1} at pH = 7.3, T = 20°C (Giuffrè et al. 2000)) is also one order of magnitude faster than NO-dissociation from the same site in the reduced state. The markedly different dissociation rates displayed by nitrite and NO from the relative CcOX adducts were indeed widely used to extract information on the inhibition pathway operating under different experimental conditions, particularly at more integrated levels, as in mitochondria and cells (Mastronicola et al. 2003).

Recently, evidence was provided in favour of a nitrite reductase activity of CcOX (Castello et al. 2006, 2008; Poyton et al. 2009). According to these studies, initially carried out on yeast mitochondria and then extended also to mitochondria from human endothelial cells, under acidic conditions and at low O_2 tension, CcOX is able to reduce nitrite to NO. Such a nitrite-reductase activity has been suggested to play a pivotal role in hypoxic cell signalling. Interestingly, even cardiolipin-bound cytochrome c can effectively reduce nitrite to NO under anoxic acidic conditions (Basu et al. 2008), that is under conditions where the cytochrome heme iron becomes pentacoordinated.

Additional experiments supporting the 'nitrite' inhibition pathway of CcOX were reported by Torres et al. (1998) and Giuffrè et al. (2000). These authors established that a fairly rapid reaction of NO with CcOX occurs not only with **O** (if devoid of chloride), but also with intermediates **P** and **F**. With these intermediates the NO reaction is slower than with the **O** species ($k \sim 10^4$ $M^{-1}s^{-1}$ vs $k = 2 \times 10^5$ $M^{-1}s^{-1}$ at 20°C), still leading to nitrite-inhibited CcOX. As for the **O** species (Cooper et al. 1997; Giuffrè et al. 1998), also in the case of intermediates **P** and **F** NO was assumed to react at Cu_B^{2+} (Torres et al. 1998; Giuffrè et al. 2000); however, a similar fast reaction of NO was reported with the intermediate **F** of the *Azotobacter vinelandii* cytochrome *bd* oxidase, which lacks Cu_B (Borisov et al. 2006). It is thus possible that NO reacts with ferryl-oxo heme a_3 of CcOX directly, as reported for myoglobin (Mb) and haemoglobin, without involving Cu_B. Notably, the rate for the reaction of NO with **O**, **P** and **F** is much slower ($>10^3$ fold) than that for NO binding to the reduced binuclear center; nevertheless, as pointed out below, this intrinsic reactivity should be confronted with the relative population of the different CcOX O_2-intermediates at the steady-state (Giuffrè et al. 2000), as imposed by the different mitochondrial metabolic state.

Thus, based on solid theoretical (Mason et al. 2006; Cooper et al. 2008; Antunes et al. 2007) and experimental evidence (Sarti et al. 2000; Brunori et al. 2006; Mason et al. 2006), CcOX can be inhibited according to two different mechanisms: a first reaction pathway yields the nitrosyl NO-bound enzyme and a second one produces nitrite-bound CcOX. A scheme depicting the two pathways is shown in Fig. 4.3: on the left side the reactions of NO with the intermediates **O**, **P** and **F**, yielding nitrite-inhibited enzyme, are detailed; on the right side, the reactions of NO with reduced heme a_3, occurring at the binuclear center in the fully, R, or partially, E, reduced state are shown. Both pathways lead to reversible inhibition of the enzyme, and CcOX can restore its activity by dissociating either NO from ferrous heme a_3, the process being slow and light-sensitive, or nitrite from ferric heme a_3, the process being more rapid and light-insensitive. As outlined above, if the 'nitrosyl' pathway is in action, inhibition is expected to be competitive with respect to O_2, because intermediate **R** is reactive towards both O_2 and NO. On the other hand, O_2-competition is not expected for the 'nitrite' pathway, as it results from the reaction of NO with CcOX intermediates (**O**, **P** and **F**) that are unreactive towards O_2.

Overall the information above paves the way to some interesting questions. What is the mechanism of CcOX inhibition by NO under turnover conditions, and particularly *in situ*? Does CcOX metabolize NO to a significant extent in the cell? What are the physiological effects of the interaction of CcOX with NO?

4.2.2.3 Evidence for the Coexistence of Two Pathways for Complex IV Inhibition

As outlined above, a distinctive feature between the two pathways is that while the slow reversal of inhibition from nitrosyl CcOX is expected to be influenced by light, activity recovery should be faster and light-insensitive when the inhibition proceeds *via* formation of the nitrite-bound enzyme. This prompted Sarti and co-workers (Sarti et al. 2000; Mastronicola et al. 2003) to investigate under a variety of experimental conditions the effect of a bright white illumination on the rate of activity recovery of CcOX from NO inhibition, after scavenging NO in solution with oxyhemoglobin. Experiments of this kind were performed at different enzyme integration levels, from isolated CcOX up to intact cells (Mastronicola et al. 2003). In those experiments, the parameter systematically varied was the so-called 'reductive pressure' on CcOX, critically affecting the electron flux through the enzyme. This parameter was controlled by selectively increasing the fraction of reduced cytochrome c upon addition of tetramethyl-p-phenylendiamine (TMPD) and excess ascorbate.

The major result of these studies was that, under conditions of low electron flux and high $[O_2]$, the 'nitrite' inhibition pathway prevails, whereas as the electron flux is increased, and the O_2 concentration reduced, the O_2-competitive 'nitrosyl' pathway tends to take over (Sarti et al. 2000; Mastronicola et al. 2003). These results were confirmed and extended in subsequent studies performed in different laboratories. Working with purified CcOX, Mason et al. (2006) determined the apparent IC_{50} for NO inhibition as a function of both the O_2 concentration and the turnover number of the enzyme. Their results support our original view that both inhibition mechanisms may occur (Sarti et al. 2000). In addition, the reported data confirm that the pathway of inhibition depends on the CcOX turnover number, with the uncompetitive 'nitrite' pathway prevailing at low electron flux and the O_2-competitive 'nitrosyl' pathway being predominant at higher electron flux (Sarti et al. 2000). Mathematical models (Cooper et al. 2008; Antunes et al. 2007) further confirmed that experimental data on CcOX inhibition by NO can be simulated only if both the competitive and uncompetitive pathways are operative, with the latter prevailing at lower electron flux and higher $[O_2]$. The whole picture seems compatible with simulations reported by our group (Giuffrè et al. 2000) showing that, at low electron flux, the overall occupancy of intermediates **O**, **P** and **F** at steady-state should increase, thereby favouring the 'nitrite' pathway under these conditions. On the other hand, in a recent report Mason et al. (2009b) failed to detect intermediates **P** and **F** at measurable levels by optically investigating CcOX intermediates at steady-state.

A point of interest is to unveil which one of the two inhibition pathways predominates when CcOX is in turnover in intact cells respiring on endogenous substrates and the enzyme encounters NO. Working with SH-SY5Y neuroblastoma cells, Mastronicola et al. (2003) found that, if the electron flux through CcOX is not artificially enhanced by TMPD, the 'nitrite' pathways is predominant at high $[O_2]$ (>100 μM), which implies that under these 'basal' conditions CcOX may provide a catabolic route for NO. Experimental evidence consistent with this view has been more recently provided in an elegant study carried out by Palacios-Callender et al. (2007a). In this work, the authors investigated the fate of NO and the redox state of CcOX in human embryonic kidney cells (engineered to generate controlled amounts of endogenous NO) while respiring toward hypoxia. Interestingly, they found that CcOX, while in turnover, metabolizes NO to nitrite, but as the cells approach hypoxic conditions, the enzyme becomes more reduced and its ability to consume NO diminishes. It is also relevant to outline that in experiments of this kind endogenous NO causes partial inhibition of CcOX, detected as an increased reduction level of the enzyme: interestingly, this occurs without affecting cell respiration, unless $[O_2]$ becomes limiting (Palacios-Callender et al. 2007a, b). This phenomenon has been related to an increase in the reduction level of c-type cytochromes that occurs in response to partial inhibition of CcOX. These redox changes tend to compensate the inhibition of CcOX, thereby maintaining essentially unvaried the velocity of O_2 consumption. This is an example of the 'cushioning' effect described more than 40 years ago by Britton Chance (1965). An important consequence of this effect is that partial inhibition of CcOX, *without inhibition of respiration*, can result into higher reduction levels of the components of the mitochondrial electron transport chain; a condition that has been suggested to trigger superoxide and, in turn, hydrogen peroxide production which is eventually implicated in cell signalling (Palacios-Callender et al. 2004).

In summary, the issue of inhibition of CcOX by NO may be summarized as follows. The O_2-competitive inhibition pathway that occurs *via* reaction of reduced heme a_3 with NO prevails under conditions of high electron flux, i.e. high reductive supply, and low O_2 concentrations; that is under condition in which the relative occupancy of **R** (and **E**) tends to increase, although in absolute terms **R** should be only poorly populated at steady-state given its reactivity towards O_2. An independent evidence supporting this conclusion has been more recently provided using intact human cells (Masci et al. 2008). On the other hand under conditions of low electron flux and high O_2 concentrations, the inhibition proceeds *via* reaction of NO with the intermediates **O**, **P** and **F** and formation of the nitrite-adduct of CcOX prevails (Fig. 4.3).

4.3 The Metabolic Role of Nitrite in the Mitochondria

Ambiguity about the bioenergetic implications of the mitochondrial NO chemistry mostly resides in the insufficient information about the metabolic pathways activated by the inhibition of the respiratory complexes I and IV. Like during hypoxia, following NO inhibition of respiration, the aerobic ATP synthesis (OXPHOS) is depressed and glycolysis takes place, but this is not the only and probably the major effect observed (Moncada and Erusalimsky 2002, Fig. 4.4). By stimulating the cGMP production, NO induces an increase of blood flow, directly *via* vasodilatation as well indirectly through activation of neo-angiogenesis (Keynes and Garthwaite 2004 and ref therein); consequently the aerobic bioenergetic depression induced in a tissue by limited, in extent and time, NO pulses is only transient, and can be even followed by an improved oxygenation capacity. In addition NO acts as a very efficient radical scavenger, though disposal of the reaction end-product (for instance peroxynitrite) may represent a cell metabolic problem. Overall the bioavailability of NO at all levels, included the mitochondrial one, is vital and relies on the efficiency of the NO releasing systems in the cell. When oxygen tension decreases in tissues, the ability of the NOSs to generate NO is compromised by the lack of the oxygen substrate; under these conditions, the anoxic environment promotes tissue acidification, favouring in turn the reduction of nitrite to NO (16). Thus, besides the role played by the NOSs, and particularly under hypoxic conditions, the tissue/cell distribution of nitrite becomes central with respect to the NO chemistry. Nitrite is not a mere inert oxidation product of NO, waiting for further oxidation to nitrate and produced directly by oxygen or catalytically (see below). In cells and tissues nitrite represents a source of NO to be utilized upon requirement (Lundberg et al. 2008; Shiva and Gladwin 2009). The concentration of nitrite in human plasma is approximately 200 nM (Lundberg et al. 2008; Stamler et al. 1992; Gladwin et al. 2000). In cell and tissues, NO_2^- can be reduced to NO, enzymatically (Lundberg et al. 2008) or by acidic disproportionation (Zweier et al. 1999; Weitzberg and Lundberg 1998), as during ischemia. Consistently, in rodents, during focal ischemia, it was found that plasma, brain and heart were depleted of nitrite, whose physiological concentration could be promptly restored by intravenous administration preventing the effects of ischemia (Bryan et al. 2007; Dezfulian et al. 2009; Shiva et al. 2007a).

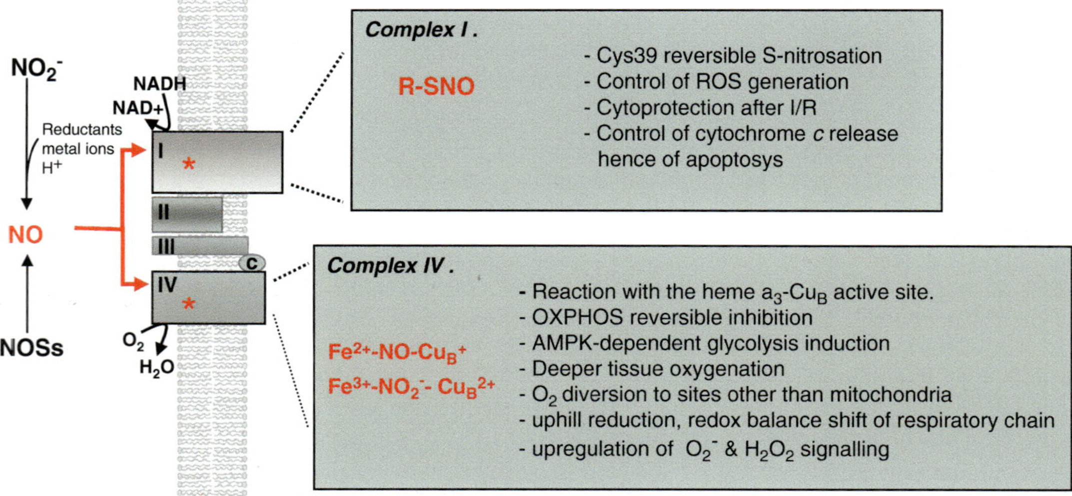

Fig. 4.4 Features and implications of the reaction of NO with mitochondrial complex I and IV The scheme summarizes the chemical targets and major cytoprotective or detrimental effects of the interaction of NO with the mitochondrial respiratory chain Complexes I and IV. I/R = Ischemia and Reperfustion

Interestingly, low doses of nitrite (~50 nM) administered to ischemic, heart-arrested mice, early during cardiopulmonary resuscitation, was shown to restore nitrite levels to near baseline, to increase the concentration of cardiac S-nitrosothiols and, most importantly, to significantly improve survival of the treated animals compared to controls (Webb et al. 2004).

4.3.1   Any Role for Oxymyoglobin?

Upon lowering oxygen, oxymyoglobin undergoes the transition to the deoxy form that promptly reacts with nitrite, generating NO (Hendgen-Cotta et al. 2008). Experiments carried out with cardiomyocites have shown that the nitrite-reductase activity of Mb can account for inhibition of complex I (Hendgen-Cotta et al. 2008; Shiva et al. 2007b; Rassaf et al. 2007). The production of nitrite by Mb is a well-known reaction extensively studied *in vitro* (Shiva et al. 2007b), and *in vivo*: of particular interest are the results of experiments carried out using $Mb^{(-/-)}$ knockout mice, undergoing an I/R injury in the absence and presence of nitrite (Hendgen-Cotta et al. 2008). Interestingly, the consequences of I/R on the $Mb^{(-/-)}$ mice were more severe than in the wild-type $Mb^{(+/+)}$ animals and the damage in the knockout mice could not be alleviated by nitrite, as it could in control animals (Hendgen-Cotta et al. 2008). Consistent with a Mb-induced NO release and the ensuing inhibition of complex I and IV, in the presence of nitrite the $Mb^{(+/+)}$ mice recovered the mitochondrial respiration efficiency more slowly than $Mb^{(-/-)}$ animals. Moreover, the detectable amount of NO-modified proteins was higher in the cardiac tissue of $Mb^{(+/+)}$ mice, whereas ROS production was significantly lower showing a direct involvement of Mb in the NO release during I/R. The average myocardial infarct size was wider in $Mb^{(-/-)}$ mice (Hendgen-Cotta et al. 2008), pointing to a cytoprotective effect of the mitochondrial nitrite/NO chemistry dependent on the presence of Mb. In synthesis, the administration of nitrite to ischemic control mice enables their cardiac deoxyMb to increase the NO bioavailability at mitochondrial level in the absence of O_2.

4.4   The Impact of the Mitochondrial NO Chemistry on Cell Physiology

Although NO reacts with a large number of targets, its reaction with mitochondrial complexes is of particular interest, as it accounts for activation of a number of reactions, following the reversible inhibition of respiration observed even in the presence of excess O_2 (Fig. 4.4).

4.4.1   Nitrosation of Mitochondria and Cytoprotection

This is a vast and still controversial issue in the field of the NO chemistry; here we will attempt to summarize a few major points. In the positive view just mentioned in the above paragraph, NO by inhibiting the respiratory complex I would limit ROS generation and oxidative protein damage, with a cytoprotective effect (Hendgen-Cotta et al. 2008; Shiva and Gladwin 2009; Webb et al. 2004). Thus, along with the mitochondrial OXPHOS inhibition, a virtuous NO pathway seems to take part to the overall cell metabolism particularly of ischemic tissues (Hendgen-Cotta et al. 2008; Dezfulian et al. 2009; Prime et al. 2009). This finding points to a new pharmacological interest in the area of ischemia; in this context, a molecular approach has been developed to generate compounds able to selectively drive the NO synthesis or release in the mitochondrion from compounds, such as S-nitrosothiols (Prime et al. 2009). The S-nitroso-2-mercaptopropionyl-glicine (SNO-MPG) has been assayed in I/R cardiomyocites, and proved to enhance mitochondrial S-nitrosation, eliciting cardioprotection (Nadtochiy et al. 2007). So that, the lipophilic triphenylphosphonium cation S-nitrosated (MitoSNO1), driven by the membrane potential, rapidly accumulates into mitochondria, where it induces protein S-nitrosation (Prime et al. 2009). A positive cell response to S-nitrosation is proved by the finding that mitochondria extracted from cardiomyocytes treated with SNO-MPG exhibit improved Ca^{2+} handling and lower ROS generation (Shiva et al. 2007a). Different nitroso compounds display different specific S-nitrosating activity. A higher concentration of nitrosoglutathione (GSNO), 100 vs 20 µM, is for instance necessary to achieve the same effect of SNO-MPG, proving a higher S-nitrosating activity of the latter compound at the mitochondrion level.

4.4.2 Pathophysiological Relevance

The reaction of NO with Complex III has been described as sluggish (Poderoso et al. 1996), whereas the reactions with Complex I and Complex IV, studied in detail, presently appear to be the most promising to elucidate the bioenergetic relevance to cell pathophysiology of the mitochondrial nitrosative stress. Only for the sake of clarity the reactions of NO with Complex I and IV have been treated separately since the *in vivo* effects of the reactions and their relative contribution to human pathophysiology are still poorly understood. A few important features, however, appear nowadays validated: based on several reports, from different groups and using different biological systems (Galkin and Moncada 2007; Cooper et al. 2008), it was shown that (i) the principal NO target on the complexes is different, i.e. the R-SH group on complex I and the binuclear active site on complex IV and, most importantly, that (ii) the kinetics of the reaction is very fast (milliseconds) for complex IV and rather slow (tens of minutes to hours) for complex I. These features, together with a fairly high NO dissociation rate from the reduced CcOX ($k_{off} = 3.9 \times 10^{-3}$ s^{-1}, at 20°C), point to a control-like function of the NO reaction at the level of Complex IV more than to a simple respiratory chain inhibition. The most evident and measurable effect of such interaction would be the ~10 fold increase of the apparent $K_{M,O2}$ measured in cells and tissues compared to CcOX in solution, i.e. ~5.0 µM *vs* ~0.5 µM (Brunori et al. 1999 and references therein). On the other hand, owing to its properties (Sect. 4.2), the reaction of NO with complex I inducing on a longer time scale a fairly stable S-nitrosation may lead to a more severe loss of function, at least in the absence of metabolites able to weaken the R-SNO bonds. Particularly for this reason it has been proposed that Complex I takes part into pathological pathways leading to chronic neurodegenerative disorders, such as Parkinson's and Huntington's diseases (Schapira 1998, 2010; Jenkins 1993; Dawson and Dawson 2003).

More complex appears the gathering of information about the pathophysiological relevance, if any, of the reaction of NO with complex IV. Since originally observed with purified CcOX in the presence of reducing substrates and O_2 (Sarti et al. 2000) and later on confirmed (Cooper 2002; Mason et al. 2006), different adducts (NO- or NO_2^--bound) are formed, depending on the electron flux level within the enzyme. As reported above, these adducts accumulate respectively at high and low concentrations of reducing equivalents, i.e. reduced cytochrome *c in situ.* (Mastronicola et al. 2003; Masci et al. 2008). This behavior has been observed by artificially modulating the fraction of reduced cytochrome *c* interacting with CcOX in the presence of NO (Mastronicola et al. 2003) and, more recently confirmed in human lymphoid cells expressing different amounts of cytochrome *c* (Masci et al. 2008, Fig. 4.5).

Any impact on cell physiology? Interestingly from the mitochondrial functional point of view the clearance of the NO-adduct is slower than that of the NO_2 – adduct, thus probably different physiological and pathological implications can be envisaged (see Cooper and Giulivi 2007; Moncada and Erusalimsky 2002; Shiva et al. 2005; Blandini et al. 2004; Erusalimsky and Moncada 2007).

A first consideration is that depending on the fraction of the NO-inhibited respiratory chain, the O_2 consumption and thereby the OXPHOS dependent synthesis of ATP may decrease. Under state

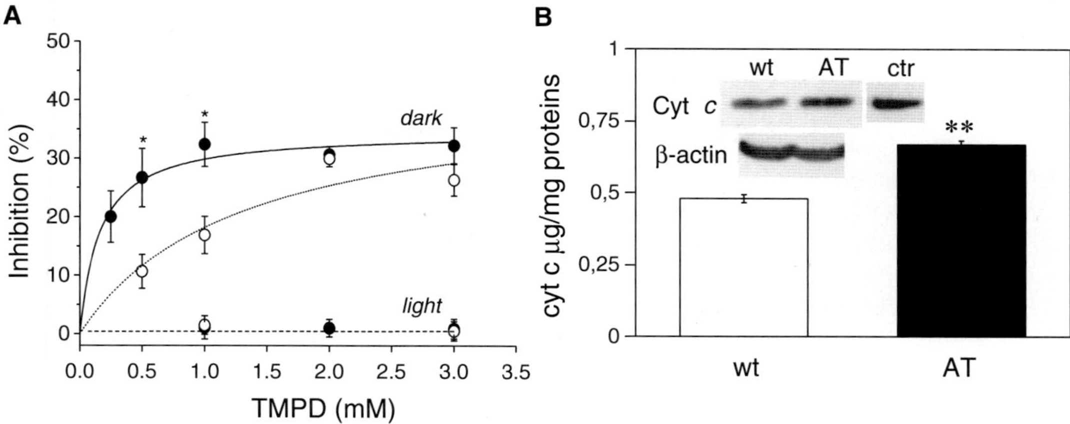

Fig. 4.5 *NO inhibition of respiration in lymphoid cells expressing different amounts of Cytochrome c.* Panel A – Residual inhibition of cell respiration by NO. Measurements have been carried out according to the protocol described in (Masci et al. 2008), i.e. in the dark to stabilize the Fe^{2+}NO-CcOX formed in the presence NO and after scavenging excess NO with hemoglobin. Upon increasing the concentration of TMPD the reduction of CcOX, thus formation of E and R species (see Sect. 4.2.2.1) is facilitated together with its nitrosylation by NO, evidently more in Ataxia Telangiectasia (●) cells than in wild type controls (○). *Light*, by destabilising the Fe^{2+}-NO bond, fully abolishes CcOX inhibition. Panel B – Immuno detection of cytochrome c in cell lysates of wild type (*wt*), and Ataxia Telangiectasia lymphoid cells (*AT*) (Modified from Masci et al. 2008)

III conditions, when $\Delta\mu_{H+}$ is used to synthesize ATP, in the presence of free NO, complex IV was found to be inhibited to a higher extent than in state IV when the electrochemical potential gradient ($\Delta\mu_{H+}$) is maximal and turnover rate minimal (Borutaite and Brown 1996; Brookes et al. 2003). If our model applies, in state III the reduced CcOX intermediates (**E, R**) are expected to be more populated than in state IV.

A second consideration is that the NO inhibition of mitochondrial O_2 consumption, when occurring, obviously results into an increase of O_2 bioavailability in the surrounding. In this respect, the NO control of mitochondrial respiration might play an important physiological role in the microcirculation network, particularly for the cells located at the boundary of capillaries. For those cells, the reduced O_2 consumption induced by NO, released at this level by the endothelial NOS, would indeed favor a deeper tissue oxygenation (Brunori et al. 2006; Poderoso et al. 1996; Thomas et al. 2001; Giulivi 2003); furthermore, this effect would synergize with the vasodilatation properties of NO, leading to a more penetrating tissue oxygenation. Further in detail, upon inhibition of CcOX by NO, a condition termed "metabolic hypoxia" is set (Moncada and Erusalimsky 2002), whereby O_2 is less used at the level of the mitochondrial respiratory chain, and becomes available for other enzymatic functions. An intriguing example of such a NO-dependent O_2 diversion from mitochondrial OXPHOS is the octapamine-dependent control of the firefly flashing: the octapamine activates the NO synthesis and thus causes the NO inhibition of cell respiration, that in turn renders O_2 more available for the light-producing luciferin-luciferase reaction (Trimmer et al. 2001).

The inactivation of the hypoxya-inducible factor (HIF, Hagen et al. 2003) pathway is another interesting example of O_2 diversion in response to NO inhibition of respiration. The HIF pathway is, indeed, inactivated by a family of prolyl hydroxylases which in an O_2-dependent manner target the HIF1α subunit for ubiquitination and degradation: an [O_2] increase elicited by NO would, therefore, lead to inactivation of the HIF pathway.

A third consideration is that mitochondria are the cell sites where important reactive signaling molecules are produced (Moncada and Erusalimsky 2002; Brookes and Darley-Usmar 2002; Brookes et al. 2002; Foster et al. 2006). In this respect it is worth recalling that the NO-inhibition of CcOX induces the accumulation of reducing equivalents upstream in the respiratory chain, and leads to an enhanced production of superoxide anion (O_2^-), eventually converted to H_2O_2 by the superoxide dismutase. Therefore, the NO-dependent modulation of complex IV might function to control the production of mitochondrial H_2O_2, an important redox-signaling molecule (Brookes and Darley-Usmar 2002). On the other hand, when a more persistent NO-inhibition of CcOX occurs, the mitochondrion likely produces an excess of O_2^- that readily reacts with NO to yield highly reactive and toxic peroxynitrite ($ONOO^-$), which in turn irreversibly damages the respiratory complexes and many other cell components (Beckman et al. 1990). These circumstances induced by $ONOO^-$ overproduction lead to a pathological impairment of the cell bioenergetics, a condition termed "nitroxia" (Shiva et al. 2005). A persistent nitroxia eventually causes cell death (Moncada and Erusalimsky 2002; Borutaite and Brown 2003), unless compensatory defense mechanisms are triggered, as observed in astrocytes but not in neurons (Almeida et al. 2001, 2004).

In conclusion, there are already clear indications that NO inhibition of respiration, particularly at the level of complex IV is set very rapidly, producing several effects that may turn from physiological to pathological depending on conditions and parameters still poorly defined. In this context, an interesting report on intact human lymphoid cells showed that, all else being equal, the fractional inhibition of complex IV induced by NO depends on the mitochondrial concentration of reduced cytochrome c (Masci et al. 2008): the higher its concentration, the deeper the complex inhibition (Fig. 4.5). This finding, fully consistent with previous theoretical and experimental reports (Sarti et al. 2000; Mason et al. 2006; Mastronicola et al. 2003), has provided the access to a measurable parameter linked to the susceptibility of cell mitochondria to nitrosative stress.

Unfortunately, owing to the experimental difficulties, the data about the actual cell mitochondria concentration of cytochrome c oxygen and NO are rather poor. This lack of information implies that quantification of the effect of NO chemistry on cell respiration *in vivo* as in our body is presently mostly speculative. One might assume that the interactions of NO with the respiratory complexes are *in vivo* as *simple* as they occur *in vitro*, so ignoring other reactions of paramount importance such as those involved in the activation of guanylate cyclase! As pointed out by Cooper and Giulivi (2007), if this was the case and all else being equal, one could predict that *in vivo* the consumption of O_2 by the mitochondrial respiratory chain should be higher in the presence of NOS inhibitors. Encouraging enough, this was often observed, though not always (ref in Cooper and Giulivi 2007), in several differently integrated systems, from cell cultures (Sarti et al. 1999) to tissue slices, cardiac or skeletal muscles, kidney or even whole animal body, keeping open the question of the patho-physiological relevance of the NO interaction with the respiratory chain.

Acknowledgments Work partially supported by Ministero dell'Istruzione, dell'Università e della Ricerca of Italy to P.S. (*PRIN* "Metabolismo Energetico dell'Ossigeno e del Monossido di Azoto: Fisiologia e Patologia").

References

Almeida A, Almeida J, Bolanos JP, Moncada S (2001) Different responses of astrocytes and neurons to nitric oxide: the role of glycolytically generated ATP in astrocyte protection. Proc Natl Acad Sci USA 98:15294–15299

Almeida A, Moncada S, Bolanos JP (2004) Nitric oxide switches on glycolysis through the AMP protein kinase and 6-phosphofructo-2-kinase pathway. Nat Cell Biol 6:45–51

Antonini E, Brunori M, Colosimo A, Greenwood C, Wilson MT (1977) Oxygen "pulsed" cytochrome c oxidase: functional properties and catalytic relevance. Proc Natl Acad Sci USA 74:3128–3132

Antunes F, Boveris A, Cadenas E (2007) On the biologic role of the reaction of NO with oxidized cytochrome c oxidase. Antioxid Redox Signal 9:1569–1579

Babcock GT (1999) How oxygen is activated and reduced in respiration. Proc Natl Acad Sci USA 96:12971–12973

Basu S, Azarova NA, Font MD, King SB, Hogg N, Gladwin MT, Shiva S, Kim-Shapiro DB (2008) Nitrite reductase activity of cytochrome c. J Biol Chem 283:32590–32597

Beckman JS, Beckman TW, Chen J, Marshall PA, Freeman BA (1990) Apparent hydroxyl radical production by peroxynitrite: implications for endothelial injury from nitric oxide and superoxide. Proc Natl Acad Sci USA 87:1620–1624

Blackmore RS, Greenwood C, Gibson QH (1991) Studies of the primary oxygen intermediate in the reaction of fully reduced cytochrome oxidase. J Biol Chem 266:19245–19249

Blandini F, Braunewell KH, Manahan-Vaughan D, Orzi F, Sarti P (2004) Neurodegeneration and energy metabolism: from chemistry to clinics. Cell Death Differ 11:479–484

Bolanos JP, Peuchen S, Heales SJ, Land JM, Clark JB (1994) Nitric oxide-mediated inhibition of the mitochondrial respiratory chain in cultured astrocytes. J Neurochem 63:910–916

Borisov VB, Forte E, Konstantinov AA, Poole RK, Sarti P, Giuffrè A (2004) Interaction of the bacterial terminal oxidase cytochrome bd with nitric oxide. FEBS Lett 576:201–204

Borisov VB, Forte E, Sarti P, Brunori M, Konstantinov AA, Giuffrè A (2006) Nitric oxide reacts with the ferryl-oxo catalytic intermediate of the CuB-lacking cytochrome bd terminal oxidase. FEBS Lett 580:4823–4826

Borisov VB, Forte E, Sarti P, Brunori M, Konstantinov AA, Giuffrè A (2007) Redox control of fast ligand dissociation from Escherichia coli cytochrome bd. Biochem Biophys Res Commun 355:97–102

Borisov VB, Forte E, Giuffrè A, Konstantinov A, Sarti P (2009) Reaction of nitric oxide with the oxidized di-heme and heme-copper oxygen-reducing centers of terminal oxidases: different reaction pathways and end-products. J Inorg Biochem 103:1185–1187

Borutaite V, Brown GC (1996) Rapid reduction of nitric oxide by mitochondria, and reversible inhibition of mitochondrial respiration by nitric oxide. Biochem J 315(Pt 1):295–299

Borutaite V, Brown GC (2003) Nitric oxide induces apoptosis via hydrogen peroxide, but necrosis via energy and thiol depletion. Free Radic Biol Med 35:1457–1468

Borutaite V, Budriunaite A, Brown GC (2000) Reversal of nitric oxide-, peroxynitrite- and S-nitrosothiol-induced inhibition of mitochondrial respiration or complex I activity by light and thiols. Biochim Biophys Acta 1459:405–412

Brookes P, Darley-Usmar VM (2002) Hypothesis: the mitochondrial NO(*) signaling pathway, and the transduction of nitrosative to oxidative cell signals: an alternative function for cytochrome C oxidase. Free Radic Biol Med 32:370–374

Brookes PS, Levonen AL, Shiva S, Sarti P, Darley-Usmar VM (2002) Mitochondria: regulators of signal transduction by reactive oxygen and nitrogen species. Free Radic Biol Med 33:755–764

Brookes PS, Kraus DW, Shiva S, Doeller JE, Barone MC, Patel RP, Lancaster JR Jr, Darley-Usmar V (2003) Control of mitochondrial respiration by NO*, effects of low oxygen and respiratory state. J Biol Chem 278:31603–31609

Brookes PS, Yoon Y, Robotham JL, Anders MW, Sheu SS (2004) Calcium, ATP, and ROS: a mitochondrial love-hate triangle. Am J Physiol Cell Physiol 287:C817–C833

Brown GC, Cooper CE (1994) Nanomolar concentrations of nitric oxide reversibly inhibit synaptosomal respiration by competing with oxygen at cytochrome oxidase. FEBS Lett 356:295–298

Brown GC, Bolanos JP, Heales SJ, Clark JB (1995) Nitric oxide produced by activated astrocytes rapidly and reversibly inhibits cellular respiration. Neurosci Lett 193:201–204

Brudvig GW, Stevens TH, Chan SI (1980) Reactions of nitric oxide with cytochrome *c* oxidase. Biochemistry 19:5275–5285

Brunori M, Giuffrè A, Sarti P, Stubauer G, Wilson MT (1999) Nitric oxide and cellular respiration. Cell Mol Life Sci 56:549–557

Brunori M, Giuffrè A, Forte E, Mastronicola D, Barone MC, Sarti P (2004) Control of cytochrome *c* oxidase activity by nitric oxide. Biochim Biophys Acta 1655:365–371

Brunori M, Forte E, Arese M, Mastronicola D, Giuffrè A, Sarti P (2006) Nitric oxide and the respiratory enzyme. Biochim Biophys Acta 1757:1144–1154

Bryan NS, Calvert JW, Elrod JW, Gundewar S, Ji SY, Lefer DJ (2007) Dietary nitrite supplementation protects against myocardial ischemia-reperfusion injury. Proc Natl Acad Sci USA 104:19144–19149

Carr GJ, Ferguson SJ (1990) Nitric oxide formed by nitrite reductase of Paracoccus denitrificans is sufficiently stable to inhibit cytochrome oxidase activity and is reduced by its reductase under aerobic conditions. Biochim Biophys Acta 1017:57–62

Castello PR, David PS, McClure T, Crook Z, Poyton RO (2006) Mitochondrial cytochrome oxidase produces nitric oxide under hypoxic conditions: implications for oxygen sensing and hypoxic signaling in eukaryotes. Cell Metab 3:277–287

Castello PR, Woo DK, Ball K, Wojcik J, Liu L, Poyton RO (2008) Oxygen-regulated isoforms of cytochrome c oxidase have differential effects on its nitric oxide production and on hypoxic signaling. Proc Natl Acad Sci USA 105:8203–8208

Chance B (1965) Reaction of oxygen with the respiratory chain in cells and tissues. J Gen Physiol 49(Suppl):163–195

Cleeter MW, Cooper JM, Darley-Usmar VM, Moncada S, Schapira AH (1994) Reversible inhibition of cytochrome c oxidase, the terminal enzyme of the mitochondrial respiratory chain, by nitric oxide. Implications for neurodegenerative diseases. FEBS Lett 345:50–54

Clementi E, Brown GC, Feelisch M, Moncada S (1998) Persistent inhibition of cell respiration by nitric oxide: crucial role of S-nitrosylation of mitochondrial complex I and protective action of glutathione. Proc Natl Acad Sci USA 95:7631–7636

Clementi E, Brown GC, Foxwell N, Moncada S (1999) On the mechanism by which vascular endothelial cells regulate their oxygen consumption. Proc Natl Acad Sci USA 96:1559–1562

Cooper CE (2002) Nitric oxide and cytochrome oxidase: substrate, inhibitor or effector? Trends Biochem Sci 27:33–39

Cooper CE, Giulivi C (2007) Nitric oxide regulation of mitochondrial oxygen consumption II: molecular mechanism and tissue physiology. Am J Physiol Cell Physiol 292:C1993–C2003

Cooper CE, Torres J, Sharpe MA, Wilson MT (1997) Nitric oxide ejects electrons from the binuclear centre of cytochrome c oxidase by reacting with oxidised copper: a general mechanism for the interaction of copper proteins with nitric oxide? FEBS Lett 414:281–284

Cooper CE, Mason MG, Nicholls P (2008) A dynamic model of nitric oxide inhibition of mitochondrial cytochrome c oxidase. Biochim Biophys Acta 1777:867–876

Dawson TM, Dawson VL (2003) Molecular pathways of neurodegeneration in Parkinson's disease. Science 302:819–822

Dezfulian C et al (2009) Nitrite therapy after cardiac arrest reduces reactive oxygen species generation, improves cardiac and neurological function, and enhances survival via reversible inhibition of mitochondrial complex I. Circulation 120:897–905

Di Lisa F, Bernardi P (2006) Mitochondria and ischemia-reperfusion injury of the heart: fixing a hole. Cardiovasc Res 70:191–199

Erusalimsky JD, Moncada S (2007) Nitric oxide and mitochondrial signaling: from physiology to pathophysiology. Arterioscler Thromb Vasc Biol 27:2524–2531

Fabian M, Wong WW, Gennis RB, Palmer G (1999) Mass spectrometric determination of dioxygen bond splitting in the "peroxy" intermediate of cytochrome c oxidase. Proc Natl Acad Sci USA 96:13114–13117

Forte E, Urbani A, Saraste M, Sarti P, Brunori M, Giuffrè A (2001) The cytochrome cbb3 from Pseudomonas stutzeri displays nitric oxide reductase activity. Eur J Biochem 268:6486–6491

Foster KA, Galeffi F, Gerich FJ, Turner DA, Muller M (2006) Optical and pharmacological tools to investigate the role of mitochondria during oxidative stress and neurodegeneration. Prog Neurobiol 79:136–171

Galkin A, Moncada S (2007) S-nitrosation of mitochondrial complex I depends on its structural conformation. J Biol Chem 282:37448–37453

Galkin A, Abramov AY, Frakich N, Duchen MR, Moncada S (2009) Lack of oxygen deactivates mitochondrial complex I: implications for ischemic injury? J Biol Chem 284(52):36055–36061

Gavrikova EV, Vinogradov AD (1999) Active/de-active state transition of the mitochondrial complex I as revealed by specific sulfhydryl group labeling. FEBS Lett 455:36–40

Gibson Q, Greenwood C (1963) Reactions of cytochrome oxidase with oxygen and carbon monoxide. Biochem J 86:541–555

Giuffrè A, Stubauer G, Brunori M, Sarti P, Torres J, Wilson MT (1998) Chloride bound to oxidized cytochrome c oxidase controls the reaction with nitric oxide. J Biol Chem 273:32475–32478

Giuffrè A, Stubauer G, Sarti P, Brunori M, Zumft WG, Buse G, Soulimane T (1999) The heme-copper oxidases of Thermus thermophilus catalyze the reduction of nitric oxide: evolutionary implications. Proc Natl Acad Sci USA 96:14718–14723

Giuffrè A, Barone MC, Mastronicola D, D'Itri E, Sarti P, Brunori M (2000) Reaction of nitric oxide with the turnover intermediates of cytochrome c oxidase: reaction pathway and functional effects. Biochemistry 39:15446–15453

Giuffrè A, Barone MC, Brunori M, D'Itri E, Ludwig B, Malatesta F, Muller HW, Sarti P (2002) Nitric oxide reacts with the single-electron reduced active site of cytochrome c oxidase. J Biol Chem 277:22402–22406

Giuffrè A, Forte E, Brunori M, Sarti P (2005) Nitric oxide, cytochrome c oxidase and myoglobin: competition and reaction pathways. FEBS Lett 579:2528–2532

Giuffrè A, Sarti P, D'Itri E, Buse G, Soulimane T, Brunori M (1996) On the mechanism of inhibition of cytochrome c oxidase by nitric oxide. J Biol Chem 271:33404–33408

Giulivi C (2003) Characterization and function of mitochondrial nitric-oxide synthase. Free Radic Biol Med 34:397–408

Gladwin MT, Shelhamer JH, Schechter AN, Pease-Fye ME, Waclawiw MA, Panza JA, Ognibene FP, Cannon RO 3rd (2000) Role of circulating nitrite and S-nitrosohemoglobin in the regulation of regional blood flow in humans. Proc Natl Acad Sci USA 97:11482–11487

Hagen T, Taylor CT, Lam F, Moncada S (2003) Redistribution of intracellular oxygen in hypoxia by nitric oxide: effect on HIF1alpha. Science 302:1975–1978

Hare JM, Keaney JF Jr, Balligand JL, Loscalzo J, Smith TW, Colucci WS (1995) Role of nitric oxide in parasympathetic modulation of beta-adrenergic myocardial contractility in normal dogs. J Clin Invest 95:360–366

Hendgen-Cotta UB et al (2008) Nitrite reductase activity of myoglobin regulates respiration and cellular viability in myocardial ischemia-reperfusion injury. Proc Natl Acad Sci USA 105:10256–10261

Hess DT, Matsumoto A, Kim SO, Marshall HE, Stamler JS (2005) Protein S-nitrosylation: purview and parameters. Nat Rev Mol Cell Biol 6:150–166

Jenkins RR (1993) Exercise, oxidative stress, and antioxidants: a review. Int J Sport Nutr 3:356–375

Keynes RG, Garthwaite J (2004) Nitric oxide and its role in ischaemic brain injury. Curr Mol Med 4:179–191

Lundberg JO, Weitzberg E, Gladwin MT (2008) The nitrate-nitrite-nitric oxide pathway in physiology and therapeutics. Nat Rev Drug Discov 7:156–167

Masci A, Mastronicola D, Arese M, Piane M, De Amicis A, Blanck TJ, Chessa L, Sarti P (2008) Control of cell respiration by nitric oxide in Ataxia Telangiectasia lymphoblastoid cells. Biochim Biophys Acta 1777:66–73

Mason MG, Nicholls P, Wilson MT, Cooper CE (2006) Nitric oxide inhibition of respiration involves both competitive (heme) and noncompetitive (copper) binding to cytochrome c oxidase. Proc Natl Acad Sci USA 103:708–713

Mason MG, Shepherd M, Nicholls P, Dobbin PS, Dodsworth KS, Poole RK, Cooper CE (2009a) Cytochrome bd confers nitric oxide resistance to Escherichia coli. Nat Chem Biol 5:94–96

Mason MG, Nicholls P, Cooper CE (2009b) The steady-state mechanism of cytochrome c oxidase: redox interactions between metal centres. Biochem J 422:237–246

Mastronicola D et al (2003) Control of respiration by nitric oxide in Keilin-Hartree particles, mitochondria and SH-SY5Y neuroblastoma cells. Cell Mol Life Sci 60:1752–1759

Moncada S, Erusalimsky JD (2002) Does nitric oxide modulate mitochondrial energy generation and apoptosis? Nat Rev Mol Cell Biol 3:214–220

Nadtochiy SM, Burwell LS, Brookes PS (2007) Cardioprotection and mitochondrial S-nitrosation: effects of S-nitroso-2-mercaptopropionyl glycine (SNO-MPG) in cardiac ischemia-reperfusion injury. J Mol Cell Cardiol 42:812–825

Palacios-Callender M, Quintero M, Hollis VS, Springett RJ, Moncada S (2004) Endogenous NO regulates superoxide production at low oxygen concentrations by modifying the redox state of cytochrome c oxidase. Proc Natl Acad Sci USA 101:7630–7635

Palacios-Callender M, Hollis V, Mitchison M, Frakich N, Unitt D, Moncada S (2007a) Cytochrome c oxidase regulates endogenous nitric oxide availability in respiring cells: a possible explanation for hypoxic vasodilation. Proc Natl Acad Sci USA 104:18508–18513

Palacios-Callender M, Hollis V, Frakich N, Mateo J, Moncada S (2007b) Cytochrome c oxidase maintains mitochondrial respiration during partial inhibition by nitric oxide. J Cell Sci 120:160–165

Pearce LL, Kanai AJ, Birder LA, Pitt BR, Peterson J (2002) The catabolic fate of nitric oxide: the nitric oxide oxidase and peroxynitrite reductase activities of cytochrome oxidase. J Biol Chem 277:13556–13562

Poderoso JJ, Carreras MC, Lisdero C, Riobo N, Schopfer F, Boveris A (1996) Nitric oxide inhibits electron transfer and increases superoxide radical production in rat heart mitochondria and submitochondrial particles. Arch Biochem Biophys 328:85–92

Poyton RO, Castello PR, Ball KA, Woo DK, Pan N (2009) Mitochondria and hypoxic signaling: a new view. Ann N Y Acad Sci 1177:48–56

Prime TA et al (2009) A mitochondria-targeted S-nitrosothiol modulates respiration, nitrosates thiols, and protects against ischemia-reperfusion injury. Proc Natl Acad Sci USA 106:10764–10769

Rassaf T, Flogel U, Drexhage C, Hendgen-Cotta U, Kelm M, Schrader J (2007) Nitrite reductase function of deoxymyoglobin: oxygen sensor and regulator of cardiac energetics and function. Circ Res 100:1749–1754

Sarti P, Lendaro E, Ippoliti R, Bellelli A, Benedetti PA, Brunori M (1999) Modulation of mitochondrial respiration by nitric oxide: investigation by single cell fluorescence microscopy. FASEB J 13:191–197

Sarti P, Giuffrè A, Forte E, Mastronicola D, Barone MC, Brunori M (2000) Nitric oxide and cytochrome c oxidase: mechanisms of inhibition and NO degradation. Biochem Biophys Res Commun 274:183–187

Sarti P, Giuffrè A, Barone MC, Forte E, Mastronicola D, Brunori M (2003) Nitric oxide and cytochrome oxidase: reaction mechanisms from the enzyme to the cell. Free Radic Biol Med 34:509–520

Schapira AH (1998) Human complex I defects in neurodegenerative diseases. Biochim Biophys Acta 1364:261–270

Schapira AH (2010) Complex I: inhibitors, inhibition and neurodegeneration. Exp Neurol 224(2):331–335

Schweizer M, Richter C (1994) Nitric oxide potently and reversibly deenergizes mitochondria at low oxygen tension. Biochem Biophys Res Commun 204:169–175

Shen W, Hintze TH, Wolin MS (1995) Nitric oxide. An important signaling mechanism between vascular endothelium and parenchymal cells in the regulation of oxygen consumption. Circulation 92:3505–3512

Shiva S, Gladwin MT (2009) Nitrite mediates cytoprotection after ischemia/reperfusion by modulating mitochondrial function. Basic Res Cardiol 104:113–119

Shiva S, Brookes PS, Patel RP, Anderson PG, Darley-Usmar VM (2001) Nitric oxide partitioning into mitochondrial membranes and the control of respiration at cytochrome c oxidase. Proc Natl Acad Sci USA 98:7212–7217

Shiva S, Oh JY, Landar AL, Ulasova E, Venkatraman A, Bailey SM, Darley-Usmar VM (2005) Nitroxia: the pathological consequence of dysfunction in the nitric oxide-cytochrome c oxidase signaling pathway. Free Radic Biol Med 38:297–306

Shiva S et al (2007a) Nitrite augments tolerance to ischemia/reperfusion injury via the modulation of mitochondrial electron transfer. J Exp Med 204:2089–2102

Shiva S et al (2007b) Deoxymyoglobin is a nitrite reductase that generates nitric oxide and regulates mitochondrial respiration. Circ Res 100:654–661

Stamler JS et al (1992) Nitric oxide circulates in mammalian plasma primarily as an S-nitroso adduct of serum albumin. Proc Natl Acad Sci USA 89:7674–7677

Stubauer G, Giuffrè A, Brunori M, Sarti P (1998) Cytochrome c oxidase does not catalyze the anaerobic reduction of NO. Biochem Biophys Res Commun 245:459–465

Stuehr DJ, Nathan CF (1989) Nitric oxide. A macrophage product responsible for cytostasis and respiratory inhibition in tumor target cells. J Exp Med 169:1543–1555

Thomas DD, Liu X, Kantrow SP, Lancaster JR Jr (2001) The biological lifetime of nitric oxide: implications for the perivascular dynamics of NO and O2. Proc Natl Acad Sci USA 98:355–360

Torres J, Darley-Usmar V, Wilson MT (1995) Inhibition of cytochrome c oxidase in turnover by nitric oxide: mechanism and implications for control of respiration. Biochem J 312:169–173

Torres J, Cooper CE, Wilson MT (1998) A common mechanism for the interaction of nitric oxide with the oxidized binuclear centre and oxygen intermediates of cytochrome c oxidase. J Biol Chem 273:8756–8766

Torres J, Sharpe MA, Rosquist A, Cooper CE, Wilson MT (2000) Cytochrome c oxidase rapidly metabolises nitric oxide to nitrite. FEBS Lett 475:263–266

Trimmer BA, Aprille JR, Dudzinski DM, Lagace CJ, Lewis SM, Michel T, Qazi S, Zayas RM (2001) Nitric oxide and the control of firefly flashing. Science 292:2486–2488

Vinogradov AD (1998) Catalytic properties of the mitochondrial NADH-ubiquinone oxidoreductase (complex I) and the pseudo-reversible active/inactive enzyme transition. Biochim Biophys Acta 1364:169–185

Webb A, Bond R, McLean P, Uppal R, Benjamin N, Ahluwalia A (2004) Reduction of nitrite to nitric oxide during ischemia protects against myocardial ischemia-reperfusion damage. Proc Natl Acad Sci USA 101:13683–13688

Weitzberg E, Lundberg JO (1998) Nonenzymatic nitric oxide production in humans. Nitric Oxide 2:1–7

Weng L, Baker GM (1991) Reaction of hydrogen peroxide with the rapid form of resting cytochrome oxidase. Biochemistry 30:5727–5733

Xie YW, Shen W, Zhao G, Xu X, Wolin MS, Hintze TH (1996) Role of endothelium-derived nitric oxide in the modulation of canine myocardial mitochondrial respiration in vitro. Implications for the development of heart failure. Circ Res 79:381–387

Zhao G, Bernstein RD, Hintze TH (1999) Nitric oxide and oxygen utilization: exercise, heart failure and diabetes. Coron Artery Dis 10:315–320

Zweier JL, Samouilov A, Kuppusamy P (1999) Non-enzymatic nitric oxide synthesis in biological systems. Biochim Biophys Acta 1411:250–262

Chapter 5
Mitochondria and Reactive Oxygen Species. Which Role in Physiology and Pathology?

Giorgio Lenaz

Abstract Oxidative stress is among the major causes of toxicity due to interaction of Reactive Oxygen Species (ROS) with cellular macromolecules and structures and interference with signal transduction pathways. The mitochondrial respiratory chain, specially from Complexes I and III, is considered the main origin of ROS particularly under conditions of high membrane potential, but several other sources may be important for ROS generation, such as mitochondrial p66[Shc], monoamine oxidase, α-ketoglutarate dehydogenase, besides redox cycling of redox-active molecules. ROS are able to oxidatively modify lipids, proteins, carbohydrates and nucleic acids in mitochondria and to activate/inactivate signalling pathways by oxidative modification of redox-active factors. Cells are endowed with several defence mechanisms including repair or removal of damaged molecules, and antioxidant systems, either enzymatic or non-enzymatic. Oxidative stress is at the basis of ageing and many pathological disorders, such as ischemic diseases, neurodegenerative diseases, diabetes, and cancer, although the underlying mechanisms are not always completely understood.

Keywords Reactive oxygen species • ROS-generating reactions • Mitochondria • Respiratory complexes • Oxidative stress • Antioxidants

5.1 Introduction

Reactive oxygen species (ROS), is a collective term including oxygen derivatives, either radical or non-radical, that are oxidizing agents and/or are easily converted into radicals (Halliwell 2006). As we shall see in detail, ROS are formed by partial reduction of molecular oxygen. It has been considered for a long time that the appearance of oxygen on the Earth has represented a challenge for living organisms, because of toxicity inherent in its inevitable partial reduction, so that living organisms have been forced to develop a number of defence strategies against them (cf. Fridovich 1998). This is certainly true in part, but does not easily explain why evolution has conserved so many specific mechanisms for ROS production: indeed, a moderate level of such species is physiological and required for

G. Lenaz (✉)
Dipartimento di Biochimica "G. Moruzzi", Università di Bologna, Via Irnerio 48,
40126 Bologna, Italy
e-mail: giorgio.lenaz@unibo.it

R. Scatena et al. (eds.), *Advances in Mitochondrial Medicine*, Advances in Experimental Medicine and Biology 942, DOI 10.1007/978-94-007-2869-1_5,

life, and nowadays ROS are recognised to be physiologically involved in cell signalling by affecting the redox state of signalling proteins (Barja 1993). Nevertheless it has been known for a long time that, when in excess, they are among the major determinants of toxicity in cells and organisms.

In healthy cells, the continuous production of ROS is balanced by various detoxification reactions operated by a number of antioxidant systems. Only excessive ROS production or defect of protective systems leads to oxidative stress and pathological conditions.

Under normal conditions, ROS concentration is maintained within narrow boundaries and contribute to the redox balance in the cell (Linnane and Eastwood 2006): redox balance, the ratio between oxidizing and reducing species, is involved in regulation of signalling pathways, including the activity of protein kinases and phosphatases and gene expression through modulation of transcription factors (Fruehauf and Meyskens 2007); glutathione redox state plays a central role in maintaining such redox homeostasis and the GSH/GSSG ratio is an estimate of cellular redox buffering capacity (Schafer and Buettner 2001).

When in excess, ROS exert their damaging effects in mainly two ways: (i) by direct modification of cellular or extracellular macromolecules that are this way altered in their function, leading to pathological effects; (ii) by alterations of their physiological action on the redox state of factors involved in signal transduction, thus leading to hyper- or hypo-functionality of the signalling pathways.

5.1.1   Chemistry of ROS

Diatomic oxygen O_2 is a radical itself because it has two unpaired electrons each located in a different π^* antibonding orbital, but both with the same spin quantum number: this parallel spin is the reason for its low reactivity with non-radical molecules. However, inverting the spin of one of the unpaired electrons by an energy input converts O_2 into the much more reactive *singlet oxygen* $^1O_2$ in which both unpaired electrons have been moved to the same π^* orbital.

If a single electron is supplied to O_2, it enters one of the π^* orbitals to form an electron pair there, thus leaving only one unpaired electron in the *superoxide* radical anion $O_2^{\bullet-}$; addition of another electron gives the *peroxide* ion, which is a weaker acid and is protonated to hydrogen peroxide H_2O_2; addition of two more electrons breaks the molecule producing water H_2O. If one single electron is added to H_2O_2 by a reduced metal ion (e.g. Fe^{2+}), the *hydroxyl radical* $OH\bullet$ is produced by the *Fenton reaction*. The hydroxyl radical is extremely reactive with a half-life of less than 1 ns, thus it reacts very close to its site of formation.

$$O_2 + 1e^- \rightarrow O_2\bullet^- \tag{5.1}$$

$$O_2\bullet^- + 1e^- + 2H^+ \rightarrow H_2O_2 \tag{5.2}$$

$$O_2 + 2e^- + 2H^+ \rightarrow H_2O_2 \tag{5.3}$$

$$H_2O_2 + 2e^- + 2H^+ \rightarrow 2H_2O \tag{5.4}$$

$$Fe^{2+} + H_2O_2 \rightarrow Fe^{3+} + OH\bullet + OH^- \ (\text{Fenton reaction}) \tag{5.5}$$

Reaction (5.1) is catalyzed in cells by several systems described in Sect. 5.2. Reaction (5.2) producing hydrogen peroxide is catalyzed by superoxide dismutases (SOD). Reaction (5.3) also generates hydrogen peroxide by two-electron reduction of O_2 catalyzed by a number of oxidases. Reaction (5.3) is catalyzed by catalase, glutathione peroxidases and other peroxidases.

Since there are other reactive species besides those of oxygen, the term RS has been expanded to include reactive nitrogen species (RNS), reactive chlorine species (RCS), etc. Among RNS is *nitric oxide* NO•, a not very reactive radical well known as a signalling molecule (Rubio and Morales-Segura 2004; Schlossmann and Hofmann 2005). If NO• reacts with O_2•⁻ the non-radical product *peroxynitrite* is formed, that is rapidly protonated at neutral pH to the aggressive peroxynitrous acid, that can further undergo homolytic fission to hydroxyl radical and nitrogen dioxide radical.

$$NO\bullet + O_2\bullet^- + H^+ \rightarrow ONOOH \tag{5.6}$$

$$ONOOH \rightarrow NO_2\bullet + OH\bullet \tag{5.7}$$

Several other radicals are produced by reaction of RS with organic compounds and macromolecules.

5.2 Sources of ROS in Mitochondria

ROS arise in cells from exogenous and endogenous sources. Exogenous sources of ROS include UV and visible light, ionizing radiation, drugs and environmental toxins. Among endogenous sources there are xanthine oxidase, cytochrome P-450 enzymes in the endoplasmic reticulum, peroxisomal flavin oxidases, plasma membrane NADPH oxidases (Lenaz and Strocchi 2009); nevertheless, the major source of ROS is usually considered to be the mitochondrial respiratory chain in the inner mitochondrial membrane, although other enzyme systems in mitochondria can be important contributors to ROS generation.

Within a cell, mitochondria largely contribute to the production of ROS via the respiratory chain (Lenaz 1998, 2001). The relevance of mitochondrial production of ROS within a cell is indirectly revealed by the results of deficiency of mitochondrial antioxidant enzymes. Mitochondria contain an isozyme of superoxide dismutase (SOD-2) and glutathione peroxidase (GPx). The lack of SOD-2 (Melov et al. 1999) and of mitochondrial GPx (Esposito et al. 2000) severely damages cells or is incompatible with life.

5.2.1 Overview of the Mitochondrial Respiratory Chain

The respiratory chain collects reducing equivalents (hydrogen atoms) from mitochondrial oxidations of the tricarboxylic acid cycle, from pyruvate oxidation, fatty acid and amino acid catabolism and other oxidative reactions, and conveys them to molecular oxygen reducing it to water (4 electron reduction). The free energy decrease accompanying electron transfer is exploited to create an electrochemical proton gradient ($\Delta\mu OH^+$) by proton translocation from the mitochondrial inner space, the matrix, to the space between the inner and outer mitochondrial membranes (Nicholls and Ferguson 2002). The proton gradient is then used as a source of energy to synthesize ATP from ADP and Pi by the ATP synthase complex (*oxidative phosphorylation*, OXPHOS), or alternatively to drive other energy-linked reactions such as $NADH/NADP^+$ transhydrogenation and up-hill ion movements across the inner membrane. The ATP synthesized is moved to the cytoplasm in exchange with ADP by the ATP/ADP translocase.

The respiratory chain consists of four major multi-subunit complexes (Lenaz and Genova 2010) designated as NADH-Coenzyme Q (CoQ) reductase (Complex I), Succinate-CoQ reductase (Complex II), Ubiquinol-Cytochrome c reductase (Complex III) and Cytochrome c oxidase (Complex IV). The respiratory complexes are functionally joined by smaller "mobile" redox components, i.e. Coenzyme Q, imbedded in the membrane lipids, and cytochrome c, located on the outer face of the inner membrane. The best fit unit stoichiometry between complexes in beef heart mitochondria is 1 Complex I : 1.3 Complex II : 3 Complex III : 6.7 Complex IV (Schägger and Pfeiffer 2001). In addition there are

0.5 ATP synthase (also called Complex V) and 3–5 units of the ADP/ATP translocase (catalyzing the equimolar exchange of ADP and ATP across the inner membrane) for each cytochrome oxidase, and there is one NADH/NADP$^+$ transhydrogenase per Complex I.

The inner membrane contains several other proteins having electron transfer activity in smaller amounts (Lenaz and Genova 2010); among these there are electron transfer flavoproteins capable of feeding electrons to the respiratory chain by pathways not involving Complex I and/or NAD, i.e.glycerol-3-phosphate dehydrogenase, electron transfer flavoprotein (ETF)-ubiquinone oxidoreductase, dihydroorotate dehydrogenase, choline dehydrogenase, besides alternative NADH dehydrogenases in mitochondria from several organisms, especially plants and fungi.

The representation of the respiratory chain as a collection of enzymes randomly distributed in the lipid bilayer according to the random collision model (Hackenbrock et al. 1986) has somewhat changed in the recent years after the discovery of respiratory supercomplexes as supramolecular functional respiratory units (see Sect. 5.3.1).

5.2.2 The Respiratory Chain as a Source of ROS

The major sites of superoxide formation in the respiratory chain are within respiratory complexes I and III. Further sites, however, may have importance and physiological relevance. It is worth noting that mitochondria from different tissues may vary conspicuously in their capacity to produce ROS using different substrates (Kwong and Sohal 1998), and this capacity is also related to animal species and age.

Murphy (2009) has carefully analyzed the thermodynamics of mitochondrial superoxide production. The standard reduction potential for the transfer of an electron to O_2 to form $O_2^{\cdot-}$ is -160 mV at pH 7, for a standard state of 1 M O_2. Tentative estimates for $[O_2^{\cdot-}]$ within the mitochondrial matrix are in the range 10–200 pM. By combining these with a plausible intramitochondrial $[O_2]$ of 25 µM, one can calculate E_h in the range 150–230 mV for the reduction of O_2 to $O_2^{\cdot-}$. Even for a low $[O_2]$ of 1 µM and a high $[O_2^{\cdot-}]$ of 200 pM, the E_h value obtained is 68 mV.

Therefore, *in vivo*, the one-electron reduction of O_2 to $O_2^{\cdot-}$ is thermodynamically favoured, even by relatively oxidizing redox couples, and a wide range of electron donors within mitochondria could potentially carry out this reaction. However, only a small proportion of mitochondrial electron carriers with the thermodynamic potential to reduce O_2 to $O_2^{\cdot-}$ do so.

5.2.2.1 Complex I

Complex I (NADH CoQ reductase) oxidizes NADH in the mitochondrial matrix and reduces CoQ in the lipid bilayer of the inner mitochondrial membrane. The reaction is accompanied by translocation of four protons from the matrix to the intermembrane space.

$$\text{NADH} + \text{H}^+ + \text{CoQ} + 4\text{H}^+ \left(\text{in}\right) \rightarrow \text{NAD}^+ + \text{CoQH}_2 + 4\text{H}^+ \left(\text{out}\right) \tag{5.8}$$

Several prosthetic groups contribute to electron transfer within the enzyme: FMN is the entry point for electrons, that are then transferred to a series of iron-sulphur clusters (Ohnishi et al. 1998). Enzymes from different sources have different numbers of iron-sulphur clusters, most of which share the same midpoint potential. N2, that is of the kind Fe_4S_4, has the highest midpoint potential (E_m between -150 and -50 mV) and is considered to be the direct electron donor to ubiquinone. N2 iron-sulphur cluster is most likely located in the connection between the peripheral and the membrane arm. The magnetic interaction with the semiquinone radical, corresponding to a distance of about 10 Å

(Ohnishi and Salerno 2005), suggests that the ubiquinone headgroup could somehow reach up into the peripheral arm as assumed by Brandt et al. (2003), who have hypothesized an amphipathic 'ramp' guiding ubiquinone into the catalytic site. Recently the arrangement of iron-sulphur clusters in the hydrophilic domain of Complex I from *T. thermophilus* has been determined by x-ray crystallography, showing a linear chain of all clusters except N1a and N7 (Hinchliffe and Sazanov 2005).

Early experiments proved the involvement of Complex I in ROS production (Takeshige and Minakami 1979); addition of NADH at low concentration led to copious ROS production detected by lipid peroxidation; addition of NADH at high concentration, but in presence of the Complex I inhibitor, rotenone, also induced peroxidation. Water-soluble CoQ homologues used as electron acceptors from isolated Complex I stimulated H_2O_2 production whereas CoQ_6 and CoQ_{10} were inactive (Cadenas et al. 1977). More recent studies confirmed that Complex I is a major source of superoxide production in several types of mitochondria. The superoxide production by Complex I is higher during the reverse electron transport from succinate to NAD^+ (Korshunov et al. 1997; Turrens 2003; Jezek and Hlavata 2005), whereas during the forward electron transport it is much lower. Reverse electron transfer-supported ROS production requires high membrane potential and is inhibited by uncouplers and by processes dissipating membrane potential (Kushnareva et al. 2002; Starkov and Fiskum 2003) . Rotenone enhances ROS formation during forward electron transfer (Herrero and Barja 2000; Genova et al. 2001) and inhibits it during reverse electron transfer (Lambert and Brand 2004; Ohnishi et al. 2005; Vinogradov and Grivennikova 2005) .

The identification of the oxygen reducing site has been the subject of extensive investigation, and several prosthetic groups in the enzyme have been suggested to be the direct reductants of oxygen. These include FMN, ubisemiquinone, and iron sulphur cluster N2 (Lenaz et al. 2006a; Fato et al. 2009). In isolated Complex I, fully reduced FMN is considered the major electron donor to oxygen to form superoxide anion (Galkin and Brandt 2005; Kussmaul and Hirst 2006; Esterházy et al. 2008). In mitochondrial membranes, however, the identification of flavin as the site of oxygen reduction is incompatible with the finding that two classes of inhibitors both acting downstream of the iron sulphur clusters in the enzyme have opposite effects, in that rotenone enhances superoxide production whereas stigmatellin inhibits it (Fato et al. 2009). Hirst et al. (2008) admit the possible presence of two oxygen-reacting sites at the two ends of the cofactor chain, ascribing the distal one to ROS generation during reverse electron transfer. A possible explanation is that two sites for oxygen reduction exist in the complex, represented by flavin and an iron-sulphur cluster; the latter site would be predominant in membrane particles whereas the former might be available after Complex I isolation.

The electron donor to the first molecule of bound ubiquinone in the Complex is most probably FeS cluster N2 (Ohnishi et al. 1998). It is likely that this centre is also the electron donor to oxygen both directly and via one-electron reduction of several exogenous quinones (Fig. 5.1). Studies in CoQ-depleted and reconstituted mitochondria indicated that endogenous CoQ is not required for superoxide generation (Genova et al. 2001). It is worth noting that reconstituted mitochondria, containing a large excess of CoQ_{10}, produce the same amount of superoxide as CoQ-depleted mitochondria, indicating that endogenous CoQ_{10} is not a source of ROS.

EPR studies (Fato et al. 2009) show that in presence of NADH in bovine heart submitochondrial particles rotenone but not stigmatellin quenches the semiquinone radical signal; on the other hand, N2 is kept reduced in presence of rotenone but is oxidized in presence of stigmatellin (unpublished data from our laboratory); overall the results are compatible with the scheme in Fig. 5.1, showing that N2 is the direct electron donor to oxygen in submitochondrial particles.

The superoxide production by Complex I is maximal during reverse electron transfer, however the site of oxygen reduction in this instance is even less well defined (Murphy 2009).

Ohnishi et al. (2010) presented a new hypothesis that the generation of superoxide reflects a dynamic balance between the flavosemiquinone (semiflavin or SF) and the CoQ semiquinone (SQ). In a purified preparation of Complex I, during catalytic electron transfer from NADH to decyl ubiquinone, the superoxide generation site was mostly shifted to the SQ. A quinone-pocket binding inhibitor

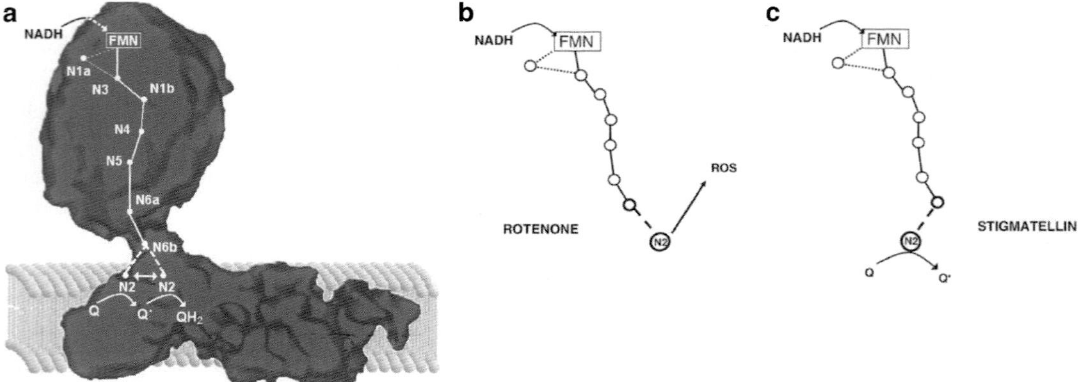

Fig. 5.1 *Proposed two step mechanism for electron transfer from NADH to quinone in Complex I.* Complex I is formed by the apposition of three different modules: a dehydrogenase domain where NADH is oxidized, containing FMN and iron-sulphur clusters N1a, N1b, N3, N4, and N5; a hydrogenase domain where CoQ is reduced, containing FeS clusters N6a, N6b and N2; and a transporter domain containing no prosthetic groups and involved in proton translocation. The *empty circles* represent the linear disposition of prosthetic groups according to Hinchliffe and Sazanov (2005) (in the order after FMN the FeS clusters N3, N1b, N4, N5, N6a, N6b, N2; centre N1a is represented in the vicinity of FMN but not in the main pathway). Superoxide formation presumably occurs at both FMN and N2 (see Fato et al. 2009) and is released in the mitochondrial matrix. (**a**) Two-step path of electron transfer in absence of inhibitors; (**b**) in presence of Class A inhibitors; (**c**) in presence of Class B inhibitors

(rotenone or piericidin A) inhibits the catalytic formation of the SQ, and it enhances the formation of SF and increases the overall superoxide generation. This suggests that if electron transfer was inhibited under pathological conditions, superoxide generation from the SF would be increased. The identification of SQ rather than N2 as the electron donor to oxygen is however in contrast with the findings reported in the previous section showing that when SQ reduction to QH_2 is blocked by stigmatellin no superoxide is produced (Fato et al. 2009). Moreover studies in CoQ-depleted and reconstituted mitochondria indicated that endogenous CoQ is not required for superoxide generation (Genova et al. 2001). It is worth noting that reconstituted mitochondria, containing a large excess of CoQ_{10}, produce the same amount of superoxide as CoQ-depleted mitochondria, indicating that endogenous CoQ_{10} is not a source of ROS.

5.2.2.2 Complex III

Complex III (ubiquinol cytochrome c reductase) represents a confluence point for reducing equivalents from various dehydrogenases: it catalyzes the transfer of electrons from ubiquinol in the lipid membrane ($CoQH_2$) to water-soluble cytochrome c on the outer surface of the inner membrane, and concomitantly links this redox reaction to translocation of protons across the membrane, converting the energy associated with electron flow into an electrochemical proton gradient.

$$CoQH_2 + 2\text{cyt. c Fe}^{3+} + 2H^+ (\text{in}) \rightarrow CoQ + 2\text{cyt. c Fe}^{2+} + 4H^+ (\text{out}) \tag{5.9}$$

The formation of superoxide in Complex III depends on the peculiar mechanism of electron transfer, the so-called Q-cycle (Crofts 2004) (Fig. 5.2). In the Q-cycle, QH_2 delivers the first electron at the outer positive site (thus called site o or P) of the inner membrane to the Rieske iron-sulphur protein and hence to cytochromes c_1 and c; the result is release of two H^+ in the inter-membrane space and formation of an unstable semiquinone anion $Q^{\circ-}$ at the Qo site, which is immediately oxidized to Q by the low-potential cytochrome b_{566} (or b_L) at the cytosolic side; the electron is then delivered to the high-potential cytochrome b_{562} (or b_H) at the internal negative side (thus called site i or N); b_H is then

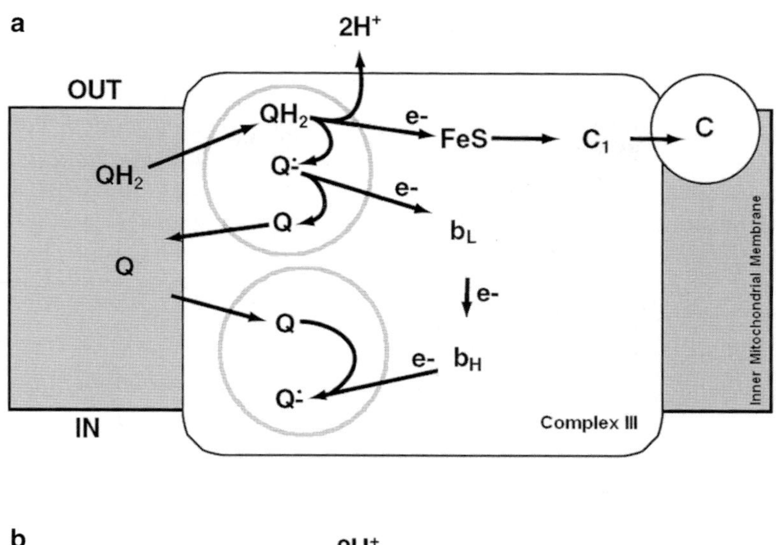

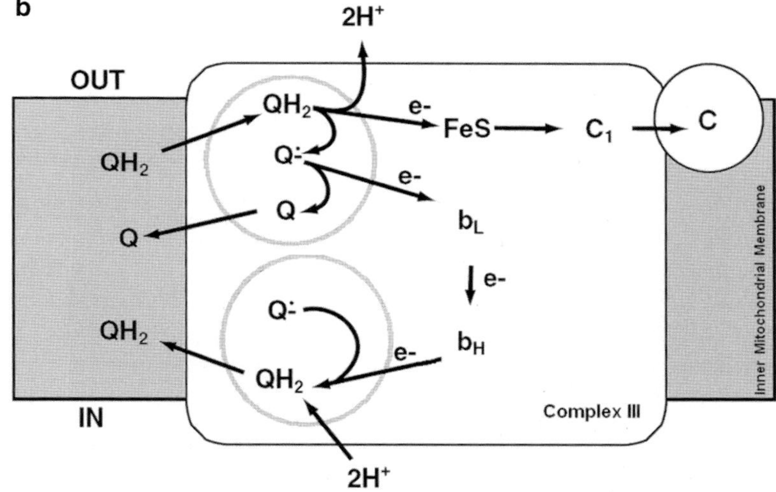

Fig. 5.2 *The Q-cycle in Complex III.* (**a**) Ubiquinol (QH_2) delivers the first electron at the outer positive site (called site o or P) of the inner membrane to the Rieske iron-sulphur protein and hence to cytochromes c_1 and c; the result is release of two protons in the inter-membrane space and formation of an unstable semiquinone anion ($Q \cdot^-$) at the Qo site, which is immediately oxidised to ubiquinone (Q) by the low-potential cytochrome b_{566} (b_L). The electron is then delivered to the high-potential cytochrome b_{562} (b_H) at the internal negative site (site i or N) then b_H is reoxidized by Q at the Qi site, forming another semiquinone. (**b**) The cycle is completed by oxidation of a second molecule of QH_2

reoxidized by CoQ at site i (Q_i) forming another semiquinone. The cycle is completed by oxidation of a second molecule of QH_2.

Since the electron transfer from cytochrome b_L to b_H occurs against the electrical gradient (from the positive to the negative side), it is strongly retarded when the electrochemical potential is high, as in the controlled state (*State 4*); this retardation prolongs the lifetime of Qo and allows reaction of the semiquinone with O_2 forming superoxide (Jezek and Hlavata 2005).

Antimycin A (AA), an inhibitor acting at the Qi site, is known not to completely inhibit electron flow from ubiquinol to cytochrome *c*: the AA-insensitive reduction of cytochrome *c* is mediated by superoxide radicals. According to the Q-cycle, AA blocks ubiquinone reduction by cytochrome b_H at center *i*, at the inner or negative side of the membrane. The antimycin-stimulated production of ROS is inhibited by the inhibitors acting at center *o* (at the outer or positive side) where ubiquinol reduces both the Rieske iron-sulfur cluster and cytochrome b_L. Thus, we may locate the site of one-electron reduction of oxygen in presence of antimycin at a component located at center o, presumably ubisemiquinone (Casteilla et al. 2001).

Myxothiazol was found to enhance ROS production using different respiratory substrates in absence of antimycin, and the effect was reversed by stigmatellin (Starkov and Fiskum 2001). Muller et al. (2003) found that *proximal* Qo site inhibitors, acting close to the b_{566} niche, induce superoxide formation in yeast submitochondrial particles supplemented with decyl-ubiquinol; the effect is not modified by antimycin, showing that the source of radicals is not at the Qi site. Muller et al. (2003) suggested that oxidation of ubiquinol at center o is biphasic, with delivery of the first electron to the Rieske iron sulfur cluster, leaving a semiquinone that in absence of further oxidation by cytochrome b_L would interact with oxygen forming superoxide.

Ubisemiquinone is relatively stable only when protein-bound, therefore the Coenzyme Q (CoQ) pool in the lipid bilayer should be no source of ROS. Exogenously administered CoQ has not been found to exert pro-oxidant effects *in vivo*: thus, the pro-oxidant species deriving from its antioxidant action (Nohl et al. 1998) would not seem to be operative in *in vivo* supplementation.

5.2.2.3 Complex II

The enzyme is also a component of the Krebs cycle (*succinate dehydrogenase*) and catalyzes the reduction of CoQ by succinate, without formation of a proton gradient.

$$\text{Succinate} + \text{CoQ} \rightarrow \text{Fumarate} + \text{CoQH}_2 \tag{5.10}$$

Mammalian Complex II is part of a class of ubiquinone-reducing enzymes containing a single b heme and anchored to the inner mitochondrial membrane by two hydrophobic subunits, SdhC (14.2 kDa) and SdhD (12.8 kDa). The soluble domain of Complex II consists of a flavoprotein subunit containing covalently linked FAD and an iron-sulphur protein subunit, both located on the matrix side of the membrane (Cecchini 2003).

The indirect evidence that often ROS production is higher when electrons are channeled through Complex II than through Complex I, while in both cases reaching Complex III, is in line with the idea that Complex II may be a source of ROS (McLennan and Degli Esposti 2000).

Ishii et al. (1998), in a study on *C. elegans*, produced evidence that a mutation in succinate dehydrogenase cytochrome b induces oxidative stress and aging. In *E. coli*, the reverse reaction, fumarate reductase (QFR), active under anaerobic conditions, is structurally analogous to Complex II (succinate-CoQ reductase, SQR), active under aerobic conditions; in contrast with Complex II, however, *E. coli* QFR has no b heme. Significantly, *E. coli* QFR is a potent source of H_2O_2 whereas SQR is not (Messner and Imlay 2002). The source of electrons to oxygen is fully reduced FAD. The difference between SQR and QFR has been ascribed to the electron-attracting capacity of cytochrome b, due to its high redox potential (Yankovskaya et al. 2003): thus, in the absence of cytochrome b, the electrons would be held preferentially on the flavin, favouring leak to oxygen.

Direct demonstration of ROS production by Complex II was obtained by Zhang et al. (1998): in purified succinate-CoQ reductase, auto-oxidation of flavin was the source of the superoxide; reconstitution with the bc1 Complex to yield an active succinate cytochrome c reductase inhibited superoxide formation.

5.2.2.4 Glycerol-3-Phosphate Dehydrogenase

The enzyme catalyzes the oxidation of glycerol-3-phosphate by CoQ:

$$\text{Glycerol} - 3 - \text{P} + \text{CoQ} \rightarrow \text{Dihydroxy acetone} - \text{P} + \text{CoQH}_2 \tag{5.11}$$

The mitochondrial enzyme (mtGPDH) is a very hydrophobic protein of the inner membrane; its catalytic centre is accessible from the outer surface of the inner membrane (Donnellan et al. 1970; Klingenberg 1970).

Besides containing FAD as prosthetic group, the presence of an iron-sulphur cluster has been suggested (Wells et al. 2001), however the putative centre has not been characterized.

A high rate of ROS production was detected in insect flight muscle mitochondria (Bolter and Chefurka 1990) and in brown adipose tissue mitochondria (Sekhar et al. 1987) when glycerol-3-phosphate was used as the respiratory substrate. This suggested that mitochondrial glycerophosphate dehydrogenase could be the source of ROS. Drahota et al.(2002) demonstrated that mtGPDH in presence of antimycin is a powerful source of hydrogen peroxide, that was strongly stimulated by addition of the one-electron acceptor ferricyanide. The ferricyanide-induced H_2O_2 production is a specific feature of mtGPDH: it is completely inhibited by mtGPDH inhibitors, and is negligible using NADH or succinate as substrates: it is reasonable that ferricyanide takes up one electron and the other is used to reduce oxygen. the observation that CoQ homologues and the hydroxyl-analog idebenone decrease superoxide formation by the enzyme in presence of ferricyanide (Drahota et al. 2002; Rauchová et al. 2006) suggests a very specific mechanism of interaction of CoQ with this enzyme, since this effect is not shared by either Complex I or Complex II.

In a study on *Drosophila* mitochondria (Miwa et al. 2003) ROS production by mtGPDH and the relative contributions of Complex I by reverse electron transfer, of centre o of Complex III, and of mtGPDH were assessed by use of specific inhibitors, demonstrating that mtGPDH was the major source of superoxide.

5.2.2.5 Dihydroorotate Dehydrogenase

Dihydroorotate dehydrogenase (DHODase, EC. 1.3.3.1) is an iron-containing 43-kDa flavoprotein (FMN) that catalyzes the oxidation of dihydroorotate to orotate, the fourth step in *de novo* pyrimidine biosyntesis (Evans and Guy 2004):

$$\text{Dihydroorotate} + \text{CoQ} \rightarrow \text{Orotate} + \text{CoQH}_2 \tag{5.12}$$

The mammalian DHODase and that isolated from *Neurospora crassa* (class 2 enzymes) are integral membrane proteins localized in the inner mitochondrial membrane with the active site facing the inter-membrane space.

The enzyme was found to be involved in the production of superoxide in liver mitochondria (Forman and Kennedy 1975) and in malarial parasite cells (Krungkrai 1991). It is worth noting that the major domain of the enzyme, carrying the carboxyl terminal, protrudes in the inter-membrane space, so that it is likely that superoxide is released in this space similarly to glycerol-3-phosphate dehydrogenase.

5.2.2.6 ETF and ETF Dehydrogenase

ETF is a small flavoprotein that accepts electrons from a variety of dehydrogenases (Beckmann and Frerman 1985), including those involved in fatty acid oxidation, in amino acid oxidation, and in choline catabolism (dimethylglycine dehydrogenase and sarcosine dehydrogenase), and is oxidized by ubiquinone by a reaction catalyzed by ETF-ubiquinone oxidoreductase (EC 1.5.5.1), a globular protein located on the matrix surface of the inner mitochondrial membrane.

$$\text{ETF}\left(\text{FADH}_2\right) + \text{CoQ} \rightarrow \text{ETF}\left(\text{FAD}\right) + \text{CoQH}_2 \tag{5.13}$$

Crystal structures of the enzyme (Zhang et al. 2006) indicate that the molecule forms a single structural domain where three closely packed functional regions bind FAD, the 4Fe4S cluster and ubiquinone.

It was observed that the oxidation of palmitoyl carnitine by mitochondria leads to production of H_2O_2 (Boveris et al. 1972). More recently St-Pierre et al. (2002) in a study on the topology of ROS production by the respiratory chain observed a copious production of H_2O_2 by rat muscle and heart, but not liver, mitochondria when oxidizing palmitoyl carnitine; since the rate was only slightly enhanced by exogenous SOD, it was suggested that superoxide production occurred at the matrix side, therefore it was generated by a site different from centre o of Complex III. The authors considered likely that the flavoproteins ETF and ETF dehydrogenase, involved in fatty acid oxidation, were the sites for generation of superoxide. In a recent paper using skeletal muscle mitochondria, Seifert et al. (2010) found that even a low supply of long chain fatty acids is associated with ROS formation in excess of that generated by NADH-linked substrates. Moreover, ROS production was evident across the physiologic range of membrane potential and was relatively insensitive to membrane potential changes. Determinations of topology and membrane potential as well as use of inhibitors revealed complex III, ETF, and ETF dehydrogenase as the likely sites of ROS production.

5.2.3 Modulation of ROS Production from the Respiratory Chain

Most of superoxide is generated at the matrix side of the inner membrane, as appears from the observation that superoxide is detected in submitochondrial particles (SMP) which are inside-out with respect to mitochondria. A study with suitable spin traps, however, demonstrated the formation of superoxide radical in mitoplasts (Han et al. 2001) indicating that a significant aliquot of this species is released at the outer face of the inner membrane (St-Pierre et al. 2002). It is likely that Complex I releases ROS in the matrix while Complex III in the intermembrane space. The superoxide anion released at the intermembrane space may be exported to the cytoplasm through an anion channel related to VDAC (Han et al. 2003).

Although the first product of oxygen reduction by the respiratory chain is superoxide, this radical has a short life and is rapidly converted into hydrogen peroxide by mitochondrial SOD or can attack other molecules, such as lipids, before being able to escape the mitochondrion. Although hydrogen peroxide is also removed by glutathione peroxidase, it is much more stable than superoxide, so that some molecules can escape the organelle and be detected outside.

Are free radicals produced by mitochondria physiologically released to the cytosol? Staniek and Nohl (2000) applied a non-invasive detecting system for hydrogen peroxide and found that isolated intact rat heart mitochondria do not produce detectable H_2O_2, unless when using succinate in presence of antimycin. Korshunov et al. (1997) also found no hydrogen peroxide formation by intact rat heart mitochondria, unless pretreated in such a way to deplete them of endogenous antioxidants. It may be inferred that under normal conditions ROS are not exported out of mitochondria. There is however overwhelming evidence that ROS production detected in different cells under pathological conditions has a mitochondrial origin.

It is not easy to demonstrate that ROS detected in cells are produced by mitochondria; the effect of respiratory inhibitors appears to be the best way to discriminate between mitochondrial and non-mitochondrial ROS. However, the effect of inhibitors is ambiguous. Although antimycin is usually found to stimulate ROS production (Boveris et al. 1972) in intact cells, as it does in mitochondria, the effect of rotenone is contradictory (Lenaz 2001). Some studies showed that rotenone enhances ROS production in intact cells whereas others showed inhibition of cellular ROS production by the same inhibitor. Since rotenone decreases ROS production by Complex III while enhancing ROS production by Complex I, the relative contribution of the two Complexes to ROS production may vary in different cells. Since ROS production by reverse flux of electrons is decreased by rotenone (Kushnareva et al. 2002), another critical point is represented by membrane potential and the contribution of reverse electron transfer in Complex I.

Mitochondrial ROS production is enhanced in State 4 and when the rate of electron transfer is lowered (Skulachev 1996). The rationale is in a more reduced state of the respiratory carriers capable of donating electrons to oxygen. To this purpose, uncoupling and release of excessive membrane proton potential may protect mitochondria from damage due to excessive free radical production. In rat hepatocytes the futile cycle of proton pumping and proton leak may be responsible for 20–25% of respiration (Brand 2000); in perfused rat muscle the value is even greater. Uncoupling may be obtained by activating proton leak through *uncoupling proteins* (Casteilla et al. 2001). In such way a tissue may dissipate a conspicuous part of the energy conserved by its mitochondria, however in such a way it keeps the mitochondrial respiratory chain under more oxidized conditions preventing the formation of damaging free radicals.

The ROS production by the respiratory chain complexes may be under physiological control; this is particularly evident for Complex I. Events leading to decrease of the rate of electron flow in the Complex also lead to overproduction of ROS; physiological states, such as cAMP-dependent subunit phosphorylation, that enhances Complex I activity, may modify its ROS generating capacity (Raha et al. 2002; Maj et al. 2004; Scacco et al. 2006). It is therefore tempting to speculate that endocrine alterations may affect the capacity of ROS formation by hyper- or hypo-phosphorylation of the Complex.

There is increasing evidence that pathological states in which Complex I activity is impaired also lead to ROS overproduction (Fato et al. 2008, 2009); in cell lines from patients with Complex I deficiency an inverse relationship was found between superoxide production and residual enzyme activity (Verkaart et al. 2007).

Mitochondrial respiration is ordinarily accompanied by low-level ROS production, but they can respond to elevated ROS concentrations by increasing their own ROS production, a phenomenon termed ROS-induced ROS release (RIRR) (Zorov et al. 2000, 2006; Brady et al. 2006). Two modes of RIRR have been described. In the first mode of RIRR, enhanced ROS leads to mitochondrial depolarization via activation of the permeability transition pore MPTP, yielding a short-lived burst of ROS originating from the mitochondrial electron transport chain (ETC). The second mode of RIRR is MPTP independent but is regulated by the mitochondrial benzodiazepine receptor (mBzR). Increased ROS in the mitochondrion triggers opening of the inner mitochondrial membrane anion channel resulting in a brief increase in ETC-derived ROS. Both modes of RIRR have been shown to transmit localized mitochondrial perturbations throughout the cardiac cell in the form of oscillations or waves but are kinetically distinct and may involve different ROS that serve as second messengers.

5.2.4 Other Mitochondrial Systems

5.2.4.1 p66[Shc]

Recently, an additional source of ROS in mitochondria (directly in the form of hydrogen peroxide) was demonstrated in the p66[Shc] protein (Migliaccio et al. 2006); p66[Shc] is a splice variant of p46[Shc]/p52[Shc], two cytoplasmic proteins involved in signal transduction from tyrosine kinases to Ras; p66[Shc] has the same modular structure of the former proteins but contains a unique N-terminal region and is not involved in Ras regulation. Its function has been recently discovered to be in the regulation of ROS metabolism and apoptosis (Migliaccio et al. 1999). P66[Shc−/−] cells are resistant to apoptosis induced by a variety of different signals (Migliaccio et al. 1999); expression of the protein is required for mitochondrial depolarization and release of cytochrome c after a variety of pro-apoptotic signals (Trinei et al. 2002). P66[Shc] deletion in mice decreases the incidence of ageing-associated diseases

(Napoli et al. 2003; Menini et al. 2006; Rota et al. 2006) and prolongs lifespan of animals (Migliaccio et al. 1999).

Pathways leading to increase of p66^{Shc} expression in oxidative stress involve p53 (Trinei et al. 2002) and PKC-β isoform (Pinton et al. 2007); moreover p66^{Shc} expression and phosphorylation is involved in stabilization of the hypoxia-inducible factor HIF1α (Bianchi et al. 2006; Carraro et al. 2007).

A fraction of p66^{Shc} has a mitochondrial localization in the intermembrane space, where it is bound in an inactive form in a high molecular weight complex including the TIM/TOM protein import system (Giorgio et al. 2005); pro-apoptotic signals dissociate the protein from the complex and activate it to a form inducing the permeability transition by opening a high conductance channel in the inner membrane, *the permeability transition pore* (Bernardi et al. 2001) involved in the events leading to apoptosis. This effect is due to the intrinsic property of p66^{Shc} to act as a redox protein accepting electrons from cytochrome c and directly producing hydrogen peroxide (Giorgio et al. 2005). Stress signals, such as UV radiation or ROS themselves, activate p66^{Shc}, which was proposed to stimulate its H_2O_2 forming activity, ultimately triggering mitochondrial disintegration (Gertz et al. 2009).

Since the reaction equilibrium of cytochrome c oxidation by p66^{Shc} is low (K_{eq}=0.1), the reaction is thermodynamically favoured when the level of cytochrome c reduction is high (Giorgio et al. 2005). This means that H_2O_2 production by this mechanism should be enhanced when cytochrome c oxidase (the enzyme catalyzing cytochrome c reoxidation by oxygen) is inhibited. The K_m of cytochrome oxidase for oxygen is very low (<1 μM), thus allowing its activity even at low oxygen tensions; however low oxygen tensions promote the activation of hypoxia-inducible factor (HIF) by a still controversial mechanism (Taylor 2008) that triggers a series of metabolic changes among which is alteration of cytochrome oxidase subunits and activity. The activation of the p66^{Shc} pathway may in part explain the paradoxical enhancement of ROS production during hypoxia (Guzy and Schumacker 2006).

Another factor leading to decrease of cytochrome oxidase activity is nitric oxide NO• that inhibits the enzyme competitively with oxygen (Sarti et al. 2000), thus elevating the K_m. The NO• inhibition may not be relevant at normal oxygen tensions (ca. 30 μM) but may become important when the oxygen tension is lowered as during ischemia.

The role of p66^{Shc} in ROS production does not appear to be restricted to mitochondria: in fact p66^{Shc} deficiency in knock-out mice causes a defect in activation of the PHOX complex of the plasma membrane NADPH oxidase, that results in decreased superoxide production (Tomilov et al. 2010).

5.2.4.2　Dihydrolipoamide Dehydrogenase

Dihydrolipoamide dehydrogenase (DLD) is a flavoprotein subunit of the α-ketoglutarate dehydrogenase and pyruvate dehydrogenase complexes situated in the mitochondrial matrix, catalyzing the reoxidation of protein bound lipoate (lipoamide) by NAD$^+$.

$$\text{Lipoamide } (SH)_2 + NAD^+ \rightarrow \text{Lipoamide} (S\text{-}S) + NADH + H^+ \tag{5.14}$$

This subunit of α-ketoglutarate dehydrogenase has been shown to be a source of superoxide by electron leak from the flavin (Starkov et al. 2004; Tretter and Adam-Vizi 2004) under State 4 conditions when the enzyme is more reduced; the contribution of the pyruvate dehydrogenase analogous subunit to superoxide formation was found 50% of that by α-ketoglutarate dehydrogenase. In *S. cerevisiae* under conditions of NAD depletion or at high NADH/NAD$^+$ ratios the contribution of α-ketoglutarate dehydrogenase to ROS formation was higher than that of the respiratory chain (Tahara et al. 2007) as demonstrated by strong ROS formation by adding α-ketoglutarate or pyruvate, but not malate, to wild type permeabilized mitochondria, and by prevention of oxidative stress in deletion mutants of the DLD gene; the oxidative stress was also prevented by calorie restriction, which is known to keep the NADH/NAD$^+$ ratio low (Lin et al. 2004).

The production of H_2O_2 by coupled bovine heart mitochondria is strongly stimulated by ammonium ion (Grivennikova et al. 2010); the ammonium-stimulated activity has been identified as dihydrolipoamide dehydrogenase (Kareyeva et al. 2011).

5.2.4.3 Monoamine Oxidase

Amine oxidases are a class of enzymes catalyzing the oxidation of amines by O_2 forming the respective aldehydes and H_2O_2; they are subdivided into FAD-dependent oxidases (monoamine oxidases, polyamine oxidases) and copper and topaquinone-dependent oxidases (Strolin Benedetti et al. 2007). Amine oxidases are involved in the oxidation of endogenous amines, such as dopamine, serotonin etc., but also of xenobiotic amines, such as tyramine and several drugs (Strolin Benedetti et al. 2006).

$$R\text{-}CH_2NH_2 + O_2 \rightarrow R\text{-}CH = NH + H_2O_2 \tag{5.15a}$$

$$R\text{-}CH = NH + H_2O \rightarrow R\text{-}CHO + NH_3 \tag{5.15b}$$

Monoamine oxidase (MAO) exists in two isoforms bound to the outer mitochondrial membrane, MAO-A and MAO-B; it is a flavoprotein (Cadenas and Davies 2000) (for a review on the molecular mechanism see Edmonson et al. 2007). MAO-A has been shown to represent an important source of ROS in rat heart (Maurel et al. 2003); oxidative stress mediated by MAO-A results in cardiomyocyte apoptosis and MAO-A inhibition reduces myocardial damage induced by ischemia-reperfusion (Bianchi et al. 2005). The increase of MAO-A activity in the heart subjected to ischemia-reperfusion has been attributed to increased availability of its substrate serotonin. Use of specific MAO inhibitors may represent a tool for cardioprotection (Di Lisa et al. 2007).

5.2.4.4 Mitochondrial Nitric Oxide Synthase

Nitric oxide synthases (NOS) are a family of enzymes including endothelial (eNOS), neuronal (nNOS) and inducible NOS (iNOS); NOS is a cytochrome P450 reductase-like enzyme that catalyzes flavin-mediated electron transfer from NADPH to a prosthetic heme group; the enzyme also requires tetrahydrobiopterin BH_4 to transfer electrons to arginine to release NO• (Bredt 1999). The reaction catalyzed by NOS is still little understood; the reaction occurs in two steps with formation of N-hydroxyarginine, but the detailed mechanism is uncertain:

$$\text{Arginine} + 2O_2 + NADPH + H^+ \rightarrow \text{Citrulline} + NO\bullet + NADP^+ \tag{5.16}$$

$NO°$ is a relatively stable radical with a half-life of 1–10 s (Brown and Borutaite 2004).

In the absence of either BH_4 or arginine, NOS uncouples, *i.e.* it reacts with oxygen generating $O_2\bullet^-$ instead of NO• (Pou et al. 1999); ROS generated by other sources are involved in a feed-forward mechanism inactivating BH_4 and leading to NOS uncoupling (Alp and Channon 2004). Simultaneous formation of NO• and $O_2\bullet^-$ would favour the production of peroxynitrite.

Although NOS is mostly a cytoplasmic enzyme, a mitochondrial isoform has been described (Ghafourifar and Sen 2007). Kanai et al. (2001) functionally demonstrated the presence of a NOS in cardiac mitochondria. This was accomplished by direct porphyrinic microsensor measurement of Ca^{2+}-dependent NO production in individual mitochondria isolated from wild-type mouse hearts. The similarity of mtNOS to the neuronal isoform was deduced by the absence of NO production in the mitochondria of knockout mice for the neuronal, but not the endothelial or inducible, isoforms. Subsequently MtNOS has been identified as the alpha isoform of nNOS, acylated at a Thr or Ser residue, and phosphorylated at the C-terminal end (Haynes et al. 2003). mtNOS-I was described to be associated with cytochrome oxidase, as proven by electron microscopic immunolocalization and co-immunoprecipitation studies (Persichini et al. 2005). Navarro and Boveris (2008) reviewed the subcellular distribution of nitric oxide synthases (NOS) emphasizing on the evidence of a mitochondrial NOS isoform (mtNOS) that exhibits a mean activity of 0.86 ± 0.09 nmol NO/min x mg protein in 13 mouse and rat organs. Brain mtNOS is the most decreased enzymatic activity upon aging; decreased levels of NO are interpreted as the cause of decreased mitochondrial biogenesis in aged brain.

The existence of mtNOS, however, is still debated (Burtwell and Brookes 2008; Lacza et al. 2009). A recent study (Venkatakrishnan et al. 2009) on ultrapure rat liver mitochondria was designed to clarify the existence of the mitochondrial NOS isoform. Linear ion trap-mass spectrometry analyses of rat liver mitochondria as well as submitochondrial particles were negative for any peptide from any NOS isoform. Also, l-[(14)C]arginine to l-[(14)C]citrulline conversion assays were negative for NOS activity. Finally, Western blot analyses of rat liver mitochondria, using NOS (neuronal or endothelial) antibodies, were negative for any NOS isoform. In conclusion, and in light of our present limits of detection, data from carefully conducted, properly controlled experiments for NOS detection, utilizing three independent yet complementary methodologies, independently as well as collectively, refute the claim that a NOS isoform exists within rat liver mitochondria.

5.2.5   Role of Electron Mediators and Redox Cycling in Mitochondria

Many physiologically active substances and xenobiotics have electron transfer functionalities, either *per se*, or more usually in their metabolites; these main groups include quinones (or phenolic precursors), metal complexes (or complexors), aromatic nitro compounds (or reduced derivatives), and conjugated imines or iminium species (Kovacic and Cooksy 2005). Many of these compounds generate ROS exploiting a mechanism of *redox cycling*.

In vivo redox cycling with oxygen can occur in a catalytic fashion giving rise to a futile cycle that regenerates the parent compound and releases ROS. Redox cycling has been suggested for several drugs, like cocaine, other abused drugs, catecholamines, and several other compounds (Halliwell and Gutteridge 1999). Electron transfer with redox cycling occurs through interference with physiological electron transfer reactions such as microsomal cytochrome P450, xanthine oxidase, and the mitochondrial respiratory chain.

The anticancer agent, *adriamycin (doxorubicin),* is endowed with severe cardiotoxicity; the toxic effect is distinct from the anticancer mechanism, and involves ROS formation, as also suggested by the protective effect of overexpressing antioxidant enzymes in transgenic animals (Sun et al. 2001).

Studies in perfused rat hearts showed that adriamycin largely localizes to mitochondria. Thus, although the drug can be reduced univalently by a variety of systems as cytochrome P450, xanthine oxidase, and mitochondrial Complex I, the oxidative activation in the heart appears to involve mainly mitochondria (Berthiaume and Wallace 2007). On the contrary, in the liver cytochrome P450 appears to account for a substantial portion of activation (Cribb et al. 2005). The mechanism of redox cycling involves initial reduction of the quinone drug to a semiquinone radical by a one-electron transfer, and then reaction with oxygen releasong superoxide and regenerating adriamycin.

Studies with physiological doses confirm that adriamycin induces acute ROS generation that occurs mainly at the level of Complex I (Salvatorelli et al. 2006). The mechanism of cardiotoxicity, however, implies long-term exposure, indicating that acute oxidative stress *per se* is not sufficient to explain cardiac failure; The major mechanisms involved in chronic toxicity also appear to involve mitochondria and are ascribed to secondary damage induced by ROS to Complex I and other mitochondrial complexes, with loss of OXPHOS efficiency, and to oxidative damage to mitochondrial DNA leading to permanent loss of the OXPHOS machinery (Berthiaume and Wallace 2007).

The activation pathway followed by carcinogenic polycyclic aromatic hydrocarbons is more complex (Luch 2005); monooxygenation by cytochrome P450 generates trans-dihydrodiols and subsequent formation of dihydrodiol epoxides that form adducts with DNA thus initiating carcinogenesis. Alternatively, trans-dihydrodiols may be converted by enzymatic oxidation into cathecols that undergo spontaneous auto-oxidation with O_2 to the corresponding o-quinones, by two one-electron steps with intermediate formation of the semiquinone anion radicals and reduction of O_2 to either $O_2{}^{\bullet-}$ or H_2O_2; both the semiquinone and the quinone forms can undergo catalytic one-electron redox cycling, being reduced by either microsomal cytochrome P450 and cytochrome b_5 reductase or mitochondrial Complex I (Luch 2005). One-electron reduction and auto-oxidation steps establish futile redox cycles in which ROS generation is amplified multiple times (Goetz and Luch 2008). Biotransformation of polycyclic hydrocarbons also leads to formation of polynuclear quinones, which also may undergo redox cycling with the corresponding quinols.

A similar mechanism has been suggested for benzene: initial metabolism occurs in the liver by cytochrome P450, with resulting formation, among other compounds, of benzene dihydrodiol which is oxidized to cathecol and then to benzoquinone (Shen et al. 1996) that undergoes redox cycling with ROS production. To this purpose, p-benzoquinone derivatives such as short-chain CoQ homologues and analogues undergo redox cycling with oxygen at the level of mitochondrial Complex I (Genova et al. 2001); the mechanism of activation involves a site close to the CoQ physiological reduction site but situated upstream of the rotenone block, presumably the iron-sulphur centre N2 (Lenaz et al. 2006a). When however the quinones are added in absence of a Complex I inhibitor but in presence of a Complex III inhibitor, thus allowing their reduction, they behave as potent antioxidants preventing ROS formation (Fato et al. 2008, 2009).

Adrenaline may undergo oxidation and cyclisation to adrenochrome in a multi-step process in which the main oxidant under physiological conditions is the superoxide anion (Bindoli et al. 1992); on the other hand adrenochrome can be reduced to the corresponding semiquinone by NADPH in liver microsomes and by mitochondrial Complex I in bovine heart (Bindoli et al. 1990); a redox cycle is then established in which the semiquinone reacts with O_2 producing superoxide and regenerating adrenochrome (Genova et al. 2006).

Since adrenochrome reduction to the semiquinone is totally insensitive to either rotenone (that acts at the level of FeS centre N2) or p-hydroxymercuribenzoate (that inhibits at the start of the iron-sulphur chain), the site of electron delivery to adrenochrome is presumably FMN. Similar events may also occur with other catecholamines such as dopamine and nor-adrenaline (Fig. 5.3). Such a redox cycle may have deep implications in the pathogenesis of Parkinson's disease (PD).

The selective loss of dopaminergic neurons in substantia nigra in PD might be due to the high content of dopamine itself (Zigmond et al. 2002). The normal enzymatic metabolism of dopamine results in the generation of hydrogen peroxide, and the nonenzymatic autoxidation of dopamine results in the formation of reactive quinones and semiquinones that react to generate hydrogen peroxide, superoxide anions, and hydroxyl radicals. These findings have provided further credence to the proposal that DA metabolism results in oxidative stress (Baumgarten and Grozganovic 2000).

The possible involvement of oxidative stress as an etiological factor of PD is further supported by studies with specific neurotoxins that are extremely potent inducers of parkinsonism in humans and animals. The best studied of these toxins are 6-hydroxydopamine (6-OHDA) and 1-methyl-4-phenylpyridinium (MPP+), the active metabolite of 1-methyl-4-phenyl-1,2,3,6-tetrahydropyridine (MPTP), which selectively destroys catecholaminergic neurons. Both toxins have been shown to generate hydroxyl radicals in the caudate of treated animals (Chiueh et al. 1993). The problem is more complex, however, since also administration of rotenone, an inhibitor of mitochondrial complex I completely unrelated to dopamine, recapitulated the major pathological features of PD, including selective loss of dopaminergic neurons and α-synuclein-positive inclusions, indicating that the inhibition of complex I might be sufficient to trigger PD pathogenesis (Betarbet et al. 2000).

Figure 5.4 summarizes the major sites of ROS production in mitochondria.

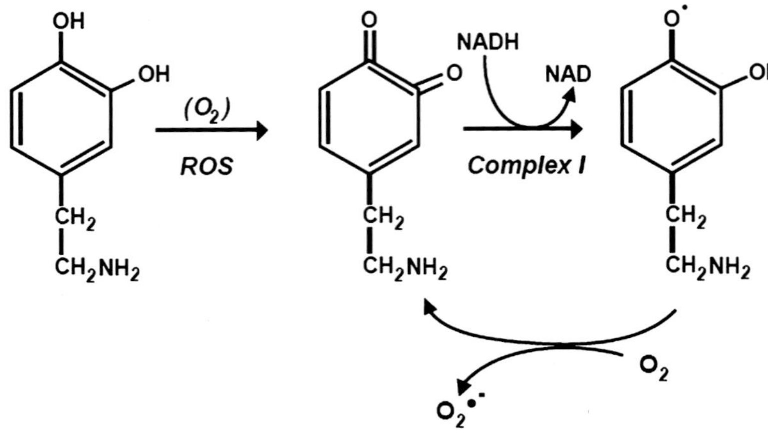

Fig. 5.3 *Redox cycling of catecholamines*: the example of dopamine is shown in the figure. Dopamine is first oxidized to dopaminochrome that is reduced by Complex I by one electron transfer to the semiquinone that auto-oxidizes generating superoxide and perpetuating the cycle

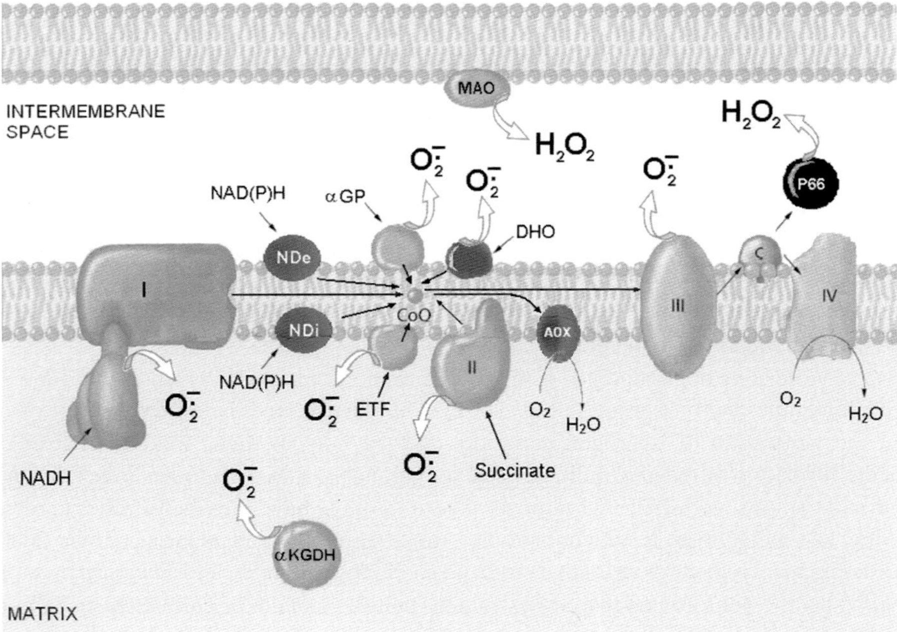

Fig. 5.4 *A schematic drawing of the major sites of ROS generation in mitochondria. I, NADH* ubiquinone oxidoreductase, *II, succinate* ubiquinone oxidoreductase, *III, ubiquinol* cytochrome *c* oxidoreductase, *IV* cytochrome oxidase, *NDi and NDe* internal and external alternative NAD(P)H dehydrogenases, *AOX* alternative oxidase, *α-GP* glycerol-3-phosphate, *ETF* electron transfer flavoprotein, *DHO* dihydroorotate, *CoQ* Coenzyme Q, *c* cytochrome c. *MAO* monoamine oxidase, *α-KGDH* α-ketoglutarate dehydrogenase. See text for details

5.3   ROS and the Supramolecular Organization of the Respiratory Chain

5.3.1   Respiratory Chain Supercomplexes

Circumstantial evidence against a random distribution of respiratory complexes came from the early investigations reporting isolation of Complex I-Complex III (Hatefi et al. 1962b) and Complex II-Complex III units (Yu et al. 1974), indicating that such units may be preferentially associated in the native membrane. The systematic resolution and reconstitution of four respiratory complexes from mitochondria was accomplished by Hatefi et al. (1962a), leading Green (Green and Tzagoloff 1966) to postulate that the overall respiratory activity is the result of both intra-complex electron transfer in solid state between redox components having fixed steric relation and, in addition, of inter-complex electron transfer ensured by rapid diffusion of the mobile components acting as co-substrates, i.e. CoQ and cytochrome c (cyt. c). This proposal was substantially confirmed over the following years, leading to the postulation by Hackenbrock et al. (1986) of the Random Diffusion Model of Electron Transfer. The organization of the respiratory chain has represented a major research subject in the 1970–1980s, culminating with acceptation of the Random Collision Model by the majority of investigators in the field. The model followed the predictions of the fluid mosaic model of membrane structure (Singer and Nicolson 1972) in which random distribution of integral membrane proteins as a two-dimensional oriented solution in the viscous phospholipid bilayer allowed high diffusional freedom in the plane of the membrane.

Much more recently new evidence of multi-complex units in yeast and mammalian mitochondria was obtained introducing Blue Native Polyacrylamide Gel Electrophoresis (BN-PAGE). (Cruciat et al. 2000; Schägger 2001; Schägger and Pfeiffer 2001). In particular, BN-PAGE in digitonin-solubilized mitochondria of *Saccharomyces cerevisiae*, which possesses no Complex I, revealed two bands with apparent masses of ~750 and 1,000 kDa containing the subunits of complexes III and IV. Similar interactions of super-complexes were investigated in bovine heart mitochondria: Complex I-III interactions were apparent from the presence of about 17% of total Complex I in the form of a I_1III_2 super-complex that was found further assembled into two major super-complexes (*respirasomes*) comprising different copy numbers of Complex IV ($I_1III_2IV_1$ and $I_1III_2IV_2$ contain 54% and 9% of total Complex I, respectively).

Only 14–16% of total Complex I was found in free form in the presence of digitonin (Schägger and Pfeiffer 2001); so it seems likely that all Complex I is bound to Complex III in physiological conditions (i.e. in the absence of detergents). Knowing the accurate stoichiometry of oxidative phosphorylation complexes according to Schägger and Pfeiffer (2001), the average ratio I:II:III:IV:V is 1.1:1.3:3:6.7:3.5 therefore it is plausible that approximately one-third of total Complex III in bovine mitochondria is not bound to monomeric Complex I. The fraction of Complex IV in free form represents >85% of total cytochrome oxidase of mitochondria. Associations of Complex II with other complexes of the OXPHOS system could not be identified under the conditions of BN-PAGE so far.

A major $I_1III_2IV_1$ supercomplex was also found in the wild type of the filamentous fungus *P. anserina*, although long-lived mutants deficient in Complex IV and overexpressing the alternative oxidase AOX had a different arrangement including a I_2III_2 supercomplex that revealed to be a major one by a gentle colourless-native PAGE (Krause et al. 2004, 2006). Interestingly, in those mutants the I_2III_2 supercomplex would release electrons from Complex I directly to the CoQ pool and Complex III would be kinetically inactive; presumably its sole function would be in stabilisation of Complex I (Krause et al. 2006).

A distinct structure was observed for all supercomplexes that were investigated, supporting the idea of highly ordered associations of the respiratory supercomplexes and discarding most doubts on artificial interactions. Three-dimensional models of the I_1III_2 supercomplex isolated from plant

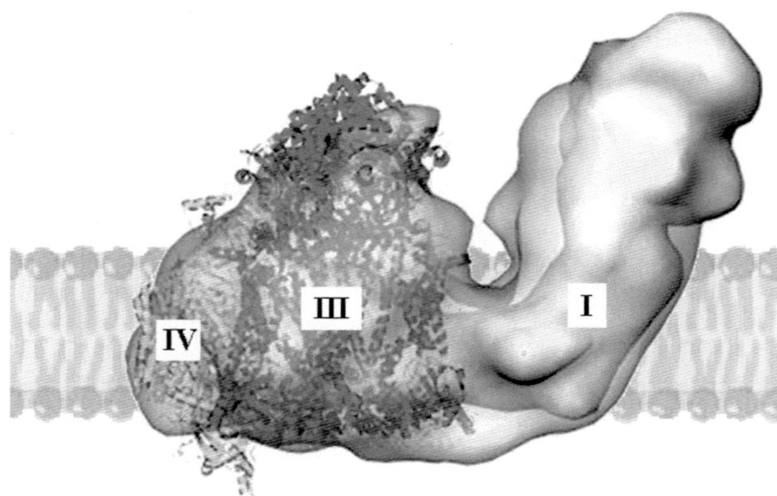

Fig. 5.5 *Model of the respiratory chain supercomplex I₁III₂IV₁ from B. Taurus.* The X-ray structures of dimeric bovine Complex III and monomeric Complex IV were filtered to 20 Å. The negative stain electron microscopy map of bovine Complex I is displayed underneath. The putative location of the membrane is visualised in the background (Redrawn with permission from Schäfer et al. 2007. Copyright © 2007, American Chemical Society)

(Dudkina et al. 2005; Peters et al. 2008) and mammalian mitochondria were generated by comparison of the 2D projection map of the supercomplex, as revealed by Electron Microscopy analysis (EM) and single particle image processing, with known EM and x-ray structures of Complex I and Complex III. In *Arabidopsis* (Dudkina et al. 2005), the specific orientation observed for the two respiratory-chain complexes indicates an interaction within the plane of the membrane whereas the matrix-exposed protein domains are in one another's vicinity but probably do not (strongly) interact. Positions and orientations of all the individual complexes were determined more in detail in a bovine supercomplex consisting of Complex I, dimeric Complex III and Complex IV ($I_1III_2IV_1$); Complex III and IV are both associated with the membrane arm of Complex I and in contact with each other and they showed that the concave face of Complex IV, which is the dimer interface in the x-ray structure, is the contact surface with the rest of the supercomplex (Schäfer et al. 2007). On the basis of the structural information gained from the 3D map (Schäfer et al. 2007), the putative mobile electron carrier (ubiquinone or cytochrome c) binding site of each complex is facing the corresponding binding site of the succeeding complex in the respiratory chain, supporting the notion of a more efficient electron transfer through the supercomplex due to the short diffusion distances of substrates. suggesting a role in substrate channelling (Vonck and Schäfer 2009) (Fig. 5.5).

It has been also proposed (Bultema et al. 2009; Strauss et al. 2008) that the OXPHOS complexes may assemble into higher types of organization, forming row-like megacomplexes composed by supercomplexes as building blocks, which seem to be important for the morphology of the inner mitochondrial membrane.

The characterisation of the super-complexes by biochemical functional analysis is still poor despite the fact that biochemical characterization is required for ascertaining a functional role of the supramolecular associations. Most evidence available has been obtained by indirect observations of deviations from "pool" behaviour of electron transfer and from studies directly aimed to prove substrate channelling by metabolic flux control analysis of electron transfer in mitochondrial membranes (Lenaz and Genova 2007; 2009a, b; 2010), while study of the kinetic properties of isolated supercomplexes is still in its infancy.

The flux control coefficients of the respiratory complexes (I, II, III, IV) were investigated using bovine heart mitochondria and submitochondrial particles devoid of substrate permeability barriers and performing titrations with specific inhibitors of each complex (Bianchi et al. 2004). Both Complex I and III were found to be highly rate-controlling over NADH oxidation ($C_I = 1.06$, $C_{III} = 0.99$), a strong kinetic evidence suggesting the existence of functionally relevant association between the two complexes. On the contrary, Complex IV appears to be randomly distributed ($C_{IV} = 0.26$), although it is possible that if any stable interaction with Complex IV exists in mammalian mitochondria, it escaped detection most likely due to a pronounced abundance of molecules in non-assembled form. Moreover, Complex II is fully rate-limiting for succinate oxidation ($C_{II} = 0.88$, $C_{III} = 0.34$, $C_{IV} = 0.20$), clearly indicating the absence of substrate channelling toward complexes III and IV (Bianchi et al. 2004).

In permeabilized mitochondria from freshly harvested potato tubers, where no activity of the so called alternative oxidase, AOX, is present at the level of ubiquinone (Affourtit et al. 2001), inhibitor titration experiments indicate that Complex III and IV are involved in the formation of a super-complex assembly comprising Complex I (Genova et al. 2008) whereas the alternative dehydrogenases, as well as the molecules of Complex II, are considered to be independent structures within the inner mitochondrial membrane.

More recently Acín-Pérez et al. (2008) in a detailed study on mouse liver mitochondria confirmed the presence of different forms of supercomplexes after solubilization in different detergents and BN-PAGE; at difference with previous studies, some supercomplexes also contained Complex II and ATP synthase (Complex V). One particular subfraction (band 3) contained all Complexes I, II, III and IV and in addition also cytochrome c and CoQ_9. The band was excised from the gel and respiration was measured with a Clark electrode, showing full respiratory activity from either NADH or succinate, that was sensitive to the specific respiratory inhibitors of all involved complexes. Very interestingly the simultaneous inclusion in the oxygen electrode chamber of the individual respiratory complexes did not allow an integrated respiration.

5.3.2 Possible Role of Supercomplex Organisation on Limiting ROS Formation

Although no direct study is available on the effect of supramolecular organisation on ROS production by the respiratory chain, indirect circumstantial evidence suggests that supercomplex assembly may limit the extent of superoxide generation by the respiratory chain. Zhang et al. (1998) showed that reconstitution of succinate CoQ reductase with the bc_1 Complex to yield an active succinate cytochrome c reductase inhibited superoxide formation. Although the relevance of a II-III supercomplex *in vivo* is questionable in the light of what discussed in section 5.3.1, the principle that a tighter organisation of the respiratory enzymes may hide auto-oxidizable prosthetic groups hindering their reaction with oxygen may have a wider application.

Similarly it has been discussed in Sect. 5.2.2.1 that two potential sites for oxygen reduction exist in Complex I, represented by FMN and iron-sulphur cluster N2; controversial results from different laboratories working either on isolated Complex I (Galkin and Brandt 2005; Kussmaul and Hirst 2006) or on mitochondrial membranes (Lenaz et al. 2006a; Fato et al. 2008, 2009) would generally indicate that N2 as a source of ROS would be predominant in membrane particles whereas FMN might become available after Complex I isolation. A reasonable hypothesis is that FMN becomes exposed to oxygen only when Complex I is dissociated from Complex III. This hypothesis is supported by direct studies in our laboratory, showing that the ROS production by Complex I is not stimulated any more by rotenone after addition of the chaotropic agent SCN-, suggesting a shift from a donor close to the rotenone site to one situated uphill (G. Barbero, E. Maranzana, M.L. Genova and G. Lenaz, unpublished).

Although the molecular structure of the individual complexes does not allow to envisage a close apposition of the matrix arm of Complex I, where FMN is localised, with either Complex III or IV (Dudkina et al. 2005; Schäfer et al. 2007; Peters et al. 2008), the actual shape of the $I_1III_2IV_1$ supercomplex from bovine heart (Schäfer et al. 2007) suggests a slightly different conformation of Complex I in the supercomplex with a smaller angle of the matrix arm with the membrane arm showing a higher bending towards the membrane (and presumably Complex III), in line with the notion that Complex I may undergo important conformational changes (Radermacher et al. 2006). Moreover, the observed destabilisation of Complex I in absence of supercomplex (D'Aurelio et al. 2006) may render the 51 kDa subunit containing the FMN more "loose" allowing it to interact with oxygen. The elevated ROS production observed in *P. anserina* respiring on AOX, where the major form of Complex I is a I_2III_2 supercomplex rather than the usual I_1III_2 supercomplex (Krause et al. 2006), is in line with this reasoning, because it is likely that the Complex I dimer may undergo a less tight interaction than a Complex I monomer with the Complex III dimer.

On the basis of their studies on rat brain mitochondria oxidizing different substrates, Panov et al. (2007) suggested that supercomplex organization of Complex I within the chain prevents excessive superoxide production on oxidation of NAD-linked substrates because the efficient channelling helps maintaining the chain in the oxidized state, whereas on succinate oxidation the backward electron flow keeps the centers in Complex I more reduced favoring production of superoxide; to this purpose it is interesting to note that Complex II is not forming a respirasome.

Additional circumstantial evidence on the role of supercomplex organisation may come from the observation that high mitochondrial membrane potential elicits ROS generation, while uncoupling strongly reduces ROS production (Lenaz 2001; Jezek and Hlavata 2005); although likely explanations have been given to these observations, they are compatible with the suggestion by Piccoli et al. (2006) that high membrane potential may dissociate the supercomplexes into the individual units.

The possibility that loss of supercomplex organisation may induce excessive ROS formation has been discussed in previous publications (Lenaz and Genova 2007; 2009a, b; Dencher et al. 2007), but still requires direct investigation.

5.4 ROS in Physiology: ROS and Cell Signalling

It is clear nowadays that ROS (and RNS) act as second messengers (Dröge 2002; Forman et al. 2008) by interfering with the expression of a number of signal transduction pathways and genes. At moderate concentrations ROS play an important role as regulatory mediators in signalling processes. Many of the ROS-mediated responses actually protect the cell against oxidative stress and re-establish redox homeostasis, but several other responses act on a number of different unrelated systems.

Because ROS are oxidants, they influence the redox state of signalling proteins: to produce a redox-dependent modification of an enzyme, enzymatic catalysis is usually required to allow the modification to occur under physiological conditions; for the same reason not all ROS are equally suitable for signal transduction, for instance the $OH°$ radical is too unspecific to undergo catalyzed reactions, while $O_2{}^{•-}$, H_2O_2 and lipid peroxidation derivatives like 4-hydroxy-2-nonenal (HNE) are widely used. Depending on their concentration, ROS can have positive responses (cell proliferation) or negative responses (cell death).

The ROS concentration within cells is largely dependent on the redox state of glutathione (GSH/GSSG) and thioredoxin (Trx) that has two critical cysteine residues. GSH reduces H_2O_2

enzymatically (glutathione peroxidase Gpx) generating the oxidized form GSSG, but the GSH/GSSG ratio also depends on disulphide exchange with proteins catalyzed by *protein disulphide isomerase* (PDI).

$$2GSH + H_2O_2 \rightarrow GSSG + 2H_2O \text{ (Gpx)} \tag{5.17}$$

$$\text{Protein-SH} + GSSG \rightarrow \text{Protein-SSG} + GSH \text{ (PDI)} \tag{5.18}$$

Also Trx is involved in disposing H_2O_2 by Trx peroxidases or *peroxiredoxins* (Prdx):

$$\text{Trx (SH)}_2 + H_2O_2 \rightarrow \text{Trx(S-S)} + 2H_2O \text{ (Prdx)} \tag{5.19}$$

Proteins may be glutathionylated by ROS by a two-step mechanism:

$$\text{Protein-S}^- + H_2O_2 \rightarrow \text{Protein-SO}^- + H_2O \tag{5.20a}$$

$$\text{Protein-SO}^- + GSH \rightarrow \text{Protein-SSG} + OH^- \tag{5.20b}$$

Glutathionylation has been proposed to act as a protective mechanism to prevent overoxidation of cysteines in signal transducing proteins.

Signalling proteins thus modified include phosphoprotein phosphatases (PTPs), Ras, large G-proteins, serine/threonine kinases of the MAPK families, transcription factors as AP-1, NFκB, p53 and others. The effect of oxidants is different with different proteins: PTPs are inhibited, nuclear transcription factors are activated (Valko et al. 2006). Thus for example activation of ERK1/2, Akt, NFκB promote cell survival, whereas activation of c-jun N-terminal kinases (JNK), p38 kinase, p53 would lead to cell cycle arrest and apoptosis. During neoplastic transformation certain signalling pathways bypass the programs leading to apoptosis and senescence.

Beneficial effects of ROS/RNS (e.g. superoxide radical and nitric oxide) occur at low/moderate concentrations and involve physiological roles in cellular responses to noxia, as for example in defence against infectious agents, in the function of a number of cellular signalling pathways, and the induction of a mitogenic response (Valko et al. 2007). Various ROS-mediated actions in fact protect cells against ROS-induced oxidative stress and re-establish or maintain "redox balance" termed also "redox homeostasis". A growing body of evidence shows that ROS within cells act as secondary messengers in intracellular signalling cascades which induce and maintain the oncogenic phenotype of cancer cells, however, ROS can also induce cellular senescence and apoptosis and can therefore function as anti-tumourigenic species.

In addition ROS appear to activate the hypoxia-inducible factor HIF-1α (Kietzmann and Gorlach 2005) by inhibiting prolyl-4-hydroxylase (that hydroxylates a critical proline directing the factor to proteolytic digestion) similarly to what happens in anoxia for lack of O_2 required for HIF hydroxylation. Although some authors believe reactive oxygen species (ROS) to be essential to activate HIF-1 (Kietzmann and Gorlach 2005), others challenge this idea (Gong and Agani 2005), therefore the role of mitochondrial ROS in the regulation of HIF-1 under hypoxia is still controversial (Bell et al. 2008). Moreover, the contribution of functional mitochondria to HIF-1 regulation has also been questioned by others (Srinivas et al. 2001; Vaux et al. 2001; Guo et al. 2008).

Numerous studies have shown that HNE at physiological concentrations stimulates cell proliferation, differentiation and cytoprotective response through affecting multiple signalling pathways: activation of protein kinase C, of the family of MAPK, and of tyrosine kinase receptors, inhibition of Ca-ATPases with consequent accumulation of Ca^{2+} in the cytoplasm, and others (Forman et al. 2008). It is beyond the scope of this chapter to provide a detailed description of the signalling pathways modified by ROS (cf e.g. Finkel (2006) for Ras signalling, also in relation to mitochondria, and Nakano et al. (2006) for the role of ROS in the interplay between nFκB and c-jun N-terminal kinase).

A special mention is needed for the role of mitochondria in relation to ROS signalling (Inoue et al. 2003; Ott et al. 2007). A cross-talk of molecular oxygen, superoxide anion and NO regulates the circulation, energy metabolism and apoptosis, and represents a major defence system against pathogens. Given the fact that mitochondrial ROS appear to be only generated at specific sites and that particular ROS species display a unique chemistry and have specific molecular targets, mitochondria-derived ROS might constitute local regulatory signals (Forkink et al. 2010).

Apoptotic stimuli induce release of protein-bound p66[Shc] (Sect. 5.2.4.1) that interacts with cytochrome c generating H_2O_2. A key player of ROS signalling is p53 that is stabilized by DNA damage by ROS and activates the apoptotic machinery in mitochondria (Liu et al. 2008): it has been shown that ROS act both as an upstream signal for p53 activation and a downstream factor that mediates apoptosis; p53 activation by ROS may be either direct or indirect *via* other signalling pathways.

A key event in apoptosis is the release of proapoptotic factors, among which cytochrome c, from the intermembrane space through permeabilization of the outer membrane. The release mechanisms include interactions of B-cell/lymphoma 2 Bcl2 family proteins with a mitochondria-specific phospholipid, cardiolipin, to cause permeabilization of the outer mitochondrial membrane. Using oxidative lipidomics, Kagan et al. (2005) showed that cardiolipin is the only phospholipid in mitochondria that undergoes early oxidation during apoptosis. The oxidation is catalyzed by a cardiolipin-specific peroxidase activity of cardiolipin-bound cytochrome c. During apoptosis, the complex induces accumulation of cardiolipin oxidation products that are essential for detachment of cyt c from the mitochondrial membrane, induction of permeability transition, and release of proapoptotic factors into the cytosol.

These results provide insight into the role of reactive oxygen species in triggering the cell-death pathway and describe an early role for cytochrome c before caspase activation, and set the basis for the molecular design of specific inhibitors (Borisenko et al. 2008).

Direct action of mitochondrial ROS within mitochondria on the apoptotic cascade can be effected through opening of the *permeability transition pore*, a large channel of the inner membrane activated by various stimuli and involved in outer membrane permeabilization and release of apoptotic factors, such as cytochrome c, from the intermembrane space (Rasola and Bernardi 2007); the pore is activated by ROS presumably via redox-sensitive cysteines (Fruehauf and Meyskens 2007). The role of oxidative stress in apoptosis is out of the scope of this chapter; for important references see Ott et al. (2007), Ryter et al. (2007). Zorov et al. (2005) postulate the presence of intracellular oxygen and ROS sensors and the possible involvement of ROS in the process of fragmentation of mitochondrial reticulum made of long mitochondrial filaments serving in the cell as "electric cables".

Finally mitochondrial damage induced by ROS or other agents and resulting in decreased membrane potential may induce a retrograde response to the nucleus to activate nuclear genes involved in compensatory mitochondrial biogenesis via a decreased mitochondrial Ca^{2+} uptake and concomitant rise in the cytosol (Butow and Avadhani 2004).

5.5 Antioxidant Defences

ROS production and ROS-mediated damage are counteracted in cells by different mechanisms (Zimniak 2008), that will be described here only in general terms.

First, cells have devised mechanisms capable of repairing damage once occurred: the best known example is represented by *DNA repair* that removes oxidative and other lesions from chromosomal and mitochondrial DNA and restores the original strands (Hazra et al. 2007); the mtDNA-repairing systems are usually considered less efficient than those operating in the nucleus (de Souza-Pinto et al. 2008).

Damaged molecules, in particular proteins, are recognized by degrading systems; oxidatively modified proteins are extensively ubiquitinated and directed to the *proteasome* where their complete digestion takes place (Grune et al. 1997; Ghazi et al. 2007). Incapability of the proteasome to digest some proteins or accumulation of insoluble protein aggregates may lead to profound alterations in cells.

Since the mitochondria is a major source of reactive oxygen species, mitochondrial proteins are especially exposed to oxidative modification and elimination of oxidized proteins is crucial for maintaining the integrity of this organelle. Hence, enzymatic reversal of protein oxidation and protein degradation are critical for protein homeostasis while protein maintenance failure has been implicated in the age-related accumulation of oxidized proteins. Within the mitochondrial matrix, the ATP-stimulated mitochondrial Lon protease (Pim-1) is believed to play an important role in the degradation of oxidized protein (Bayot et al. 2010) and age-associated impairment of Lon-like protease activity has been suggested to contribute to oxidized protein build up in the mitochondria. (Bulteau et al. 2006; Ugarte et al. 2009).

Oxidized protein repair in mitochondria is limited to certain oxidation products of the sulfur-containing amino-acids cysteine and methionine. Oxidized protein repair systems, thioredoxin/thioredoxin reductase or glutaredoxin/glutathione/glutathione reductase that catalytically reduce disulfide bridges or sulfenic acids and methionine sulfoxide reductase that reverse methionine sulfoxide back to methionine within proteins, are present in the mitochondrial matrix (Ugarte et al. 2009).

Cellular structures and organelles undergo turnover and after a suitable life time are directed to *autophagy* by lysosomal digestion (Bergamini 2006; Chen and Gibson 2008); autophagy systems recognize damaged organelles, as mitochondria, and preferentially address them to digestion. The term *mitoptosis* was suggested (Skulachev 2006) to define the removal of oxidatively damaged mitochondria.

In a way, *apoptosis* is an extreme devise to eliminate cells where extensive damage has taken place, rather than allowing them to propagate the oxidative stress to other cells, *e.g.* by different kinds of plasma membrane NAD(P)H oxidases (Lambeth 2007; Cho and Morré 2009). The notion that ROS may activate apoptosis through p53 and the mitochondrial permeability transition is in line with this assumption.

Other defence mechanisms operate to reduce ROS production. In mitochondria, UCPs have been suggested to fulfil this function producing mild uncoupling and limiting ROS generation by the respiratory chain. Also substrate supply down-regulation and decrease of pO_2 would limit ROS production (Barja 2007).

An opposite strategy of defence is biosynthesis of macromolecules resistant to oxidative stress (Pamplona and Barja 2007). For instance, the presence of less unsaturated fatty acyl chains in membrane lipids represents a powerful defence against lipid peroxidation. Likewise, lowering the amount of components highly susceptible to oxidation, as methionine in proteins and guanine in nucleic acids render them more resistant to alteration. On the other hand, the presence of a non essential methionine in proteins may represent a sink against ROS damage (Levine et al. 1996): it was shown that a mtDNA polymorphism (mt5178C $\rightarrow$ A) substituting Leu with Met at position 237 in Complex I subunit ND2 confers a longevity trait (Tanaka et al. 1998) possibly by reducing oxidative damage to other more functional amino acids.

Finally, cells and body fluids contain molecules that neutralize or scavenge ROS, collectively termed *antioxidants*. Antioxidants may be divided into antioxidant enzymes that neutralize ROS by forming less toxic species, and antioxidant small molecules: the latter may either be endogenous metabolites and biosynthesised cofactors, or exogenous molecules taken up from the diet. Certain antioxidants are able to regenerate other antioxidants establishing an *antioxidant network* (Sies et al. 2005).

5.5.1 *Enzymatic Antioxidants*

Superoxide dismutase catalyzes the dismutation of superoxide to H_2O_2 and oxygen (Eq. 5.2); it exists in three isoforms in humans: cytosolic Cu,Zn-SOD, mitochondrial Mn-SOD, and extracellular SOD (Landis and Tower 2005). SOD must work in concomitance with enzymes removing H_2O_2, otherwise accumulation of the latter in presence of reduced metal ions would activate the Fenton reaction (Eq. 5.5).

The systems capable of removing H_2O_2 are represented by catalase and peroxidases. *Catalase* (Mates et al. 1999) is localized in peroxisomes and is very efficient having one of the highest turnover numbers known for an enzyme:

$$2H_2O_2 \rightarrow 2H_2O + O_2 \tag{5.21}$$

Although mitochondria in most cells appear to lack catalase (Bai and Cederbaum 2001), the enzyme has been detected in mitochondria from rat heart (Radi et al. 1991) and rat liver (Salvi et al. 2007); overexpression of mitochondrial catalase in a HepG2 cell line was able to protect cells from oxidative injury induced by hydrogen peroxide and antimycin A (Bai and Cederbaum 2001).

Among the arsenal of antioxidants and detoxifying enzymes existing in mitochondria, mitochondrial glutathione (mGSH) emerges as the main line of defense for the maintenance of the appropriate mitochondrial redox environment to avoid or repair oxidative modifications leading to mitochondrial dysfunction and cell death. mGSH importance is based not only on its abundance, but also on its versatility to counteract hydrogen peroxide, lipid hydroperoxides, or xenobiotics, mainly as a cofactor of enzymes such as glutathione peroxidase or glutathione-S-transferase (GST) (Marí et al. 2009).

Glutathione peroxidase (GPx) exists in two main forms, one selenium-dependent and the other not (Mates et al. 1999); humans have four different Se-GPx. The enzyme catalyzes Eq. 5.17 using H_2O_2 as an oxidant for GSH, but can also use organic peroxides:

$$2GSH + ROOH \rightarrow GSSG + ROH + H_2O \tag{5.22}$$

GSH must be regenerated by *glutathione reductase* (GR) using NADPH as the reductant; the major source of NADPH for cytosolic GR is the pentose phosphate pathway, while in mitochondria is energy linked $NADH/NADP^+$ transhydrogenation.

$$GSSG + NADPH + H^+ \rightarrow 2\ GSH + NADP^+ \tag{5.23}$$

Perhaps peroxiredoxins (Prdx), catalyzing reaction in Eq. 5.19, are the most important peroxide-removing systems (Rhee et al. 2005). *Trx reductase* is a Se-enzyme that regenerates reduced Trx and exists in two isoforms, one cytosolic and the other mitochondrial (Conrad 2009).

5.5.2　Non-enzymatic Antioxidants

Some of these are water-soluble and act in the cell's soluble fraction or in plasma, others being lipid-soluble act within membranes, while amphipathic molecules can act in both environments.

Vitamin C (ascorbic acid) is water-soluble and cooperates with lipid-soluble Vitamin E to regenerate α-tocopherol from tocopheroxyl radical produced during the Vitamin E radical scavenging activity; the product of the reaction is a very stable ascorbate radical ($Asc^{\circ-}$).

Although excessive doses of ascorbate may be pro-oxidant, physiological amounts have always been proven to be antioxidant even in presence of metal ions (Valko et al. 2006).

Vitamin E includes eight different derivatives, of which *α-tocopherol* is the most potent in humans; it is the most important lipid-soluble antioxidant, that is distributed in all cellular membranes including mitochondria as a function of lipid content (Saito et al. 2009) and mainly prevents lipid peroxidation; its dietary supplementation is beneficial, however high doses may be pro-oxidant (Valko et al. 2006). Its reaction with lipid radicals (mainly peroxyl radicals) generates the α-tocopheroxyl radical that can be re-reduced to α-tocopherol by ascorbate in the water phase or by *reduced Coenzyme Q* ($CoQH_2$) in the lipid phase. $CoQH_2$ can also directly scavenge radicals like LOO° generating its semiquinone form (Ernster and Dallner 1995)

$$QH_2 + LOO^\circ \rightarrow Q^{\circ-} + LOOH \tag{5.24}$$

Coenzyme Q (ubiquinone, CoQ) is an essential electron carrier in the mitochondrial respiratory chain, but is also present in serum lipoproteins, endomembranes and the plasma membrane (Turunen et al. 2004). Chemically, CoQ is constituted by a benzoquinone ring and a lipid side chain with several isoprenoid units, its number being species specific. Its redox reactions can be driven either by the simultaneous transfer of two electrons in a single step, or by two sequential steps of one electron transfer through a partially reduced semiquinone intermediate. CoQ is the only lipidic antioxidant that is synthesized in mammals, and its biosynthesis is a complex process which involves the participation of at least eight gene products.

Besides the mitochondrial respiratory chain, several enzymes catalyze CoQ reduction to achieve its antioxidant reduced state in eukaryotic cells. *NADH-cytochrome b_5 reductase* can reduce CoQ through a one-electron reaction mechanism (Arroyo et al. 1998). The soluble enzyme *NAD(P) H:quinone oxidoreductase 1 (NQO1, DT-diaphorase)* can reduce quinones by a two-electron reaction and maintains the reduced state of CoQ_{10} *in vitro* (Beyer et al. 1996). A distinct cytosolic *NADPH-CoQ reductase* different from NQO1 has been also described (Takahashi et al. 1995).

Glutathione GSH besides scavenging H_2O_2 enzymatically can also scavenge radicals directly forming thiyl radicals that can dimerize generating oxidised glutathione GSSG:

$$GSH + R^\circ \rightarrow GS^\circ + RH \tag{5.25}$$

$$GS^\circ + GS^\circ \rightarrow GSSG \tag{5.26}$$

GSH is also able to regenerate vitamins C and E to their active forms.

Another dithiol antioxidant is *lipoic acid* in its reduced form dihydrolipoic acid: it is able to quench ROS and to regenerate other antioxidants as described above.

Finally there is a great number of *dietary antioxidants* contained in fruit and vegetables that are not vitamins or part of coenzymes, such as *carotenoids* and *flavonoids*. They may act as quenchers of singlet oxygen and peroxyl radicals forming more stable radicals that do not propagate and may act as chain terminators by reacting with other radicals (Valko et al. 2006).

To the end of 2011 PubMed counts 4478 reviews on dietary antioxidants. Nutritional compounds which display anti-inflammatory and antioxidant effects have specific applications in preventing oxidative stress induced injury which characterizes their pathogenesis (Soory 2009). Patient control over diet and disease has been demonstrated in diabetes mellitus, cardiovascular disease, rheumatology, carcinogenesis and other diseases. Polyphenolic compounds are ubiquitous dietary components, mainly flavonoids and tannins. Specific polyphenols are effective in scavenging reactive oxygen and reactive nitrogen species. Their overall effect is protective in overcoming damaging effects of chronic diseases and in delaying the degenerative effects of ageing.

Antioxidants are able to modulate genes associated with metabolism, stress defence, drug metabolizing enzymes, detoxification and transporter proteins. Nutrients interact with the human genome (*Nutrigenetics*) to modulate molecular pathways that may become disrupted, resulting in an increased risk of developing various chronic diseases (El-Sohemy 2007). Genetic polymorphisms affect the metabolism of dietary factors, which in turn affects the expression of genes involved in a number of important metabolic processes. Genetic polymorphisms in the targets of nutrient action such as receptors, enzymes or transporters could alter molecular pathways that influence the physiological response to dietary interventions. Among the candidate genes with functional variants that affect nutrient metabolism are those that code for xenobiotic-metabolizing enzymes (also called drug-metabolizing enzymes). These enzymes are involved in the phase I and II biotransformation reactions that produce metabolites with either increased or decreased biological activity compared to the parent compound. A number of dietary factors are known to alter the expression of these genes that, in turn, metabolize a vast array of foreign chemicals including dietary factors such as antioxidants, vitamins, phytochemicals, caffeine, sterols, fatty acids and alcohol.

5.6   ROS in Pathology

5.6.1   Effects of ROS on Cellular Molecules and Cellular Structures with Particular Emphasis on Mitochondria

All biomolecules in the cell are targets of ROS and undergo chemical modifications that accumulate with age (Diplock 1994; Lenaz 1998): protein carbonylation and methionine oxidation, advanced glycation end-products (AGE), lipid peroxidation, and nucleotide modifications. However, it is not completely understood which species are responsible for the damage *in vivo* and how the increased availability of ROS translates into the accumulation of specific oxidative damage (Schoneich 1999): for instance some proteins are better targets than others for oxidative damage.

The damages induced by ROS depend on the extent and specificity of their reactivity (Halliwell 2006): if two free radicals meet, they can join their unpaired electrons to form non-radical products; this may lead to loss of reactivity, but in some cases the products may be even more dangerous than the reactants, *e.g.* the reaction of $O2\bullet^-$ and $NO\bullet$ generates the toxic peroxynitrite (Eq. 5.6).

When a radical meets a non-radical species, several options are possible (Halliwell 2006). If the radical is reactive enough it attacks the non-radical generating a new radical and initiating a chain reaction. There are several types of reaction: (i) The radical can add to the non-radical, forming an adduct still having an unpaired electron. (ii) The radical may behave as a reductant, donating a single electron to the non-radical. (iii) The radical may be an oxidant, taking a single electron from the non-radical. (iv) A radical may abstract a hydrogen atom from a C–H bond, for example $OH\bullet$ can abstract $H\bullet$ from a hydrocarbon forming water and a carbon-centred radical.

5.6.1.1   Lipid Peroxidation

The polyunsaturated fatty acyl chains of phospholipids are very sensitive to oxidation by ROS (Balazy and Nigam 2003). Since subcellular membranes contain high amounts of polyunsaturated fatty acids (PUFA), formation of carbon-centred radicals within membranes results in peroxidation of fatty acids.

The overall process of lipid peroxidation can be divided into three stages: (a) *Initiation, i.e.* extraction of hydrogen from allylic or bis-allylic positions of PUFA; carbon radicals in presence of O_2 generate peroxyl radicals ($LOO\bullet$) and random mixtures of cyclic peroxides and hydroperoxides. The initiating species may be the $OH\bullet$ radical, but also a Fe^{2+}-O_2-Fe^{3+} complex or a ADP-Fe^{2+} complex (Valko et al. 2006). (b) *Radical chain propagation*: Peroxyl radicals may react with side chains of PUFA, yielding hydroperoxides ROOH and other carbon radicals, thus initiating a chain reaction. Phospholipid hydroperoxides may be cleaved by phospholipase A_2 to yield the free fatty acid hydroperoxides (Williams and Gottlieb 2002). In addition, hydroperoxides can further degrade to alkoxyl ($LO\bullet$), alkyl ($L\bullet$) or $OH\bullet$ radicals, thereby initiating another cycle of chain reactions. (c) *Termination:* when a radical meets another radical or an antioxidant the chain reaction is terminated. However peroxyl radicals can react with O_2 by cyclisation to produce a cyclic peroxide, that can undergo a second cyclisation to form a bicyclic peroxide and then an endoperoxide; the latter is cleaved to produce aldehyde products, the major being *malondialdehyde (MDA)* and *4-hydroxy-2-nonenal (4-HNE)*, but including also alkadienals, crotonaldehyde, acrolein etc., all cumulatively designated as *advanced lipid peroxidation end products (ALE)* (Negre-Salvayre et al. 2008). Oxidation of ω-6 PUFA yields 4-HNE, while oxidation of ω-3 PUFA yields 4-hydroxy-2-hexanal.

MDA is a volatile molecule that reacts via Schiff base formation with amino groups of protein, lipid, and DNA. In addition MDA also reacts with DNA bases forming adducts that are mutagenic (Marnett 1999). 4-HNE is more reactive than MDA with proteins; in addition the modified proteins are not degraded efficiently by the proteasome (Friguet and Szweda 1997).

Other non-enzymatic products of arachidonic acid oxidation are *isoprostanes* that are formed *in situ* within phospholipids and are then removed by action of phospholipase A2; isoprostanes are similar to prostaglandins, exert numerous biological functions, but also may form protein adducts with lysine side chains. Isoprostanes are used as indicators of oxidative stress (Morrow 2005; Dalle Donne et al. 2006).

Another class of reactive ALE precursors is represented by α-oxoaldehydes (methylglyoxal and glyoxal); they are basically derived from sugars in hyperglycaemic conditions, however they are also generated from lipid peroxidation (glyoxal) or the catabolism of glycerol and ketone bodies (methylglyoxal) (Negre-Salvayre et al. 2008). Methylglyoxal metabolism is also linked to ROS production both in the generation and in the degradation of this compound (Kalapos 2008).

The initial H• abstraction from polyunsaturated fatty acids can occur at different points of the carbon chain; thus the peroxidation of arachidonic acid (20:4) gives 6 lipid hydroperoxides, eicosapentaenoic acid (20:5) can give 8, and docosahexaenoic acid (22:6) 10, plus high numbers of cyclic peroxides and isoprostanes (Halliwell 2006).

Cholesterol can be peroxidised at different positions (5α, 6α, 6β, 7α, 7β) by free radical or singlet oxygen attack. Subsequent breakage of the B ring will produce aldehydes (secosterols), that induce protein misfolding (Bieschke et al. 2006). A common product in atherosclerotic plaques is 27-hydroxy-cholesterol.

Metal ions may split lipid hydroperoxides to produce alkoxyl (LO•) and more peroxyl (LOO•) radicals, that will continue the chain reaction.

$$LOOH + Fe^{2+} \rightarrow Fe^{3+} + LO\bullet + OH^- \tag{5.27}$$

$$LOOH + Fe^{3+} \rightarrow Fe^{2+} + LOO\bullet + H^+ \tag{5.28}$$

Lipid hydroperoxides have relatively long lifetimes, compared with lipid radicals; for this reason they can easily translocate to relatively long distances (Girotti 2008); a well known example is the transbilayer movement of peroxidized phosphatidyl serine in cells destined to apoptosis; in addition ROOH can move from one to another membrane within a single cell, or from the plasma membrane of a cell to that of another cell or to a lipoprotein (Girotti 2008). Movement of peroxides from one membrane to another may greatly expand their range of toxic damage, particularly if they move to a compartment richer in iron and/or poor in antioxidants (Vila et al. 2000).

A distinct lipid modification is the reaction of the *cis* double bonds of arachidonic acid with the nitrogen dioxide radical (•NO$_2$) forming nitroeicosanoid derivatives that can then split to four different *trans* isomers; these compounds have a number of biological effects, including induction of apoptosis, and may be regarded as selective biomarkers of nitro-oxidative stress (Balazy and Chemtob 2008).

At the cellular level lipid peroxidation induces changes in cell membranes with modification of their permeability and alterations of lipid-dependent enzymes. This latter effect is well studied in mitochondria where oxidation of cardiolipin induces decrease of activity of respiratory complexes (Paradies et al. 2000, 2002) and loss of super-complex organization (Lenaz et al. 2007, 2010; Lenaz and Genova 2010). Wenz et al. (2009) suggest that cardiolipin stabilizes respiratory supercomplex formation by neutralizing the charges of lysine residues in the vicinity of the presumed interaction domain between cytochrome bc$_1$ complex and cytochrome c oxidase. Even moderate oxidative stress by hypoxia/reoxygenation causes a decrease in cardiolipin that is paralleled by a decrease in active respiration of isolated rat heart mitochondria.(Wiswedel et al. 2010).

5.6.1.2 Protein Oxidation

Hydroxyl radicals produced by ionizing radiation or by the Fenton reaction are able to attack the polypeptide backbone of proteins to form a carbon-centred radical which may react with O$_2$ to form peroxyl radical (Stadtman 1992, 2004). The peroxyl radical is then converted to alkyl peroxide by reaction with protonated superoxide $\cdot HO_2$. The alkoxyl derivatives of proteins may then undergo peptide bond cleavage. In absence of radiation or metal ions, superoxide and H_2O_2 would be inactive.

The side chains of all amino acids in proteins are susceptible to oxidation; however some residues like proline, histidine, arginine, lysine, and cysteine are highly sensitive to oxidation by metal ions; thus it is believed that Fe^{2+} binding to the above residues undergoes the Fenton reaction with H_2O_2 to yield $OH\cdot$ at those specific sites.

The amino acid residues that are most vulnerable to attack by ROS are arginine, glutamate, histidine, tyrosine, valine, cysteine, proline, threonine and methionine (Stadtman 2004). Cysteine and methionine residues are particularly susceptible to oxidation by ROS. The oxidation of methionine residues by ROS forms methionine sulphoxide Met-SO. The oxidation of the amino acid residues, as well as the glycation of lysine groups (cf Sect. 3.3) generates carbonyl groups: protein carbonylation is the most widely used marker of protein oxidation both *in vitro* and in pathological conditions (Dalle Donne et al. 2006).

Peroxynitrite formed by reaction of $NO\cdot$ with $O_2\cdot^-$ may react with cysteine SH groups, oxidizes methionine to methionine sulphoxide, and reacts with tyrosine forming 3-nitrotyrosine (another important marker of oxidative protein damage).

Protein oxidation by ROS is associated with the formation of many different kinds of inter- and intra-protein cross-linkages, such as by addition of a lysine amino group to a carbonyl group of the oxidized protein, by interaction of two carbon-centred radicals of polypeptide backbones, by oxidation of cysteine residues to form S-S cross-links, or by oxidation of tyrosine residues to form tyr-tyr cross-links. The cysteine S-S cross-links are reversible since they can be repaired by disulphide exchange reactions. Oxidation of cysteine residues can also lead to reversible formation of mixed disulphides particularly with glutathione (GSH) (S-glutathionylation); S-glutathionylated proteins accumulate under conditions of oxidative stress (Dalle Donne et al. 2005).

Besides being altered by direct oxidation by ROS, proteins may be *covalently* modified by products of lipid peroxidation, such as the reactive aldehydes described in Sect. 5.6.1.1 (Bieschke et al. 2006).

High levels of free radicals produced by the mitochondrial respiratory chain, with subsequent damage to mitochondria have been implicated in a large and growing number of diseases. The underlying pathology of these diseases is oxidative damage to mitochondrial DNA, lipids and proteins which accumulate over time to produce a metabolic deficiency. Murray et al. (2008) developed an antibody based immunocapture array for many important mitochondrial proteins involved in free radical production, detoxification and mitochondrial energy production, and analyzed the proteomic differences in oxidative phosphorylation enzymes between human heart and liver tissues, cells grown in media promoting aerobic versus anaerobic metabolism, and the catalytic/proteomic effects of mitochondria exposed to oxidative stress. Protein oxidation is identified as carbonyl formation arising from reactive oxygen species and 3-nitrotyrosine as a marker of reactive nitrogen species.

A recent proteomic study has been aimed to detect modified mitochondrial proteins in Alzheimer disease (AD), an age-related neurodegenerative disorder, characterized histopathologically by the presence of senile plaques (SP), neurofibrillary tangles and synapse loss in selected brain regions. In the mitochondria isolated from AD brain, Abeta oligomers that correlated with the reported increased oxidative stress markers in AD have been reported. The markers of oxidative stress have been localized in the brain regions of AD that show pathological hallmarks of this disease, suggesting the possible role of Abeta in the initiation of the free-radical mediated process and consequently to the build up oxidative stress and AD pathogenesis. Using redox proteomics Sultana and Butterfield (2009) found a number of oxidatively modified brain proteins that are directly in or are associated with the mitochondrial proteome, consistent with a possible involvement of the mitochondrial targeted oxidatively modified proteins in AD progression or pathogenesis.

5.6.1.3 Advanced Glycation end Products (AGE)

AGE are a group of heterogeneous compounds that form constantly in the body but are markedly increased in conditions of hyperglycaemia and oxidative stress (Vlassara 2005). AGE are the end-products of the *Maillard reaction* between sugars and proteins: a sugar reacts with a protein amino group to form a Schiff base then stabilized in the form of an Amadori product and its subsequent rearrangement leads to formation of stable and irreversible AGE compounds.

The final step of the Maillard reaction is driven by oxidative stress, and AGEs accelerate oxidation, thus favouring their own production. Protein adducts also arise from lipid oxidation and are often included among AGE, although they should be more properly called ALE.

For the process of AGE formation glucose is the predominant substrate, but other sugars as fructose, glucose-6-phosphate, glyceraldehyde-3-phosphate, ascorbate, and methylglyoxal may react with proteins and produce chemically distinct AGE (Bohlender et al. 2004; Soskic et al. 2008). AGE-modified proteins are recognized by specific receptors (RAGE) whose activation is responsible for the cellular effects of AGE and their pathological consequences (Wendt et al. 2003). Binding and activation of RAGE can promote further oxidative stress and AGE formation via the NADPH oxidase pathway (Peppa et al. 2008).

The diet is a major source of AGE and dietary AGE are called glycotoxins: exaggerated intake of thermally treated food may exert oxidative stress and pathological consequences (Vlassara and Striker 2007).

AGE are also formed in mitochondria. Hamelin et al. (2007) observed a significant decrease in the respiratory activity of rat liver mitochondria with aging, and an increase in the advanced glycation endproduct-modified protein level in the mitochondrial matrix. Western blot analysis of the glycated protein pattern after 2D electrophoresis revealed that only a restricted set of proteins was modified. Within this set they identified, by mass spectrometry, proteins connected with the urea cycle, and especially glutamate dehydrogenase, which is markedly modified in older animals. Moreover, mitochondrial matrix extracts exhibited a significant decrease in glutamate dehydrogenase activity and altered allosteric regulation with age. Altogether, these results showed that advanced glycation endproduct modifications selectively affect mitochondrial matrix proteins, particularly glutamate dehydrogenase, a crucial enzyme at the interface between tricarboxylic acid and urea cycles. Furthermore, these results suggest a role for such intracellular glycation in age-related dysfunction of mitochondria.

5.6.1.4 DNA Damage

The hydroxyl radical reacts with all components of the DNA molecule damaging the purine and pyrimidine bases and the deoxyribose backbone (Dizdaroglu et al. 2002; Cooke et al. 2003): permanent modifications of genetic material are the first step involved in mutagenesis, cancerogenesis and ageing. To date more than 100 products have been identified from the oxidation of DNA, including single- or double-strand DNA breaks, purine, pyrimidine and deoxyribose modifications, and DNA cross-links (Valko et al. 2006). DNA damage can result in either arrest or induction of transcription, induction of signal transduction pathways, replication errors and genome instability.

The OH• radical is able to add to double bonds of DNA bases and to abstract an H atom from the methyl group of thymine and each of the C atoms of deoxyribose; the formation of *8-hydroxydeoxy-guanine* (8-OH-dG) is the most prominent example among over 20 base modifications.

8-OH-dG is the most easily formed base alteration, is mutagenic and carcinogenic and is a good biomarker of oxidative DNA damage; this modification occurs in one in 10^5 G residues in normal cells, but increases in oxidative stress, ageing and a number of diseases (Halliwell and Gutteridge 1999). Mitochondrial DNA is more susceptible than nuclear DNA to oxidative damage (Ott et al. 2007) due to the close proximity of the respiratory chain and the lack of protective histones; the incidence of 8-OH-dG is 10-20-fold higher in mtDNA than in nuclear DNA. The oxidative damage to mtDNA can lead to deletions or other rearrangements (Meissner 2007). In particular the 4,977 base pair deletion ("*common deletion*") has been studied in many tissues and found to increase with ageing (Lenaz et al. 2006b).

Also products of lipid peroxidation as MDA can react with DNA bases forming adducts (Marnett 1999).

The "*Mitochondrial Theory of Aging*" (Linnane et al. 1989) is based on the hypothesis that mitochondrial DNA somatic mutations, caused by accumulation of oxygen radicals damage, induce alterations of the OXPHOS machinery culminating in an energetic failure that is at the basis of cellular senescence. Moreover a *vicious circle* (Ozawa 1997) can be established since the accumulated damage to the respiratory chain would enhance ROS generation. Many reports (reviewed in Lenaz et al. 2006b) demonstrate that the rate of production of ROS from mitochondria increases with age in mammalian tissues and in fibroblasts during replicative cell senescence, considered to represent a plausible model of in vivo aging (Hayflick 2003).

Compelling evidence for the mitochondrial theory of aging derives from several observations: the strong negative correlation existing between expected lifespan and rate of ROS production of different species (Sohal et al. 1995; Barja and Herrero 2000), within the same species under different activity conditions (Yan and Sohal 2000), and between lifespan and membrane lipid unsaturation (Pamplona et al. 2002). Furthermore the demonstration that caloric restriction while prolonging lifespan in mammals reduces ROS production (Barja 2004) provides additional points in favour of the role of ROS in aging.

A large number of large-scale deletions, point mutations, and tandem duplications have been observed in tissues of aged individuals (Ozawa 1997; Lee and Wei 1997; Wei and Lee 2002). Michikawa et al. (1999) reported that a T414G transversion in the D-loop of mtDNA is accumulated in skin fibroblasts from old subjects, while two different point mutations (A189G and T408A) accumulate in the D-loop in muscle of old individuals (Wang et al. 2001). These mutations are located in the control region of mtDNA and may impair its replication and transcription.

A minimal threshold level of 50–95% mutated mtDNA is usually necessary to impair respiratory chain function, depending on the type of mutation and the tissue affected (Rossignol et al. 2003). Since the proportions of mutated mtDNA within aging human tissues rarely exceed 1%, it has been questioned how these levels may cause significant bioenergetic effects. Hayakawa et al. (1996) using 180 kinds of PCR primers found that mtDNA in elderly subjects is extensively fragmented in minicircles with different sizes. As a result, the amount of mtDNA mutations may reach such a high level to cause significant impairment of OXPHOS. Furthermore, mutated mtDNA molecules may be distributed unevenly among the cells of affected tissues in a mosaic pattern of mtDNA segregation (Linnane et al. 1995) . Exponential accumulation of mutated mtDNA during life suggests that there is a preferential replication of the mutant genomes.

Point mutations and deletions of mtDNA accumulate in a variety of tissues during ageing in humans, monkeys and rodents (Wallace 2005; Lenaz et al. 2006b) are unevenly distributed and can accumulate clonally in certain cells, causing a mosaic pattern of respiratory chain deficiency in tissues such as heart, skeletal muscle and brain. In terms of the ageing process, their possible causative effects have been intensely debated because of their low abundance and purely correlative connection with ageing. This question was addressed experimentally by creating homozygous knock-in mice that express a proof-reading-deficient version of PolgA, the nucleus-encoded catalytic subunit of mtDNA polymerase (Trifunovic et al. 2004), showing that the knock-in mice develop an mtDNA mutator phenotype with a threefold to fivefold increase in the levels of point mutations, as well as increased amounts of deleted mtDNA. This increase in somatic mtDNA mutations is associated with reduced lifespan and premature onset of ageing-related phenotypes thus providing a causative link between mtDNA mutations and ageing phenotypes in mammals. Even if these mice do not have an enhanced

ROS production (Trifunovic 2006; Trifunovic and Larsson 2008), it is likely that this effect results from the severe extent of mutation in the mutator mice, while the *natural* way to induce mutations is ROS attack.

5.6.2 Involvement of Mitochondrial ROS in Pathology

An overwhelming body of evidence accumulated in the last decades has demonstrated that mitochondria have a central role in the development of the aging process and in the etiology and pathogenesis of most major chronic diseases (Lenaz 1998; Balaban et al. 2005; Wallace 2005; Chan 2006; Lenaz et al. 2006a; McFarland et al. 2007; Zeviani and Carelli 2007; Di Mauro and Schon 2008; Reeve et al. 2008); the involvement of mitochondria in disease, that has generated the term "Mitochondrial Medicine" (Di Mauro et al. 2006; Smeitink et al. 2006; Koene and Smeitink 2009), has been ascribed to their central role in production of ROS and to the damaging effect of ROS on these organelles. In particular, damage to mitochondrial DNA (mtDNA) would induce alterations of the polypeptides encoded by mtDNA in the respiratory complexes, with consequent decrease of electron transfer activity, leading to further production of ROS, and thus establishing a vicious circle of oxidative stress and energetic decline (Ozawa 1997; Lenaz et al. 1999). This fall of mitochondrial energetic capacity is considered to be the cause of ageing and age-related degenerative diseases (Wallace 2005; Lenaz et al. 2006a; Kukat and Trifunovic 2009; Gruber et al. 2008), although the picture is further complicated by the complex interplay and cross-talk with nuclear DNA and the rest of the cell (Calabrese et al. 2004; Ryan and Hoogenraad 2007). This vicious circle might be broken by agents capable to prevent a chain reaction of ROS formation and damage, such as CoQ in its reduced form (Ernster and Dallner 1995).

It is easy to foresee a deep implication of super-complex organization as a missing link between oxidative stress and energy failure (Lenaz and Genova 2007). It is tempting in fact to speculate that oxidative stress induces dissociation of Complex I-III interactions, with loss of facilitated electron channeling and resumption of the less efficient pool behavior of the free ubiquinone molecules. In such regard, the loss of efficient electron transfer observed in experimental heart failure together with the loss of super-complex organization (Rosca et al. 2008) appears as a clear indication of the deleterious consequence of lack of supramolecular organization.

As predicted by Lenaz and Genova (2007), dissociation of super-complexes might have further deleterious consequences, such as disassembly of Complex I and loss of electron transfer and/or proton translocation; it cannot be excluded that the consequent alteration of electron transfer may elicit further induction of ROS generation. The numerous observations that Complex III (and Complex IV) alterations prevent proper assembly of Complex I (Stroh et al. 2004; Schägger et al. 2004; Acin-Perez et al. 2004; Blakely et al. 2005; D'Aurelio et al. 2006; Diaz et al. 2006) has therefore deep pathological implications beyond the field of genetic mitochondrial cytopathies. Following this line of thought, the different susceptibility of different types of cells and tissues to ROS damage may depend, among other reasons, on the extent and tightness of super-complex organization of their respiratory chains, that depend on their hand on phospholipids content and composition of their mitochondrial membranes (Lenaz et al. 2010). In this regard, cardiolipin appears an essential prerequisite for supercomplex stabilization (Lange et al. 2001; Zhang et al. 2002; Pfeiffer et al. 2003). It has been shown that respiratory supercomplexes are destabilized in Barth syndrome, a genetic disease characterized by a disturbance of cardiolipin metabolism (McKenzie et al. 2006).

These changes may have deep metabolic consequences, as depicted in the scheme in Fig. 5.6: an initial enhanced ROS generation due to different possible reasons and originating in different districts of the cell besides mitochondria would induce super-complex disorganization eventually leading to possible decrease of Complex I assembly; both the lack of efficient electron channeling and the loss of Complex I would decrease NAD-linked respiration and ATP synthesis.

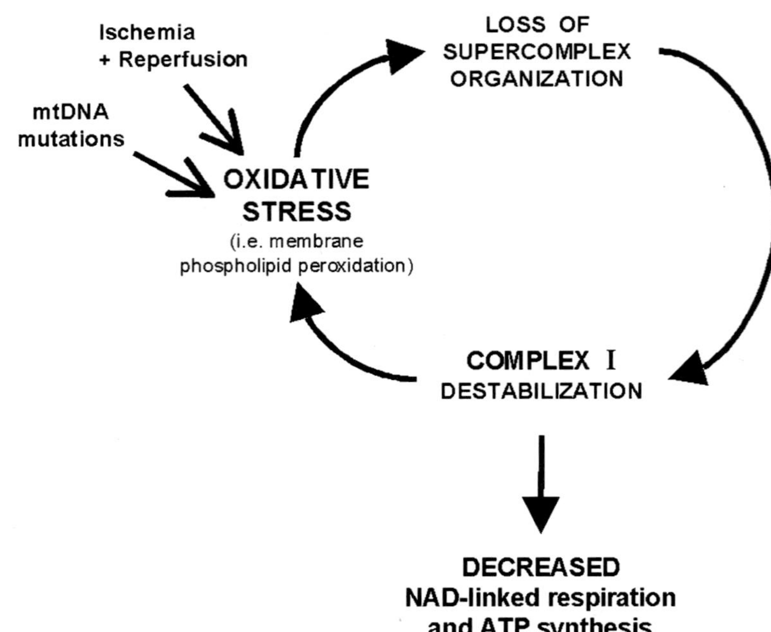

Fig. 5.6 *Scheme showing the possible effects of loss of supercomplex organisation on mitochondrial function.* Membrane phospholipid peroxidation and consequent loss of supercomplex organisation may occur due to oxidative stress induced by genetic changes (i.e. mitochondrial DNA mutations) or by exogenous factors (i.e. ischemia and reperfusion); the ensuing destabilization of Complex I results in OXPHOS deficiency and further oxidative stress. As a consequence of these changes, cells may be forced to rely on glycolysis for energy production. See text for explanations

A study on human neutrophil mitochondria (Van Raam et al. 2008) clearly points out the consequences of lack of super-complex organization. In neutrophils, mitochondria are present but their respiration with NAD-linked substrates is not apparently used for ATP synthesis; the activity of individual complexes is present although rather low for complexes I, III, and IV; it was shown that the individual complexes were present only in non-assembled form with complete absence of super-complex organization. On the other hand, the super-complexes are present in the myeloid cell line HL-60, but during differentiation to neutrophil-like cells, HL-60 loose super-complex organization with consequent lack of respiration.

Similarly clear indications were obtained in a study (Rosca et al. 2008) on canine cardiac mitochondria in heart failure induced experimentally by micro-embolization. Although the activity of individual complexes I, III and IV was normal, respiration with NAD-linked substrates in State 3 or after treatment with uncoupler was severely affected; BN-PAGE showed a similar severe reduction of supramolecular organization with particular decrease of the major $I_1III_2IV_1$ super-complex. Clearly the OXPHOS defect was to be ascribed to alteration of the supramolecular assembly rather than to the individual components of the respiratory chain; the reason for such diminished assembly was not discussed in the paper by Rosca et al. (2008), although it is tempting to speculate that enhanced ROS production due to ischemia and reperfusion in the micro-embolized vessels modifies the membrane environment as a consequence of lipid peroxidation, thus disrupting super-complex assembly.

A recent study in aged rat heart (Gómez et al. 2009) showed by BN-PAGE and proteomic analysis that super-complexes decline with age, although the amounts of individual complexes stay steady. This finding may provide a rationale to the observed decline in respiration and ATP synthesis during aging (Lenaz et al. 2006a).

Further evidence on the role of super-complex disruption in pathology is provided by a recent study from our laboratory on *K-ras*-transformed fibroblasts (Baracca et al. 2010).

In order to critically analyze the molecular basis of the change of carbon metabolism in cancer cells, we compared two cell lines that had been previously characterized (Chiaradonna et al. 2006a, b), that is NIH3T3 mouse fibroblasts and NIH3T3 cells transformed by an activated form of the *K-ras* oncogene. Ras proteins are intracellular switches whose activation state (i.e. their binding to GDP or GTP) controls downstream pathways leading to cell growth and differentiation. Mutation of the *ras* gene is a critical event in the onset of different malignant phenotypes (Bos 1989). Cells harboring *K-ras* mutations were consistently found to have an increased expression of the glucose transporter GLUT1 and an enhanced glycolytic rate, presumably as a compensation to glucose deprivation (Yun et al. 2009). We showed that the major phenotypic change of transformed fibroblasts is a dramatic loss of activity and content of respiratory Complex I (50% approx.), resulting in a strong decrease of both NAD-linked respiration and ATP synthesis rate (Baracca et al. 2010). Accordingly, a significant change in the expression of several genes encoding subunits of the mitochondrial OXPHOS complexes, and in particular a decrease of Complex I, was observed in neoplastic cells.

It has been shown that Complex I is unstable and becomes disassembled in absence of super-complex organization (see above). To this purpose, it was evident from 2D-electrophoresis that the low residual amount of Complex I in transformed fibroblasts is mostly in isolated form rather than assembled with Complex III and Complex IV in high molecular weight super-complexes. In particular, the larger super-complex detected in control cells is almost absent in *ras*-transformed fibroblasts. In addition, *ras*-transformed fibroblasts also have an enhanced production of ROS (Chiaradonna et al. 2006b). We have previously discussed evidence that enhanced ROS generation induces dissociation of the I-III super-complex with consequent lack of efficient electron channeling from Complex I to Complex III; moreover the concomitant disruption of Complex I assembly induced by super-complex dissociation might also account for the decrease of NAD-linked respiration and ATP synthesis. The OXPHOS dysfunction in *K-ras* transformed cells might then lead to compensatory enhancement of glycolysis to overcome the energetic deficiency.

Several other observations from the literature may find a reasonable explanation in the existence of super-complexes and their pathological alterations. The loss of Complex I content and activity reported in several pathological conditions accompanied by oxidative stress, such as Parkinson's disease (Fato et al. 2008), schizophrenia (Ben-Shachar 2009), non-alcoholic fatty liver (Petrosillo et al. 2007), aging (Ventura et al. 2002; Petrosillo et al. 2009), ischemia and reperfusion (Paradies et al. 2004), and diabetes (Bonnard et al. 2008; Ritov et al. 2009) should be investigated in terms of organization of the respiratory chain. The involvement of cardiolipin oxidation reported in some of these changes (Petrosillo et al. 2007, 2009; Paradies et al. 2004) further strengthens this hypothesis.

In a cell line obtained from a thyroid oncocytoma, although a strong decrease of Complex I activity is a likely direct consequence of a point mutation in the mitochondrial gene for Complex I subunit ND1 (Bonora et al. 2006), both the presence of a concomitant heteroplasmic mutation in cytochrome *b* of Complex III and an extremely high ROS production together with loss of super-complex organization were also noticed (Genova et al. 2008; Bonora et al. 2006), in line with the above working hypothesis.

Super-complex organization should be also discussed in terms of therapeutic interventions (Lenaz and Genova 2009b).

Strong evidence exists that exogenous CoQ_{10} administration is beneficial in several disease states, e.g. in genetic CoQ_{10} deficiency (Rötig et al. 2000; Di Giovanni et al. 2001), cardiac failure (Rosenfeldt et al. 2005), Parkinson's disease (Shults et al. 2002; Matthews et al. 1998; Beal 2004) and Friedreich ataxia (Hart et al. 2005). There is evidence, mainly indirect, that orally administered CoQ_{10} may be incorporated into mitochondria, at least in conditions of partial CoQ tissue deficiency, where it may enhance electron transfer and ATP synthesis, besides exerting an antioxidant effect in its reduced form.

The existence of I-III super-complexes where only inter-complex bound CoQ is active by channeling electrons from Complex I to Complex III is apparently incompatible with a dose-dependent effect of added CoQ_{10}, but the notion that inter-complex bound CoQ is in chemical equilibrium with CoQ in the pool (Lenaz and Genova 2009a, b) may explain the improved cell bioenergetics upon addition of exogenous CoQ_{10}. Nevertheless, the increasing evidence previously discussed in this section that super-complex assembly may be disrupted under several pathological conditions, and the demonstration that electron transfer between Complex I and Complex III may occur through CoQ pool behavior suggest that the beneficial effect of exogenous CoQ_{10} may be in supporting electron transfer by collision-mediated interactions when channeling within the super-complex is hampered.

References

Acin-Perez R, Bayona-Bafaluy MP, Fernandez-Silva P, Moreno-Loshuertos R, Perez-Martos A, Bruno C, Moraes CT, Enriquez JA (2004) Respiratory complex III is required to maintain complex I in mammalian mitochondria, *Mol. Cell* 13:805–815

Acín-Pérez R, Fernández-Silva P, Peleato ML, Pérez-Martos A, Enriquez JA (2008) Respiratory active mitochondrial supercomplexes. Mol Cell 32:529–539

Affourtit C, Krab K, Moore AL (2001) Control of plant mitochondrial respiration. Biochim Biophys Acta 504:58–69

Alp NJ, Channon KM (2004) Regulation of endothelial nitric oxide synthase by tetrahydrobiopterin in vascular disease. Arterioscler Thromb Vasc Biol 24:413–420

Arroyo A, Navarro F, Navas P, Villalba JM (1998) Ubiquinol regeneration by plasma membrane ubiquinone reductase. Protoplasma 205:107–113

Bai J, Cederbaum AI (2001) Mitochondrial catalase and oxidative injury. Biol Signals Recept 10:189–199

Balaban RS, Nemoto S, Finkel T (2005) Mitochondria, oxidants and aging. Cell 120:483–495

Balazy M, Chemtob S (2008) Trans-arachidonic acids: new mediators of nitro-oxidative stress. Pharmacol Ther 119:275–290

Balazy M, Nigam S (2003) Aging, lipid modifications and phospholipases–new concepts. Ageing Res Rev 2:191–209

Baracca A, Chiaradonna F, Sgarbi G, Solaini G, Alberghina L, Lenaz G (2010) Mitochondrial Complex I decrease is responsible for bioenergetic dysfunction in K-ras transformed fibroblasts. Biochim Biophys Acta 1797:314–323

Barja G (1993) Oxygen radicals, a failure or a success of evolution? Free Radic Res Commun 18:63–70

Barja G (2004) Aging in vertebrates, and the effect of caloric restriction: a mitochondrial free radical production-DNA damage mechanism? Biol Rev Camb Philos Soc 79:235–251

Barja G (2007) Mitochondrial oxygen consumption and reactive oxygen species production are independently modulated: implications for aging studies. Rejuvenation Res 10:215–223

Barja G, Herrero A (2000) Oxidative damage to mitochondrial DNA is inversely related to maximum life span in the heart and brain of mammals. FASEB J 14:312–318

Baumgarten HG, Grozganovic Z (2000) 6-Hydroxydopamine. In: Spencer PS (ed) Experimental and clinical neurotoxicology. Oxford University Press, New York, pp 659–667

Bayot A, Gareil M, Rogowska-Wrzesinska A, Roepstorff P, Friguet B, Bulteau AL (2010) Identification of novel oxidized protein substrates and physiological partners of the mitochondrial ATP-dependent Lon-like protease Pim1. J Biol Chem 285(15):11445–11457, Epub 11 Feb 2010

Beal MF (2004) Mitochondrial dysfunction and oxidative damage in Alzheimer's and Parkinson's diseases and Coenzyme Q10 as a potential treatment. J Bioenerg Biomembr 36:381–386

Beckmann JD, Frerman FE (1985) Reaction of electron-transfer flavoprotein with electron-transfer flavoprotein-ubiquinone oxidoreductase. Biochemistry 24:3922–3925

Bell EL, Klimova T, Chandel NS (2008) Targeting the mitochondria for cancer therapy: regulation of hypoxia-inducible factor by mitochondria. Antioxid Redox Signal 10:635–640

Ben-Shachar D (2009) The interplay between mitochondrial complex I, dopamine and Sp1 in schizophrenia. J Neural Transm 116:1383–1396

Bergamini E (2006) Autophagy: a cell repair mechanism that retards ageing and age-associated diseases and can be intensified pharmacologically. Mol Aspects Med 27:403–410

Bernardi P, Petronilli V, Di Lisa F, Forte M (2001) A mitochondrial perspective of cell death. Trends Biochem Sci 26:112–117

Berthiaume JM, Wallace KB (2007) Adriamycin-induced oxidative mitochondrial cardiotoxicity. Cell Biol Toxicol 23:15–25

Betarbet R, Sherer TB, MacKenzie G, Garcia-Osuna M, Panov AV, Greenamyre JT (2000) Chronic systemic pesticide exposure reproduces features of Parkinson's disease. Nat Neurosci 3:1301–1306

Beyer RE, Segura-Aguilar J, Di Bernardo S, Cavazzoni M, Fato R, Fiorentini D, Galli M, Setti M, Landi L, Lenaz G (1996) The role of DT-diaphorase in the maintenance of the reduced antioxidant form of coenzyme Q in membrane systems. Proc Natl Acad Sci USA 93:2528–2532

Bianchi C, Genova ML, Parenti Castelli G, Lenaz G (2004) The mitochondrial respiratory chain is partially organized in a supercomplex assembly: kinetic evidence using flux control analysis. J Biol Chem 279:36562–36569

Bianchi P, Kunduzova O, Masini E, Cambon C, Bani D, Raimondi L, Seguelas MH, Nistri S, Colucci W, Leducq N, Parini A (2005) Oxidative stress by monoamine oxidase mediates receptor-independent cardiomyocyte apoptosis by serotonin and postischemic myocardial injury. Circulation 112:3297–3305

Bianchi G, Di Giulio C, Rapino C, Antonucci A, Castaldi A (2006) p53 and p66 proteins compete for hypoxia-inducible factor 1 alpha stabilization in young and old rat hearts exposed to intermittent hypoxia. Gerontology 52:17–23

Bieschke J, Zhang Q, Bosco DA, Lerner RA, Powers ET, Wentworth P Jr, Kelly JW (2006) Small molecule oxidation products trigger disease-associated protein misfolding. Acc Chem Res 39:611–619

Bindoli A, Deeble DJ, Rigobello MP, Galzigna L (1990) Direct and respiratory chain- mediated redox cycling of adrenochrome. Biochim Biophys Acta 1016:349–356

Bindoli A, Rigobello MP, Deeble DJ (1992) Biochemical and toxicological properties of the oxidation products of catecholamines. Free Radic Biol Med 13:391–405

Blakely EL, Mitchell AL, Fisher N, Meunier B, Nijtmans LG, Schaefer AM, Jackson MJ, Turnbull DM, Taylor RW (2005) A mitochondrial cytochrome b mutation causing severe respiratory chain enzyme deficiency in humans and yeast. FEBS J 272:3583–3592

Bohlender JM, Franke S, Stein G, Wolf G (2004) Advanced glycation end products and the kidney. Am J Physiol Renal Physiol 289:F645–F659

Bolter CJ, Chefurka W (1990) Extramitochondrial release of hydrogen peroxide from insect and mouse liver mitochondria using the respiratory inhibitors phosphine, myxothiazol, and antimycin and spectral analysis of inhibited cytochromes. Arch Biochem Biophys 278:65–72

Bonnard C, Durand A, Peyrol S, Chanseaume E, Chauvin MA, Morio B, Vidal H, Rieusset J (2008) Mitochondrial dysfunction results from oxidative stress in the skeletal muscle of diet-induced insulin-resistant mice. J Clin Invest 118:789–800

Bonora E, Porcelli AM, Gasparre G, Biondi A, Ghelli A, Carelli V, Baracca A, Tallini G, Martinuzzi A, Lenaz G, Rugolo M, Romeo G (2006) Defective oxidative phosphorylation in thyroid oncocytic carcinoma is associated with pathogenic mitochondrial DNA mutations affecting complexes I and III. Cancer Res 66:6087–6096

Borisenko GG, Kapralov AA, Tyurin VA, Maeda A, Stoyanovsky DA, Kagan VE (2008) Molecular design of new inhibitors of peroxidase activity of cytochrome c/cardiolipin complexes: fluorescent oxadiazole-derivatized cardiolipin. Biochemistry 47:13699–13710

Bos JL (1989) Ras oncogenes in human cancer: a review. Cancer Res 49:4682–4689

Boveris A, Oshino N, Chance B (1972) The cellular production of hydrogen peroxide. Biochem J 128:617–630

Brady NR, Hamacher-Brady A, Westerhoff HV, Gottlieb RA (2006) A wave of reactive oxygen species (ROS)-induced ROS release in a sea of excitable mitochondria. Antioxid Redox Signal 8:1651–1665

Brand MD (2000) Uncoupling to survive? The role of mitochondrial inefficiency in ageing. Exp Gerontol 35:811–820

Brandt U, Kerscher S, Drose S, Zwicker K, Zickermann V (2003) Proton pumping by NADH:ubiquinone oxidoreductase. A redox driven conformational change mechanism? FEBS Lett 545:9–17

Bredt DS (1999) Endogenous nitric oxide synthesis: biological functions and pathophysiology. Free Radic Res 31:577–596

Brown GC, Borutaite V (2004) Inhibition of mitochondrial Complex I by nitric oxide, peroxynitrite and S-nitrosothiols. Biochim Biophys Acta 1658:44–49

Bulteau AL, Szweda LI, Friguet B (2006) Mitochondrial protein oxidation and degradation in response to oxidative stress. Exp Gerontol 41:653–657

Bultema JB, Braun HP, Boekema EJ, Kouril R (2009) Megacomplex organization of the oxidative phosphorylation system by structural analysis of respiratory supercomplexes from potato. Biochim Biophys Acta 1787(1):60–67

Burtwell LYS, Brookes PS (2008) Mitochondria as a target for the cardioprotective effects of nitric oxide in ischemia-reperfusion injury. Antioxid Redox Signal 10:579–599

Butow RA, Avadhani NG (2004) Mitochondrial signalling: the retrograde response. Mol Cell 14:1–15

Cadenas E, Davies KJA (2000) Mitochondrial free radical generation, oxidative stress, and aging. Free Radic Biol Med 29:222–230

Cadenas E, Boveris A, Ragan CI, Stoppani AOM (1977) Production of superoxide radicals and hydrogen peroxide by NADH-ubiquinone reductase and ubiquinol-cytochrome c reductase from beef heart mitochondria. Arch Biochem Biophys 180:248–257

Calabrese V, Scapagnini G, Ravagna A, Colombrita C, Spadaro F, Butterfield DA, Giuffrida Stella AM (2004) Increased expression of heat shock proteins in rat brain during aging: relationship with mitochondrial function and glutathione redox state. Mech Ageing Dev 125:325–335

Carraro F, Pucci A, Pellegrini M, Pelicci PG, Baldari CT, Naldini A (2007) p66[Shc] is involved in promoting HIF-1-alpha accumulation and cell death in hypoxic T cells. J Cell Physiol 211:439–447

Casteilla L, Rigoulet M, Pénicaud L (2001) Mitochondrial ROS metabolism: modulation by uncoupling proteins. IUBMB Life 52:181–188

Cecchini G (2003) Function and structure of complex II of the respiratory chain. Annu Rev Biochem 72:77–109

Chan DC (2006) Mitochondria: dynamic organelles in disease, aging, and development. Cell 125:1241–1252

Chen Y, Gibson SB (2008) Is generation of reactive oxygen species a trigger for autophagy? Autophagy 4:246–248

Chiaradonna F, Sacco E, Manzoni R, Giorgio M, Vanoni M, Alberghina L (2006a) Ras-dependent carbon metabolism and transformation in mouse fibroblasts. Oncogene 25:5391–5404

Chiaradonna F, Gaglio D, Vanoni M, Alberghina L (2006b) Expression of transforming K-Ras oncogene affects mitochondrial functions and morphology in mouse fibroblasts. Biochim Biophys Acta 1757:1338–1356

Chiueh CC, Miyake H, Peng MT (1993) Role of dopamine autoxidation, hydroxyl radical generation, and calcium overload in underlying mechanisms involved in MPTP-induced parkinsonism. Adv Neurol 60:251–258

Cho N, Morré DJ (2009) Early developmental expression of a normally tumour-associated and drug-inhibited cell surface-located NADH oxidase (ENOX2) in non-cancer cells. Cancer Immunol Immunother 58:547–552

Conrad M (2009) Transgenic mouse models for the vital selenoenzymes cytosolic thioredoxin reductase, mitochondrial thioredoxin reductase and glutathione peroxidase 4. Biochim Biophys Acta 1790:1575–1585

Cooke MS, Evans MD, Dizdaroglu M, Lunec J (2003) Oxidative DNA damage: mechanisms, mutation and disease. FASEB J 17:1195–1214

Cribb AE, Peynou M, Muruganandan S, Schneider L (2005) The endoplasmic reticulum in xenobiotic toxicity. Drug Metab Rev 37:405–442

Crofts AR (2004) Proton-coupled electron transfer at the Qo-site of the bc1 complex controls the rate of ubihydroquinone oxidation. Biochim Biophys Acta 1655:77–92

Cruciat CM, Brunner S, Baumann F, Neupert W, Stuart RA (2000) The cytochrome bc1 and cytochrome c oxidase complexes associate to form a single supracomplex in yeast mitochondria. J Biol Chem 275:18093–18098

D'Aurelio M, Gajewski CD, Lenaz G, Manfredi G (2006) Respiratory chain supercomplexes set the threshold for respiration defects in human mtDNA mutant cybrids. Hum Mol Genet 15:2157–2169

Dalle Donne I, Rossi R, Giustarini D, Colombo R, Milzani A (2005) Is there a role for S- glutathionylation of proteins in human disease? IUBMB Life 57:189–192

Dalle Donne I, Rossi R, Colombo R, Giustarini D, Milzani A (2006) Biomarkers of oxidative damage in human disease. Clin Chem 52:601–623

de Souza-Pinto N, Wilson DM III, Stevnsner TV, Bohr VA (2008) Mitochondrial DNA, base excision repair and neurodegeneration. DNA Repair 7:1098–1109

Dencher NA, Frenzel M, Reifschneider NH, Sugawa M, Krause F (2007) Proteome alterations in rat mitochondria caused by aging. Ann N Y Acad Sci 1100:291–298

Di Giovanni S, Mirabella M, Spinazzola A, Crociati P, Silvestri G, Broccolini A, Tonali P, Di Mauro S, Servidei S (2001) Coenzyme Q10 reverses pathological phenotype and reduces apoptosis in familial CoQ10 deficiency. Neurology 57:375–376

Di Lisa F, Canton M, Menabò R, Kaludercic N, Bernardi P (2007) Mitochondria and cardioprotection. Heart Fail Rev 12:249–260

Di Mauro S, Schon EA (2008) Mitochondrial disorders in the nervous system. Annu Rev Neurosci 31:91–123

Di Mauro S, Hirano M, Schon EA (eds) (2006) Mitochondrial medicine. Informa Healthcare, London

Diaz F, Fukui H, Garcia S, Moraes CT (2006) Cytochrome c oxidase is required for the assembly/stability of respiratory complex I in mouse fibroblasts. Mol Cell Biol 26:4872–4881

Diplock AT (1994) Antioxidants and disease prevention. Mol Aspects Med 15:293–376

Dizdaroglu M, Jaruga P, Birincioglu M, Rodriguez H (2002) Free radical-induced damage to DNA: mechanisms and measurement. Free Radic Biol Med 32:1102–1115

Donnellan JF, Barker MD, Wood J, Beechey RB (1970) Specificity and locale of the L-3-glycerophosphate-flavoprotein oxidoreductase of mitochondria isolated from the flight muscle of Sarcophaga barbata thoms. Biochem J 120:467–478

Drahota Z, Chowdhury SK, Floryk D, Mracek T, Wilhelm J, Rauchova H, Lenaz G, Houstek J (2002) Glycerophosphate-dependent hydrogen peroxide production by brown adipose tissue mitochondria and its activation by ferricyanide. J Bioenerg Biomembr 34:105–113

Dröge W (2002) Free radicals in the physiological control of cell function. Physiol Rev 82:47–95

Dudkina NV, Eubel H, Keegstra W, Boekema EJ, Braun HP (2005) Structure of a mitochondrial supercomplex formed by respiratory-chain complexes I and III. Proc Natl Acad Sci USA 102:3225–3229

Edmonson DE, Binda C, Mattevi A (2007) Structural insights into the mechanism of amine oxidation by monoamine oxidases A and B. Arch Biochem Biophys 464:269–276

El-Sohemy A (2007) Nutrigenetics. Forum Nutr 60:25–30

Ernster L, Dallner G (1995) Biochemical, physiological and medical aspects of ubiquinone function. Biochim Biophys Acta 1271:195–204

Esposito LA, Kokoszka JE, Waymire KG, Cottrell B, MacGregor GR, Wallace DC (2000) Mitochondrial oxidative stress in mice lacking the glutathione peroxidase-1 gene. Free Radic Biol Med 28:754–766

Esterházy D, King MS, Yakovlev G, Hirst J (2008) Production of reactive oxygen species by complex I (NADH:ubiquinone oxidoreductase) from Escherichia coli and comparison to the enzyme from mitochondria. Biochemistry 47: 3964–3971

Evans DR, Guy HI (2004) Mammalian pyrimidine biosynthesis: fresh insights into an ancient pathway. J Biol Chem 279:33035–33038

Fato R, Bergamini C, Leoni S, Strocchi P, Lenaz G (2008) Generation of reactive oxygen species by mitochondrial Complex I: implications in neurodegeneration. Neurochem Res 33:2487–2501

Fato R, Bergamini C, Bortolus M, Maniero AL, Leoni S, Ohnishi T, Lenaz G (2009) Differential effects of Complex I inhibitors on production of reactive oxygen species. Biochim Biophys Acta 1767:384–392

Finkel T (2006) Intracellular redox regulation by the family of small GTPases. Antioxid Redox Signal 8:1857–1863

Forkink M, Smeitink JA, Brock R, Willems PH, Koopman WJ (2010) Detection and manipulation of mitochondrial reactive oxygen species in mammalian cells. Biochim Biophys Acta 1797(6–7):1034–1044, Epub 25 Jan 2010

Forman HJ, Kennedy J (1975) Superoxide production and electron transport in mitochondrial oxidation of dihydroorotic acid. J Biol Chem 250:4322–4326

Forman HJ, Fukuto JM, Miller T, Zhang H, Rinna A, Levy S (2008) The chemistry of cell signalling by reactive oxygen and nitrogen species and 4-hydroxynonenal. Arch Biochem Biophys 477:183–195

Fridovich I (1998) Oxygen toxicity: a radical explanation. J Exp Biol 201:1203–1209

Friguet B, Szweda LI (1997) Inhibition of the multicatalytic proteinase by 4-hydroxy-2- nonenal cross-linked protein. FEBS Lett 405:21–25

Fruehauf JP, Meyskens FL Jr (2007) Reactive oxygen species: a breath of life or death? Clin Cancer Res 13:789–794

Galkin A, Brandt U (2005) Superoxide radical formation by pure complex I (NADH:ubiquinone oxidoreductase) from Yarrowia lipolytica. J Biol Chem 280:30129–30135

Genova ML, Ventura B, Giuliano G, Bovina C, Formiggini G, Parenti CG, Lenaz G (2001) The site of production of superoxide radical in mitochondrial Complex I is not a bound ubisemiquinone but presumably iron-sulfur cluster N2. FEBS Lett 505:364–368

Genova ML, Abd-Elsalam NM, Mahdy ES, Bernacchia A, Lucarini M, Peduli GF, Lenaz G (2006) Redox cycling of adrenaline and adrenochrome catalysed by mitochondrisal Complex I. Arch Biochem Biophys 447:167–173

Genova ML, Baracca A, Biondi A, Casalena G, Faccioli M, Falasca AI, Formiggini G, Sgarbi G, Solaini G, Lenaz G (2008) Is supercomplex organization of the respiratory chain required for optimal electron transfer activity? Biochim Biophys Acta 1777:740–746

Gertz M, Fischer F, Leipelt M, Wolters D, Steegborn C (2009) Identification of Peroxiredoxin 1 as a novel interaction partner for the lifespan regulator protein p66Shc. Aging (Albany NY) 1:254–265

Ghafourifar P, Sen CK (2007) Mitochondrial nitric oxide synthase. Front Biosci 12:1072–1078

Ghazi A, Henis-Korenblit S, Kenyon C (2007) Regulation of Caenorhabditis elegans lifespan by a proteasomal E3 ligase complex. Proc Natl Acad Sci USA 104:5947–5952

Giorgio M, Migliaccio E, Orsini F, Paolucci D, Moroni M, Contursi C, Pelliccia G, Luzi L, Minacci S, Marcaccio M, Pinton P, Rizzuto R, Bernardi P, Paolucci F, Pelicci PG (2005) Electron transfer between cytochrome c and p66Shc generates reactive oxygen species that trigger mitochondrial apoptosis. Cell 122:221–233

Girotti AW (2008) Translocation as a means of disseminating lipid hydroperoxide-induced oxidative damage and effector action. Free Radic Biol Med 44:956–968

Goetz ME, Luch A (2008) Reactive species: a cell damaging rout assisting to chemical carcinogens. Cancer Lett 266:73–83

Gómez LA, Monette JS, Chavez JD, Maier CS, Hagen TM (2009) Supercomplexes of the mitochondrial electron transport chain decline in the aging rat heart. Arch Biochem Biophys 490:30–35

Gong Y, Agani FH (2005) Oligomycin inhibits HIF-1α expression in hypoxic tumor cells. Am J Physiol Cell Physiol 288:C1023–C1029

Green DE, Tzagoloff A (1966) The mitochondrial electron transfer chain. Arch Biochem Biophys 116:293–304

Grivennikova VG, Kareyeva AV, Vinogradov AD (2010) What are the sources of hydrogen peroxide production by heart mitochondria? Biochim Biophys Acta 1797:939–944

Gruber J, Schaffer S, Halliwell B (2008) The mitochondrial free radical theory of ageing–where do we stand? Front Biosci 13:6554–6579

Grune T, Reinheckel T, Davies KJA (1997) Degradation of oxidized proteins in mammalian cells. FASEB J 11:526–534

Guo S, Bragina O, Xu Y, Cao Z, Chen H, Zhou B, Morgan M, Lin Y, Jiang BH, Liu KJ, Shi H (2008) Glucose upregulates HIF-1 alpha expression in primary cortical neurons in response to hypoxia through maintaining cellular redox status. J Neurochem 105:1849–1860

Guzy RD, Schumacker PT (2006) Oxygen sensing by mitochondria at Complex III: the paradox of increased reactive oxygen species during hypoxia. Exp Physiol 91:807–819

Hackenbrock CR, Chazotte B, Gupte SS (1986) The random collision model and a critical assessment of diffusion and collision in mitochondrial electron transport. J Bioenerg Biomembr 18:331–368

Halliwell B (2006) Oxidative stress and neurodegeneration: where are we now? J Neurochem 97:1634–1658

Halliwell B, Gutteridge JMC (1999) Free radicals in biology and medicine. Oxford University Press, New York

Hamelin M, Mary J, Vostry M, Friguet B, Bakala H (2007) Glycation damage targets glutamate dehydrogenase in the rat liver mitochondrial matrix during aging. FEBS J 274:5949–5961

Han D, Williams E, Cadenas E (2001) Mitochondrial respiratory chain-dependent generation of superoxide anion and its release into the intermembrane space. Biochem J 353:411–416

Han D, Antunes F, Canali R, Rettori D, Cadenas E (2003) Voltage-dependent anion channels control the release of the superoxide anion from mitochondria to cytosol. J Biol Chem 278:5557–5563

Hart PE, Lodi R, Rajagopalan B, Bradley JL, Crilley JG, Turner C, Blamire AM, Manners D, Styles P, Schapira AH, Cooper JM (2005) Antioxidant treatment of patients with Friedreich ataxia: four-year follow-up. Arch Neurol 62:621–626

Hatefi Y, Haavik AG, Fowler LR, Griffiths DE (1962a) Studies on the electron transfer system. XLII. Reconstitution of the electron transfer system. J Biol Chem 237:2661–2669

Hatefi Y, Haavik AG, Griffiths DE (1962b) Studies on the electron transfer system. XL. Preparation and properties of mitochondrial DPNH-Coenzyme Q reductase. J Biol Chem 237:1676–1680

Hayakawa M, Katsumata K, Yoneda M, Tanaka M, Sugiyama S, Ozawa T (1996) Age-related extensive fragmentation of mitochondrial DNA into minicircles. Biochem Biophys Res Commun 226:369–377

Hayflick L (2003) Living forever and dying in the attempt. Exp Gerontol 38:1231–1241

Haynes V, Elfering SL, Squires RJ, Traaseth N, Solien J, Ettl A, Giulivi C (2003) Mitochondrial nitric-oxide synthase: role in pathophysiology. IUBMB Life 55:599–603

Hazra TK, Das A, Das S, Choudhury S, Kow YW, Roy R (2007) Oxidative DNA damage repair in mammalian cells: a new perspective. DNA Repair 6:470–480

Herrero A, Barja G (2000) Localization of the site of oxygen radical generation inside the Complex I of heart and non-synaptic brain mammalian mitochondria. J Bioenerg Biomembr 32:609–616

Hinchliffe P, Sazanov LA (2005) Organization of iron-sulfur clusters in respiratory complex I. Science 309:71–74

Hirst J, King MS, Pryde KR (2008) The production of reactive oxygen species by complex I. Biochem Soc Trans 36:976–980

Inoue M, Sato EF, Nishikawa M, Park A-M, Kira Y, Imada I, Utsumi K (2003) Mitochondrial generation of reactive oxygen species and its role in aerobic life. Curr Med Chem 10:2495–2505

Ishii N, Fujii M, Hartman PS, Tsuda M, Yasuda K, Senoo-Matsuda N, Yanase S, Ayusawa D, Suzuki K (1998) A mutation in succinate dehydrogenase cytochrome b causes oxidative stress and ageing in nematodes. Nature 394:694–697

Jezek P, Hlavata L (2005) Mitochondria in homeostasis of reactive oxygen species in cell, tissues, and organism. Int J Biochem Cell Biol 37:2478–2503

Kagan VE, Tyurin VA, Jiang J, Tyurina YY, Ritov VB, Amoscato AA, Osipov AN, Belikova NA, Kapralov AA, Kini V, Vlasova II, Zhao Q, Zou M, Di P, Svistunenko DA, Kurnikov IV, Borisenko GG (2005) Cytochrome c acts as a cardiolipin oxygenase required for release of proapoptotic factors. Nat Chem Biol 1:223–232

Kalapos MP (2008) The tandem of free radicals and methylglyoxal. Chem Biol Interact 171:251–271

Kanai AJ, Pearce LL, Clemens PR, Birder LA, VanBibber MM, Choi SY, de Groat WC, Peterson J (2001) Identification of a neuronal nitric oxide synthase in isolated cardiac mitochondria using electrochemical detection. Proc Natl Acad Sci USA 98:14126–14131

Kareyeva AV, Grivennikova VG, Cecchini G, Vinogradov AD (2011) Molecular identification of the enzyme responsible for the mitochondrial NADH-supported ammonium-dependent hydrogen peroxide production. FEBS Lett 585: 385–389

Kietzmann T, Gorlach A (2005) Reactive oxygen species in the control of hypoxia-inducible factor-mediated gene expression. Semin Cell Dev Biol 16:474–486

Klingenberg M (1970) Localization of the glycerol-phosphate dehydrogenase in the outer phase of the mitochondrial inner membrane. Eur J Biochem 13:247–252

Koene S, Smeitink J (2009) Mitochondrial medicine: entering the era of treatment. J Intern Med 265:193–209

Korshunov SS, Skulachev VP, Starkov AA (1997) High protonic potential actuates a mechanism of production of reactive oxygen species in mitochondria. FEBS Lett 416:15–18

Kovacic P, Cooksy AL (2005) Unifying mechanism for the toxicity and addiction by abused drugs: electron transfer and reactive oxygen species. Med Hypotheses 64:357–366

Krause F, Scheckhuber CQ, Werner A, Rexroth S, Reifschneider NH, Dencher NA, Osiewacz HD (2004) Supramolecular organization of cytochrome c oxidase- and alternative oxidase-dependent respiratory chains in the filamentous fungus Podospora anserina. J Biol Chem 279:26453–26461

Krause F, Scheckhuber CQ, Werner A, Rexroth S, Reifschneider NH, Dencher NA, Osiewacz HD (2006) OXPHOS Supercomplexes: respiration and life-span control in the aging model Podospora anserina. Ann N Y Acad Sci 1067: 106–115

Krungkrai J (1991) Malarial dihydroorotate dehydrogenase mediates superoxide radical production. Biochem Int 24:833–839

Kukat A, Trifunovic A (2009) Somatic mtDNA mutations and aging–facts and fancies. Exp Gerontol 44:101–105

Kushnareva Y, Murphy AN, Andreyev A (2002) Complex I-mediated reactive oxygen species generation: modulation by cytochrome c and NAD(P)+oxidation-reduction state. Biochem J 368:545–553

Kussmaul L, Hirst J (2006) The mechanism of superoxide production by NADH:ubiquinone oxidoreductase (complex I) from bovine heart mitochondria. Proc Natl Acad Sci USA 103:7607–7612

Kwong LK, Sohal RS (1998) Substrate and site specificity of hydrogen peroxide generation in mouse mitochondria. Arch Biochem Biophys 350:118–126

Lacza Z, Pankotai E, Busija DW (2009) Mitochondrial nitric oxide synthase: current concepts and controversies. Front Biosci 14:4436–4443

Lambert AJ, Brand MD (2004) Inhibitors of the quinone-binding site allow rapid superoxide production from mitochondrial NADH:ubiquinone oxidoreductase (complex I). J Biol Chem 279:39414–39420

Lambeth JD (2007) Nox enzymes, ROS, and chronic disease: an example of antagonistic pleiotropy. Free Radic Biol Med 43:332–347

Landis GN, Tower J (2005) Superoxide dismutase evolution and life span regulation. Mech Ageing Dev 126:365–379

Lange C, Nett JH, Trumpower BL, Hunte C (2001) Specific roles of protein-phospholipid interactions in the yeast cytochrome bc1 complex structure. EMBO J 20:6591–6600

Lee HC, Wei YH (1997) Mutation and oxidative damage of mitochondrial DNA and defective turnover of mitochondria in human aging. J Formos Med Assoc 96:770–778

Lenaz G (1998) Role of mitochondria in oxidative stress and aging. Biochim Biophys Acta 1366:53–67

Lenaz G (2001) The mitochondrial production of reactive oxygen species: mechanisms and implications in human pathology. IUBMB Life 52:159–164

Lenaz G, Genova ML (2007) Kinetics of integrated electron transfer in the mitochondrial respiratory chain: random collisions vs. solid state electron channeling. Am J Physiol Cell Physiol 292:C1221–C1239

Lenaz G, Genova ML (2009a) Mobility and function of Coenzyme Q (ubiquinone) in the mitochondrial respiratory chain. Biochim Biophys Acta 1787:563–573

Lenaz G, Genova ML (2009b) Structural and functional organization of the mitochondrial respiratory chain: a dynamic super-assembly. Int J Biochem Cell Biol 41:1750–1772

Lenaz G, Genova ML (2010) Structure and organization of mitochondrial respiratory complexes: a new understanding of an old subject. Antioxid Redox Signal 12(8):961–1008, Epub 15 Feb 2010

Lenaz G, Strocchi P (2009) Reactive oxygen species in the induction of toxicity. In: Ballantyne B, Marrs T, Syversen T (eds) General and applied toxicology, vol 1. Wiley, Chichester, chapter 15

Lenaz G, Bovina C, Formiggini G, Parenti Castelli G (1999) Mitochondria, oxidative stress, and antioxidant defences. Acta Biochim Pol 46:1–21

Lenaz G, Baracca A, Fato R, Genova ML, Solaini G (2006a) New insights into structure and function of mitochondria and their role in aging and disease. Antioxid Redox Signal 8:417–437

Lenaz G, Fato R, Genova ML, Bergamini C, Bianchi C, Biondi A (2006b) Mitochondrial Complex I: structural and functional aspects. Biochim Biophys Acta 1757:1406–1420

Lenaz G, Fato R, Formiggini G, Genova ML (2007) The role of Coenzyme Q in mitochondrial electron transport. Mitochondrion 7:S8–S33

Lenaz G, Baracca A, Barbero G, Bergamini C, Dalmonte ME, Del Sole M, Faccioli M, Falasca A, Fato R, Genova ML, Sgarbi G, Solaini G (2010) Mitochondrial respiratory chain super-complex I-III in physiology and pathology. Biochim Biophys Acta 1797(6–7):633–640, Epub 30 Jan 2010

Levine RL, Mosoni L, Berlett BS, Stadtman ER (1996) Methionine residues as endogenous antioxidants in proteins. Proc Natl Acad Sci USA 93:15036–15040

Lin SJ, Ford E, Hagis M, Liszt G, Guarente L (2004) Calorie restriction extends life span by lowering the level of NADH. Genes Dev 18:12–16

Linnane AW, Eastwood H (2006) Cellular redox regulation and prooxidant signalling systems: a new perspective on the free radical theory of aging. Ann NY Acad Sci 1067:47–55

Linnane AW, Marzuki S, Ozawa T, Tanaka M (1989) Mitochondrial DNA mutations as an important contributor to ageing and degenerative diseases. Lancet 1:642–645

Linnane AW, Degli Esposti M, Generowicz M, Luff AR, Nagley P (1995) The universality of bioenergetic disease and amelioration with redox therapy. Biochim Biophys Acta 1271:191–194

Liu B, Chen Y, St. Clair DK (2008) ROS and p53: a versatile partnership. Free Radic Biol Med 44:1529–1535

Luch A (2005) The carcinogenic effects of polycyclic aromatic hydrocarbons. Imperial College Press, London

Maj MC, Raha S, Myint T, Robinson BH (2004) Regulation of NADH/CoQ oxidoreductase: do phosphorylation events affect activity? Protein J 23:25–32

Marí M, Morales A, Colell A, García-Ruiz C, Fernández-Checa JC (2009) Mitochondrial glutathione, a key survival antioxidant. Antioxid Redox Signal 11:2685–2700

Marnett LJ (1999) Lipid peroxidation – DNA damage by malondialdehyde. Mutat Res 424:83–95

Mates JM, Perez-Gomez C, De Castro IN (1999) Antioxidant enzymes and human diseases. Clin Biochem 32:595–603

Matthews RT, Yang L, Browne S, Baik M, Beal MF (1998) Coenzyme Q10; administration increases brain mitochondrial concentrations and exerts neuroprotective effects. Proc Natl Acad Sci USA 95:8892–8897

Maurel A, Hernandez C, Kunduzova O, Bompart G, Cambon C, Parini A, Frances B (2003) Age-dependent increase in hydrogen peroxide production by cardiac monoamine oxidase A in rats. Am J Physiol Heart Circ Physiol 284:H1460–H1467

McFarland R, Taylor RW, Turnbull DM (2007) Mitochondrial disease–its impact, etiology, and pathology. Curr Top Dev Biol 77:113–155

McKenzie M, Lazarou M, Thorburn DR, Ryan MT (2006) Mitochondrial respiratory chain supercomplexes are destabilized in Barth syndrome patients. J Mol Biol 361:462–469

McLennan H, Degli Esposti M (2000) The contribution of mitochondrial respiratory complexes in the production of reactive oxygen species. J Bioenerg Biomembr 32:153–162

Meissner C (2007) Mutations of mitochondrial DNA: cause or consequence of the ageing process? Z Gerontol Geriatrie 40:325–333

Melov S, Coskun P, Patel M, Tuinstra M, Cottrell B, Jun AS, Zastawny TH, Dizdaroglu M, Goodman SI, Huang TT, Miziorko H, Epstein CJ, Wallace DC (1999) Mitochondrial disease in superoxide dismutase 2 mutant mice. Proc Natl Acad Sci USA 96:846–851

Menini S, Amadio L, Oddi G, Ricci C, Pesce C, Pugliese F, Giorgio M, Migliaccio E, Pelicci PG, Iacobini C, Pugliese G (2006) Deletion of p66Shc longevity gene protects against experimental diabetic glomerulopathy by preventing diabetes-induced oxidative stress. Diabetes 55:1642–1650

Messner KR, Imlay JA (2002) Mechanism of superoxide and hydrogen peroxide formation by fumarate reductase, succinate dehydrogenase, and aspartate oxidase. J Biol Chem 277:42563–42571

Michikawa Y, Mazzucchelli F, Bresolin N, Scarlato G, Attardi G (1999) Aging-dependent large accumulation of point mutations in the human mtDNA control region for replication. Science 286:774–779

Migliaccio E, Giorgio M, Mele S, Pelicci G, Reboldi P, Pandolci PP, Lanfrancone L, Pelicci PG (1999) The p66shc adaptor protein controls oxidative stress response and life span in mammals. Nature 402:309–313

Migliaccio E, Giorgio M, Pelicci PG (2006) Apoptosis and aging: role of p66Shc protein. Antioxid Redox Signal 8:600–608

Miwa S, St-Pierre J, Partridge L, Brand MD (2003) Superoxide and hydrogen peroxide production in *Drosophila* mitochondria. Free Radic Biol Med 35:938–948

Morrow JD (2005) Quantification of isoprostanes as indices of oxidant stress and the risk of atherosclerosis in humans. Arterioscler Thromb Vasc Biol 25:279–286

Muller FL, Roberts AG, Bowman NK, Kramer DM (2003) Architecture of the Qo site of the cytochrome bc1 complex probed by superoxide production. Biochemistry 42:6493–6499

Murphy MP (2009) How mitochondria produce reactive oxygen species. Biochem J 417:1–13

Murray J, Oquendo CE, Willis JH, Marusich MF, Capaldi RA (2008) Monitoring oxidative and nitrative modification of cellular proteins; a paradigm for identifying key disease related markers of oxidative stress. Adv Drug Deliv Rev 60:1497–1503

Nakano H, Nakajima A, Sakon-Komazawa S, Piao J-H, Xue X, Okumura K (2006) Reactive oxygen species mediate cross-talk between nFκB and JNK. Cell Death Differ 13:730–737

Napoli C, Martin-Padura I, De Nigris F, Giorgio M, Mansueto G, Somma P, Condorelli M, Sica G, De Rosa G, Pelicci PG (2003) Deletion of the p66Shc longevity gene reduces systemic and tissue oxidative stress, vascular cell apoptosis, and early atherogenesis in mice fed a high-fat diet. Proc Natl Acad Sci USA 18:2112–2116

Navarro A, Boveris A (2008) Mitochondrial nitric oxide synthase, mitochondrial brain dysfunction in aging, and mitochondria-targeted antioxidants. Adv Drug Deliv Rev 60:1534–1544

Negre-Salvayre A, Coatrieux C, Ingueneau C, Salvayre R (2008) Advanced lipid peroxidation end products in oxidative damage to proteins. Potential role in diseases and therapeutic prospects for the inhibitors. Br J Pharmacol 153:6–20

Nicholls DG, Ferguson SJ (2002) Bioenergetics, 3rd edn. Academic, London

Nohl H, Gille L, Kozlov AV (1998) Antioxidant-derived prooxidant formation from ubiquinol. Free Radic Biol Med 25:666–675

Ohnishi T, Salerno JC (2005) Conformation-driven and semiquinone-gated proton-pump mechanism in the NADH-ubiquinone oxidoreductase (complex I). FEBS Lett 579:4555–4561

Ohnishi T, Sled VD, Yano T, Yagi T, Burbaev DS, Vinogradov AD (1998) Structure-function studies of iron-sulfur clusters and semiquinones in the NADH-Q oxidoreductase segment of the respiratory chain. Biochim Biophys Acta 1365:301–308

Ohnishi ST, Ohnishi T, Muranaka S, Fujita H, Kimura H, Uemura K, Yoshida K, Utsumi K (2005) A possible site of superoxide generation in the complex I segment of rat heart mitochondria. J Bioenerg Biomembr 37:1–15

Ohnishi ST, Shinzawa-Itoh K, Ohta K, Yoshikawa S, Ohnishi T (2010) New insights into the superoxide generation sites in bovine heart NADH-ubiquinone oxidoreductase (Complex I): the significance of protein-associated ubiquinone and the dynamic shifting of generation sites between semiflavin and semiquinone radicals. Biochim Biophys Acta 1797:1901–1909

Ott M, Gogvadze V, Orrenius S, Zhivotovsky B (2007) Mitochondria, oxidative stress and cell death. Apoptosis 12:913–922

Ozawa T (1997) Genetic and functional changes in mitochondria associated with aging. Physiol Rev 77:425–464

Pamplona R, Barja G (2007) Highly resistant macromolecular components and low rate of generation of endogenous damage: two key traits of longevity. Ageing Res Rev 6:189–210

Pamplona R, Barja G, Portero-Otin M (2002) Membrane fatty acid unsaturation, protection against oxidative stress, and maximum life span: a homeoviscous-longevity adaptation? Ann N Y Acad Sci 959:475–490

Panov A, Dikalov S, Shalbuyeva N, Hemendinger R, Greenamyre JT, Rosenfeld J (2007) Species- and tissue-specific relationships between mitochondrial permeability transition and generation of ROS in brain and liver mitochondria of rats and mice. Am J Physiol Cell Physiol 292:C708–C718

Paradies G, Petrosillo G, Pistolese M, Ruggiero FM (2000) The effect of reactive oxygen species generated from the mitochondrial electron transport chain on the cytochrome c oxidase activity and on the cardiolipin content in bovine heart submitochondrial particles. FEBS Lett 466:323–326

Paradies G, Petrosillo G, Pistolese M, Ruggiero FM (2002) Reactive oxygen species affect mitochondrial electron transport complex I activity through oxidative cardiolipin damage. Gene 286:135–141

Paradies G, Petrosillo G, Pistolese M, Di Venosa N, Federici A, Ruggiero FM (2004) Decrease in mitochondrial complex I activity in ischemic/reperfused rat heart: involvement of reactive oxygen species and cardiolipin. Circ Res 94:53–59

Peppa M, Uribarri J, Vlassara H (2008) Aging and glycoxidant stress. Hormones (Athens) 7:123–132

Persichini T, Mazzone V, Policelli F, Moreno S, Venturini G, Clementi E, Colasanti M (2005) Mitochondrial type I nitric oxide synthase physically interacts with cytochrome c oxidase. Neurosci Lett 384:254–259

Peters K, Dudkina NV, Jänsch L, Braun HP, Boekema EJ (2008) A structural investigation of complex I and I+III2 supercomplex from Zea mays at 11-13 A resolution: assignment of the carbonic anhydrase domain and evidence for structural heterogeneity within complex I. Biochim Biophys Acta 1777:84–93

Petrosillo G, Portincasa P, Grattagliano I, Casanova G, Matera M, Ruggiero FM, Ferri D, Paradies G (2007) Mitochondrial dysfunction in rat with nonalcoholic fatty liver Involvement of complex I, reactive oxygen species and cardiolipin. Biochim Biophys Acta 1767:1260–1267

Petrosillo G, Matera M, Moro N, Ruggiero FM, Paradies G (2009) Mitochondrial complex I dysfunction in rat heart with aging: critical role of reactive oxygen species and cardiolipin, *Free Radic*. Biol Med 46:88–94

Pfeiffer K, Gohil V, Stuart RA, Hunte C, Brandt U, Greenberg ML, Schägger H (2003) Cardiolipin stabilizes respiratory chain supercomplexes. J Biol Chem 278:52873–52880

Piccoli C, Scrima R, Boffoli D, Capitanio N (2006) Control by cytochrome c oxidase of the cellular oxidative phosphorylation system depends on the mitochondrial energy state. Biochem J 396:573–583

Pinton P, Rimessi A, Marchi S, Orsini F, Migliaccio E, Giorgio M, Contursi C, Minucci S, Mantovani F, Wieckowski MR, Del Sal G, Pelicci PG, Rizzato R (2007) Protein kinase Cβ and prolyl isomerase 1 regulate mitochondrial effects of the life-span determinant p66Shc. Science 315:659–663

Pou S, Keaton L, Surichamorn W, Rosen GM (1999) Mechanism of superoxide generation by neuronal nitric oxide synthase. J Biol Chem 274:9573–9580

Radermacher M, Ruiz T, Clason T, Benjamin S, Brandt U, Zickermann V (2006) The three-dimensional structure of complex I from Yarrowia lipolytica: a highly dynamic enzyme. J Struct Biol 154:269–279

Radi R, Turrens JF, Chang LY, Bush KM, Crapo JD, Freeman BA (1991) Detection of catalase in rat heart mitochondria. J Biol Chem 266:22028–22034

Raha S, Myint AT, Johnstone L, Robinson BH (2002) Control of oxygen free radical formation from mitochondrial complex I: roles for protein kinase A and pyruvate dehydrogenase kinase. Free Radic Biol Med 32:421–430

Rasola A, Bernardi P (2007) The mitochondrial permeability transition pore and its involvement in cell death and in disease pathogenesis. Apoptosis 12:815–833

Rauchová H, Vrbacký M, Bergamini C, Fato R, Lenaz G, Houstek J, Drahota Z (2006) Inhibition of glycerophosphate-dependent H2O2 generation in brown fat mitochondria by idebenone. Biochem Biophys Res Commun 339: 362–366

Reeve AK, Krishnan KJ, Turnbull DM (2008) Age related mitochondrial degenerative disorders in humans. Biotechnol J 3:750–756

Rhee SG, Chae HZ, Kim K (2005) Peroxiredoxins: a historical overview and speculative preview of novel mechanisms and emerging concepts in cell signalling. Free Radic Biol Med 38:1543–1552

Ritov VB, Menshikova EV, Azuma K, Wood RJ, Toledo FG, Goodpaster BH, Ruderman NB, Kelley DE (2009) Deficiency of electron transport chain in human skeletal muscle mitochondria in type 2 diabetes mellitus and obesity. Am J Physiol Endocrinol Metab 298(1):E49–E58, Epub 3 Nov 2009

Rosca MG, Vazquez EJ, Kerner J, Parland W, Chandler MP, Stanley W, Sabbah HN, Hoppel CL (2008) Cardiac mitochondria in heart failure: decrease in respirasomes and oxidative phosphorylation. Cardiovasc Res 80:30–39

Rosenfeldt F, Marasco S, Lyon W, Wowk M, Sheeran F, Bailey M, Esmore D, Davis B, Pick A, Rabinov M, Smith J, Nagley P, Pepe S (2005) Coenzyme Q10 therapy before cardiac surgery improves mitochondrial function and in vitro contractility of myocardial tissue. J Thorac Cardiovasc Surg 129:25–32

Rossignol R, Faustin B, Rocher C, Malgat M, Mazat JP, Letellier T (2003) Mitochondrial threshold effects. Biochem J 370:751–762

Rota M, LeCapitaine N, Hosoda T, Boni A, De Angelis A, Padin-Iruegas ME, Esposito G, Vitale S, Urbanek K, Casarsa C, Giorgio M, Luscher TF, Pelicci PG, Anversa P, Leri A, Kajstura J (2006) Diabetes promotes cardiac stem cell aging and heart failure, which are prevented by deletion of the p66Shc gene. Circ Res 99:42–52

Rötig A, Appelkvist EL, Geromel V, Chretien D, Khadom N, Edery P, Lebideau M, Dallner G, Munnich A, Ernster L, Rustin P (2000) Quinone-responsive multiple respiratory chain dysfunction due to widespread coenzyme Q10 deficiency. Lancet 356:391–395

Rubio AR, Morales-Segura MA (2004) Nitric oxide, an iceberg in cardiovascular physiology: far beyond vessel tone control. Arch Med Res 35:1–11

Ryan MT, Hoogenraad NJ (2007) Mitochondrial-nuclear communications. Annu Rev Biochem 76:701–722

Ryter SW, Kim HP, Hoetzel A, Park JW, Nakahira K, Wang X, Choi AMK (2007) Mechanisms of cell death in oxidative stress. Antioxid Redox Signal 9:49–89

Saito Y, Fukuhara A, Nishio K, Hayakawa M, Ogawa Y, Sakamoto H, Fujii K, Yoshida Y, Niki E (2009) Characterization of cellular uptake and distribution of coenzyme Q10 and vitamin E in PC12 cells. J Nutr Biochem 20:350–357

Salvatorelli E, Guarnieri S, Menna P, Liberi G, Calafiore AM, Mariggiò MA, Mordente A, Gianni L, Minotti G (2006) Detective one- or two-electron reduction of the anticancer anthracycline epirubicin in human heart. Relative importance of vesicular sequestration and impaired efficiency of electron addition. J Biol Chem 281:10990–11001

Salvi M, Battaglia V, Brunati AM, La Rocca N, Tibaldi E, Pietrangeli P, Marcocci L, Mondovì B, Rossi CA, Toninello A (2007) Catalase takes part in rat liver mitochondria oxidative stress defense. J Biol Chem 282:24407–24415

Sarti P, Giuffré A, Forte E, Mastronicola D, Barone MC, Brunori M (2000) Nitric oxide and cytochrome oxidase: mechanisms of inhibition and NO degradation. Biochem Biophys Res Commun 274:183–187

Scacco S, Petruzzella V, Bestini E, Luso A, Papa F, Bellomo F, Signorile A, Torraco A, Papa S (2006) Mutations in structural genes of complex I associated with neurological diseases. Ital J Biochem 55:254–262

Schafer FQ, Buettner GR (2001) Redox environment of the cell as viewed through the redox state of the glutathione disulfide/glutathione couple. Free Radic Biol Med 30:1191–1212

Schäfer E, Dencher NA, Vonck J, Parcej DN (2007) Three-dimensional structure of the respiratory chain supercomplex $I_1III_2IV_1$ from bovine heart mitochondria. Biochemistry 46:12579–12585

Schägger H (2001) Respiratory chain supercomplexes. IUBMB Life 52:119–128

Schägger H, Pfeiffer K (2001) The ratio of oxidative phosphorylation complexes I-V in bovine heart mitochondria and the composition of respiratory chain supercomplexes. J Biol Chem 276:37861–37867

Schägger H, de Coo R, Bauer MF, Hofmann S, Godinot C, Brandt U (2004) Significance of respirasomes for the assembly/stability of human respiratory chain complex I. J Biol Chem 279:36349–36353

Schlossmann JU, Hofmann F (2005) cGMP-dependent protein kinases in drug discovery. Drug Discov Today 10:627–634

Schoneich C (1999) Reactive oxygen species and biological aging: a mechanistic approach. Exp Gerontol 34:19–34

Seifert EL, Estey C, Xuan JY, Harper ME (2010) Electron transport chain-dependent and -independent mechanisms of mitochondrial H2O2 emission during long-chain fatty acid oxidation. J Biol Chem 285:5748–5758

Sekhar BS, Kurup CK, Ramasarma T (1987) Generation of hydrogen peroxide by brown adipose tissue mitochondria. J Bioenerg Biomembr 19:397–407

Shen Y, Shen HM, Shi CY, Ong CN (1996) Benzene metabolites enhance reactive oxygen species generation in HL60 human leukaemia cells. Hum Exp Toxicol 15:422–427

Shults CW, Oakes D, Kieburtz K, Beal MF, Haas R, Plumb S, Juncos JL, Nutt J, Shoulson I, Carter J, Kompoliti K, Perlmutter JS, Reich S, Stern M, Watts RL, Kurlan R, Molho E, Harrison M, Lew M, Parkinson Study Group (2002) Effects of Coenzyme Q10 in early Parkinson's disease: evidence of slowing of the functional decline. Arch Neurol 59:1541–1550

Sies H, Stahl W, Sevanian A (2005) Nutritional, dietary and post-prandial oxidative stress. J Nutr 135:969–972

Singer SJ, Nicolson GL (1972) The fluid mosaic model of the structure of cell membranes. Science 175:720–731

Skulachev VP (1996) Role of uncoupled and non-coupled oxidations in maintenance of safely low levels of oxygen and its one-electron reductants. Q Rev Biophys 29:169–202

Skulachev VP (2006) Bioenergetic aspects of apoptosis, necrosis and mitoptosis. Apoptosis 11:473–485

Smeitink JA, Zeviani M, Turnbull DM, Jacobs HT (2006) Mitochondrial medicine: a metabolic perspective on the pathology of oxidative phosphorylation disorders. Cell Metab 3:9–13

Sohal RS, Sohal BH, Orr WC (1995) Mitochondrial superoxide and hydrogen peroxide generation, protein oxidative damage, and longevity in different species of flies. Free Radic Biol Med 19:499–504

Soory M (2009) Relevance of nutritional antioxidants in metabolic syndrome, ageing and cancer: potential for therapeutic targeting. Infect Disord Drug Targets 9:400–414

Soskic V, Groebe K, Schrattenholz A (2008) Nonenzymatic posttranslational protein modifications in ageing. Exp Gerontol 43:247–257

Srinivas V, Leshchinsky I, Sang N, King MP, Minchenko A, Caro J (2001) Oxygen sensing and HIF-1 activation does not require an active mitochondrial respiratory chain electron-transfer pathway. J Biol Chem 276:21995–21998

Stadtman ER (1992) Protein oxidation and aging. Science 257:1220–1224

Stadtman ER (2004) Role of oxidant species in aging. Curr Med Chem 11:1105–1112

Staniek K, Nohl H (2000) Are mitochondria a permanent source of reactive oxygen species? Biochim Biophys Acta 1460:268–275

Starkov AA, Fiskum G (2001) Myxothiazol induces H_2O_2 production from mitochondrial respiratory chain. Biochem Biophys Res Commun 281:645–650

Starkov AA, Fiskum G (2003) Regulation of brain mitochondrial H_2O_2 production by membrane potential and NAD(P)H redox state. J Neurochem 86:1101–1107

Starkov AA, Fiskum G, Chinopoulos C, Lorenzo BJ, Browne SE, Patel MS, Beal MF (2004) Mitochondrial alpha-ketoglutarate dehydrogenase complex generates reactive oxygen species. J Neurosci 24:7779–7788

St-Pierre J, Buckingham JA, Roebuck SJ, Brand MD (2002) Topology of superoxide production from different sites in the mitochondrial electron transfer chain. J Biol Chem 277:44784–44790

Strauss M, Hofhaus G, Schröder RR, Kühlbrandt W (2008) Dimer ribbons of ATP synthase shape the inner mitochondrial membrane. EMBO J 27:1154–1160

Stroh A, Anderka O, Pfeiffer K, Yagi T, Finel M, Ludwig B, Schägger H (2004) Assembly of respiratory complexes I, III, and IV into NADH oxidase supercomplex stabilizes complex I in Paracoccus denitrificans. J Biol Chem 279:5000–5007

Strolin Benedetti M, Whomsley R, Baltes E (2006) Involvement of enzymes other than cytochrome P450 in the oxidative metabolism of xenobiotics. Expert Opin Drug Metab Toxicol 2:895–921

Strolin Benedetti M, Tipton KF, Whomsley R (2007) Amine oxidases and monooxygenases in the in vivo metabolism of xenobiotic amines in humans: has the involvement of amine oxidases been neglected? Fundam Clin Pharmacol 21:467–479

Sultana R, Butterfield DA (2009) Oxidatively modified, mitochondria-relevant brain proteins in subjects with Alzheimer disease and mild cognitive impairment. J Bioenerg Biomembr 41:441–446

Sun X, Zhou Z, Kang YI (2001) Attenuation of doxorubicin chronic toxicity in metallothionein-overexpressing transgenic mouse heart. Cancer Res 61:3382–3387

Tahara EB, Barros MH, Oliveira GA, Netto LES, Kowaltowski AJ (2007) Dihydrolipoyl dehydrogenase as a source of reactive oxygen species inhibited by caloric restriction and involved in *Saccharomyces cerevisiae* aging. FASEB J 21:274–283

Takahashi T, Yamaguchi T, Shitashige M, Okamoto T, Kishi T (1995) Reduction of ubiquinone in membrane lipids by rat liver cytosol and its involvement in the cellular defence system against lipid peroxidation. Biochem J 309:883–890

Takeshige K, Minakami S (1979) NADH and NADPH-dependent formation of superoxide anions by bovine heart submitochondrial particles and NADH-ubiquinone reductase preparation. Biochem J 180:129–135

Tanaka M, Gong JS, Zhang J, Yoneda M, Yagi K (1998) Mitochondrial genotype associated with longevity. Lancet 351:185–186

Taylor CT (2008) Mitochondria and cellular oxygen sensing in the HIF pathway. Biochem J 409:19–26

Tomilov AA, Bicocca V, Schoenfeld RA, Giorgio M, Migliaccio E, Ramsey JJ, Hagopian K, Pelicci PG, Cortopassi GA (2010) Decreased superoxide production in macrophages of long-lived p66Shc knock-out mice. J Biol Chem 285:1153–1165

Tretter L, Adam-Vizi V (2004) Generation of reactive oxygen species in the reaction catalyzed by alpha-ketoglutarate dehydrogenase. J Neurosci 24:7771–7778

Trifunovic A (2006) Mitochondrial DNA and ageing. Biochim Biophys Acta 1757:611–617

Trifunovic A, Larsson NG (2008) Mitochondrial dysfunction as a cause of ageing. J Intern Med 263:167–178

Trifunovic A, Wredenberg A, Falkenberg M, Spelbrink JN, Rovio AT, Bruder CE, Bohlooly-Y M, Gidlöf S, Oldfors A, Wibom R, Törnell J, Jacobs HT, Larsson NG (2004) Premature ageing in mice expressing defective mitochondrial DNA polymerase. Nature 429:417–423

Trinei M, Giorgio M, Cicalese A, Barozzi S, Ventura A, Migliaccio E, Milia E, Padura IM, Raker VA, Maccarana M, Petronilli V, Minucci S, Bernardi P, Lanfrancone L, Pelicci PG (2002) A p53-p66Shc signalling pathway controls intracellular redox status, levels of oxidation-damaged DNA and oxidative stress-induced apoptosis. Oncogene 21:3872–3878

Turrens JF (2003) Mitochondrial formation of reactive oxygen species. J Physiol 552:335–344

Turunen M, Olsson J, Dallner G (2004) Metabolism and function of coenzyme Q. Biochim Biophys Acta 1660:171–199

Ugarte N, Petropoulos I, Friguet B (2010) Oxidized mitochondrial protein degradation and repair in aging and oxidative stress. Antioxid Redox Signal 13(4):539–549, Epub 3 Dec 2009

Valko M, Rhodes CJ, Moncol J, Izakovic M, Mazur M (2006) Free radicals, metals and antioxidants in oxidative stress-induced cancer. Chem Biol Interact 160:1–40

Valko M, Leibfritz D, Moncol J, Cronin MT, Mazur M, Telser J (2007) Free radicals and antioxidants in normal physiological functions and human disease. Int J Biochem Cell Biol 39:44–84

Van Raam BJ, Sluiter W, de Wit E, Roos D, Verhoeven AJ, Kuijpers TW (2008) Mitochondrial membrane potential in human neutrophils is maintained by complex III activity in the absence of supercomplex organisation. PLoS One 3:e2013

Vaux EC, Metzen E, Yeates KM, Ratcliffe PJ (2001) Regulation of hypoxia-inducible factor is preserved in the absence of a functioning mitochondrial respiratory chain. Blood 198:296–302

Venkatakrishnan P, Nakayasu ES, Almeida IC, Miller RT (2009) Absence of nitric-oxide synthase in sequentially purified rat liver mitochondria. J Biol Chem 284:19843–19855

Ventura B, Genova ML, Bovina C, Formiggini G, Lenaz G (2002) Control of oxidative phosphorylation by Complex I in rat liver mitochondria: implications for aging. Biochim Biophys Acta 1553:249–260

Verkaart S, Koopman WJH, van Ernst-de Vries SE, Nijtmans LGJ, van den Heuvel LWPJ, Smeitink JAM, Willems PHGM (2007) Superoxide production is inversely related to Complex I activity in inherited Complex I deficiency. Biochim Biophys Acta 1772:373–381

Vila A, Korytowsky W, Girotti AW (2000) Dissemination of peroxidative stress via intermembrane transfer of lipid peroxides: model studies with cholesterol hydroperoxides. Arch Biochem Biophys 380:208–218

Vinogradov AD, Grivennikova VG (2005) Generation of superoxide-radical by the NADH:ubiquinone oxidoreductase of heart mitochondria. Biochemistry (Moscow) 70:120–127

Vlassara H (2005) Advances glycation in health and disease: role of the modern environment. Ann NY Accad. Sci. 1043: 452–460

Vlassara H, Striker G (2007) Glycotoxins in the diet promote diabetes and diabetic complications. Curr Diab Rep 7:235–241

Vonck J, Schäfer E (2009) Supramolecular organization of protein complexes in the mitochondrial inner membrane. Biochim Biophys Acta 1793:117–124

Wallace DC (2005) A mitochondrial paradigm of metabolic and degenerative diseases, aging, and cancer: a dawn for evolutionary medicine. Annu Rev Genet 39:359–407

Wang Y, Michikawa Y, Mallidis C, Bai Y, Woodhouse L, Yarasheski KE, Miller CA, Askanas V, Engel WK, Bhasin S, Attardi G (2001) Muscle-specific mutations accumulate with aging in critical human mtDNA control sites for replication. Proc Natl Acad Sci USA 98:4022–4027

Wei Y-H, Lee H-C (2002) Oxidative stress, mitochondrial DNA mutation, and impairment of antioxidant enzymes in aging. Exp Biol Med 227:671–682

Wells WW, Xu DP, Washburn MP, Cirrito HK, Olson LK (2001) Polyhydroxybenzoates inhibit ascorbic acid activation of mitochondrial glycerol-3-phosphate dehydrogenase: implications for glucose metabolism and insulin secretion. J Biol Chem 276:2404–2410

Wendt T, Tanji N, Guo J, Hudson BI, Bierhaus A, Ramasamy R, Arnold B, Nawroth PP, Yan SF, d'Agati V, Schmidt AM (2003) Glucose, glycation and RAGE: implications for amplification of cellular dysfunction in diabetic nephropathy. J Am Soc Nephrol 14:1383–1395

Wenz T, Hielscher R, Hellwig P, Schägger H, Richers S, Hunte C (2009) Role of phospholipids in respiratory cytochrome bc(1) complex catalysis and supercomplex formation. Biochim Biophys Acta 1787:609–616

Williams SD, Gottlieb RA (2002) Inhibition of mitochondrial calcium-independent phospholipase A2 (iPLA2) attenuates mitochondrial phospholipid loss and is cardioprotective. Biochem J 362:23–32

Wiswedel I, Gardemann A, Storch A, Peter D, Schild L (2010) Degradation of phospholipids by oxidative stress–exceptional significance of cardiolipin. Free Radic Res 44:135–145

Yan LJ, Sohal RS (2000) Prevention of flight activity prolongs the life span of the housefly, Musca domestica, and attenuates the age-associated oxidative damamge to specific mitochondrial proteins. Free Radic Biol Med 29:1143–1150

Yankovskaya V, Horsefield R, Tornroth S, Luna-Chavez C, Miyoshi H, Léger C, Byrne B, Cecchini G, Iwata S (2003) Architecture of succinate dehydrogenase and reactive oxygen species generation. Science 299:700–704

Yu A, Yu L, King TE (1974) Soluble cytochrome b-c1 complex and the reconstitution of succinate-cytochrome c reductase. J Biol Chem 249:4905–4910

Yun J, Rago C, Cheong I, Pagliarini R, Angenendt P, Rajagopalan H, Schmidt K, Willson JK, Markowitz S, Zhou S, Diaz LA Jr, Velculescu VE, Lengauer C, Kinzler KW, Vogelstein B, Papadopoulos N (2009) Glucose deprivation contributes to the development of KRAS pathway mutations in tumor cells. Science 325:1555–1559

Zeviani M, Carelli V (2007) Mitochondrial disorders. Curr Opin Neurol 20:564–571

Zhang L, Yu L, Yu CA (1998) Generation of superoxide anion by succinate cytochrome c reductase from bovine heart mitochondria. J Biol Chem 273:33972–33976

Zhang M, Mileykovskaya E, Dowhan W (2002) Gluing the respiratory chain together. Cardiolipin is required for supercomplex formation in the inner mitochondrial membrane. J Biol Chem 277:43553–43556

Zhang J, Frerman FE, Kim JJ (2006) Structure of electron transfer flavoprotein-ubiquinone oxidoreductase and electron transfer to the mitochondrial ubiquinone pool. Proc Natl Acad Sci USA 103:16212–16217

Zigmond MJ, Hastings TG, Perez RG (2002) Increased dopamine turnover after partial loss of dopaminergic neurons: compensation or toxicity? Parkinsonism Relat Disord 8:389–393

Zimniak P (2008) Detoxification reactions: relevance to aging. Aging Res Rev 7:281–300

Zorov DB, Filburn CR, Klotz LO, Zweier JL, Sollott SJ (2000) Reactive oxygen species (ROS)-induced ROS release: a new phenomenon accompanying induction of the mitochondrial permeability transition in cardiac myocytes. Exp Med 192:1001–1014

Zorov DB, Bannikova SY, Belousov VV, Vyssokikh MY, Zorova LD, Isaev NK, Krasnikov BF, Plotnikov EY (2005) Reactive oxygen and nitrogen species: friends or foes? Biochemistry (Moscow) 70:215–221

Zorov DB, Juhaszova M, Sollott SJ (2006) Mitochondrial ROS-induced ROS release: an update and review. Biochim Biophys Acta 1757:509–517

Chapter 6
Uncoupling Proteins: Molecular, Functional, Regulatory, Physiological and Pathological Aspects

Francis E. Sluse

Abstract Uncoupling proteins are a subfamily of the mitochondrial anion carrier family. They are widespread in the whole eukaryotic world with a few exceptions and present tissue specific isoforms in higher organisms. They mediate purine nucleotide-sensitive free fatty acid-activated proton inward flux through the inner mitochondrial membrane. This proton flux occurs at the expense of the proton motive force build up by the respiration and weakens the coupling between respiration and ATP synthesis. In this chapter we describe current and reliable knowledge of uncoupling proteins. A new methodology allowing study of their activity and regulation during phosphorylating respiration is described. It has entitled us to assert that all uncoupling proteins share common mechanisms of activation and regulation. This is of the utmost importance in order to understand the physiological roles of UCPs as well as their participation in pathological processes since every role of the UCPs in every cell is an integral part of their function and regulation. The central role of reduction level of ubiquinone in the control of their regulation is well-argued. Their potential and reliable roles in thermogenesis, reactive oxygen species prevention and energy flow are discussed as well as their role in some pathological disorders.

Keywords Partitioning of proton electrochemical gradient • Physiological roles of uncoupling proteins (UCP) • Reactive oxygen species prevention and energy metabolism balance • Pathological implications of UCPs linked to their physiological roles • Regulation mechanisms of UCP activity • Widespread distribution of UCPs

6.1 Introduction

Mitochondria are the respiring entities of eukaryotic cells. They are the centre of oxidative metabolism in cells, coupling catabolic pathways to the respiration first and second, respiration to the synthesis of ATP. Terminal catabolism occurs in mitochondria providing, the respiratory chain with reducing cofactors (NADH and FADH2). During the transfer of electrons from cofactors to molecular oxygen

F.E. Sluse (✉)
Laboratory of Bioenergetics and Cellular Physiology, Department of Life Sciences,
Faculty of Sciences, University of Liege, B4000 Liege, Belgium
e-mail: F.Sluse@ulg.ac.be

R. Scatena et al. (eds.), *Advances in Mitochondrial Medicine*, Advances in Experimental
Medicine and Biology 942, DOI 10.1007/978-94-007-2869-1_6,
© Springer Science+Business Media B.V. 2012

which is catalysed by the respiratory chain (RC), an H^+ electrochemical gradient is generated across the inner membrane. This H^+ electrochemical gradient is used for many purposes, not only for ATP synthesis (see below).

6.1.1   *Respiration as a H^+ Electrochemical Gradient Generator*

The respiratory chain, or electron transport chain, consists of respiratory enzyme complexes containing numerous electrons carriers (redox centers). These complexes have an appropriate orientation in the membrane in order to catalyse a vectorial H^+ movement outward the mitochondrial matrix which is coupled to the oxidoreduction reactions. This vectorial H^+ pumping generates an H+ gradient across the membrane (ΔpH, acidic outside). The net transport of H^+ across the membrane (in to out) and the net movement of electrons inside the complexes (out to in) generate also an electrical potential difference ($\Delta\psi$ negative inside). Both ΔpH, H^+ concentration difference, and $\Delta\psi$, electrical potential difference, constitute the "protonmotive force" (pmf or $\Delta\mu H^+$ or Δp) which is the primary form of redox reaction energy conversion (Mitchell 1961). Once created the $\Delta\mu H^+$ represents a thermodynamic constraint which controls the electron flow in the respiratory chain. The free energy contained in the H^+ electrochemical gradient is available for various "works".

6.1.2   *H^+ Electrochemical Gradient Sharing*

Once produced the protonmotive force is mainly used to perform the ATP synthesis process. Consequently the pmf couples respiration and ATP synthesis. This overall energy conversion implies that oxidoreduction reactions in the respiratory chain and ATP hydrolysis are both coupled to H^+ pumping, thus ATP synthase must be a reversible H^+ ATPase. This coupling between respiration and ATP synthesis implies that the H^+ are free to diffuse in the aqueous phase on both sides of the membrane creating a delocalized H^+ circuit between RC proton pumps and ATP synthase and requires the inner membrane to have a low H^+ conductance (Saraste 1999). As the coupling is delocalized the pmf may be used to drive other processes. Thus the pmf can be shared, among others, between ATP synthase, ion carriers, metabolite carriers and uncoupling proteins.

6.1.3   *Outline of the Chapter*

The aim of this chapter is to gather updated understanding of uncoupling proteins. The discovery of "PUMP" a plant UCP in potato mitochondria, by A. Vercesi in 1995 (Vercesi et al. 1995) has terminated the long solo life of brown fat UCP (now UCP1). Since then UCP's have been discovered widespread distributed in eukaryotic cells. The so-called UCP1 analogues are still believed to be different from UCP1 in their activation and regulation processes (Azzu et al. 2010). Some evidences of the contrary are described below and the UCPs potential physiological roles are discussed. It is also stressed that the precise knowledge of UCP activity-regulation mechanisms are of utmost importance to understand the physiological roles of UCPs as well as their participation in pathological processes. UCP1 is not unique by itself (see below) it has just been discovered first in a specialized mammalian tissue devoted to heat production, the brown adipose tissue (BAT).

6.2   Uncoupling Protein Family

Uncoupling proteins form a sub-family in the mitochondrial anion carrier family (MACP)

6.2.1 Mitochondrial Anion Carrier Family (MACF)

The metabolic compartmentalization within eukaryotic cells requires an intense traffic of metabolites across the membrane of organelles closely linking metabolic pathways between organelles and the cytosol and between the different organelles. This traffic of metabolites is operated by trans-membrane proteins, sharing similar structure, called carriers or translocators (Sluse 1996; el Moualij et al. 1997). As such metabolites are mainly polar molecules and sometimes have to move against a concentration gradient, free energy is required for their movement across the mitochondrial inner membrane. The activity of the members of MACF is linked with the H^+ electrochemical gradient built up by the respiration. All members of MACF rely on the pmf for their activity, directly or indirectly, whatever their transport mode is: electrophoretic uniport or antiport, electroneutral H^+ compensated or electroneutral exchanges. For example carriers directly involved in oxidative phosphorylation (OXPHOS) are free energy consuming: inorganic phosphate import is electroneutral $1H^+$ compensated and export of ATP^{4-} in exchange of ADP^{3-} is electrophoretic, total cost for both: $1H^+$ reentry. Uncoupling protein which belongs to the MACF is proposed to catalyze the export of anionic free fatty acid (FFA^-) at the expense of electrical potential gradient (1 charge) through a FFA recycling process: translocated FFA^- is protonated in the cytosol and crosses back the membrane by diffusion into the matrix where it is deprotonated (Garlid et al. 1996). This cycle results in a net H^+ reuptake that consumes the pmf and can affect the coupling between respiration and ATP synthesis.

6.2.2 Widespread Distribution

For more than 20 years UCP1 of BAT was believed to be unique and a late evolutionary acquisition of mammals devoted to thermogenesis in newborn, cold-acclimated and hibernating animals (Klingenberg 1990; Nicholls and Rial 1999; Klingenberg and Echtay 2001). Currently we know that UCP1 analogues are widespread in various tissues and in the 4 eukaryotic kingdoms: animals, plants, fungi and protists (Sluse and Jarmuszkiewicz 2002). The discovery of UCP in *Acanthamoeba castellanii* (Jarmuszkiewicz et al. 1999) proves that UCPs emerged as specialized proteins for H^+ recycling soon during phylogenesis before the major radiation of phenotypic diversity in eukaryotes more than 10^9 years ago! Since 15 years the presence of UCP1 analogues has been evidenced in several unicellular eukaryotes as amoeboid and parasitic protists, non-fermentative yeast and filamentous fungi (Jarmuszkiewicz et al. 2000b). "New UCP" were discovered throughout mammalian tissues (UCP2 in several tissues, UCP3 in muscles and BAT, UCP4-5 in brain) (Ricquier and Bouillaud 2000) and are also quite ubiquitous in plant tissues with several isoforms evidenced, for review see (Vercesi et al. 2006). Then a critical question has arose: are all these UCPs doing the same thing (increase H+ conductance of the membrane) in the same way (activation, inhibition, regulation) for the same purpose?

6.2.3 Brown Fat UCP1 as a Reference?

In brown adipose tissue UCP1 is very abundant and is by far the most studied and the best characterized for a review see (Cannon and Nedergaard 2004). UCP1 sustains a FFA-induced purine-nucleotide-inhibited H^+ conductance that importantly decreases the pmf and therefore is responsible (by removal of the thermodynamic constraint) for a strong increase of the BAT mitochondrial respiration rate.

FFAs originate from the stimulation of lipolysis under the control of hormonal stimulus (noradrenaline). Thus UCP1 takes advantage of a peculiar situation into cells sensitive to sympathomimetic stimulation of their beta3-adrenergic receptors. In addition to the high UCP1 content BAT mitochondria also exhibit peculiar properties namely, a high capacity of the respiratory chain relative to a low capacity of ATP synthase. In such a way, under hormonal stimulation BAT mitochondria are almost non-phosphorylating entities. On the contrary UCP1-analogues present a low abundance in their respective cell or tissue. Activation by FFA is well documented in reconstituted systems but still debated in isolated mitochondria and inhibition by purine nucleotides (PN), which is considered as a diagnostic of UCP activity, even if observed in reconstituted proteoliposomes is rarely observed with isolated mitochondria under non-phosphorylating conditions. From such considerations it has been assumed that UCP1 and its analogues were not subjected to the same molecular regulation and perhaps did not share the same mechanism of uncoupling. However as UCP1-analogues are found in basically phosphorylating mitochondria, perhaps their study has not been undertaken in the appropriate respiratory conditions?

6.3 Energy Dissipating Systems

Energy dissipation is believed to be necessary for the maintenance of metabolic homeostasis by allowing adjustments in energy metabolic balance. Indeed energy dissipation could have a subtle role in energy metabolism control working as safety valves in conditions where excess of reducing power or in phosphate potential occur (Jarmuszkiewicz et al. 2001). This point will be discussed in Sect. 6.3.

6.3.1 Proton and Electron Leaks

UCPs are not the only proteins that can dissipate free energy. Two types of catalysed leaks can occur at the level of the respiratory chain: electron leak and proton leak. According the cell both systems are present or only H^+ leak occurs. It must be pointed out that they are not independent as electron leak finally leads to a decrease in the rate of H^+ electrochemical gradient building. In plant mitochondria, both energy dissipation coexist (Sluse and Jarmuszkiewicz 2000) thanks to -peripheral NADH-ubiquinol oxido-reductases and ubiquinol-oxygen oxidoreductase (alternative oxidase: AOX) that allow electrons to bypass Complex I and Complexes III+CIV respectively -and to uncoupling protein that catalyses H+ leak. Interestingly both UCP and AOX are present at the same time but UCP is activated by FFA whereas AOX is inhibited (Sluse et al. 1998a). Animals have lost AOX and peripheral NADH dehydrogenases but have retained UCP during evolution as both types of energy dissipating proteins are present in microorganisms like fungi, trypanosomes, and amoeba. The only obvious physiological function of both AOX and UCP occur in specialized plant and animal thermogenic tissues as heat generation related to increase in temperature of a tissue or of the body (thermogenesis): as already mentioned UCP in BAT during cold acclimation and AOX in spadices of *Araceae* during reproductive processes (Meeuse 1975). In other types of tissues and in unicellular organisms they should play no significant role in thermogenesis due to their low abundance and in microorganisms due to the high surface/volume ratio that excludes any steady-state local heating because heat diffusion rate is too fast due to the important thermal conductivity of the medium.

6.3.2 Uncoupling Protein 1 as a Heat Generator

UCP1 is not a thermal molecular machine: it does not produce heat by simply dissipating the H^+ electrochemical gradient built up by the respiratory chain. Indeed thermogenesis is not only restricted by a lower-size limit but also by the actual effect of activation of energy dissipating systems on heat production rate at a given overall steady-state metabolic activity *in vivo*. This last point requires that different oxidative pathways have large differences in enthalpy changes, more exothermic for AOX-sustained and UCP-sustained respirations compared to ADP-sustained respiration (phosphorylating state 3 respiration). This is not the case as combined calorimetric and respirometric data (Breidenbach et al. 1997) invalidate large difference in enthalpy change supposed above because the enthalpy of ATP hydrolysis is included in the balance. It would be different *in vitro* with isolated mitochondria devoid of ATP consuming processes. Nevertheless no local mitochondrial increase in temperature could be detected (size limit). These thermodynamic reflections apply to UCP1-sustained thermogenesis that depends on a net increase in overall steady-state oxygen uptake rate through metabolic and cellular up-regulations. This is well illustrated in BAT during cold acclimation for example: stimulation of adrenergic receptors stimulates lipolysis producing FFAs that activate UCP1 and are consumed (metabolic response), and leads to up-regulation of UCP1 expression together with recruitment of BAT cells (cellular response) that increase the weight of BAT. As the capacity of the respiratory chain is large, a strong increase in respiration rate (burst) occurs immediately after UCP1 activation. During acclimation an up-regulation of expression of UCP1 occurs (20 fold) together with respiratory chain complexes (10 fold) and upstream catabolic pathways (beta-oxidation and Krebs cycle) that provide the respiratory chain with reduced co-enzymes (Navet et al. 2007). Thus thermogenesis hinges on increase of oxygen (combustive) uptake: "more fuel+ more combustive=more fire=more heat".

6.3.3 Other UCP's

Low abundance of UCP1 analogues seems to exclude them from thermogenic processes. Nevertheless they are all H^+ electrochemical gradient spendthrift as it will be shown below and when studied in phosphorylating mitochondria they exhibit a PN-sensitivity like UCP1 (Jarmuszkiewicz et al. 2004b). Moreover their activation decreases the oxidative phosphorylation efficiency.

6.4 Measurement of H+ Partitioning *In Vitro*

Most researches have focused on the activation of UCPs in non-phosphorylating respiring mitochondria, i.e. at a maximal state 4 pmf. In this way the FFA-activated PN-inhibited H^+ conductance which is considered as a diagnostic of an activation of a UCP was always tested in state 4 through a so-called force/flow titration or proton-conductance curve (Voltage dependence of electron flux in the respiratory chain). Two characteristics can be tested by such titrations. First, the protonophoric effect of the addition of FFA on non-phosphorylating respiration rate and second the PN-sensitivity of this effect. Force/flow titrations with BAT mitochondria exhibit the canonical behavior of UCP1 when respiratory rate state 4 is progressively inhibited and $\Delta\psi$ is measured in the presence or in the absence of a constant FFA concentration and in the presence or the absence of PN: an equidistant curve (state 4 rate versus $\Delta\psi$) is obtained in the presence of FFA corresponding to a roughly constant drop in electrical potential difference (in the non-ohmic part of the titration) which is cancelled in the presence of PN. Force/flow

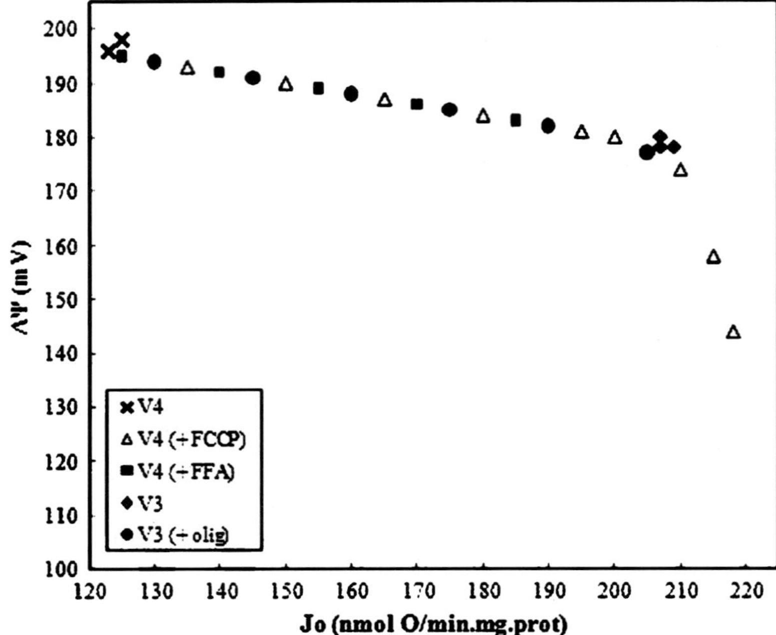

Fig. 6.1 Relation between $\Delta\psi$ and mitochondrial respiration rate Jo (Force/Flow relationship). Phosphorylating respiration i.e. full state 3 rate V3 (♦); State 4 rate V4 (x); State 4 titration with increasing concentrations of FFA (■); State 4 titration with increasing concentrations of uncoupler FCCP (carbonyl cyanide p-trifluoromethoxyphenylhydrazone) (Δ); State 3 titration with increasing concentrations of oligomycin (●)

titrations with other mitochondria containing UCP1 analogues permit only to prove the protonophoric effect of increasing concentrations of FFA that is not distinguishable from the effect of a well known protonophore like FCCP (Jarmuszkiewicz et al. 1999, 2000b). This single (FFA and FCCP) force/flow relationship (Fig. 6.1) indicates that FFA does not interact with the respiratory chain and has a pure protonophoric effect. Titration with constant FFA concentration exhibits also a drop in $\Delta\psi$ but is not convincingly reversed by PN. The use of non-phosphorylating conditions in order to study the regulation properties of UCP1 analogues may limit the understanding of their *in vitro* and *in vivo* regulation as they are located in mitochondria which are basically phosphorylating entities contrarily to UCP1. Thus another approach must be delineated in order to investigate the properties of these "new" UCPs. This method hinges on the partitioning of H⁺ electrochemical gradient between ATP synthase and UCP1 analogues which affects indeed the OXPHOS yield *i.e.* the ADP/O ratio.

6.4.1 The ADP/O Method Applied to UCP1 Analogues

In 1996 a new method has been designed to determine the contributions of two processes in sustaining total respiration on isolated mitochondria (Jarmuszkiewicz et al. 1996). This method was first applied to evaluate the contributions (electron partitioning) of AOX (energy dissipating, see above) and cytochrome pathways (energy conserving) in overall respiration of *Acanthamoeba castellanii* isolated mitochondria and was based on their respective effect on the oxidative phosphorylation yield, *i.e.*, the ADP/O ratio during a state 3 respiration (phosphorylating) titration with an inhibitor of the oxidizable substrate uptake. The ADP/O method, based on the non-phosphorylating property of AOX, involves pair measurements of ADP/O ratios in the presence and in the absence of AOX inhibitor and measurements of the overall respiration rate in state 3. Since 1998 the ADP/O method is applied to measure the H^+ partitioning between ATP synthase and uncoupling protein with FFA-depleted mitochondria of several organisms: tomato (Jarmuszkiewicz et al. 1998, 2000a; Sluse et al. 1998b), *Acanthamoeba castellanii* (Jarmuszkiewicz et al. 1999), rat muscle (Jarmuszkiewicz et al. 2004b), potato (Navet et al. 2005). To apply this method several conditions must be fulfilled merely: (1) $\Delta\mu H^+$ dissipation in the presence of FFA to activate UCP occurs only through UCP activity, (2) FFA has no effect on the intrinsic stoichiometries of oxidative phosphorylation (H^+/O and ATP/H^+) and (3) $\Delta\psi$ is constant into the titration range. Then, the two following equations can be used to calculate both contributions (part of respiration sustained by ATP synthesis, $V_{cyt\ path}$ and part of respiration sustained by UCP activity, V_{UCP}):

$$V_{cyt\ path} = V_3 \times (ADP/O)/(ADP/O)_{-FFA} \tag{6.1}$$

$$V_{UCP} = V_3 - V_{cytpath} \tag{6.2}$$

Where $(ADP/O)_{-FFA}$ is the ratio measured in the absence of FFA, (ADP/O) is the ration measured in the presence of FFA (UCP activated) and $V3$ is the overall steady state 3 respiration rate in the presence of FFA. Equations 6.1 and 6.2 can be rearranged to give:

$$V_3 \times (ADP/O) = (ADP/O)_{-FFA} \times (V_3 - V_{UCP}) \tag{6.3}$$

This equation predicts a linear relationship (Fig. 6.2b) between the rate of ATP synthesis ($J_p = V_3 \times (ADP/O)$) and the overall state 3 respiration rate ($J_o = V_3$) provided that V_{UCP} remains constant when V_3 is decreased by inhibition of substrate uptake as it has been verified (see ref. above). The linear relationship can be extrapolated to abscissa and crosses the origin if there is no basal H^+ leak during state 3 respiration (like in plant and protist mitochondria), then the measured $(ADP/O)_{-FFA}$ ratio is constant during titration and corresponds to the intrinsic (ADP/O) ratio (ratio of fixed intrinsic H^+/O and ATP/H^+ stoichiometric ratios). In mammal mitochondria it is not the case as the linear relationship between J_p and J_o crosses the abscissa axis on the right of the origin indicating that a part of the state 3 respiration rate of FFA-depleted mitochondria is sustained by a constant endogenous (or basal) H^+ leak. Thus Eq. 6.3 becomes:

$$J_P = (ADP/O)_{intrinsic} \times (J_o - J_{o\ basal\ leak}) = (ADP/O)_{measured} \times J_o \tag{6.4}$$

Then the measured ADP/O is decreasing when V_3 is decreased by inhibition of substrate uptake. However the slope of the straight line remains the intrinsic ADP/O ratio.

6.4.2   *Activation of UCP1 Analogues by FFA*

Activation of UCP analogues by FFA at low concentrations (μM range) is observed during J_p/J_o titration (Fig. 6.2b) for every type of mitochondria tested (plant, protist, animal): straight line relationships are observed between J_p and J_O in the absence and in the presence of given concentrations of FFA. All the straight lines have the same slope proving that the intrinsic stoichiometric ADP/O ratio remains unchanged in the presence of FFA. However with increasing the FFA concentration, the abscissa axis intercept is shifted to the right (size of the shift = V_{UCP}) indicating a FFA-concentration dependence of the UCP activity. Thus a set of parallel straight lines strongly suggest not only that FFA has no effect on H^+ pumps employed in oxidative phosphorylation but also that the H^+ conduction rate via UCP does not change with respiration rates. All these observation strongly suggest that UCP1 analogues can be activated *in vitro* by FFA alone and that this activation does not require lipid peroxidation products (Considine et al. 2003; Echtay et al. 2003).

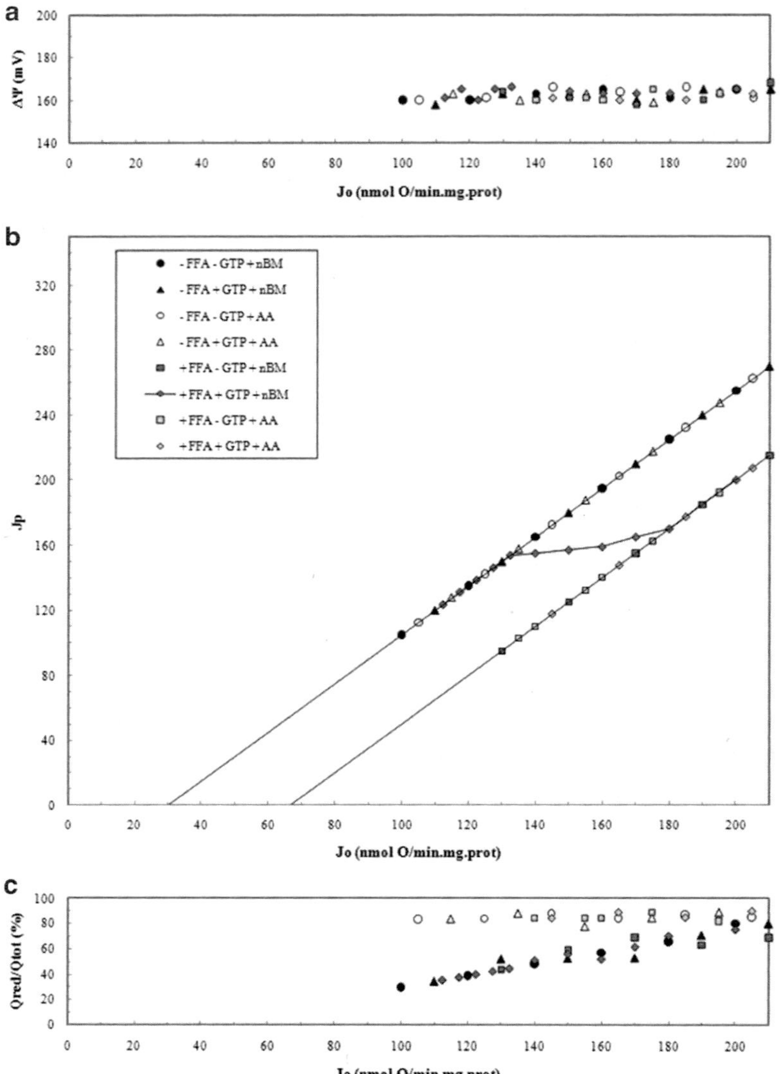

Fig. 6.2 Effect of purine nucleotide (GTP) in phosphorylating mitochondria when QH_2-oxidizing or Q-reducing pathways are inhibited. Relationships between $\Delta\psi$ (**a**), rate of ADP phosphorylation (J_p) (**b**), Q reduction level (**c**) and the rate of oxygen consumption during state 3 respiration (J_O). All the conditions are indicated by different symbols in the *inset*

6.4.3 The Paradox of GTP Inhibition

Purine nucleotide inhibition is a diagnostic of UCP activity. The binding of PN to a high affinity binding site of UCP1 inhibits the H^+ conductance triggered by FFA (Gonzalez-Barroso et al. 1996). As already mentioned above, conflicting results were obtained with UCP1 analogues. In reconstituted proteoliposomes, UCP2, UCP3 and plant UCP are inhibited by PN (Jaburek et al. 1999; Borecky et al. 2001; Zackova et al. 2003) and their affinity to PN is in the μM range like UCP1 (Klingenberg and Echtay 2001; Jekabsons et al. 2002). However results obtained with isolated mitochondria showed that FFA-activated H+ conductance was poorly sensitive to PN under non-phosphorylating conditions (Jarmuszkiewicz et al. 1998; Rial et al. 1999; Zhang et al. 1999; Hourton-Cabassa et al. 2002). Only a so-called "superoxide-activated" state of UCP homologues has been shown to be PN sensitive in state 4 respiration (Echtay et al. 2002; Considine et al. 2003; Echtay et al. 2003). Anyway a paradox exists concerning PN inhibition of UCPs and PN concentration in the cell. Indeed, if the measured PN affinity is true then no UCP including UCP1 could be activated *in vivo* because of the large concentrations of PN present in the cell (mM range). Thus a physiologically relevant mechanism must exist to allow H+ conductance through UCPs to be regulated by PN.

6.4.4 Central Role of Q Reduction State

With the help of the ADP/O method it has been possible to clarify the PN-inhibition paradox and to show that PN are also very efficient inhibitors of FFA-activated UCP1 analogues (Jarmuszkiewicz et al. 2004b, 2005; Navet et al. 2005). Indeed, in 2004 (Jarmuszkiewicz et al. 2004b) it was shown in well-defined conditions that, with rat skeletal muscle mitochondria during state 3 respiration titration by n-butylmalonate (inhibitor of succinate uptake) in the presence or the absence of linoleic acid (LA) and of GTP (PN), we could observe at full state 3 rate no effect of GTP but, together with the decrease of state 3 rate, the appearance of an inhibitory effect of GTP on the LA-induced H^+ conductance (Fig. 6.2b). This inhibitory effect was total at about 50% inhibition of phosphorylating state 3 respiration rate. The same titration range of respiration with antimycin A (inhibitor of complex III of RC) did not lead to the appearance of an inhibitory effect by PN. At the same time the membrane $\Delta\psi$ (Fig. 6.2a) and the redox state of ubiquinone were monitored (Fig. 6.2c). Membrane electrical potential did not change in the respiration titration range and could not explain the progressive inhibition of LA-induced H+ conductance by GTP. On the other hand ubiquinone (Q) reduction level (Q_R/Q_T, i.e. the ratio reduced ubiquinone versus total ubiquinone in the membrane) decreased importantly during respiration titration with n-butylmalonate when GTP inhibition occurred. On the contrary inhibition with antimycin A (AA), which increased lightly the Q reduction level, did not lead to an inhibion by GTP during AA titration. Thus, the reduction level of coenzyme Q appears to monitor the PN inhibition of muscle UCP in phosphorylating mitochondria. Coenzyme Q or ubiquinone is a redox intermediate of the respiratory chain translocating electrons from dehydrogenases (electron entry) to the cytochrome pathway (in animals) and alternative oxidase (in plants and protists) thus playing a central role as crossroads of electrons in the RC. The Q reduction level seems to be too high in non-phosphorylating (state 4 respiration) mitochondria to observe an inhibition of H+ conductance by PN. Similar results as those given in Fig. 6.2 were obtained with mitochondria from the protist *Acanthamoebe castellanii* using succinate and external NADH as oxidizable substrates: no inhibition of FFA-induced H+ conductance by PN in full state 3 and state 4 but appearance of progressive inhibition related to the decrease in Q reduction level in inhibited state 3 at the side of electron entry. Even much better illustration of the role of Q reduction level in PN inhibition control was given by experiment on potato mitochondria, although the starting situation (in full state 3 respiration rate) was different, the results were in perfect accordance with those obtained with rat and protist mitochondria. Indeed, as the initial Q reduction level of full state 3 respiration rate was quite low in potato mitochondria, a full inhibition of FFA-induced UCP activity by PN was observed without n-butylmalonate (that still decreased more the Q reduction level). However, an inhibition of state 3 respiration rate with AA that increases the Q reduction level progressively cancelled the PN inhibition which could be restored by the further titration of state 3 respiration rate with n-butylmalonate. These results strongly suggest that the reduction level of Q is a "metabolic sensor" that modulates the inhibition of FFA-induced UCP1-analogue activity by PN in phosphorylating mitochondria (Sluse et al. 2006). Interestingly, in the case of UCP1,

UCP2 and UCP3, Q has been shown to be an obligatory factor for their active reconstitution in proteoliposomes (Echtay et al. 2000, 2001). The finding that in phosphorylating mitochondria the reduction level of Q modulates the sensitivity to PN of the FFA-induced UCP1 analogue activity is very important as it provides not only a new key-feature of the UCP activity regulation in phosphorylating mitochondria but also an explanation of how UCPs could be activated in vivo despite the large concentrations of PN present in the cell. This regulation also reconciles the conflicting results obtained with reconstituted systems and isolated mitochondria as it means the PN binding site operational in proteoliposomes and the unlike PN inhibition in non-phosphorylating mitochondria. Last but not least, the occurrence of this feature in mammals, plants and protists supports the universality of this new regulatory mechanism.

6.4.5 *UCP1 Is Also Under the Control of Q Reduction Level*

If the reduction level of Q modulates universally the PN sensitivity of the FFA-induced UCP1-analogue activity, then the following questions arise: has UCP1 the same regulatory feature implying Q or has UCP1 lost this feature and is able to overcome its PN inhibition simply by its interaction with FFA? As the study of UCP1 H^+ conductance and its regulation in BAT mitochondria during phosphorylating respiration is seemingly impossible task two ways have been used: (1) forget state 3 respiration and try to show in force/flow titration experiments in state 4 that FFA-induced H+ conductance is sensitive to Q reduction state and/or (2) Study PN sensitivity regulation in state 3 with a heterologous yeast expression system containing low amount of rat UCP1 in its mitochondria. Both studies have been realized recently (Swida-Barteczka et al. 2009) and led to very interesting and convincing results. First on the yeast mitochondria expressing UCP1 at 1 µg of UCP1 per mg of mitochondrial protein (Douette et al. 2006) force/flow titration with malonate (inhibitor of succinate uptake and oxidation) exhibits the classical profile as in BAT mitochondria, *i.e.* a nearly equidistant shift towards lower $\Delta\psi$ on the addition of oleic acid (OA) which is cancelled by 2 mM GTP (Fig. 6.3a). During these titrations the reduction level of Q decreases from 82% to 43%. However when the reduction state of Q is increased from 83% to 98% during the titrations with cyanide the inhibitory effect of GTP on FFA-induced UCP1-sustained H^+ leak is decreased progressively (Fig. 6.3b) and is almost cancelled for the lowest $\Delta\psi$ (around 160 mV). This observation suggests that the effect of Q reduction level on PN sensitivity threshold can be detected with UCP1 too. When the ADP/O method is used with phosphorylating yeast mitochondria containing low amount of UCP1 the classical J_p/J_O relationship is observed (straight line through the origin), oleic acid inducing a equidistant shift to the right corresponding to the OA-induced UCP1-catalysed proton leak-sustained respiration rate as it can be inhibited by GTP during n-butylmalonate titration (decreasing Q reduction level from 60% to 30%) but not during antimycin A titration (increasing Q reduction level from 60% to 95%). Thus with heterologously low-expressed UCP1 it is possible to evidence that the reduction level of Q modulates the PN-inhibition of FFA-induced H^+ conductance of mitochondria both in state 3 and state 4 respirations. The challenge was then to show that in native situation (in BAT mitochondria) it was also possible to detect during non-phosphorylating respiration a Q-reduction level-dependence of the PN-inhibition of FFA-induced UCP1-sustained H^+ conductance (never observed before). This has been shown by force/flow titrations in state 4+GTP with malonate compared with cyanide: cyanide titration curve with respect to malonate titration curve progressively shifts to the left indicating a partial alleviation of PN inhibition of UCP1-sustained H^+ conductance: Q reduction level decreases from 80% to 74% with malonate but increases to 86% with cyanide (Swida-Barteczka et al. 2009). Thus even in BAT mitochondria Q reduction level can modulate detectibly the PN-sensitivity of FFA-induced UCP1-sustained proton conductance. This regulatory feature of UCPs is then proved to be universal.

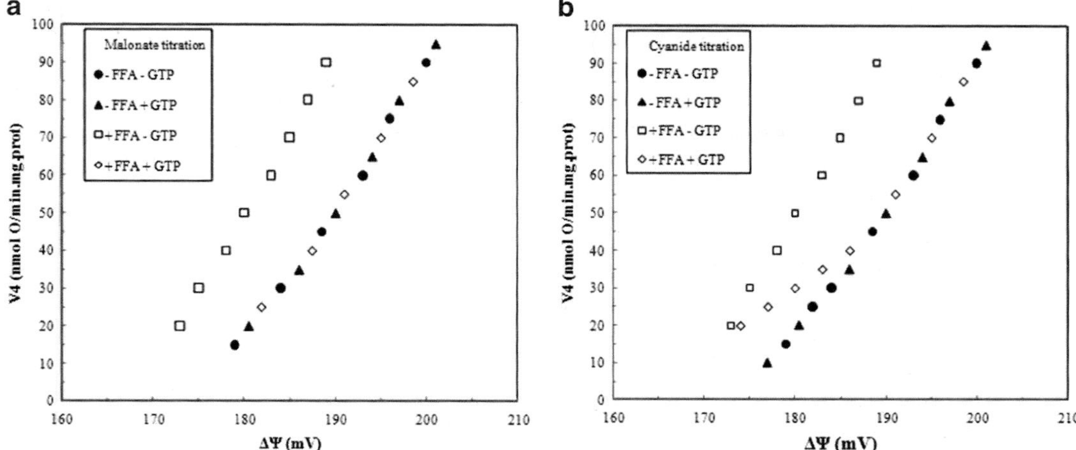

Fig. 6.3 Kinetics of proton leak in state 4 respiration (V4 versus $\Delta\psi$): effect of GTP when Q-reducing pathway is inhibited with malonate (**a**) or QH2-oxidizing pathway is inhibited with cyanide (**b**). All the conditions are indicated by different symbols in the *insets*

6.5 Mechanism of Regulation of All UCP's

Universal does not mean unique. All UCPs seem to be activated by FFA, inhibited by PN and the latter inhibition be modulated by the reduction level of Q. However many papers in the literature report activations of UCPs by superoxide anion, other reactive oxygen species (ROS) or products of lipoperoxidation (Echtay 2007). In fact, there is even not yet agreement with the way FFA "activate" UCP! Three models are currently evoked to explain the FFA-dependence of the protonophoric activity of UCPs. Firstly, FFA act as co-factors by adding their carboxyl groups inside UCP playing a role as relay for binding and releasing H^+, in this model UCPs are H^+ carriers (Klingenberg and Winkler 1985). Secondly, as described under Sect. 6.2.1, UCPs participate in a FFA cycle by exporting anionic FFA from the matrix and do not translocate protons, in this model UCPs are anion carrier (Garlid et al. 1996). Thirdly, since FFA and PN seem to affect H^+ conductance through a simple competitive kinetics, FFA could not be directly required in UCP protonophoric activity and act as allosteric activators, in this model UCPs are proton carriers (Shabalina et al. 2004). However this competition (mutual exclusion) cannot exclude anionic FFA as substrate because it is quite possible that the PN-allosteric binding site interacts with the anionic FFA-substrate binding site with as a consequence an apparent mutual competition between the allosteric negative effector and the substrate. This, of course, does not mean that FFAs are positive allosteric effectors. Concerning activation of UCPs by superoxide and its byproducts it remains quite controversial (Nicholls 2006). This model is based on the observation that some UCPs can be activated by both superoxide (Echtay et al. 2002) and lipid peroxydation products such as hydroxynonenal (Echtay et al. 2003). This suggests that superoxide reacts with membrane phospholipids generating the final activator hydroxynonenal (Murphy et al. 2003).

6.5.1 The Activation by ROS

The current model pathway for UCP activation by superoxide anion assumes that it occurs indirectly through peroxidation of polyunsaturated fatty acid side chain of membrane lipids. Superoxide anion is the product of reduction of O_2 by a single electron at the level of the respiratory chain when pmf is high and then electron carriers very reduced. Its dismutation in H_2O_2 is catalysed by SOD and then hydrogen peroxide may be either reduced into water via glutathione and thioredoxine paths or in the presence of ferrous ions be the source of a highly reactive hydroxyl radical: ·OH. Then the lipid per-oxydation can proceed through a cascade of reaction with successive formation of carbon-centred lipid radical, peroxyl radical, hydroperoxide, alkoxyl radical (in the presence of Fe^{2+}), cyclic hydroper-oxide and hydroxynonenal (HNE, starting from arachidinic acid). Activation of UCPs by lipid per-oxydized derivatives (such as HNE and structurally related compounds like *trans*-retinoic acid, *trans*-retinal and 2-alkenals (Rial et al. 1999; Smith et al. 2004) as well as by superoxide itself (with added superoxide anion and H_2O_2 generating systems (Echtay et al. 2002)) is quite appealing possibil-ity. Indeed if we consider the irrefutable fact that reactive oxygen species (ROS) prevention (see below) is a role of UCPs which is an obligatory outcome of their biochemical function (decrease of pmf which increases electron flux to oxygen and by the fact decreases the reduction state of elec-tron carrier, namely coenzyme Q, important source of superoxide anion) a retro-positive control of UCP activity (stimulation) by ROS could be save for the cell components and life. However, the nature of the path(s) by which ROS could activate UCPs remains unknown. Moreover this would mean that the system of prevention would start to work effectively when damage are already done. Then concern about that possibility may be expressed except if we do not consider an acute ROS-activation of the protonophoric function of UCPs but a ROS-initiated up-regulation of UCP expression level and protein concentration.

6.5.2 Connecting ROS and Q Reduction Level: A Logical Model

Nevertheless, function and regulation of UCPs are completely "surrounded" by PN, FFA and ROS or ROS source (Q reduction level). PN-inhibition is a diagnostic of H^+ conductance through UCPs and can be currently considered as a certain property of UCPs. If FFA^- activation is not the only acute activation way, it is nevertheless a universal feature for all UCPs. Acute ROS-activation is currently very much debated as well as the pathways they could use to activate UCPs. Q reduction level (QH_2 is an important source of superoxide and derived ROS through the semiquinone form Q^- (reduced by a single electron)), is now proved to play an important role in the modulation of PN-inhibition of UCP1 and every-kingdom UCP analogues. So it is tempting to try to propose a model of UCP regula-tion that puts together all the reliable information extracted from the huge amount of researches pub-lished on UCPs. This attempt is not pointless (Fig. 6.4) as every physiological role of the UCPs in every cell is an integral part of their function and regulation. To sum up: -UCPs are activated by FFA and some ROS (superoxide anion or lipid peroxidized derivatives) and inhibited by purine nucle-otides;- UCPs activity decreases the protonmotive force allowing an acceleration of electron flux in the respiratory chain and consequently a decrease of the reduction level of electron carriers;-This decrease is itself responsible of a lower level of superoxide anion production and of derived peroxi-dised lipids together with a lower level of QH_2;-The ROS decrease could result in a UCP deactivation;-Instead of acting directly on activity the decrease of QH_2 level allows PN to inhibit UCPs. The latter mechanism could be faster decreasing UCP activity. Thus both could be complementarily working in sequence: immediate inhibition by PN through increase in Q reduction level and progressive decline of the ROS-activated UCP activity. The model just described above corresponds to acute regulation of UCP activity (temporally speaking). However long term regulation of activity also occurs in which ROS could also play a role by acting as messengers to increase UCP expression level. Thus it appears clearly that UCP level and activity are tightly regulated via several ways, most of which originate in the Q reduction level.

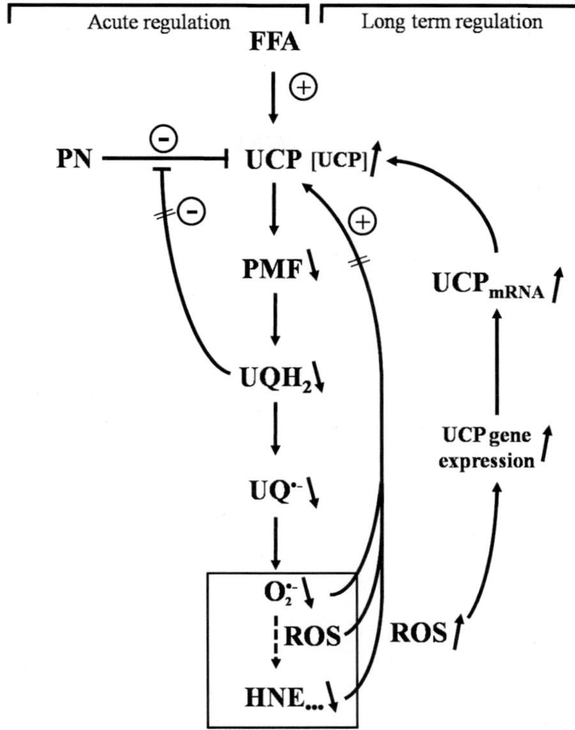

Fig. 6.4 Schematic model of UCP regulation: acute regulation on UCP activity and long term regulation on UCP concentration

6.6   Physiological Roles of UCPs

According to their localization (cells, tissues, animals, plants, fungi, protists) UCPs could have various physiological roles even if they share common functional properties. In contrast to UCP1 the physiological roles of UCP analogues are still under debate or completely unknown. In general the physiological role of UCPs can fall into various categories: adaptive non-shivering thermogenesis (NST), prevention of mitochondrial ROS production, response to stress (wide meaning) and regulation of energy metabolism balance.

6.6.1   UCPs and Thermogenesis

Only UCP1 in BAT is implicated in adaptive non-shivering thermogenesis in a way described above (under Sect. 6.3.2), for a review see (Cannon and Nedergaard 2004). UCP1 ablation in mice has revealed not only the expected results, like absence of non-shivering thermogenesis (Enerback et al. 1997) and loss of cold tolerance, but also an apparent role in body weight keeping. Indeed if the UCP1-ablated mice are hold at thermoneutrality (30°C) they become obese (Feldmann et al. 2009), contrarily obesity is not observed at 20–22°C (Enerback et al. 1997). Thus the absence of thermal stress in UCP1-ablated mice creates a situation that leads to attribute to UCP1 a role in body weight control. Due to their molecular and functional similarities with UCP1, UCP2 and UCP3 were also believed to be thermogenic. However their very low level of expression that could be 1,000-fold less than UCP1 expression indicates that they do not play a significant role in non-shivering thermogenesis and in adaptive response to cold. This is sustained by several studies with UCP-ablated mice. No phenotypic difference was evidenced between UCP1-ablated mice and *Ucp 1,3* double knockouts (Gong et al. 2000). The effect of starvation in rat muscle where gene expression of *Ucp 2 and 3* increases (Cadenas et al. 1999) together with the normal responses to cold exposure and absence of obesity of *Ucp2* and *Ucp3* knock-out mice (Gong et al. 2000; Vidal-Puig et al. 2000) provide evidences against a role of these UCP analogues in body temperature and mass control in normal conditions. UCP5 mRNA is abundant in brain (Sanchis et al. 1998) and testis whereas UCP4 mRNA is present only in brain (Mao et al. 1999). The uncoupling function of UCP4 and 5 are not yet well established and their role in local thermogenesis requires further studies. Plant uncoupling proteins (PUMP: plant uncoupling mitochondrial protein) form a group of 6 members in *Arabidopsis*, some are ubiquitous and others are tissue-specific, for a review see: (Vercesi et al. 2006). PUMPS are present in low amounts and probably play no role in thermogenesis even in thermogenic plant tissue (spadice of *Arum*) where heat production is related to the increase of AOX activity (see above Sect. 6.3.1). Uncoupling proteins from unicellular eukaryotes are up-regulated under low temperature (Jarmuszkiewicz et al. 2009) but this cannot be related to thermogenesis as already discussed (see above Sect. 6.3.2).

6.6.2 UCPs and Prevention of ROS Production

Skulachev has demonstrated that the production of ROS by mitochondria is tightly related to the $\Delta\psi$: up to the $\Delta\psi$ corresponding to the phosphorylating state 3 respiration the ROS production remains low and constant but increases with $\Delta\psi$ when it moves to higher values corresponding to the non-phosphorylating state 4 respiration (Skulachev 1991; Korshunov et al. 1997). Thus it is tempting, if pmf is such a key factor modulating the superoxide anion production at complex I and III, to postulate that a crucial factor moderating ROS production at this level would be the activity of UCPs. A possible physiological role of UCPs is a precise monitoring of $\Delta\psi$ in order to maintain optimal oxidative phosphorylation and minimal ROS production, ultimately attenuating the cellular damage caused by mitochondrial ROS production. In favor of this proposal it has been shown that inhibition of UCP2 by GDP increased $\Delta\psi$ and mitochondrial ROS production (Negre-Salvayre et al. 1997). Again regulation of expression have brought interesting information: mitochondria from *Ucp3* KO mice show higher ROS production and increased levels of oxidative damage (Brand et al. 2002) and myotubes over-expressing *Ucp3* show reduced production of ROS (MacLellan et al. 2005). However there are some discrepant results with transgenic animals (Echtay 2007). For instance mice over-expressing UCP3 have the same level of oxidative damage if compared to WT strain (Brand et al. 2002). Over-expression of mitochondrial MnSOD which decreases ROS in mouse muscle mitochondria does not change GDP-sensitive proton conductance compared to WT. This would mean that expression of muscle UCP are not regulated by the level of ROS! Nevertheless it seems that a major role of UCP2 and UCP3 is to moderate the ROS production by mitochondria *in vitro* and *in vivo*. Indeed, in vitro experiments have clearly demonstrated that activation of UCP3 is protective against superoxide anion production by rat skeletal muscle mitochondria. Superoxide anion generation and impairment of oxidative phosphorylation yield (ADP/O ratio) were studied in mitochondria submitted to anoxia/reoxygenation (Navet et al. 2006). Production of superoxide anion increases with the number of anoxia/reoxygenation cycles (A/R) together with a decrease of phosphorylating state 3 respiration rates and ADP/O ratios measured after A/R (9 cycles). The latter was proved to result from a proton leak. The addition of palmitic acid during A/R cycles was responsible for a dose-dependent inhibition of superoxide anion production as well as a protection of the ADP/O ratio. The decrease of ADP/O ratios after A/R cycles was inhibited by cyclosporine A indicating that the proton leak after A/R was due to the activation of the permeability transition induced by superoxide anion produced during A/R cycles (Di Lisa and Bernardi 1998) as it was cancelled by the spin trap (POBN), which scavenges superoxide anion and by palmitic acid, which activates UCP3. Thus palmitic acid-activated UCP3-sustained proton leak cancels superoxide anion production during A/R and as a consequence prevents the occurrence of superoxide anion-induced permeability transition-mediated proton leak after A/R. The ROS/proton leak couple can play an important role in cell protection not only against ROS but also against energy wasting (Brookes 2005). Indeed in the Navet's work it is shown that, on one hand ROS generated during A/R leads to energy wasting proton leak after A/R through a cyclosporine sensitive pathway (permeability transition) and on the other hand, the FFA-induced UCP3-sustained proton leak during A/R decreases A/R-induced superoxide anion production and consequently cancels the A/R-induced detrimental proton leak that impairs the ADP/O ratio after A/R. Thus, here the ROS-activated system is not UCP. It has been shown that heterologous expression of UCP1 in yeast affects oxygen free radical production (Douette et al. 2006). Indeed it was found that most of the proteins involved in the cellular response to ectopically expressed UCP1 are related to energy metabolism (increase in oxidative metabolism) and that the cellular H_2O_2 release depends on the amount of ectopic UCP1. The results suggest that UCP1 has a dual influence on ROS generation, on one side FFA-activated UCP1 decreases the superoxide anion production (obligatory outcome of UCP activation even in a heterologous context) inhibited by PN, on the other side, an increase in UCP1 content is concomitant with an increase in the basal release of superoxide anion by mitochondria (inhibited by PN) as a consequence of the overall increase in energy metabolism, for review see (Douette and Sluse 2006; Sluse et al. 2006). Thus in this heterologous system two outcomes of the presence of UCP are observed: increase in upstream metabolism and increase in ROS production (even if activation of UCP1 diminishes ROS production). In plant mitochondria UCPs are supposed to prevent ROS generation by the respiratory chain. In unicellular eukaryotes, such as amoeba, it has been shown that FFA-induced proton-conductance sustained respiration can prevent ROS formation (Czarna and Jarmuszkiewicz 2005). This role becomes important when amoebae are grown in stress conditions. Indeed it has been shown that in *Acanthamoeba castellanii* grown in cold the mitochondrial UCP protein content and activity is higher (Jarmuszkiewicz et al. 2004a) likely accompanying a higher ROS production (Avery et al. 1994).

6.6.3   UCPs and Energy Flow

Tightly regulated uncoupling of mitochondria through FFA-activated PN-inhibited UCP-mediated proton conductance may influence the flow in upstream catabolic pathways. Of course UCP1 activation in BAT is concomitant with a well-known huge burst in catabolic activity which was also evidenced at the mitoproteomic level after cold acclimation (Navet et al. 2007): upregulation of expression of enzymes of the β-oxidation, Krebs cycle and CR complex I and III. This was also observed in UCP1 ectopically-expressed yeast at the mitoproteomic level (Douette et al. 2006): specific UCP1 dose/response upregulation of Krebs cycle enzymes, RC complex III, ATP synthase but decrease in fermentation. It is tempting to allocate similar role to UCP2 and UCP3 at a much lower level due to their lower abundance. However they could manage a little uncoupling between respiration and ATP synthesis that could allow increase activity of Krebs cycle in order to improve its anaplerotic role necessary to anabolic pathway. For example it was shown that UCP2 is upregulated in hepatocytes of hyperphagic obese ob/ob mice (Chavin et al. 1999). Mitoproteomic study of these mice (Douette et al. 2005) versus control has shown upregulation in enzyme expression of Krebs cycle, β-oxidation, ketogenesis, gluconeogenesis and RC complex I and ETF oxidoreductase. All these changes are proposed to lead to a higher Q reduction state disabling PN inhibition of UCP2 which together with high FFA availability and increase in UCP2 content could result in an increase in respiration uncoupling. Thus UCP2 would act as an energy spendthrift to promote reducing substrate turnover and to control the upstream energetic flux. It is noteworthy that this increased metabolic turnover leads to higher ROS production at higher $\Delta\psi$ in obese hepatocytes even though UCP2 is upregulated (Yang et al. 2000).

The same type of modulation of the coupling between Krebs cycle activity and ATP synthesis has been observed with plant (potato) UCP in anabolic demand conditions (Smith et al. 2004): increase in UCP content leads to an increase in Krebs cycle flux. Expression of UCP genes is strongly modified during fruit ripening suggesting a developmental stage specific regulation of plant UCP (Considine et al. 2001). Studies on tomato ripening have shown that AOX and UCP are efficient under distinct physiological conditions [for review see (Vercesi et al. 2006)]. The tissue and temporal specific expressions of each UCP isoforms suggest they have different roles during development of plant tissues. In unicellular eukaryotes UCP is believed to play a role in the regulation of energy metabolism during cell growth cycle (Jarmuszkiewicz et al. 2009).

6.7 Physiopathological Aspects

As mentioned above the two well-documented physiological roles of the UCPs (apart from thermogenesis) are prevention of ROS formation and balance of energy metabolism. All implications of UCPs in physiopathology is obligatory linked not only to their biochemical function and regulation, their physiological roles but also to the energetic and the metabolic status of the peculiar cells and tissues implicated in the pathology. Then physiological disorders exhibiting either an increase of ROS production or an impairment of the metabolic balance are suspected to be potentially linked to UCP. A large number of studies show some implication of UCP2 and UCP3 in a broad range of pathological processes like obesity, type 2 diabetes, insulin resistance and insufficiency, autoimmune diseases, atherosclerosis, tumor formation and aging, for review see (Azzu et al. 2010; Echtay 2007). The role of UCP1 in the control of body weight (against-obesity appearance) is mainly sustained by the study of *Ucp1* knockout mice at thermoneutrality (see under Sect. 6.1). The ablation of UCP1 creates a situation in which the brown adipose tissue loses its metabolic properties, i.e. its ability to consume a large amount of metabolites. This combined with the absence of caloric demand for the maintenance of body temperature leads to an overall metabolic imbalance responsible for the weight gain which is diet dependant. Role of UCP2 in glucose sensing-cells is well documented but remains debated. UCP2 activity can attenuate insulin secretion by the pancreas through the peculiar role of mitochondrial metabolism in glucose-stimulated insulin secretion (GSIS). The very low level of lactate dehydrogenase in pancreatic β cells makes that most of the pyruvate produced by the glycolysis is catabolized in the mitochondria and that metabolism of glucose is supported by mitochondria. Thus as a direct consequence, the elevation of the glucose concentration leads to a higher reducing equivalent production that leads to an elevation of the intracellular ATP/ADP ratio. This is important in the GSIS process since it reduces the opening probability of the plasma membrane K_{ATP} channel responsible of the depolarization of the membrane and the subsequent opening of the voltage gated Ca^{2+} channel with influx of Ca^{2+} triggering insulin secretion. Then UCP2 can decrease insulin secretion in two ways: by lowering ATP production by OXPHOS and by decreasing the production of ROS which are important signals for GSIS (Leloup et al. 2009). This negative feedback loop would prevent an over secretion of insulin and contribute to blood glucose homeostasis. Overexpression of *Ucp2* attenuates GSIS supporting this negative regulatory effect (Chan et al. 1999). Conversely, in *Ucp2* knockout mice pancreatic islets have increased insulin secretion, clearly showing the regulatory role of UCP2 in GSIS (Zhang et al. 2001). Downregulation of UCP2 could then improve the diabetic phenotype. However the absence of UCP2 could also impair β cell function because permanent oxidative stress (Pi et al. 2009). In type 2 diabetes, a prolonged exposition to high glucose and lipid content severely impairs β-cells functions and promotes UCP2 expression. Thus it can be assumed that UCP-2 activation in hyperglycemic animals would impair GSIS by reducing phosphate potential and severely contribute to enhance insulin resistance. Consequently, in this situation, the classical "beneficial" effect of the uncoupling protein activation on ROS prevention and metabolic turnover would constitute an important drawback. Numerous studies have shown that UCP2 play a role in cytoprotection and its absence enhances colon tumor induction (Derdak et al. 2006) and atherosclerosis (Moukdar et al. 2009). Role of UCP3 in ROS protection is supported by the fact that its over-expression neutralizes oxidative stress in mouse myotubes (Barreiro et al. 2009), decrease ROS production in skeletal muscle during exercise (Jiang et al. 2009) and in heart and skeletal muscles during aging (Nabben and Hoeks 2008). Conversely UCP3 under-expression in mice leads to higher oxidative damage in skeletal muscle mitochondria (Brand et al. 2002). UCP3 could also be involved in fatty acid metabolism as its over-expression in mice increases fatty acid transport and oxidation (Bezaire et al. 2005) and moreover decreases diet-induced obesity and insulin resistance (Son et al. 2004). Insulin resistance in skeletal muscle is a major cause of type 2 diabetes that can be promoted by obesity and aging. The link between mitochondrial uncoupling and aging has been carefully reviewed recently (Mookerjee et al. 2010). According the free radical theory of aging, ROS production and oxidative damage cause aging. Therefore to counteract aging long life span animals should maintain low level of ROS through either ROS production prevention or improved antioxidant activity or increased resistance to ROS or all together (Lambert et al. 2007). As UCPs are widely recognized as ROS production preventing systems they could be suspected to play an important role in lifespan. However no consistent role for uncoupling in lifespan has been evidenced. This could be due to either the multifactorial character of lifespan and/or the inadequacy of experimental approaches. Indeed overall methodologies are necessary to undertake this kind of very complex study.

6.8 Concluding Comments

Study of uncoupling proteins is a very hot topic in Bioenergetics (boiling) since 15 years and UCP1 is studied since the sixties. Amazingly, their mode of action and regulation are still debated and their physiological roles and pathological implications are mostly not understood. This situation hampers the development of fundamental knowledge in the field and therapeutic aspects in molecular medicine. Modern overall methodologies should be introduced in this wide research field.

Acknowledgments The author wants to thank Dr. Rachel Navet, Dr. Gregory Mathy and PhD student Arnaud Blomme for their invaluable help during the preparation of this chapter.

References

Avery SV, Harwood JL et al (1994) Low temperature-induced adaptations in lipid metabolism and physiological function in Acanthamoeba castellanii cultures of different ages. Biochem Soc Trans 22(3):257S

Azzu V, Jastroch M et al (2010) The regulation and turnover of mitochondrial uncoupling proteins. Biochim Biophys Acta 1797(6–7):785–791

Barreiro E, Garcia-Martinez C et al (2009) UCP3 overexpression neutralizes oxidative stress rather than nitrosative stress in mouse myotubes. FEBS Lett 583(2):350–356

Bezaire V, Spriet LL et al (2005) Constitutive UCP3 overexpression at physiological levels increases mouse skeletal muscle capacity for fatty acid transport and oxidation. FASEB J 19(8):977–979

Borecky J, Maia IG et al (2001) Functional reconstitution of Arabidopsis thaliana plant uncoupling mitochondrial protein (AtPUMP1) expressed in Escherichia coli. FEBS Lett 505(2):240–244

Brand MD, Pamplona R et al (2002) Oxidative damage and phospholipid fatty acyl composition in skeletal muscle mitochondria from mice underexpressing or overexpressing uncoupling protein 3. Biochem J 368(Pt 2):597–603

Breidenbach RW, Saxton MJ et al (1997) Heat generation and dissipation in plants: can the alternative oxidative phosphorylation pathway serve a thermoregulatory role in plant tissues other than specialized organs? Plant Physiol 114(4):1137–1140

Brookes PS (2005) Mitochondrial H(+) leak and ROS generation: an odd couple. Free Radic Biol Med 38(1):12–23

Cadenas S, Buckingham JA et al (1999) UCP2 and UCP3 rise in starved rat skeletal muscle but mitochondrial proton conductance is unchanged. FEBS Lett 462(3):257–260

Cannon B, Nedergaard J (2004) Brown adipose tissue: function and physiological significance. Physiol Rev 84(1):277–359

Chan CB, MacDonald PE et al (1999) Overexpression of uncoupling protein 2 inhibits glucose-stimulated insulin secretion from rat islets. Diabetes 48(7):1482–1486

Chavin KD, Yang S et al (1999) Obesity induces expression of uncoupling protein-2 in hepatocytes and promotes liver ATP depletion. J Biol Chem 274(9):5692–5700

Considine MJ, Daley DO et al (2001) The expression of alternative oxidase and uncoupling protein during fruit ripening in mango. Plant Physiol 126(4):1619–1629

Considine MJ, Goodman M et al (2003) Superoxide stimulates a proton leak in potato mitochondria that is related to the activity of uncoupling protein. J Biol Chem 278(25):22298–22302

Czarna M, Jarmuszkiewicz W (2005) Activation of alternative oxidase and uncoupling protein lowers hydrogen peroxide formation in amoeba Acanthamoeba castellanii mitochondria. FEBS Lett 579(14):3136–3140

Derdak Z, Fulop P et al (2006) Enhanced colon tumor induction in uncoupling protein-2 deficient mice is associated with NF-kappaB activation and oxidative stress. Carcinogenesis 27(5):956–961

Di Lisa F, Bernardi P (1998) Mitochondrial function as a determinant of recovery or death in cell response to injury. Mol Cell Biochem 184(1–2):379–391

Douette P, Sluse FE (2006) Mitochondrial uncoupling proteins: new insights from functional and proteomic studies. Free Radic Biol Med 40(7):1097–1107

Douette P, Navet R et al (2005) Steatosis-induced proteomic changes in liver mitochondria evidenced by two-dimensional differential in-gel electrophoresis. J Proteome Res 4(6):2024–2031

Douette P, Gerkens P et al (2006) Uncoupling protein 1 affects the yeast mitoproteome and oxygen free radical production. Free Radic Biol Med 40(2):303–315

Echtay KS (2007) Mitochondrial uncoupling proteins–what is their physiological role? Free Radic Biol Med 43(10):1351–1371

Echtay KS, Winkler E et al (2000) Coenzyme Q is an obligatory cofactor for uncoupling protein function. Nature 408(6812):609–613

Echtay KS, Winkler E et al (2001) Uncoupling proteins 2 and 3 are highly active H(+) transporters and highly nucleotide sensitive when activated by coenzyme Q (ubiquinone). Proc Natl Acad Sci USA 98(4):1416–1421

Echtay KS, Roussel D et al (2002) Superoxide activates mitochondrial uncoupling proteins. Nature 415(6867):96–99

Echtay KS, Esteves TC et al (2003) A signalling role for 4-hydroxy-2-nonenal in regulation of mitochondrial uncoupling. EMBO J 22(16):4103–4110

el Moualij B, Duyckaerts C et al (1997) Phylogenetic classification of the mitochondrial carrier family of Saccharomyces cerevisiae. Yeast 13(6):573–581

Enerback S, Jacobsson A et al (1997) Mice lacking mitochondrial uncoupling protein are cold-sensitive but not obese. Nature 387(6628):90–94

Feldmann HM, Golozoubova V et al (2009) UCP1 ablation induces obesity and abolishes diet-induced thermogenesis in mice exempt from thermal stress by living at thermoneutrality. Cell Metab 9(2):203–209

Garlid KD, Orosz DE et al (1996) On the mechanism of fatty acid-induced proton transport by mitochondrial uncoupling protein. J Biol Chem 271(5):2615–2620

Gong DW, Monemdjou S et al (2000) Lack of obesity and normal response to fasting and thyroid hormone in mice lacking uncoupling protein-3. J Biol Chem 275(21):16251–16257

Gonzalez-Barroso MM, Fleury C et al (1996) Activation of the uncoupling protein by fatty acids is modulated by mutations in the C-terminal region of the protein. Eur J Biochem 239(2):445–450

Hourton-Cabassa C, Mesneau A et al (2002) Alteration of plant mitochondrial proton conductance by free fatty acids. Uncoupling protein involvement. J Biol Chem 277(44):41533–41538

Jaburek M, Varecha M et al (1999) Transport function and regulation of mitochondrial uncoupling proteins 2 and 3. J Biol Chem 274(37):26003–26007

Jarmuszkiewicz W, Sluse-Goffart C et al (1996) Determination of the respective contributions of the cytochrome and alternative oxidase pathways in Acanthamoeba castellanii mitochondria. Biothermokinetics of the living cell. BioThemoKinetics Press, Amsterdam, pp 31–34

Jarmuszkiewicz W, Almeida AM et al (1998) Linoleic acid-induced activity of plant uncoupling mitochondrial protein in purified tomato fruit mitochondria during resting, phosphorylating, and progressively uncoupled respiration. J Biol Chem 273(52):34882–34886

Jarmuszkiewicz W, Sluse-Goffart CM et al (1999) Identification and characterization of a protozoan uncoupling protein in Acanthamoeba castellanii. J Biol Chem 274(33):23198–23202

Jarmuszkiewicz W, Almeida AM et al (2000a) Proton re-uptake partitioning between uncoupling protein and ATP synthase during benzohydroxamic acid-resistant state 3 respiration in tomato fruit mitochondria. J Biol Chem 275(18):13315–13320

Jarmuszkiewicz W, Milani G et al (2000b) First evidence and characterization of an uncoupling protein in fungi kingdom: CpUCP of Candida parapsilosis. FEBS Lett 467(2–3):145–149

Jarmuszkiewicz W, Sluse-Goffart CM et al (2001) Alternative oxidase and uncoupling protein: thermogenesis versus cell energy balance. Biosci Rep 21(2):213–222

Jarmuszkiewicz W, Antos N et al (2004a) The effect of growth at low temperature on the activity and expression of the uncoupling protein in Acanthamoeba castellanii mitochondria. FEBS Lett 569(1–3):178–184

Jarmuszkiewicz W, Navet R et al (2004b) Redox state of endogenous coenzyme q modulates the inhibition of linoleic acid-induced uncoupling by guanosine triphosphate in isolated skeletal muscle mitochondria. J Bioenerg Biomembr 36(5):493–502

Jarmuszkiewicz W, Swida A et al (2005) In phosphorylating Acanthamoeba castellanii mitochondria the sensitivity of uncoupling protein activity to GTP depends on the redox state of quinone. J Bioenerg Biomembr 37(2):97–107

Jarmuszkiewicz W, Woyda-Ploszczyca A et al (2009) Mitochondrial uncoupling proteins in unicellular eukaryotes. Biochim Biophys Acta 1797(6–7):792–799

Jekabsons MB, Echtay KS et al (2002) Nucleotide binding to human uncoupling protein-2 refolded from bacterial inclusion bodies. Biochem J 366(Pt 2):565–571

Jiang N, Zhang G et al (2009) Upregulation of uncoupling protein-3 in skeletal muscle during exercise: a potential antioxidant function. Free Radic Biol Med 46(2):138–145

Klingenberg M (1990) Mechanism and evolution of the uncoupling protein of brown adipose tissue. Trends Biochem Sci 15(3):108–112

Klingenberg M, Echtay KS (2001) Uncoupling proteins: the issues from a biochemist point of view. Biochim Biophys Acta 1504(1):128–143

Klingenberg M, Winkler E (1985) The reconstituted isolated uncoupling protein is a membrane potential driven H+ translocator. EMBO J 4(12):3087–3092

Korshunov SS, Skulachev VP et al (1997) High protonic potential actuates a mechanism of production of reactive oxygen species in mitochondria. FEBS Lett 416(1):15–18

Lambert AJ, Boysen HM et al (2007) Low rates of hydrogen peroxide production by isolated heart mitochondria associate with long maximum lifespan in vertebrate homeotherms. Aging Cell 6(5):607–618

Leloup C, Tourrel-Cuzin C et al (2009) Mitochondrial reactive oxygen species are obligatory signals for glucose-induced insulin secretion. Diabetes 58(3):673–681

MacLellan JD, Gerrits MF et al (2005) Physiological increases in uncoupling protein 3 augment fatty acid oxidation and decrease reactive oxygen species production without uncoupling respiration in muscle cells. Diabetes 54(8):2343–2350

Mao W, Yu XX et al (1999) UCP4, a novel brain-specific mitochondrial protein that reduces membrane potential in mammalian cells. FEBS Lett 443(3):326–330

Meeuse B (1975) Thermogenic respiration in Aroids. Annu Rev Plant Physiol 26:117–126

Mitchell P (1961) Coupling of phosphorylation to electron and hydrogen transfer by a chemi-osmotic type of mechanism. Nature 191:144–148

Mookerjee SA, Divakaruni AS et al (2010) Mitochondrial uncoupling and lifespan. Mech Ageing Dev 131(7–8):463–472

Moukdar F, Robidoux J et al (2009) Reduced antioxidant capacity and diet-induced atherosclerosis in uncoupling protein-2-deficient mice. J Lipid Res 50(1):59–70

Murphy MP, Echtay KS et al (2003) Superoxide activates uncoupling proteins by generating carbon-centered radicals and initiating lipid peroxidation: studies using a mitochondria-targeted spin trap derived from alpha-phenyl-N-tert-butylnitrone. J Biol Chem 278(49):48534–48545

Nabben M, Hoeks J (2008) Mitochondrial uncoupling protein 3 and its role in cardiac- and skeletal muscle metabolism. Physiol Behav 94(2):259–269

Navet R, Douette P et al (2005) Regulation of uncoupling protein activity in phosphorylating potato tuber mitochondria. FEBS Lett 579(20):4437–4442

Navet R, Mouithys-Mickalad A et al (2006) Proton leak induced by reactive oxygen species produced during in vitro anoxia/reoxygenation in rat skeletal muscle mitochondria. J Bioenerg Biomembr 38(1):23–32

Navet R, Mathy G et al (2007) Mitoproteome plasticity of rat brown adipocytes in response to cold acclimation. J Proteome Res 6(1):25–33

Negre-Salvayre A, Hirtz C et al (1997) A role for uncoupling protein-2 as a regulator of mitochondrial hydrogen peroxide generation. FASEB J 11(10):809–815

Nicholls DG (2006) The physiological regulation of uncoupling proteins. Biochim Biophys Acta 1757(5–6):459–466

Nicholls DG, Rial E (1999) A history of the first uncoupling protein, UCP1. J Bioenerg Biomembr 31(5):399–406

Pi J, Bai Y et al (2009) Persistent oxidative stress due to absence of uncoupling protein 2 associated with impaired pancreatic beta-cell function. Endocrinology 150(7):3040–3048

Rial E, Gonzalez-Barroso M et al (1999) Retinoids activate proton transport by the uncoupling proteins UCP1 and UCP2. EMBO J 18(21):5827–5833

Ricquier D, Bouillaud F (2000) The uncoupling protein homologues: UCP1, UCP2, UCP3, StUCP and AtUCP. Biochem J 345(Pt 2):161–179

Sanchis D, Busquets S et al (1998) Skeletal muscle UCP2 and UCP3 gene expression in a rat cancer cachexia model. FEBS Lett 436(3):415–418

Saraste M (1999) Oxidative phosphorylation at the fin de siecle. Science 283(5407):1488–1493

Shabalina IG, Jacobsson A et al (2004) Native UCP1 displays simple competitive kinetics between the regulators purine nucleotides and fatty acids. J Biol Chem 279(37):38236–38248

Skulachev VP (1991) Fatty acid circuit as a physiological mechanism of uncoupling of oxidative phosphorylation. FEBS Lett 294(3):158–162

Sluse FE (1996) Mitochondrial metabolite carrier family, topology, structure and functional properties: an overview. Acta Biochim Pol 43(2):349–360

Sluse FE, Jarmuszkiewicz W (2000) Activity and functional interaction of alternative oxidase and uncoupling protein in mitochondria from tomato fruit. Braz J Med Biol Res 33(3):259–268

Sluse FE, Jarmuszkiewicz W (2002) Uncoupling proteins outside the animal and plant kingdoms: functional and evolutionary aspects. FEBS Lett 510(3):117–120

Sluse FE, Almeida AM et al (1998a) Free fatty acids regulate the uncoupling protein and alternative oxidase activities in plant mitochondria. FEBS Lett 433(3):237–240

Sluse FE, Jarmuszkiewicz W et al (1998b) Determination of actual contribution of energy-dissipating pathways to mitochondrial respiration: the ADP/O method. In: Plant mitochondria: from gene to function. Backhuys Publisher, Leiden

Sluse FE, Jarmuszkiewicz W et al (2006) Mitochondrial UCPs: new insights into regulation and impact. Biochim Biophys Acta 1757(5–6):480–485

Smith AM, Ratcliffe RG et al (2004) Activation and function of mitochondrial uncoupling protein in plants. J Biol Chem 279(50):51944–51952

Son C, Hosoda K et al (2004) Reduction of diet-induced obesity in transgenic mice overexpressing uncoupling protein 3 in skeletal muscle. Diabetologia 47(1):47–54

Swida-Barteczka A, Woyda-Ploszczyca A et al (2009) Uncoupling protein 1 inhibition by purine nucleotides is under the control of the endogenous ubiquinone redox state. Biochem J 424(2):297–306

Vercesi AE, Martins LS et al (1995) PUMPing plants. Nature 375(6526):24-24

Vercesi AE, Borecky J et al (2006) Plant uncoupling mitochondrial proteins. Annu Rev Plant Biol 57:383–404

Vidal-Puig AJ, Grujic D et al (2000) Energy metabolism in uncoupling protein 3 gene knockout mice. J Biol Chem 275(21):16258–16266

Yang S, Zhu H et al (2000) Mitochondrial adaptations to obesity-related oxidant stress. Arch Biochem Biophys 378(2):259–268

Zackova M, Skobisova E et al (2003) Activating omega-6 polyunsaturated fatty acids and inhibitory purine nucleotides are high affinity ligands for novel mitochondrial uncoupling proteins UCP2 and UCP3. J Biol Chem 278(23): 20761–20769

Zhang CY, Hagen T et al (1999) Assessment of uncoupling activity of uncoupling protein 3 using a yeast heterologous expression system. FEBS Lett 449(2–3):129–134

Zhang CY, Baffy G et al (2001) Uncoupling protein-2 negatively regulates insulin secretion and is a major link between obesity, beta cell dysfunction, and type 2 diabetes. Cell 105(6):745–755

Chapter 7
The Mitochondrial Pathways of Apoptosis

Jérome Estaquier, François Vallette, Jean-Luc Vayssiere, and Bernard Mignotte

Abstract Apoptosis is a process of programmed cell death that serves as a major mechanism for the precise regulation of cell numbers, and as a defense mechanism to remove unwanted and potentially dangerous cells. Studies in nematode, *Drosophila* and mammals have shown that, although regulation of the cell death machinery is somehow different from one species to another, it is controlled by homologous proteins and involves mitochondria. In mammals, activation of caspases (cysteine proteases that are the main executioners of apoptosis) is under the tight control of the Bcl-2 family proteins, named in reference to the first discovered mammalian cell death regulator. These proteins mainly act by regulating the release of caspases activators from mitochondria. Although for a long time the absence of mitochondrial changes was considered as a hallmark of apoptosis, mitochondria appear today as the central executioner of apoptosis. In this chapter, we present the current view on the mitochondrial pathway of apoptosis with a particular attention to new aspects of the regulation of the Bcl-2 proteins family control of mitochondrial membrane permeabilization: the mechanisms implicated in their mitochondrial targeting and activation during apoptosis, the function(s) of the oncosuppressive protein p53 at the mitochondria and the role of the processes of mitochondrial fusion and fission.

Keywords Apoptosis • Mitochondria • Bcl-2 family proteins • p53

J. Estaquier
Faculté Créteil Henri Mondor, Institut National de la Sante et de la Recherche Médicale, U955, 8 Rue du Général Sarrail, 94010 Créteil, France

F. Vallette
Centre de Recherche en Cancérologie Nantes Angers (UMR 892 INSERM et 6299 CNRS/Université de Nantes), 9 Quai Moncousu, 44007 Nantes, France

J.-L. Vayssiere • B. Mignotte (✉)
Laboratoire de Génétique et Biologie Cellulaire, EA4589, Université Versailles St-Quentin, Ecole Pratique des Hautes Etudes, 45 av des Etats-Unis, 78035 Versailles cedex, France
e-mail: bernard.mignotte@uvsq.fr

R. Scatena et al. (eds.), *Advances in Mitochondrial Medicine*, Advances in Experimental Medicine and Biology 942, DOI 10.1007/978-94-007-2869-1_7, © Springer Science+Business Media B.V. 2012

Abbreviations

ANT	adenine nucleotide translocase
Bcl-2	B-cell lymphoma 2
BH	Bcl-2 homology
BOP	BH3 only protein
CARD	caspase activation and recruitment domain
caspase	cysteine aspartase
CED	cell death
DED	death effector domain
Dronc	*Drosophila* nedd-2 like caspase
EGL-1	egg-laying-1
IAP	inhibitor of apoptosis protein
MOMP	mitochondrial outer membrane permeabilization
PTP	permeability transition pore
TOM	translocase of the outer membrane
VDAC	voltage-dependent anion channel

7.1   Introduction

Soon after it was recognized that organisms are made of cells, cell death was discovered as an important part of life. First observed during amphibian metamorphosis, normal cell death was soon found to occur in many developing tissues in both invertebrates and vertebrates (reviews: Clarke 1990; Clarke and Clarke 1996). The term "programmed cell death" (PCD) was used to describe cell deaths that occur in predictable places and at predictable times during development, to emphasize that death can be somewhat programmed into the development plan of the organism. Subsequently it has been established that PCD also serves as a major mechanism for the precise regulation of cell numbers and as a defense mechanism to remove unwanted and potentially dangerous cells, such as self-reactive lymphocytes, cells that have been infected by viruses and tumor cells. In addition to the beneficial effects of PCD, the inappropriate activation of cell death may cause or contribute to a variety of diseases, including acquired immunodeficiency syndrome (AIDS), neurodegenerative diseases, and ischemic strokes. Conversely, a defect in PCD activation could be responsible for some autoimmune diseases and is also involved in oncogenesis. For a recent overview on PCD in development and disease see the review of Fuchs and Steller (2011)).

Apoptosis is a process whereby cells activate an intrinsic cell suicide program that is one of the potential cellular responses, such as differentiation and proliferation. It has been defined in 1972 by Kerr et al. in contrast to necrosis, which is a cell death generally due to aggressions from the external medium (Kerr et al. 1972). The apoptotic process is associated with characteristic morphological and biochemical changes, such as membrane blebbing, cell shrinkage, chromatin condensation, DNA cleavage and fragmentation of the cell into membrane-bound apoptotic bodies whose surface expresses potent triggers for phagocytosis. However, it must be kept in mind that although apoptosis is the most common form of PCD, dying cells may follow other morphological types (Bredesen et al. 2006). This chapter reviews our current knowledge on the mitochondrial pathway of apoptosis with a particular emphasis to new aspects of the regulation of the Bcl-2 proteins family control of mitochondrial membrane permeabilization (MOMP) and the mechanisms implicated in their mitochondrial targeting and activation, the function(s) of the oncosuppressive protein p53 at the mitochondria and the role of the processes of mitochondrial fusion and fission.

7.2 The Various Roles of Mitochondria in Apoptosis

7.2.1 Insights from Studies in Invertebrate Models

Genetic screens performed in *C. elegans* have allowed the discovery of a genetic control of PCD and elucidation of the signaling cascade leading to cell death (for review see Lettre and Hengartner 2006). At the heart of this pathway is the *ced-3* gene, which encodes a member of a family of cysteine proteases that cleave proteins at specific aspartyl residues called caspases, whose activation is under the control of the caspase activator CED-4. In living cells, CED-4 is constantly sequestered by CED-9 on the mitochondrial outer membrane. Upon a proapoptotic stimuli, EGL-1 is transcriptionally activated and binds to CED-9 to displace CED-4 (Fig. 7.1). CED-4 and CED-3 can then interact through their CARD (caspase recruitment domain) domains to form a complex called apoptosome that leads to CED-3 activation (Fig. 7.1). Apoptosome formation and activation constitute key events for cell death execution in worm in a step controlled by EGL-1 and CED-9. Activated CED-3 will then cleave cellular components leading to cell destruction and engulfing. Subsequent studies, performed in various species, have shown that caspases are also instrumental to the execution of apoptosis in other species. These enzymes are expressed in cells as inactive or low-activity zymogens that require oligomerization and/or cleavage for activation. In *C. elegans*, CED-3 is able to autocatalyze its own cleavage

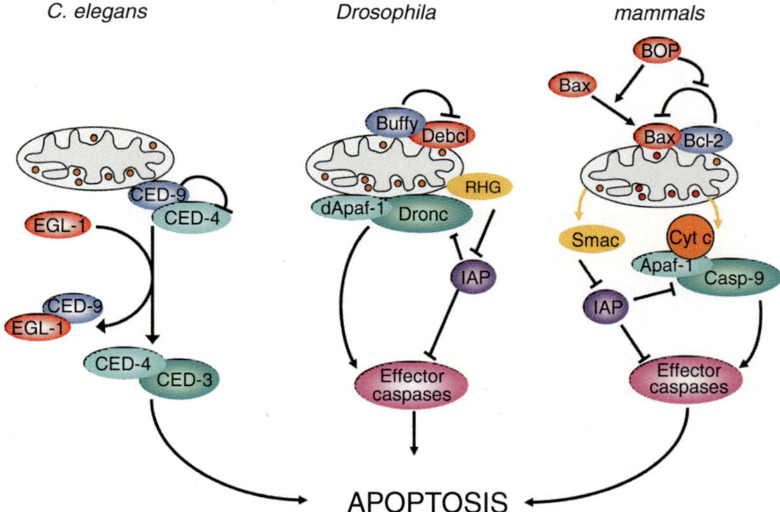

Fig. 7.1 Main regulators of the mitochondrial apoptotic pathway in *C. elegans*, *Drosophila* and *mammals*. In all these species, this apoptotic pathway relies on caspase activation into an apoptosome. The apoptosome contains at least an oligomer of caspase activator (*CED-4, Dapaf-1 or Apaf-1*) and several copies of a CARD-carrying initiator caspase (*CED-3, DRONC or Caspase-9*). In mammals, cytochrome c is an additional co-factor required for apoptosome formation. In these three clades, Bcl-2 family members, which are either proapoptotic (*EGL-1, Debcl, BOP or Bax*) or antiapoptotic (*CED-9, Buffy, Bcl-2*) regulate each other at the level of the mitochondria and are involved in the regulation of apoptosome activation. Nonetheless, their mode of action differs: in the nematode, the antiapoptotic protein CED-9 prevents apoptosome formation by direct binding to CED-4, and EGL-1 promotes apoptosome formation by releasing CED-4 from CED-9. In *Drosophila*, Bcl-2 proteins are localized to mitochondria and the proapoptotic Debcl induces an apoptosome-dependent cell death, in which the role of cytochrome c remains unclear. In mammals, proteins of the Bcl-2 family either promote (such as Bax or BH3-only proteins) or inhibit (such as Bcl-2) the release of apoptogenic factors from the mitochondrial intermembrane space to the cytosol, one of which being the Apaf-1 co-factor, cytochrome c. In both mammals and *Drosophila*, apoptosome activity can be limited by *IAPs*

(Hugunin et al. 1996). As CED-3 is the only apoptotic caspase in the worm, it plays a central role in apoptosis execution in this organism (Ellis and Horvitz 1986; Shaham et al. 1999).

Studies performed in *Drosophila* with p35 (a baculovirus caspases inhibitor) have shown that caspases are also involved in apoptosis in fruit flies. However, regulation of caspase activation in flies appears to be mainly controlled at another level. A genetic screen of a deletion mutant library showed that the H99 deletion abolishes almost all cell death during embryogenesis in *Drosophila* (White et al. 1994). This phenotype is the consequence of the loss of three genes: *Reaper*, *Hid*, and *Grim*, collectively called RHG proteins. In healthy cells, IAPs, caspase inhibitor proteins that contain a RING domain and Baculoviral IAP repeat (BIR) motifs such as DIAP1 cause the ubiquitylation of procaspases, thereby inactivating them (for a recent review, see Bergmann 2010). In response to an apoptotic stimulus, RHG proteins are activated, leading to the RHG protein-dependent ubiquitylation and proteosomal degradation of DIAP1 (Chai et al. 2003; Goyal et al. 2000; Wilson et al. 2002; Yoo et al. 2002). Overexpression of any one of the RHG genes triggers excessive cell death, indicating that the inhibition of IAP is sufficient to induce caspase activation and apoptosis. Consistently, DIAP1 deficiency leads to spontaneous apoptosis in most fly cells (Goyal et al. 2000; Yoo et al. 2002). These data led to the concept that *Drosophila* caspases might not require activation, but simply relief from potent inhibitors of caspases. However, the *Drosophila* initiator caspase DRONC contains in its aminoterminal region a long prodomain that carries a CARD motif which mediates DRONC binding to Dark/Dapaf-1, the *Drosophila* homologue of the nematode CED-4 caspase activator, and the formation of the fly apoptosome (Daish et al. 2004; Xu et al. 2005). Furthermore, analysis of the *Drosophila* genome allowed the discovery of two homologues of CED-9 (*i.e.* Debcl and Buffy), which are constitutively located at the mitochondria (Fig. 7.1). The first one is a proapoptotic member called Debcl (Colussi et al. 2000; Brachmann et al. 2000; Igaki et al. 2000), and the second is the antiapoptotic Buffy (Quinn et al. 2003). These data show that regulation of caspases activation is somehow conserved between worms and *Drosophila* and suggest that critical events take place at the mitochondrial level.

7.2.2 The Mitochondrial Pathway of Apoptosis in Mammals

In mammals, apoptosis induction also usually leads to caspase activation even though not all of caspase activities are linked to cell death commitment and apoptosis can proceed in some instances without caspase activity (Godefroy et al. 2004). Caspases can be classified into two subgroups: the first one is constituted by effector caspases which present a short prodomain and whose activating cleavage is performed by other proteases (such as caspases or calpain). The second group is constituted by initiator or apical caspases, which present a long prodomain carrying a protein/protein interaction motif dubbed "death domain" (Park et al. 2007). This motif can either be a CARD (Caspase Activation and Recruitment Domain) or a DED (Death Effector Domain) domain. Initiator caspases are characterized by their ability to autoactivate within specialized complexes (Bao and Shi 2007; Ho and Hawkins 2005; Stennicke and Salvesen 2000). Two main pathways lead to caspase activation during apoptosis in mammals. The first one involves transmembrane receptors at the plasma membrane and is thus termed extrinsic pathway or death-receptor pathway (for review: Guicciardi and Gores 2009). The second one, which is more similar to the worm death pathway, is termed intrinsic or mitochondrial pathway and places mitochondria at the core of the signaling cascade (for review: Wang and Youle 2009).

However, for a long time the absence of mitochondrial changes was considered as a hallmark of PCD (Kerr et al. 1972; Kerr and Harmon 1991) and it was thus postulated that apoptosis is controlled at the nuclear level. This theory was however challenged during the 1990s by several lines of evidence. First, the Bcl-2 protooncogene, responsible for B cell follicular lymphomas due to t(14;18) chromosomal translocations, and other Bcl-2 related proteins like Bcl-xL, were found to be negative regulators of cell death, able to prevent cells from undergoing apoptosis induced by various stimuli in a wide variety of cell types (Korsmeyer 1992; Zhong et al. 1993). Although, the mechanism(s) by which proteins of the Bcl-2 family modulate apoptosis was not known, it was observed that most members of the Bcl-2 family proteins are localized to the nuclear envelope, the endoplasmic reticulum and the outer mitochondrial membrane. Furthermore, this membrane association seemed of functional significance, as mutant Bcl-2 molecules lacking this membrane anchorage capacity were found less effective at preventing apoptosis in some systems (Borner et al. 1994; Nguyen et al. 1994; Zhu et al. 1996). Second, several changes in mitochondrial biogenesis and function were found associated with the commitment to apoptosis. A fall of the membrane potential ($\Delta\Psi$m) occurs before the fragmentation of the DNA in oligonucleosomal fragments (Vayssiere et al. 1994; Petit et al. 1995; Zamzami et al. 1995). This drop of $\Delta\Psi$m is responsible for changes in mitochondrial biogenesis and activity (Vayssiere et al. 1994). These data showed that the nuclear fragmentation is a late event as compared to mitochondrial changes. Last, translocation of cytochrome c from mitochondria to cytosol has been shown to be a crucial step in the activation of the apoptosis machinery in various cell death models and in a cell-free system using *Xenopus* egg extracts or dATP-primed cytosol of growing cells (Liu et al. 1996; Kluck et al. 1997b). Once released, cytochrome c, in interaction with the apoptosis protease-activating factor 1 (Apaf-1), triggers the initiator caspases-9 activation, which leads to the subsequent characteristic features of apoptosis, including chromatin condensation and nuclear fragmentation, cleavage of fodrin, PARP and Lamin B$_1$. Remarkably, part of the sequence of Apaf-1 shows a striking similarity to that of CED-4, with the two proteins aligning over most of the CED-4 sequence. Finally, a decisive observation was that release of cytochrome c is blocked by overexpression of Bcl-2 (Kluck et al. 1997a; Yang et al. 1997). These data firmly established an active role of mitochondrial outer membrane permeabilization (MOMP) in apoptosis. Soon after this discovery, mitochondria was found to release many other proteins that could participate in apoptosis. Smac/DIABLO was identified simultaneously by its ability to enhance cytochrome c-mediated caspase-3 activation (Du et al. 2000) and by its interaction with XIAP (Verhagen et al. 2000). It facilitates caspase activation by binding to IAPs, and removing their inhibitory activity in a way similar to that of *Drosophila* RHG proteins. Soon after, HtrA2/Omi was found to be another XIAP-binding protein (Hegde et al. 2002; Martins et al. 2002; Suzuki et al. 2001) released from mitochondria during apoptosis and exhibiting proapoptotic activity (van Loo et al. 2002). These data showed that, although regulation of caspase activation within the apoptosome is different to some extent between worm, *Drosophila* and mammals, it is controlled by homologous proteins (Table 7.1) and involves mitochondria (for review: Colin et al. 2009b; Wang and Youle 2009). Moreover, apart from this pivotal role of mitochondria in the control of caspases activation, it should be noticed that reactive oxygen species (ROS) produced by the mitochondria (see Chap. 5) can be involved in apoptosis signaling (for reviewed: Fleury et al. 2002) and that Bcl-2 has been shown to regulate mitochondrial respiration and the level of different ROS (for review : Chen and Pervaiz 2009a), at least in part through a control of cytochrome c oxidase activity (Chen and Pervaiz 2009b).

7.2.3 Evolution of the Mitochondrial Pathway of Apoptosis

In mammals, since apoptosome activation requires the release of cytochrome c from the mitochondrial intermembrane space to the cytosol, it is therefore subjected to the regulation of cytochrome c location. Two major models that are not mutually exclusive have been proposed to explain the Bcl-2 family proteins control of the MOMP (for review Desagher and Martinou 2000; Kroemer et al. 2007). The first model involves a regulation of the opening of the PTP (Permeability Transition Pore), a macromolecular channel which includes ANT, VDAC, cyclophilin D and other variable components, Opening of PTP leads to matrix swelling, decrease of $\Delta\Psi$m, subsequent rupture of the outer membrane, and nonselective release of proteins located in the intermembrane space. *In vitro* experiments as well as experiments on isolated mitochondria indicate that both antiapoptotic and proapoptotic Bcl-2 family proteins could regulate the PTP opening. However, genetic analysis of mice KO for VDAC or ANT suggests that in most cases PTP opening might rather be a consequence of apoptosis.

Table 7.1 Conservation during evolution of proteins involved in the mitochondrial pathway of caspases activation

		Nematode	*Drosophila*	Mammals
Caspases	Initiator caspases	CED-3	DRONC	Casp-9, -8…
	Effector caspases	CED-3	DrIce, DREDD …	Casp-3, -7…
	Adaptators	CED-4	Dark	Apaf-1
Bcl-2 family	Antiapoptotic proteins	CED-9	Buffy	Bcl-2, Bcl-xL…
	Multidomain Proapoptotic proteins		Debcl*	Bax, Bak
	Proapoptotic BH3 only proteins (BOP)	EGL-1		BID, BIM, PUMA…
	Inhibitors of caspases	CSP-3**	DIAP1, DIAP2…	c-IAP1, c-IAP2…
	Disruptors of the anti-caspase activity of IAPs		RPR, HID, GRIM, SICKLE	Smac/Diablo, Omi/HtrA2

Three families of proteins involved in the core of the apoptotic machinery have been identified in nematodes, Drosophila and mammals: CED-3, –4, –9 are homologous to caspases, caspase activators (such as Apoptosis activating factor 1, Apaf-1) and proteins of the Bcl-2 (B Cell Lymphoma 2) family. In Drosophila and mammals, caspase inhibitors (IAPs, Inhibitor of Apoptosis Proteins) and proteins able to abrogate this inhibition also participate in the control of caspase activity (Smac/Diablo, RPR, HID, GRIM…). *: Since Debcl does not seem to promote MOMP by itself and is required for the proapoptotic function of mammalian Bax heterologously expressed in Drosophila (Galindo et al. 2009), it not yet clear whether it really belong to the multidomain proapoptotic proteins or could act as a BH3 only proteins (BOP). **: In *C. elegans* CED-3 can be inhibited by CSP-3, a partial caspase homologue unrelated to IAPs, to prevent CED-3 auto-activation (review: (Brady and Duckett 2009))

The second model relies on the formation in the mitochondrial outer membrane of channels formed by some proapoptotic members of the Bcl-2 family allowing the release of proteins of the intermembrane space into the cytosol. In this model other members of the family can either activate or inhibit the formation of these channels. Recently, as reviewed in Sect. 7.5, a third model, involving proteins involved in the regulation of mitochondrial shape and dynamics, has also been proposed (see also: Jourdain and Martinou 2009; Wasilewski and Scorrano 2009; Autret and Martin 2009). However, whatever the model, antiapoptotic members of the Bcl-2 family impair release of apoptogenic factors in the cytosol while proapoptotic ones favor this relocation.

In contrast to the mammalian apoptosome, the *Drosophila* apoptosome activation, although supposed to occur at or nearby mitochondria, has been shown to be mainly regulated by modulating its inhibition by IAP proteins. In fact, apoptosis induction leads to the release of the apoptosome from DIAP1 mediated inhibition (Muro et al. 2002). In this process of apoptosome activation, cytochrome c is clearly not crucial. In addition, although mammalian Bcl-2 inhibits apoptosis induced by various stimuli in *Drosophila* (Gaumer et al. 2000; Brun et al. 2002), *Drosophila* Bcl-2 family members do not seem to be key regulators of developmental apoptosis. Indeed, Debcl has a limited role in developmental apoptosis (Galindo et al. 2009) but could be important for stress-induced cell death (Sevrioukov et al. 2007). Moreover, the way this protein family regulates the *Drosophila* apoptosome is still unclear. Nevertheless, it seems that the apoptotic cascade is inverted between flies and worm/mammals. Indeed, contrarily to what happens in these two organisms, in which apoptosis regulators are relocated from mitochondria to the cytosol, it seems that *Drosophila* apoptosis regulators use an opposite relocation to concentrate at or around mitochondria during apoptosis. Indeed, RHG proteins relocalize to mitochondria and form multimeric complexes required for their full proapoptotic activity (Claveria et al. 2002; Olson et al. 2003; Freel et al. 2008; Sandu et al. 2010). In the nematode, it seems that a third mode of apoptosome control has been selected. Once more, Bcl-2 family members are important for regulation of apoptosome activity but this regulation, although involving CED-4 release from mitochondria-bound CED-9, occurs directly without involving mitochondrial membrane permeabilization as a decisive step. Taken together, studies of apoptosome activation in these different species show that the way Bcl-2 family proteins bound to mitochondria regulate caspase activity has evolved during evolution.

7.3 The Bcl-2 Family

The discovery that Bcl-2 was the functional homolog of *C. elegans* cell survival protein CED-9 (Hengartner and Horvitz 1994) and could prevent apoptosis in many systems led to the discoveries of homologous proteins exhibiting structures similar to Bcl-2 albeit not identical functions. Members of this family of proteins (hence dubbed the Bcl-2 family protein) share homologies restricted to 1 to 4 domains. Proteins with 4 Bcl-2 Homology domains (BH1-4) are anti apoptotic (*i.e.* Bcl-2, Bcl-xL, Mcl-1…), other members of this family are proapoptotic (Chipuk et al. 2010). Proapoptotic proteins are divided between multidomain proapoptotic proteins (Bax, Bak…), which exhibit a BH1-3 domains homology and proteins with homology essentially restricted to the BH3 domain and thus called the BH3 only proteins (BOPs) (Chipuk et al. 2010). Apoptosis is tightly controlled, at early stages, by the interaction between members of the Bcl-2 family. If it has been clearly established that proteins such as Bax and Bak are responsible for the mitochondrial apoptotic permeability and that survival proteins like Bcl-2 are inhibitors of the latter processes, the role of BOPs is still a matter of a vivid debate (Chipuk et al. 2010; Giam et al. 2008). BOPs have been shown to fall into two categories, a group of proteins, which interact with all multidomain antiapoptotic proteins (*i.e.* BID, BIM and PUMA), while a second group exhibits distinct affinities toward antiapoptotic proteins of the family (*i.e.* BIK, BMF, BAD, NOXA, HRK…) (Fig. 7.2). Several models depicting the roles of the members of the

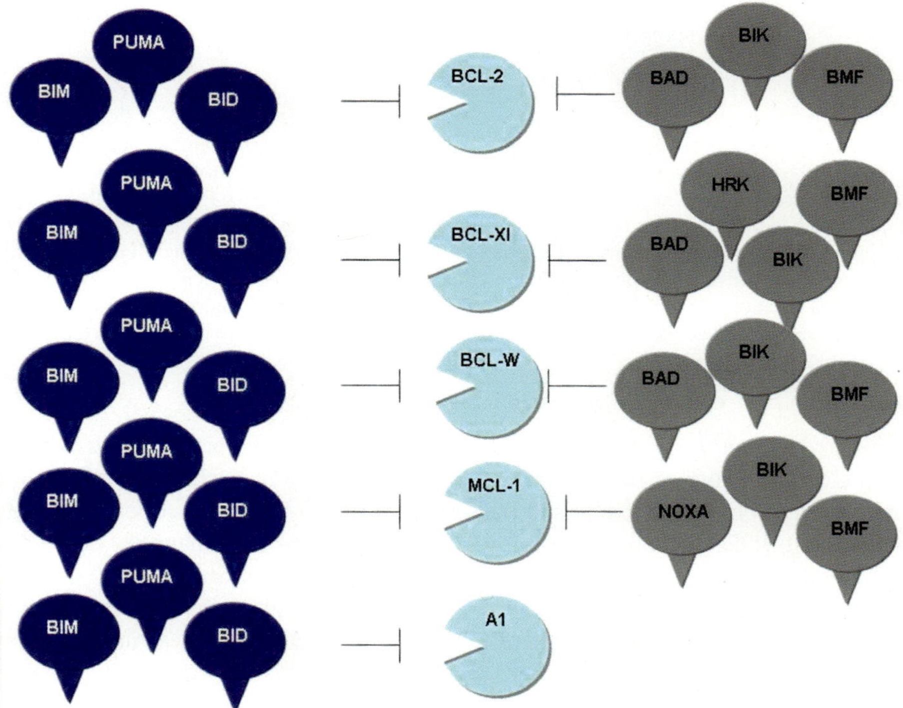

Fig. 7.2 Interaction between BH3 only proteins and survival members of the *Bcl-2* family. A class of BOP (*i.e. BIM, PUMA* and *BID*) binds to all survival Bcl-2 like proteins (and most likely to the proapoptotic ones) while other *BOPs* only bind to a subset of these proteins. Apoptosis can only be triggered when selective interactions occur following activation of specific signals. A complete database on the BCL-2 family can be found at http://bcl2db.ibcp.fr/

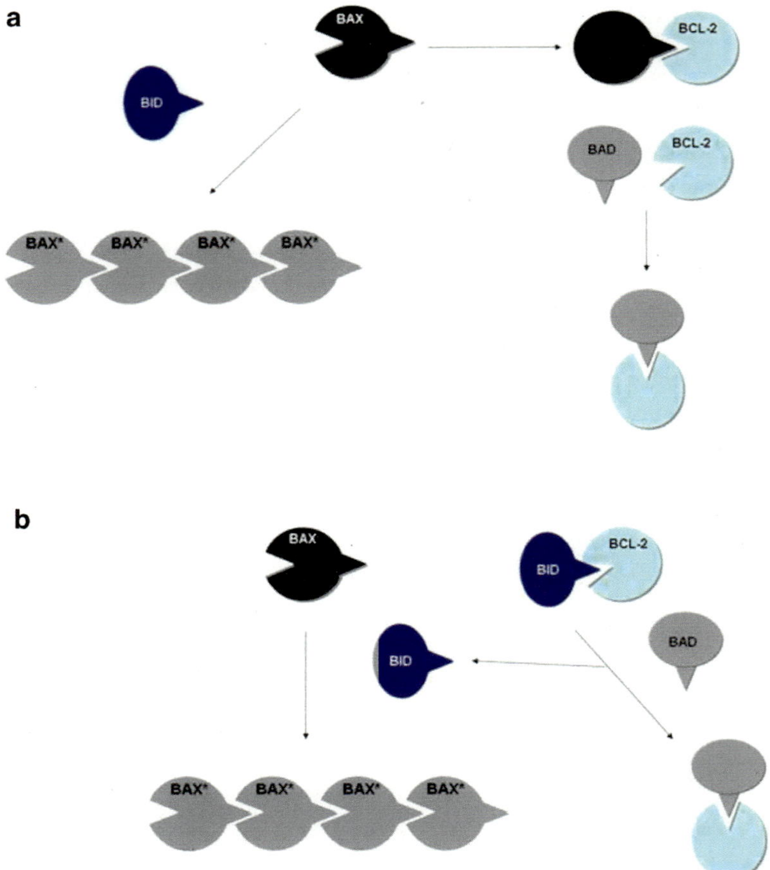

Fig. 7.3 Two models of activation of *BAX* and *BAK*. (**a**) For Bax activation, the primary event in the activation of apoptosis is a change of conformation induced by the transient interaction with *BID* (or PUMA or BIM) which leads to a change of conformation that facilitates the insertion of Bax into mitochondria. The inhibition of Bax by *Bcl-2* or other prosurvival proteins of the BCL-2 family is prevented by a competitive inhibition with BOPs with the specificity depicted in Fig. 7.1. Bak activation is roughly similar to Bax's, (**b**) In this model, BOPs intervention is divided into two steps: firstly, BOPs liberate PUMA/BID/BIM complexed to prosurvival proteins and secondly, the liberated PUMA/BID/BIM are thus able to activate Bax or Bak

Bcl-2 family in the control of Bax/Bak activation have been proposed but after a decade of exciting but somehow contradictory results, the remaining questions point to the existence of a direct or indirect activation of proapoptotic Bax and Bak by BOPs (Fig. 7.3). Two theories are still discussed: one postulates that BOPs directly activate Bax or Bak and induce their change of conformation and mitochondrial integration by a "kiss and run" mechanism (Youle and Strasser 2008). This has been shown for at least BID and BIM (Chipuk et al. 2010), and appears to be also the case for PUMA (Cartron et al. 2004; Kim et al. 2009). Other BOPs act as mere inhibitors of antiapoptotic proteins (a property also shared by activators of Bax/Bak) (Fig. 7.2). It is not surprising that activators of Bax and Bak can also bind all the antiapoptotic members of the Bcl-2 family (cf Figs. 7.1 and 7.2). Indeed, the activity of this class of BOPs might require both features (Merino et al. 2009). The specificity of other BOPs for subclasses of survival proteins of the Bcl-2 family are supposed to be link to the specificity of these proteins to intervene in apoptosis. These BOPs are the most upstream apoptotic sensors because of their early and selective activation by tissue restricted and/or stress signals. For example, it has been shown that BAD was especially responsive to growth factors withdrawal and/or the impairment of glucose metabolism (Danial 2008). Similarly, proteins like PUMA and NOXA are sensors of DNA damage in a p53 manner while BID is specifically activated by the Fas pathway (Youle and Strasser 2008). However, in the past years, it has become evident that these proteins could also be involved in other cellular functions as diverse as cell cycle regulation, DNA repair and metabolism. For example, BAD resides in and controls the formation of a glucokinase complex that regulates mitochondria respiration (Danial et al. 2003). BAD is active in this complex as a phosphorylated protein and a glucose deficit triggers dephosphorylation of BAD and disassembly of the complex, which thus in turn amplifies BAD-induced death signal (Danial et al. 2003). This function appears to be playing an important role in the insulin secretion in beta cells, favoring physiological adaption of these cells to high fat diet (Danial et al. 2008). Proapoptotic BOP activity has been particularly studied in the case of BID, which upon cleavage by caspase 8 becomes tBID, a very efficient direct activator of BAX and BAK (Luo et al. 1998; Li et al. 1998). As such, tBID conveys the apoptotic signal form cell surface death receptors to mitochondria (Youle and Strasser 2008). However, it should be noted that BID, under its native form, has been involved in "life" functions and more particularly in cell cycle progression into S phase (Yin 2006; Gross 2006). It is thus likely that other functions of BOPs, especially mitochondrial ones, will be revealed in the future. One might suggest that members of the Bcl-2 family have evolved and adapted from specific functions to the control of apoptosis.

Mitochondria have been considered to be passive actors during apoptosis beyond the activation of PTP. However, in the past years, it has become obvious that this organelle could play an active role in its BAX/BAK-mediated permeabilization. Kuwana et al. (2002) using a simple liposome system, have suggested that mitochondrial proteins are dispensable for BID-mediated insertion of Bax, as long as cardiolipin, a lipid mainly located in the inner membrane of the mitochondria, was added in important proportion. Cardiolopin is important for the insertion of BID in liposomes or mitochondria in conjunction with mitochondrial carrier homolog 2, a mitochondrial inner membrane transporter (Grinberg et al. 2005; Schug and Gottlieb 2009). In that respect, it is important to note that this cardiolipin requirement was not found with BIM or oligomerized BAX (Schafer et al. 2009), suggesting that other agents such as proteins are needed in this process as discussed in Petit et al. (2009). Indeed, several groups have postulated the existence of mitochondrial proteins involved in the docking and/or the insertion of Bax into mitochondria (reviewed in Petit et al. 2009).

The majority of mitochondrial proteins is encoded in the nucleus and thus is imported into mitochondria *via* different translocation complexes such as the translocase of the outer membrane (called the TOM complex) and the translocase of the inner membrane (called the TIM complex), as well as the sorting and the assembly machinery (the SAM complex) (Becker et al. 2009). The question of the involvement of the TOM complex in the docking of BAX during apoptosis has been raised by recent studies (Petit et al. 2009; Ott et al. 2009). This point is of importance as the signal of Bax addressing has not been clearly established yet (Petit et al. 2009). Nevertheless, several proteins of the Bcl-2 family have been shown to interact with proteins of the TOM complex namely Bcl-2 with TOM20 (Schleiff et al. 1997; Motz et al. 2002), Mcl-1 with TOM70 (Chou et al. 2006) and Bax with TOM22 (Bellot et al. 2007; Colin et al. 2009a) and TOM40 (Ott et al. 2007; Cartron et al. 2008). It should be noted that an unnatural C–terminal mutant of Bax (*i.e.* Bax Ser184Val) constitutively associates with mitochondria and does not interact with the TOM complex during TNF alpha-induced apoptosis (Ross et al. 2009). This result suggests that either the forced localization of Bax through mutations abrogated the requirement for TOM complex or that BAX interaction with TOM depends on the nature of the apoptotic signal. The exact implication of mitochondrial translocases during apoptosis remains thus to be established as well as its impact with mitochondrial physiology.

Contrary to BAX, which is a cytosolic protein in resting cells, BAK permanently resides at the mitochondrion. Cheng et al. (2003) have found that Bak complexes with a low abundant isoform of VDAC (VDAC2) in viable cells and that this association keeps BAK inactive. This step might provide a connection between the PTP and the Bcl-2 family members.

7.4   Functions of p53 on Mitochondria

The p53 protein, first described about 30 years ago, was characterized as a tumor suppressor at the beginning of 1990 decade, and is nowadays the subject of almost 50,000 articles.[1] The p53 tumor suppressor protein plays a central role in the regulation of apoptosis, cell cycle and senescence as a response to a broad range of stresses such as DNA damage, oncogene activation and hypoxia; *p53* gene or its product was found to be inactivated in more than 50% of all human cancers. The crucial tumor suppressor activity of p53 involves both transcription-dependent and -independent mechanisms (Fridman and Lowe 2003). Thus, p53 activates the transcription of genes that encode apoptotic effectors, such as PUMA, NOXA, BID, Bax, p53AIP1 proteins (Miyashita and Reed 1995; Oda et al. 2000), and it represses the transcription of antiapoptotic genes such as *bcl-2* and *survivin* (Shen and Shenk 1994; Hoffman et al. 2002). Beside these well-known activities, p53 has lately been described as regulating a wide spectrum of processes such as the metabolism (glycolysis, ROS homeostasis), autophagy, cell invasion and motility, angiogenesis, bone remodeling, etc. (for review see Vousden and Lane 2007). For more than a decade now, many papers emerged describing the transcription-independent proapoptotic activities of p53, and its capacity to regulate the function of proteins involved in apoptosis commitment. Indeed, transactivation-incompetent p53 mutants can induce apoptosis in human cells as efficiently as wild type p53 (Caelles et al. 1994; Kakudo et al. 2005). Moreover, p53 can promote apoptosis when the nuclear import of p53 (and thereby its transcriptional activity) is inhibited (Chipuk et al. 2004). Transcription-independent pathways induced by p53 could play a primary role in gamma irradiation-induced apoptosis in mouse (Erster et al. 2004). Similarly, it was shown that upregulation of proapoptotic targets can be insufficient to induce apoptosis and requires further transcription-independent p53 signaling (Johnson et al. 2008).

The intensive study of these surprising pathways has identified mitochondria as a major site of transcriptional-independent apoptotic activity of p53. Indeed, numerous publications report that p53 itself relocates and induces apoptosis directly at mitochondria, *via* the interaction with members of the Bcl-2 family (Marchenko et al. 2000; Moll and Zaika 2001). Moreover, some data suggest that p53 could also act in altering mitochondrial physiology to promote apoptosis. Last but not least, recent studies have revealed the importance of p53 under conditions of apparent normal growth and development, *i.e.* in the absence of chronic or severe stress (Vousden and Lane 2007). For example, basal or low levels of p53 were shown to contribute to the maintenance and the activity of mitochondria (Bensaad and Vousden 2007), in part through nuclear transcription-dependent mechanisms.

7.4.1   *Mitochondrial Localization of p53 in Stress Condition*

A new paradigm for the transcription-independent apoptotic activities of p53 first emerged with the evidence of the possible accumulation of p53 in the cytosol or mitochondria in response to stress (Green and Kroemer 2009). It was reinforced by the demonstration that p53 could activate the intrinsic apoptotic pathway by directly inducing mitochondrial outer membrane permeabilization (MOMP) and triggering the release of proapoptotic factors from the intermembrane space. Indeed, the accumulation of mitochondrial p53 was described in a variety of experimental systems - from transformed cell lines to animal models - and was shown to correlate with transcription-independent mechanisms. For example, irradiation of mice or ischemic damage of the brain promotes the translocation of p53 to the mitochondrion. Similarly, *in vitro* studies illustrated the ability of p53 to interact with isolated mitochondria and to promote MOMP.

Numerous data suggest that the transcription-independent activity of p53 at the mitochondrial level is dependent on a primary interaction with members of the Bcl-2 family that leads to the induction of

---

[1] A search in PubMed database, with "p53" as query target, returns more than 52,000 results as of February 2010.

MOMP; p53 acting somehow as a BH3 only protein. The direct or indirect activation of Bak and Bax proapoptotic members plays a central role in this mechanism. Binding of p53 to Bak, an intrinsic outer mitochondrial membrane, was found to catalyze Bak activation and cytochrome c release (Leu et al. 2004). Characterization of the p53–Bak interaction revealed the crucial importance of the DNA-binding domain of p53 for interacting and oligomerizing with Bak (Leu et al. 2004; Pietsch et al. 2008). However, some results indicate that binding of p53 to Bak is not sufficient to induce apoptosis *in vivo*. Indeed, overexpression in human cancer cell lines of a transcriptionally impaired p53 showed that although p53 was able to bind to Bak it did not exhibit apoptotic activity (Mihara et al. 2003; Pietsch et al. 2008). Cytosolic accumulation of p53 was also shown to promote transcription-independent activation of Bax *in vivo* (Tan et al. 2005; Speidel et al. 2006; Akhtar et al. 2006; Geng et al. 2007) according to a 'hit-and-run' model involving the proline-rich domain of p53 that is located near its N-terminus (Chipuk et al. 2004). In addition to the interactions with Bax and Bak, p53 was reported to bind with the antiapoptotic Bcl-2 family proteins Bcl-xL and Bcl-2 through its DNA-binding domain (Petros et al. 2004; Tomita et al. 2006; Sot et al. 2007). Mutations within this domain abolish the binding of p53 to Bcl-xL/Bcl-2 (Mihara et al. 2003). Distinct models have been proposed to explain the function of the Bcl-xL/Bcl-2–p53 interactions. Some data suggest that binding of p53 to these proteins counteracts their inhibitory action on proapoptotic members of the Bcl-2 family (Bak and Bax) (Mihara et al. 2003). In this way, p53 mutants that are defective in the ability to bind Bcl-xL/Bcl-2 also lack apoptotic activity, which is in agreement with the fact that p53 abolishes the antiapoptotic function ability of Bcl-2 and Bcl-xL (Jiang et al. 2006; Fletcher et al. 2008). Conversely, other results point to a model in which complexes between p53 and antiapoptotic Bcl-2 proteins are rather a sequestering mechanism that inhibits apoptotic functions of p53. Indeed, apoptosis induction has correlated with disruption of the Bcl-xL –p53 complex rather than an increase in its formation (Chipuk et al. 2005). Expression of a Bcl-xL unable to bind proapoptotic Bcl-2 members inhibited p53-induced apoptosis suggesting that Bcl-xL can inhibit apoptotic function of p53.

The importance of p53 activity at the mitochondrial level was underscored by the observed effect of pifithrin-μ, a drug that reduces the binding of p53 to mitochondria but has no apparent effect on p53-dependent transactivation (Strom et al. 2006). This drug probably blocks the interaction of p53 with anti- and proapoptotic Bcl-2 family members. Pifithrin-μ can protect thymocytes from otherwise lethal irradiation although the upregulation of p53 target genes was not affected. In the same way, this drug reduces apoptosis of human embryonic stem cells upon UV irradiation (Qin et al. 2007). Conversely, it was shown that the proapoptotic effect of a drug as CP-31398 correlated with the translocation of p53 to mitochondria and the induction of a p53-dependent MOMP (Tang et al. 2007).

Several studies have confirmed the *in vivo* and physiological relevance of transcription-independent mechanisms in p53-mediated apoptosis. It has been shown that upregulation of proapoptotic p53 target genes is not sufficient to induce apoptosis following irradiation of mouse fibroblasts. The transcription-independent signaling, *i.e.* the activation of Bax by cytosolic p53, provides the decisive signal for the onset of cell death (Speidel et al. 2006). Similarly, mouse embryo fibroblasts expressing a p53 variant that was transcriptionally active but unable to interact with Bax were resistant to genotoxic stress although proapoptotic target genes were strongly activated (Johnson et al. 2008). Furthermore, it was described that the onset of apoptosis correlated with the translocation of p53 to mitochondria in sensitive tissues after gamma irradiation of mice (Erster et al. 2004).

Besides the evidences of a direct proapoptotic action of p53 on mitochondria, some results add complexity to the significance of the mitochondrial location of p53 in stress condition. First, mitochondrial p53 has been detected not only in apoptotic conditions but also associated to a growth arrest response to drug treatment; however the connection between the two events is not yet well established (Mahyar-Roemer et al. 2004; Essmann et al. 2005). Second, most data indicate that p53 is located to, or near, the outer membrane where it interacts with proteins of the Bcl-2 family to promote MOMP and apoptosis, but some publications suggest that a part of p53 is found within the mitochondria, in the matrix or associated to the inner membrane. Localization of p53 into the mitochondrion could be correlated to a transcription-independent role of p53 in the maintenance and stability of the mitochondrial genome. Indeed, p53 was shown to directly interact with mtDNA polymerase γ and to consequently enhance the DNA replication function of polymerase γ (Achanta et al. 2005). Moreover, p53 could bind directly to the mitochondrial base excision repair machinery (mtBER) (Chen et al. 2006) to remove damaged bases and stimulate repair mechanisms. Moreover, p53 is also able to bind the mitochondrial transcription factor A (mtTFA) in order to regulate both transcription and repair of mtDNA (Yoshida et al. 2003). Altogether, these data suggest that p53 can also exert a protective effect on mitochondria thanks to mechanisms that are independent of its nuclear transcriptional activities. In this model, p53 would reduce the risk of mtDNA mutations and mitochondrial malfunctions in the presence of ROS or DNA-damaging agents. This would explain both the increased genetic instability associated with the loss of p53 function in the late stage of cancer development and that mtDNA mutations promote aggressive tumor behavior (Petros et al. 2005; Shidara et al. 2005).

7.4.2 Mitochondrial Localization of p53 in the Absence of Stress

If the localization of p53 in conditions of stress is now relatively well documented, there are few literature data concerning the localization of p53 in the absence of stress. In this condition, p53 is assumed to be maintained at a basal protein level *via* Mdm2-induced poly-ubiquitination and degradation (Haupt et al. 1995; Grossman et al. 2003). Some studies have shown that Mdm2-mediated mono-ubiquitination leads to the export of p53 from the nucleus to the cytoplasm (Li et al. 2002; Brooks and Gu 2006). Once in the cytoplasm the major part of p53 is degraded by the proteasome. However, low levels of p53 are still present in normal tissues. According to the authors, in such conditions p53 is exclusively localized either in the nucleus or in the cytoplasm, depending on the cell status (normal or tumor/transformed cells). Some data suggest a cytoskeleton associated location of wild type p53 either with the actin filaments (Katsumoto et al. 1995), or with the microtubule network (Giannakakou et al. 2000). The interaction with microtubules is mediated by a motor protein (dynein), which in conditions of stress participates to the transport of p53 toward the nucleus using the microtubule network as a "highway". In certain human cancers such as breast cancers, colon cancers and neuroblastoma, wild type p53 is only detected in the cytoplasm (Moll et al. 1995; Bosari et al. 1995). Shuttling the protein out of the nucleus is an efficient way to control the activity of a tumor suppressor protein that acts as a transcription factor. Cytoplasmic sequestration of wild type p53 in these cancers has been associated with their poor response to chemotherapy and radiation therapy. In this case, proteins such as Parc have been shown to be cytoplasmic anchors for wild type p53, that prevent p53 transport to the nucleus (Nikolaev et al. 2003). Nevertheless, cytoplasmic sequestration of p53 can also be associated to a physiological occurrence in some cell types such as in the mammary gland during lactation (Moll et al. 1992) or in embryonic stem cells (Aladjem et al. 1998) to permit transient proliferation.

Furthermore, some data indicate that p53 could be located at mitochondria in the absence of stress. A first report showed a direct positive influence of a mitochondria targeted p53 on mitochondrial biogenesis and function (Donahue et al. 2001). We demonstrate that wild type p53 can be localized at mitochondria in living and proliferative cells issued from different species and regardless of the cell status (tumor, immortalized or primary cells) (Ferecatu et al. 2009). This mitochondrial localization of p53 in normal conditions agrees with recent observations of a direct positive influence of p53 on the biogenesis and the activity of mitochondria in part through nuclear transcription-dependent mechanisms (Bensaad and Vousden 2007).

Besides a role in mitochondria biogenesis, we cannot rule out the possibility that mitochondrial p53 represents a pool of p53 at the outer membrane; which could induce outer membrane permeabilization through physical interaction with members of the Bcl-2 family members following induction of apoptosis. Organelle location of p53 may also represent a way to sequestrate the tumor suppressor under normal conditions.

7.4.3 *Mitochondrial Targeting of p53*

p53 stabilization and activation depend on a series of post-translational modifications that include phosphorylation, acetylation, methylation, ubiquitination, sumoylation neddylation, glycosylation and rybosylation. Post-translational modifications also provide key signals for the cellular trafficking of p53 between organelles, although interaction with specific factors may also be involved in this process. Because p53 seems to be primarily a nuclear protein, its nuclear export and abundance in the cytosol could determine its ability to interact with mitochondria.

p53's ubiquitination is crucial in its nucleo-cytoplasmic shuttling, and is mediated by the Mdm2 protein. p53 is ubiquitinated by Mdm2 within the nucleus, unmasking the nuclear export signal (NES) of p53 and permitting p53 exit through the nuclear pores into the cytoplasm (Gottifredi and Prives 2001; Geyer et al. 2000). Mdm2 alone only catalyzes monoubiquitination of p53 (at one or multiple sites) and p53 poly-ubiquitination, which addresses p53 to the proteasome, involves a cytosolic cofactor, p300, which mediates the formation of a complex containing both p53 and the proteasome (Grossman et al. 2003; Lai et al. 2001). Moreover, low levels of Mdm2 induce monoubiquitination and nuclear export of p53 whereas high levels of Mdm2 promote polyubiquitination and degradation by nuclear proteasomes (Li et al. 2002).

Acetylation regulates both the stability of p53 by inhibiting Mdm2-induced ubiquitination as they occur at the same sites (Li et al. 2002) and the sub-cellular localization of p53. It was shown that p53 hyperacetylation prevents p53 oligomerization and determines the cytoplasmic accumulation of p53 by exposing the NES (Kawaguchi et al. 2006). The acetylation of more than four lysines promotes p53 export to the cytoplasm but no functional role has yet been associated to such hyperacetylation of p53.

Since the structure of p53 does not harbor a typical mitochondrial targeting sequence, the mechanisms responsible for p53 mitochondrial localization remain unclear. Only few studies concern signals that address p53 to mitochondria in conditions of stress and that govern its interaction with members of the Bcl-2 family members to promote MOMP. Post-translational modifications have been studied as putative mitochondria translocation signals. Primary data indicate that neither acetylation nor phosphorylation seems to be involved in p53 targeting to mitochondria (Mahyar-Roemer et al. 2004; Nemajerova et al. 2005). However, it was recently shown that Ser15 phosphorylation contributes to p53 interaction with Bcl2 and Bcl-xL (Park et al. 2005) and that Lys120 acetylation promotes the binding of p53 to Mcl-1 (Sykes et al. 2009). Up to this date, there is no data about p53 mitochondrial targeting in proliferative and living cells.

Monoubiquitylation of p53 was recently described as a possible mechanism for mitochondrial translocation (Marchenko and Moll 2007). Upon arrival at mitochondria, p53 undergoes deubiquitination by HAUSP, a process essential for complex formation with Bcl-2 family members, because only non-ubiquitinated p53 forms such complexes. The formation of these complexes and consequently the ability of p53 to associate with mitochondria are also conditioned by the status of its binding partners. Notably, post-translational modification of these partners could play an important role; for example, dephosphorylation of Bcl-2 was shown to enhance the formation of the Bcl-2–p53 complex (Deng et al. 2006, 2009). Moreover, non-Bcl-2 proteins could also interfere with mitochondrial binding of p53 and apoptosis induction. Indeed, hepatic IGFBP1 was found to bind to Bak, thus preventing Bak interaction with p53 and apoptosis (Leu et al. 2007). Similarly, ASC (Ohtsuka et al. 2004), clusterin (Zhang et al. 2005) and humanin (Guo et al. 2003) were shown interacting with Bax and Bak and affecting their activation, possibly through the inhibition of their interaction with p53.

Most results concerning the mitochondrial localization of p53 assumed that Bcl-2 family members are crucial mediators of p53 binding to mitochondria, more precisely at the outer membrane, and of its transcription-independent apoptotic activity. However, some studies indicate on the one hand that p53 could localize at a more inner compartment to prevent stress damages and, on the other hand, that p53 could be tightly associated to mitochondria in living and proliferative cells. Clearly, the study of mechanisms which regulate p53 mitochondrial targeting is one of the key areas in the field that requires further work.

7.5 Mitochondrial Dynamics and Apoptosis

7.5.1 Mitochondrial Fission and Apoptosis

There is compelling evidence that the eukaryotic organelles, chloroplasts and mitochondria, are evolutionarily derived from bacteria (Gray 1993; Lutkenhaus 1998). Mitochondria are dynamic organelles that continually move, fuse and divide. Thus, the distribution of mitochondria to daughter cells during cell division is an essential feature of cell proliferation and cell survival. These dynamic processes are also believed to ensure an adequate provision of ATP to those cytoplasmic regions where energy consumption is particularly high. Indeed, mitochondria are essential in ensuring ATP production, the usable energy molecule that is required for most of the endoergonic processes (Ernster and Schatz 1981). This highly efficient process is provided by the oxidative phosphorylation, and allows the generation of an electrochemical gradient across the inner mitochondrial membrane. ATP synthase generates ATP from ADP and phosphate. Tubular mitochondrial network can be also engaged in calcium signaling. Therefore, perturbations of mitochondrial dynamics have tremendous consequences on cell metabolism and therefore on cell life (Benard et al. 2007; Westermann 2008). In many senescent cell types, an extensive elongation of mitochondria occurs (Mai et al. 2010), and mice defective in mitochondrial fusion cannot sustain development and die (Wakabayashi et al. 2009; Ishihara et al. 2009). Yeast mutants also defective in mitochondrial fusion lose their mitochondrial DNA and cannot run oxidative phosphorylations (Okamoto and Shaw 2005; Dimmer et al. 2002). Similar perturbations of human cell mitochondria dynamics lead to numerous disorders such as Charcot-Marie-Tooth 2A or 4A or autosomal dominant optic atrophy.

The dynamic nature of mitochondria appears to be dependent upon the cytoskeleton and mechanoenzymes, including kinesins and dynamins (Yoon and McNiven 2001). Dynamins are a family of GTPases that participate in multiple membrane transport processes, and some of them such as Dnm1p or Mgm1p control mitochondrial morphology. Interestingly, homologs of these GTPases have been identified in higher eukaryotes, including flies, worms and mammalian cells, indicating that this process of mitochondrial morphology maintenance is evolutionarily conserved (Hales and Fuller 1997; Labrousse et al. 1999; Pitts et al. 1999; Smirnova et al. 1998; Bleazard et al. 1999). Another non-dynamin GTPase called Fzo1p was demonstrated to function in mitochondrial morphogenesis (Yoon and McNiven 2001). In mammalian cells, at least two proteins, DLP1 and Fis1, are required for fission. The dynamin-related protein DLP1 is a large cytosolic GTPase that is translocated to the mitochondria, where it couples GTP hydrolysis with scission of the mitochondrial tubule (Smirnova et al. 2001). Fis1p is anchored in the outer mitochondrial membrane with its amino-terminus exposed to the cytoplasm and a short carboxy-terminal tail protruding into the mitochondrial intermembrane space (Yoon et al. 2003). When the normal function of DLP1 was inhibited in cultured mammalian cells, mitochondrial tubules became elongated and entangled, collapsing around the nucleus. Further insights have come from work on the *C. elegans* homolog DRP1 showing that DRP1 functions in fission of the mitochondrial outer membrane (MOM).

Post-translational modifications are rapid, effective and reversible ways to regulate protein stability, localization, function, and their interactions with other molecules. Post-translational modifications usually occur as chemical modifications at amino acid residues, including for example, phosphorylation, SUMOylation, and S-nitrosylation. It has been shown that Drp1 phosphorylation participates in the control of mitochondrial shape integrating cAMP and calcium signals (Taguchi et al. 2007; Chang and Blackstone 2007; Cribbs and Strack 2007; Han et al. 2008). The modification of proteins by the small ubiquitin-like modifier (SUMO) is known to regulate an increasing array of cellular processes. Ubc9 and Sumo1 are specific DRP1-interacting proteins and DRP1 is a Sumo1 substrate (Harder et al. 2004). SUMOylation of DRP1 stimulates mitochondrial fission. Furthermore, the mitochondrial-anchored protein ligase (MAPL), the first mitochondrial-anchored SUMO E3 ligase, was shown to link MAPL and the fission machinery (Braschi et al. 2009). Prominent among these post-translational modifications are the addition of ubiquitin moieties that confer new binding surfaces and conformational states on the modified proteins. MARCH5, a mitochondrial E3 ubiquitin ligase has been identified as a molecule that binds mitochondrial Fis1 and mitofusin 2 (Nakamura et al. 2006; Karbowski et al. 2007). MARCH5 RNA interference induces an abnormal elongation and interconnection of mitochondria. Other clues suggest a role of Drp1 in neurodegenerative diseases. Indeed, mutations in PTEN-induced kinase 1 (PINK1) or PARKIN are the most frequent causes of recessive Parkinson's disease. Genetic studies in *Drosophila* indicate that PINK1 acts upstream of Parkin in a common pathway that influences mitochondrial integrity. Thus, the loss of the E3 ubiquitin ligase Parkin or the serine/threonine kinase PINK1 promotes mitochondrial fission and/or inhibits fusion (Poole et al. 2008; Deng et al. 2008). Notably, Pink1 interacts with Drp1, and knocking down Pink1 increases the ratio of mitochondrial fission over fusion proteins, leading to fragmented mitochondria (Cui et al. 2010).

Because it remains unclear how the MOM is permeabilized during apoptosis, several models potentially accounting for MOMP have been put forward. Based on the discovery that fragments of the mitochondrial network associated with remodeling of the cristae are generated during cell death, it has been proposed that the actors of the fission machinery regulate cell death (Bossy-Wetzel et al. 2003; Frank et al. 2001; Karbowski et al. 2002). Interestingly, mitochondrial fragmentation has also been reported during apoptosis of *Drosophila* cells (Goyal et al. 2007; Abdelwahid et al. 2007). However, other observations are disagreeing with the view that mitochondrial fission/fragmentation is important for apoptosis. Studies of mitochondrial dynamics during apoptosis suggest that mitochondrial fragmentation follows, rather than precedes, mitochondrial cytochrome c release after ActD treatment (Arnoult et al. 2005a). Inhibition of *Drp1* expression failed to block apoptosis in response to a number of proapoptotic stimuli (Parone et al. 2006; Estaquier and Arnoult 2007). Inhibition of *Fis1* expression, another major regulator of mitochondrial fission, has been reported either to inhibit apoptosis (Lee et al. 2004) or to have little effect on this process (Parone et al. 2006). Furthermore, Ced-9, the *C. elegans* Bcl-2 homolog, promotes mitochondrial fusion upon overexpression in mammalian cells, but failed to prevent cytochrome c release or apoptosis (Delivani et al. 2006). Similarly a chemical inhibitor of DRP1, mdivi-1 (for mitochondrial division inhibitor) uncouples mitochondrial fission and apoptosis (Cassidy-Stone et al. 2008).

7.5.2   *Mitochondrial Fusion and Apoptosis*

Mitochondrial fusion in mammalian cells involves a different set of proteins: the large transmembrane GTPase mitofusins (Mfn1, Mfn2) anchored to the MOM and the dynamin-like GTPase OPA1 (optic atrophy 1, Mgm1p) located in the IMS (Ishihara et al. 2004; Chen et al. 2003; Cipolat et al. 2004; Griparic et al. 2004). Despite a high level of homology, Mfn1 and Mfn2 show functional differences. Mfn1 has a center role in mitochondrial docking and fusion, while Mfn2 could participate in the stabilization of the interaction between adjacent mitochondria (Chen et al. 2003; Koshiba et al. 2004). Mice lacking *Mfn1* are viable and display no major defects. On the contrary, *Mfn2* knockout mouse present a degeneration of Purkinje cells (Chen et al. 2007). In yeast, Ugo1p – an adaptor protein – is required to couple fusion of the outer membrane, mediated by the Mfns orthologue Fzo1p, and that of the inner membrane, which also requires the Opa1 orthologue Mgm1p (Sesaki and Jensen 2004). Opa1 is so far the only dynamin-related protein targeted to the inner membrane of mitochondria, via a specific N-terminal targeting sequence, followed by a hydrophobic stretch that allows its insertion into the membrane (Olichon et al. 2002). Mutations in Opa1 are associated with Dominant Optic Atrophy (DOA), the Kjer optic neuropathy, a non-syndromic neurological disease specifically affecting the retinal ganglion cells (RGCs), leading to reduced visual acuity, and sometimes to legal blindness (Delettre et al. 2000; Alexander et al. 2000). Opa1 exists in eight splice variants in humans (five in mouse) (Akepati et al. 2008; Delettre et al. 2001) and is further regulated by posttranslational cleavage that generates short and long forms of the protein. OPA1 contributes to the Inner Mitochondrial Membrane (IMM) structures, i.e. cristae, cristae junction and domains of interaction with the OMM. Strong evidences suggest that OPA1 is required in maintaining respiratory chain integrity. Thus, OPA1 was recently found physically interacting with Complex-I, Complex-II and Complex-III, but not Complex-IV of the respiratory chain, suggesting a possible connection between cristae structure and organization of the respiratory chain C-I to C-III that exchange electrons through the membrane, while electron transfer from C-III to C-IV occurs out of the IMM via cytochrome c (Zanna et al. 2008). Interestingly, fibroblast strains with deleterious OPA1 mutation showed a coupling defect of oxidative phosphorylation as well as a faint decrease in ATP production driven by C-I substrates (Zanna et al. 2008). Therefore, a central OPA1 function consists in maintaining IMM integrity to prevent proton leakage and to facilitate efficient electron transport inside this membrane between respiratory chain complexes. Moreover, OPA1 down-regulation evidenced perturbation of the IMM structure and induces drastic fragmentation of the network (Misaka et al. 2006; Olichon et al. 2007; Legros et al. 2002) that correlated to a strong dissipation of the membrane potential (Olichon et al. 2003, 2007). OPA1 has been shown to interact with the mitofusins MFN1 and MFN2 (Cipolat et al. 2006; Guillery et al. 2008). In *Caenorhabditis elegans*, mutation in the *eat-3* gene, the *OPA1* orthologue, induces mitochondrial fragmentation, and shorter and scarce cristae. These worms are smaller, grow slower and show oxidative phosphorylation defects (Kanazawa et al. 2008). In *Drosophila melanogaster*, mutations in *dOpa1* cause haploinsufficiency and heterozygous flies show no discernable phenotype, but a reduced life span (Tang et al. 2009).

Several proteolytic machineries have been implicated in the cleavage of OPA1. Rhomboids are among the most conserved family of polytopic membrane proteins known to date, sequenced in bacterial, archaeal and eukaryotic genomes (Koonin et al. 2003). In mammalian cells, Parl – for presenilin-associated rhomboid-like protein – was discovered following a yeast two-hybrid screening using as bait Presenilin-2 (PSEN2), a proapoptotic familial Alzheimer's disease protein (Wolozin et al. 1996). Subsequent studies indicated, however, that the reported interaction between Parl and the presenilin proteins was artifactual (Pellegrini et al. 2001). Parl is localized in the inner mitochondrial membrane, with the N-terminus exposed to the matrix and the C-terminus to the IMS (Jeyaraju et al. 2006). In *S. cerevisiae*, two rhomboid genes exist, *Rbd1* and *Rbd2* (Esser et al. 2002). *Rbd1*, encodes a mitochondrial rhomboid protease, which is required for the processing of cytochrome c peroxidase (Ccp1p). Ablation of *Pcp1/Rbd1* activity has a profound effect on mitochondrial shape. Yeast lacking Pcp1p are missing the 90-kDa short-Mgm1 (OPA1) form but have the 100 kDa long-Mgm1 form (Esser et al. 2002). Mice lacking Parl die between weeks 8 and 12 from cachexia sustained by multisystemic atrophy. However, Parl[+/−] mice do not show any obvious phenotype, suggesting the existence of compensatory mechanisms to gene dosage effects. Moreover, *Parl* ablation did not alter the morphology of the mitochondrial reticulum or mitochondrial respiration, irrespective of the substrate used by the organelle; loss of *Parl* expression did not affect mitochondria fusion (Cipolat et al. 2006).

Although some groups have proposed that in steady state conditions the function of Parl is to execute the cleavage of Opa1 which is dependent on ATP, to either directly or indirectly liberate an IMS-soluble form of the protein (IMS-Opa1) that assembles in macromolecular complexes with Parl and with the uncleaved IMM-bound form of Opa1 (Herlan et al. 2003; Lemberg et al. 2005; Cipolat et al. 2006), other groups have reported a lack of PARL involvement in OPA1 processing and have implicated other metalloproteases – the m-AAA proteases (matrix of mitochondria oriented; homo- or heteromeric complexes containing paraplegin and/or Afg3L1 and Afg3L2 subunits) and the i-AAA protease Yme1L (intermembrane space oriented) (Griparic et al. 2007; Ishihara et al. 2006; Song et al. 2007). Thus, the bivalent metal chelator, 10-phenanthroline (o-phe) was reported to inhibit m-AAA proteases and OPA1 processing (Ishihara et al. 2006). However, the effects of paraplegin siRNA were modest in preventing OPA1 processing (Duvezin-Caubet et al. 2007). Thus, down-regulation of individual subunits of m-AAA protease isoenzymes did not affect the processing of OPA1. Some confusion may have also arisen from the fact that OPA1 is controlled by complex patterns of alternative splicing and proteolysis. Thus, the scenario proposed is that the i-AAA protease Yme1L generates the short form of OPA1 (S-OPA1) whereas the remaining isoforms – the long isoforms of OPA1 (L-OPA1)– are normally not cleaved by m-AAA proteases. S-and L-OPA1 are both required for fusion. There is also evidence suggesting that a decrease in mitochondrial ATP levels upon inhibition of the F1F0-ATP synthase with oligomycin or upon the dissipation of $\Delta\Psi$m with the uncoupler CCCP, is crucial in the control of L-OPA1 processing (Baricault et al. 2007). Thus, it has been proposed that another protease mediates processing and degradation of the L-OPA1 isoforms. Two other groups have recently identified another peptidase, OMA1 (Oma1 for overlapping activity with m-AAA protease 1) (Head et al. 2009; Ehses et al. 2009). Mammalian OMA1 is similar in sequence to the yeast mitochondrial Oma1 (Kaser et al. 2003). Interestingly, down-regulation of OMA1 before the addition of CCCP or oligomycin inhibits L-OPA1 processing. However, the implication of OMA1 merits further analysis. Indeed, the substrate specificity of OMA1 is distinct in mammalian and yeast (Duvezin-Caubet et al. 2007). Furthermore, no OMA1-like peptidase can be found in *Caenorhabditis elegans* and *Drosophila melanogaster,* although mitochondrial morphology depends on OPA1 in both organisms. Finally, down-regulation of OMA1 does not affect mitochondrial morphology suggesting that OMA1 is dispensable for the formation of S- and L-OPA1 isoforms (Ehses et al. 2009). Thus, OMA1 should be responsible for stress-induced OPA1 cleavage. Thus, it is likely that several proteases participate in the regulation of OPA1 processing.

Prohibitin complexes assemble with *m*-AAA proteases in the mitochondrial inner membrane, increasing the complexity of protein interaction controlling mitochondrial dynamics (Steglich et al. 1999). PHB complex acts as a chaperone for newly synthesized mitochondrial proteins and is required for a correct yeast replicative lifespan (Coates et al. 1997; Nijtmans et al. 2000). Thus, the sequence similarity of prohibitins to lipid raft–associated proteins of the SPFH family (Browman et al. 2007) is consistent with a scaffolding function of prohibitin complexes in the inner membrane. Multiple copies of two homologous subunits, PHB1 (BAP32, often simply termed prohibitin) and PHB2 (BAP37, REA), form large complexes within the mitochondria (Ikonen et al. 1995; Coates et al. 1997; Berger and Yaffe 1998). PHB2 is a highly conserved, ubiquitously expressed protein and its homologs are found in bacteria, yeast, plants, *Drosophila* and mammals (Nijtmans et al. 2000). Interestingly, it has been shown an essential role of the prohibitin complex for the processing of OPA1 within mitochondria that results in impaired cell proliferation, resistance toward apoptosis, and mitochondrial cristae morphogenesis. Deletion of *PHB2* leads to the selective loss of L-OPA1 isoforms (Merkwirth et al. 2008). Finally, although prohibitins are required for embryonic development in mice, *Caenorhabditis elegans*, and *Drosophila melanogaster*, deletion of prohibitin genes in yeast leads to premature ageing but does not affect cell survival (Merkwirth et al. 2008). Recently, SLP-2 has been identified as a mitochondrial member of a superfamily of putative scaffolding proteins (Da Cruz et al. 2003; Morrow and Parton 2005). SLP-2 interacts with MFN2 (Hajek et al. 2007) and with PHB1/2 (Da Cruz et al. 2008). In SLP-2-deficient stressed cells, mitochondria are fragmented, and it has been proposed that SLP-2 is required for stress-induced mitochondrial hyperfusion (Tondera et al. 2009).

Growing evidences suggest that proteins involved in the control of fusion are also key actors in the control of apoptosis. Thus, fuzzyonions/Mitofusins are reported to antagonize cytochrome c release and to inhibit apoptosis upon transient overexpression (Lee et al. 2004; Sugioka et al. 2004; Jahani-Asl et al. 2007). However, the role of cristae remodeling in the full release of cytochrome c and cell death is also much debated (Parone et al. 2006; Yamaguchi et al. 2008; Sheridan et al. 2008). The downregulation of OPA1 or its cleavage by PARL favors the release of cytochrome c by inducing mitochondrial fragmentation and remodeling of the cristae (Arnoult et al. 2005a; Cipolat et al. 2006; Frezza et al. 2006; Olichon et al. 2003). However, it has been suggested that mitochondrial fission/fragmentation occurs as a consequence of apoptosis-associated permeabilization of MOM and subsequent loss of intermembrane space proteins, such as Opa1, Arnoult et al. (2005a, b). Moreover, Youle and colleagues have found that Bax/Bak-deficient cells show constitutive defects in mitochondrial morphology and contain mitochondria that are shorter than normal (Karbowski et al. 2006). Thus, in these different models mitochondrial fragmentation is uncoupled with apoptosis. OMA1 siRNA slows the onset of apoptosis associated with the absence of L-OPA1 processing. This preventive effect on OPA1 cleavage was stronger for ActD than for Staurosporine-mediated apoptosis. Intriguingly, OMA1 siRNA prevents cytochrome C release and cell death following ActD treatment. This may appear paradoxical given that loss of OPA1 is more a consequence of MOMP-mediated by ActD (Sheridan et al. 2008). Like *OPA1* knockout cells, *PHB2* deficient cells are more sensitive to apoptotic stimuli involving both the intrinsic and the extrinsic pathways (Merkwirth et al. 2008). Altogether, these observations suggest that mitochondrial fragmentation is not the main driving force *per se*, but the absence of or defect in those proteins within the mitochondria increases mitochondria sensitivity to apoptotic insults.

Because as mentioned Bax/Bak are the gate keepers controlling mitochondria, it remains unclear whether Bax/Bak is required for mitochondrial fragmentation, given that this process is systematically reported during Bax/Bak-dependent apoptosis (Arnoult et al. 2005a; Parone et al. 2006; Yamaguchi et al. 2008; Sheridan et al. 2008). Several groups have described Bax/Bak-independent release of cytochrome c (Scorrano et al. 2003; Claveria et al. 2004; Lei et al. 2006; Majewski et al. 2004; Mizuta et al. 2007). Thus, whether defective expression of *OPA1* or *PHB2* sensitizes cells to apoptotic insults that do not depend on Bax and Bak proteins could be an interesting question.

7.6 Concluding Remarks

In conclusion, mitochondria appears today at the heart of apoptosis signaling. However, although MOMP appears as a decisive step during mammalian cells apoptosis, the role of mitochondria in nematodes and flies remains more elusive. Moreover, in spite of the growing amount of data concerning the mechanisms and regulations of MOMP in mammals, several concurrent non-exclusive hypotheses still coexist and a unifying model (if pertinent) remains to be established. Mechanisms involved in Bcl-2 family proteins mitochondrial translocation and activation, as well as their relationship with other proteins constitutively or transiently located to mitochondria that are critical for the survival/death behavior of cell populations remain to be fully understood. The answers to these questions should allow designing new chemotherapeutic drugs for cancer and other apoptosis-related diseases treatment.

Acknowledgments We gratefully acknowledge Sébastien Gaumer for his critical reading of the manuscript. The work of the authors was supported in part by grants from the "Association pour la Recherche Contre le Cancer" and the "Ligue Nationale Contre le Cancer".

References

Abdelwahid E, Yokokura T, Krieser RJ, Balasundaram S, Fowle WH, White K (2007) Mitochondrial disruption in Drosophila apoptosis. Dev Cell 12:793–806
Achanta G, Sasaki R, Feng L, Carew JS, Lu W, Pelicano H, Keating MJ, Huang P (2005) Novel role of p53 in maintaining mitochondrial genetic stability through interaction with DNA Pol gamma. EMBO J 24:3482–3492

Akepati VR, Muller EC, Otto A, Strauss HM, Portwich M, Alexander C (2008) Characterization of OPA1 isoforms isolated from mouse tissues. J Neurochem 106:372–383

Akhtar RS, Geng Y, Klocke BJ, Roth KA (2006) Neural precursor cells possess multiple p53-dependent apoptotic pathways. Cell Death Differ 13:1727–1739

Aladjem MI, Spike BT, Rodewald LW, Hope TJ, Klemm M, Jaenisch R, Wahl GM (1998) ES cells do not activate p53-dependent stress responses and undergo p53-independent apoptosis in response to DNA damage. Curr Biol 8:145–155

Alexander C, Votruba M, Pesch UE, Thiselton DL, Mayer S, Moore A, Rodriguez M, Kellner U, Leo-Kottler B, Auburger G, Bhattacharya SS, Wissinger B (2000) OPA1, encoding a dynamin-related GTPase, is mutated in autosomal dominant optic atrophy linked to chromosome 3q28. Nat Genet 26:211–215

Arnoult D, Grodet A, Lee YJ, Estaquier J, Blackstone C (2005a) Release of OPA1 during apoptosis participates in the rapid and complete release of cytochrome c and subsequent mitochondrial fragmentation. J Biol Chem 280:35742–35750

Arnoult D, Rismanchi N, Grodet A, Roberts RG, Seeburg DP, Estaquier J, Sheng M, Blackstone C (2005b) Bax/Bak-dependent release of DDP/TIMM8a promotes Drp1-mediated mitochondrial fission and mitoptosis during programmed cell death. Curr Biol 15:2112–2118

Autret A, Martin SJ (2009) Emerging role for members of the Bcl-2 family in mitochondrial morphogenesis. Mol Cell 36:355–363

Bao Q, Shi Y (2007) Apoptosome: a platform for the activation of initiator caspases. Cell Death Differ 14:56–65

Baricault L, Segui B, Guegand L, Olichon A, Valette A, Larminat F, Lenaers G (2007) OPA1 cleavage depends on decreased mitochondrial ATP level and bivalent metals. Exp Cell Res 313:3800–3808

Becker T, Gebert M, Pfanner N, van der Laan M (2009) Biogenesis of mitochondrial membrane proteins. Curr Opin Cell Biol 21:484–493

Bellot G, Cartron PF, Er E, Oliver L, Juin P, Armstrong LC, Bornstein P, Mihara K, Manon S, Vallette FM (2007) TOM22, a core component of the mitochondria outer membrane protein translocation pore, is a mitochondrial receptor for the proapoptotic protein Bax. Cell Death Differ 14:785–794

Benard G, Bellance N, James D, Parrone P, Fernandez H, Letellier T, Rossignol R (2007) Mitochondrial bioenergetics and structural network organization. J Cell Sci 120:838–848

Bensaad K, Vousden KH (2007) p53: new roles in metabolism. Trends Cell Biol 17:286–291

Berger KH, Yaffe MP (1998) Prohibitin family members interact genetically with mitochondrial inheritance components in Saccharomyces cerevisiae. Mol Cell Biol 18:4043–4052

Bergmann A (2010) The role of ubiquitylation for the control of cell death in Drosophila. Cell Death Differ 17:61–67

Bleazard W, McCaffery JM, King EJ, Bale S, Mozdy A, Tieu Q, Nunnari J, Shaw JM (1999) The dynamin-related GTPase Dnm1 regulates mitochondrial fission in yeast. Nat Cell Biol 1:298–304

Borner C, Martinou I, Mattmann C, Irmler M, Schaerer E, Martinou JC, Tschopp J (1994) The protein bcl-2 alpha does not require membrane attachment, but two conserved domains to suppress apoptosis. J Cell Biol 126:1059–1068

Bosari S, Viale G, Roncalli M, Graziani D, Borsani G, Lee AK, Coggi G (1995) p53 gene mutations, p53 protein accumulation and compartmentalization in colorectal adenocarcinoma. Am J Pathol 147:790–798

Bossy-Wetzel E, Barsoum MJ, Godzik A, Schwarzenbacher R, Lipton SA (2003) Mitochondrial fission in apoptosis, neurodegeneration and aging. Curr Opin Cell Biol 15:706–716

Brachmann CB, Jassim OW, Wachsmuth BD, Cagan RL (2000) The Drosophila bcl-2 family member dBorg-1 functions in the apoptotic response to UV-irradiation. Curr Biol 10:547–550

Brady GF, Duckett CS (2009) A caspase homolog keeps CED-3 in check. Trends Biochem Sci 34:104–107

Braschi E, Zunino R, McBride HM (2009) MAPL is a new mitochondrial SUMO E3 ligase that regulates mitochondrial fission. EMBO Rep 10:748–754

Bredesen DE, Rao RV, Mehlen P (2006) Cell death in the nervous system. Nature 443:796–802

Brooks CL, Gu W (2006) p53 ubiquitination: Mdm2 and beyond. Mol Cell 21:307–315

Browman DT, Hoegg MB, Robbins SM (2007) The SPFH domain-containing proteins: more than lipid raft markers. Trends Cell Biol 17:394–402

Brun S, Rincheval V, Gaumer S, Mignotte B, Guenal I (2002) reaper and bax initiate two different apoptotic pathways affecting mitochondria and antagonized by bcl-2 in Drosophila. Oncogene 21:6458–6470

Caelles C, Helmberg A, Karin M (1994) p53-dependent apoptosis in the absence of transcriptional activation of p53-target genes. Nature 370:220–223

Cartron PF, Gallenne T, Bougras G, Gautier F, Manero F, Vusio P, Meflah K, Vallette FM, Juin P (2004) The first alpha helix of Bax plays a necessary role in its ligand-induced activation by the BH3-only proteins Bid and PUMA. Mol Cell 16:807–818

Cartron PF, Bellot G, Oliver L, Grandier-Vazeille X, Manon S, Vallette FM (2008) Bax inserts into the mitochondrial outer membrane by different mechanisms. FEBS Lett 582:3045–3051

Cassidy-Stone A, Chipuk JE, Ingerman E, Song C, Yoo C, Kuwana T, Kurth MJ, Shaw JT, Hinshaw JE, Green DR, Nunnari J (2008) Chemical inhibition of the mitochondrial division dynamin reveals its role in Bax/Bak-dependent mitochondrial outer membrane permeabilization. Dev Cell 14:193–204

Chai J, Yan N, Huh JR, Wu JW, Li W, Hay BA, Shi Y (2003) Molecular mechanism of Reaper-Grim-Hid-mediated suppression of DIAP1-dependent Dronc ubiquitination. Nat Struct Biol 10:892–898

Chang CR, Blackstone C (2007) Cyclic AMP-dependent protein kinase phosphorylation of Drp1 regulates its GTPase activity and mitochondrial morphology. J Biol Chem 282:21583–21587

Chen ZX, Pervaiz S (2009a) BCL-2: pro-or anti-oxidant? Front Biosci (Elite Ed) 1:263–268

Chen ZX, Pervaiz S (2009b) Involvement of cytochrome c oxidase subunits Va and Vb in the regulation of cancer cell metabolism by Bcl-2. Cell Death Differ. doi:10.1038/cdd.2009.132

Chen H, Detmer SA, Ewald AJ, Griffin EE, Fraser SE, Chan DC (2003) Mitofusins Mfn1 and Mfn2 coordinately regulate mitochondrial fusion and are essential for embryonic development. J Cell Biol 160:189–200

Chen D, Yu Z, Zhu Z, Lopez CD (2006) The p53 pathway promotes efficient mitochondrial DNA base excision repair in colorectal cancer cells. Cancer Res 66:3485–3494

Chen H, McCaffery JM, Chan DC (2007) Mitochondrial fusion protects against neurodegeneration in the cerebellum. Cell 130:548–562

Cheng EH, Sheiko TV, Fisher JK, Craigen WJ, Korsmeyer SJ (2003) VDAC2 inhibits BAK activation and mitochondrial apoptosis. Science 301:513–517

Chipuk JE, Kuwana T, Bouchier-Hayes L, Droin NM, Newmeyer DD, Schuler M, Green DR (2004) Direct activation of Bax by p53 mediates mitochondrial membrane permeabilization and apoptosis. Science 303:1010–1014

Chipuk JE, Bouchier-Hayes L, Kuwana T, Newmeyer DD, Green DR (2005) PUMA couples the nuclear and cytoplasmic proapoptotic function of p53. Science 309:1732–1735

Chipuk JE, Moldoveanu T, Llambi F, Parsons MJ, Green DR (2010) The BCL-2 family reunion. Mol Cell 37:299–310

Chou CH, Lee RS, Yang-Yen HF (2006) An internal EELD domain facilitates mitochondrial targeting of Mcl-1 via a Tom70-dependent pathway. Mol Biol Cell 17:3952–3963

Cipolat S, de Brito OM, Dal Zilio B, Scorrano L (2004) OPA1 requires mitofusin 1 to promote mitochondrial fusion. Proc Natl Acad Sci USA 101:15927–15932

Cipolat S, Rudka T, Hartmann D, Costa V, Serneels L, Craessaerts K, Metzger K, Frezza C, Annaert W, D'Adamio L, Derks C, Dejaegere T, Pellegrini L, D'Hooge R, Scorrano L, de Strooper B (2006) Mitochondrial rhomboid PARL regulates cytochrome c release during apoptosis via OPA1-dependent cristae remodeling. Cell 126:163–175

Clarke PG (1990) Developmental cell death: morphological diversity and multiple mechanisms. Anat Embryol (Berl) 181:195–213

Clarke PGH, Clarke S (1996) Nineteenth century research on naturally occuring cell death and related phenomena. Anat Embryol 193:81–99

Claveria C, Caminero E, Martinez AC, Campuzano S, Torres M (2002) GH3, a novel proapoptotic domain in *Drosophila* Grim, promotes a mitochondrial death pathway. EMBO J 21:3327–3336

Claveria C, Martinez AC, Torres M (2004) A Bax/Bak-independent mitochondrial death pathway triggered by *Drosophila* Grim GH3 domain in mammalian cells. J Biol Chem 279:1368–1375

Coates PJ, Jamieson DJ, Smart K, Prescott AR, Hall PA (1997) The prohibitin family of mitochondrial proteins regulate replicative lifespan. Curr Biol 7:607–610

Colin J, Garibal J, Mignotte B, Guenal I (2009a) The mitochondrial TOM complex modulates bax-induced apoptosis in Drosophila. Biochem Biophys Res Commun 379:939–943

Colin J, Gaumer S, Guenal I, Mignotte B (2009b) Mitochondria, Bcl-2 family proteins and apoptosomes: of worms, flies and men. Front Biosci 14:4127–4137

Colussi PA, Quinn LM, Huang DC, Coombe M, Read SH, Richardson H, Kumar S (2000) Debcl, a proapoptotic Bcl-2 homologue, is a component of the Drosophila melanogaster cell death machinery. J Cell Biol 148:703–714

Cribbs JT, Strack S (2007) Reversible phosphorylation of Drp1 by cyclic AMP-dependent protein kinase and calcineurin regulates mitochondrial fission and cell death. EMBO Rep 8:939–944

Cui M, Tang X, Christian WV, Yoon Y, Tieu K (2010) Perturbations in mitochondrial dynamics induced by human mutant PINK1 can be rescued by the mitochondrial division inhibitor mdivi-1. J Biol Chem 285:11740–11752

da Cruz S, Xenarios I, Langridge J, Vilbois F, Parone PA, Martinou JC (2003) Proteomic analysis of the mouse liver mitochondrial inner membrane. J Biol Chem 278:41566–41571

da Cruz S, Parone PA, Gonzalo P, Bienvenut WV, Tondera D, Jourdain A, Quadroni M, Martinou JC (2008) SLP-2 interacts with prohibitins in the mitochondrial inner membrane and contributes to their stability. Biochim Biophys Acta 1783:904–911

Daish TJ, Mills K, Kumar S (2004) *Drosophila* caspase DRONC is required for specific developmental cell death pathways and stress-induced apoptosis. Dev Cell 7:909–915

Danial NN (2008) BAD: undertaker by night, candyman by day. Oncogene 27(Suppl 1):S53–S70

Danial NN, Gramm CF, Scorrano L, Zhang CY, Krauss S, Ranger AM, Datta SR, Greenberg ME, Licklider LJ, Lowell BB, Gygi SP, Korsmeyer SJ (2003) BAD and glucokinase reside in a mitochondrial complex that integrates glycolysis and apoptosis. Nature 424:952–956

Danial NN, Walensky LD, Zhang CY, Choi CS, Fisher JK, Molina AJ, Datta SR, Pitter KL, Bird GH, Wikstrom JD, Deeney JT, Robertson K, Morash J, Kulkarni A, Neschen S, Kim S, Greenberg ME, Corkey BE, Shirihai OS,

Shulman GI, Lowell BB, Korsmeyer SJ (2008) Dual role of proapoptotic BAD in insulin secretion and beta cell survival. Nat Med 14:144–153

Delettre C, Lenaers G, Griffoin JM, Gigarel N, Lorenzo C, Belenguer P, Pelloquin L, Grosgeorge J, Turc-Carel C, Perret E, Astarie-Dequeker C, Lasquellec L, Arnaud B, Ducommun B, Kaplan J, Hamel CP (2000) Nuclear gene OPA1, encoding a mitochondrial dynamin-related protein, is mutated in dominant optic atrophy. Nat Genet 26:207–210

Delettre C, Griffoin JM, Kaplan J, Dollfus H, Lorenz B, Faivre L, Lenaers G, Belenguer P, Hamel CP (2001) Mutation spectrum and splicing variants in the OPA1 gene. Hum Genet 109:584–591

Delivani P, Adrain C, Taylor RC, Duriez PJ, Martin SJ (2006) Role for CED-9 and Egl-1 as regulators of mitochondrial fission and fusion dynamics. Mol Cell 21:761–773

Deng X, Gao F, Flagg T, Anderson J, May WS (2006) Bcl2's flexible loop domain regulates p53 binding and survival. Mol Cell Biol 26:4421–4434

Deng H, Dodson MW, Huang H, Guo M (2008) The Parkinson's disease genes pink1 and parkin promote mitochondrial fission and/or inhibit fusion in Drosophila. Proc Natl Acad Sci USA 105:14503–14508

Deng X, Gao F, May WS (2009) Protein phosphatase 2A inactivates Bcl2's antiapoptotic function by dephosphorylation and up-regulation of Bcl2-p53 binding. Blood 113:422–428

Desagher S, Martinou JC (2000) Mitochondria as the central control point of apoptosis. Trends Cell Biol 10:369–377

Dimmer KS, Fritz S, Fuchs F, Messerschmitt M, Weinbach N, Neupert W, Westermann B (2002) Genetic basis of mitochondrial function and morphology in Saccharomyces cerevisiae. Mol Biol Cell 13:847–853

Donahue RJ, Razmara M, Hoek JB, Knudsen TB (2001) Direct influence of the p53 tumor suppressor on mitochondrial biogenesis and function. FASEB J 15:635–644

Du C, Fang M, Li Y, Li L, Wang X (2000) Smac, a mitochondrial protein that promotes cytochrome c-dependent caspase activation by eliminating IAP inhibition. Cell 102:33–42

Duvezin-Caubet S, Koppen M, Wagener J, Zick M, Israel L, Bernacchia A, Jagasia R, Rugarli EI, Imhof A, Neupert W, Langer T, Reichert AS (2007) OPA1 processing reconstituted in yeast depends on the subunit composition of the m-AAA protease in mitochondria. Mol Biol Cell 18:3582–3590

Ehses S, Raschke I, Mancuso G, Bernacchia A, Geimer S, Tondera D, Martinou JC, Westermann B, Rugarli EI, Langer T (2009) Regulation of OPA1 processing and mitochondrial fusion by m-AAA protease isoenzymes and OMA1. J Cell Biol 187:1023–1036

Ellis HM, Horvitz HR (1986) Genetic control of programmed cell death in the nematode C. elegans. Cell 44:817–829

Ernster L, Schatz G (1981) Mitochondria: a historical review. J Cell Biol 91:227s–255s

Erster S, Mihara M, Kim RH, Petrenko O, Moll UM (2004) In vivo mitochondrial p53 translocation triggers a rapid first wave of cell death in response to DNA damage that can precede p53 target gene activation. Mol Cell Biol 24: 6728–6741

Esser K, Tursun B, Ingenhoven M, Michaelis G, Pratje E (2002) A novel two-step mechanism for removal of a mitochondrial signal sequence involves the mAAA complex and the putative rhomboid protease Pcp1. J Mol Biol 323:835–843

Essmann F, Pohlmann S, Gillissen B, Daniel PT, Schulze-Osthoff K, Janicke RU (2005) Irradiation-induced translocation of p53 to mitochondria in the absence of apoptosis. J Biol Chem 280:37169–37177

Estaquier J, Arnoult D (2007) Inhibiting Drp1-mediated mitochondrial fission selectively prevents the release of cytochrome c during apoptosis. Cell Death Differ 14:1086–1094

Ferecatu I, Bergeaud M, Rodriguez-Enfedaque A, le Floch N, Oliver L, Rincheval V, Renaud F, Vallette FM, Mignotte B, Vayssiere JL (2009) Mitochondrial localization of the low level p53 protein in proliferative cells. Biochem Biophys Res Commun 387:772–777

Fletcher JI, Meusburger S, Hawkins CJ, Riglar DT, Lee EF, Fairlie WD, Huang DC, Adams JM (2008) Apoptosis is triggered when prosurvival Bcl-2 proteins cannot restrain Bax. Proc Natl Acad Sci USA 105:18081–18087

Fleury C, Mignotte B, Vayssiere JL (2002) Mitochondrial reactive oxygen species in cell death signaling. Biochimie 84:131–141

Frank S, Gaume B, Bergmann-Leitner ES, Leitner WW, Robert EG, Catez F, Smith CL, Youle RJ (2001) The role of dynamin-related protein 1, a mediator of mitochondrial fission, in apoptosis. Dev Cell 1:515–525

Freel CD, Richardson DA, Thomenius MJ, Gan EC, Horn SR, Olson MR, Kornbluth S (2008) Mitochondrial localization of Reaper to promote inhibitors of apoptosis protein degradation conferred by GH3 domain-lipid interactions. J Biol Chem 283:367–379

Frezza C, Cipolat S, De Brito OM, Micaroni M, Beznoussenko GV, Rudka T, Bartoli D, Polishuck RS, Danial NN, De Strooper B, Scorrano L (2006) OPA1 controls apoptotic cristae remodeling independently from mitochondrial fusion. Cell 126:177–189

Fridman JS, Lowe SW (2003) Control of apoptosis by p53. Oncogene 22:9030–9040

Fuchs Y, Steller H (2011) Programmed cell death in animal development and disease. Cell 147:742–758

Galindo KA, Lu WJ, Park JH, Abrams JM (2009) The Bax/Bak ortholog in Drosophila, Debcl, exerts limited control over programmed cell death. Development 136:275–283

Gaumer S, Guenal I, Brun S, Theodore L, Mignotte B (2000) Bcl-2 and Bax mammalian regulators of apoptosis are functional in Drosophila. Cell Death Differ 7:804–814

Geng Y, Akhtar RS, Shacka JJ, Klocke BJ, Zhang J, Chen X, Roth KA (2007) p53 transcription-dependent and -independent regulation of cerebellar neural precursor cell apoptosis. J Neuropathol Exp Neurol 66:66–74

Geyer RK, Yu ZK, Maki CG (2000) The MDM2 RING-finger domain is required to promote p53 nuclear export. Nat Cell Biol 2:569–573

Giam M, Huang DC, Bouillet P (2008) BH3-only proteins and their roles in programmed cell death. Oncogene 27(Suppl 1): S128–S136

Giannakakou P, Sackett DL, Ward Y, Webster KR, Blagosklonny MV, Fojo T (2000) p53 is associated with cellular microtubules and is transported to the nucleus by dynein. Nat Cell Biol 2:709–717

Godefroy N, Lemaire C, Renaud F, Rincheval V, Perez S, Parvu-Ferecatu I, Mignotte B, Vayssiere JL (2004) p53 can promote mitochondria- and caspase-independent apoptosis. Cell Death Differ 11:785–787

Gottifredi V, Prives C (2001) Molecular biology. Getting p53 out of the nucleus. Science 292:1851–1852

Goyal L, McCall K, Agapite J, Hartwieg E, Steller H (2000) Induction of apoptosis by *Drosophila reaper*, *hid* and *grim* through inhibition of IAP function. EMBO J 19:589–597

Goyal G, Fell B, Sarin A, Youle RJ, Sriram V (2007) Role of mitochondrial remodeling in programmed cell death in Drosophila melanogaster. Dev Cell 12:807–816

Gray MW (1993) Origin and evolution of organelle genomes. Curr Opin Genet Dev 3:884–890

Green DR, Kroemer G (2009) Cytoplasmic functions of the tumour suppressor p53. Nature 458:1127–1130

Grinberg M, Schwarz M, Zaltsman Y, Eini T, Niv H, Pietrokovski S, Gross A (2005) Mitochondrial carrier homolog 2 is a target of tBID in cells signaled to die by tumor necrosis factor alpha. Mol Cell Biol 25:4579–4590

Griparic L, van der Wel NN, Orozco IJ, Peters PJ, van der Bliek AM (2004) Loss of the intermembrane space protein Mgm1/OPA1 induces swelling and localized constrictions along the lengths of mitochondria. J Biol Chem 279: 18792–18798

Griparic L, Kanazawa T, van der Bliek AM (2007) Regulation of the mitochondrial dynamin-like protein Opa1 by proteolytic cleavage. J Cell Biol 178:757–764

Gross A (2006) BID as a double agent in cell life and death. Cell Cycle 5:582–584

Grossman SR, Deato ME, Brignone C, Chan HM, Kung AL, Tagami H, Nakatani Y, Livingston DM (2003) Polyubiquitination of p53 by a ubiquitin ligase activity of p300. Science 300:342–344

Guicciardi ME, Gores GJ (2009) Life and death by death receptors. FASEB J 23:1625–1637

Guillery O, Malka F, Landes T, Guillou E, Blackstone C, Lombes A, Belenguer P, Arnoult D, Rojo M (2008) Metalloprotease-mediated OPA1 processing is modulated by the mitochondrial membrane potential. Biol Cell 100:315–325

Guo B, Zhai D, Cabezas E, Welsh K, Nouraini S, Satterthwait AC, Reed JC (2003) Humanin peptide suppresses apoptosis by interfering with Bax activation. Nature 423:456–461

Hajek P, Chomyn A, Attardi G (2007) Identification of a novel mitochondrial complex containing mitofusin 2 and stomatin-like protein 2. J Biol Chem 282:5670–5681

Hales KG, Fuller MT (1997) Developmentally regulated mitochondrial fusion mediated by a conserved, novel, predicted GTPase. Cell 90:121–129

Han XJ, Lu YF, Li SA, Kaitsuka T, Sato Y, Tomizawa K, Nairn AC, Takei K, Matsui H, Matsushita M (2008) CaM kinase I alpha-induced phosphorylation of Drp1 regulates mitochondrial morphology. J Cell Biol 182:573–585

Harder Z, Zunino R, McBride H (2004) Sumo1 conjugates mitochondrial substrates and participates in mitochondrial fission. Curr Biol 14:340–345

Haupt Y, Rowan S, Shaulian E, Vousden KH, Oren M (1995) Induction of apoptosis in HeLa cells by trans-activation-deficient p53. Genes Dev 9:2170–2183

Head B, Griparic L, Amiri M, Gandre-Babbe S, van der Bliek AM (2009) Inducible proteolytic inactivation of OPA1 mediated by the OMA1 protease in mammalian cells. J Cell Biol 187:959–966

Hegde R, Srinivasula SM, Zhang Z, Wassell R, Mukattash R, Cilenti L, Dubois G, Lazebnik Y, Zervos AS, Fernandes-Alnemri T, Alnemri ES (2002) Identification of Omi/HtrA2 as a mitochondrial apoptotic serine protease that disrupts inhibitor of apoptosis protein-caspase interaction. J Biol Chem 277:432–438

Hengartner MO, Horvitz HR (1994) *C. elegans* cell survival gene *ced-9* encodes a functional homolog of the mammalian proto-oncogene *bcl-2*. Cell 76:665–676

Herlan M, Vogel F, Bornhovd C, Neupert W, Reichert AS (2003) Processing of Mgm1 by the rhomboid-type protease Pcp1 is required for maintenance of mitochondrial morphology and of mitochondrial DNA. J Biol Chem 278: 27781–27788

Ho PK, Hawkins CJ (2005) Mammalian initiator apoptotic caspases. FEBS J 272:5436–5453

Hoffman WH, Biade S, Zilfou JT, Chen J, Murphy M (2002) Transcriptional repression of the anti-apoptotic survivin gene by wild type p53. J Biol Chem 277:3247–3257

Hugunin M, Quintal LJ, Mankovich JA, Ghayur T (1996) Protease activity of in vitro transcribed and translated Caenorhabditis elegans cell death gene (ced-3) product. J Biol Chem 271:3517–3522

Igaki T, Kanuka H, Inohara N, Sawamoto K, Nunez G, Okano H, Miura M (2000) Drob-1, a Drosophila member of the Bcl-2/CED-9 family that promotes cell death. Proc Natl Acad Sci USA 97:662–667

Ikonen E, Fiedler K, Parton RG, Simons K (1995) Prohibitin, an antiproliferative protein, is localized to mitochondria. FEBS Lett 358:273–277

Ishihara N, Eura Y, Mihara K (2004) Mitofusin 1 and 2 play distinct roles in mitochondrial fusion reactions via GTPase activity. J Cell Sci 117:6535–6546

Ishihara N, Fujita Y, Oka T, Mihara K (2006) Regulation of mitochondrial morphology through proteolytic cleavage of OPA1. EMBO J 25:2966–2977

Ishihara N, Nomura M, Jofuku A, Kato H, Suzuki SO, Masuda K, Otera H, Nakanishi Y, Nonaka I, Goto Y, Taguchi N, Morinaga H, Maeda M, Takayanagi R, Yokota S, Mihara K (2009) Mitochondrial fission factor Drp1 is essential for embryonic development and synapse formation in mice. Nat Cell Biol 11:958–966

Jahani-Asl A, Cheung EC, Neuspiel M, Maclaurin JG, Fortin A, Park DS, McBride HM, Slack RS (2007) Mitofusin 2 protects cerebellar granule neurons against injury-induced cell death. J Biol Chem 282:23788–23798

Jeyaraju DV, Xu L, Letellier MC, Bandaru S, Zunino R, Berg EA, McBride HM, Pellegrini L (2006) Phosphorylation and cleavage of presenilin-associated rhomboid-like protein (PARL) promotes changes in mitochondrial morphology. Proc Natl Acad Sci USA 103:18562–18567

Jiang P, Du W, Heese K, Wu M (2006) The Bad guy cooperates with good cop p53: Bad is transcriptionally up-regulated by p53 and forms a Bad/p53 complex at the mitochondria to induce apoptosis. Mol Cell Biol 26:9071–9082

Johnson TM, Meade K, Pathak N, Marques MR, Attardi LD (2008) Knockin mice expressing a chimeric p53 protein reveal mechanistic differences in how p53 triggers apoptosis and senescence. Proc Natl Acad Sci USA 105: 1215–1220

Jourdain A, Martinou JC (2009) Mitochondrial outer-membrane permeabilization and remodelling in apoptosis. Int J Biochem Cell Biol 41:1884–1889

Kakudo Y, Shibata H, Otsuka K, Kato S, Ishioka C (2005) Lack of correlation between p53-dependent transcriptional activity and the ability to induce apoptosis among 179 mutant p53s. Cancer Res 65:2108–2114

Kanazawa T, Zappaterra MD, Hasegawa A, Wright AP, Newman-Smith ED, Buttle KF, Mcdonald K, Mannella CA, Van Der Bliek AM (2008) The C. elegans Opa1 homologue EAT-3 is essential for resistance to free radicals. PLoS Genet 4:e1000022

Karbowski M, Lee YJ, Gaume B, Jeong SY, Frank S, Nechushtan A, Santel A, Fuller M, Smith CL, Youle RJ (2002) Spatial and temporal association of Bax with mitochondrial fission sites, Drp1, and Mfn2 during apoptosis. J Cell Biol 159:931–938

Karbowski M, Norris KL, Cleland MM, Jeong SY, Youle RJ (2006) Role of Bax and Bak in mitochondrial morphogenesis. Nature 443:658–662

Karbowski M, Neutzner A, Youle RJ (2007) The mitochondrial E3 ubiquitin ligase MARCH5 is required for Drp1 dependent mitochondrial division. J Cell Biol 178:71–84

Kaser M, Kambacheld M, Kisters-Woike B, Langer T (2003) Oma1, a novel membrane-bound metallopeptidase in mitochondria with activities overlapping with the m-AAA protease. J Biol Chem 278:46414–46423

Katsumoto T, Higaki K, Ohno K, Onodera K (1995) Cell-cycle dependent biosynthesis and localization of p53 protein in untransformed human cells. Biol Cell 84:167–173

Kawaguchi Y, Ito A, Appella E, Yao TP (2006) Charge modification at multiple C-terminal lysine residues regulates p53 oligomerization and its nucleus-cytoplasm trafficking. J Biol Chem 281:1394–1400

Kerr JFR, Harmon BV (1991) Definition and incidence of apoptosis: an historical perspective. In: Tomei LD, Cope FO (eds) Apoptosis: the molecular basis of cell death. Cold Spring Harbor Laboratory Press, New York, pp 5–29

Kerr JF, Wyllie AH, Currie AR (1972) Apoptosis: a basic biological phenomenon with wide-ranging implications in tissue kinetics. Br J Cancer 26:239–257

Kim H, Tu HC, Ren D, Takeuchi O, Jeffers JR, Zambetti GP, Hsieh JJ, Cheng EH (2009) Stepwise activation of BAX and BAK by tBID, BIM, and PUMA initiates mitochondrial apoptosis. Mol Cell 36:487–499

Kluck RM, Bossy-Wetzel E, Green DR, Newmeyer DD (1997a) The release of cytochrome c from mitochondria: a primary site for Bcl-2 regulation of apoptosis. Science 275:1132–1136

Kluck RM, Martin SJ, Hoffman B, Zhou JS, Green DR, Newmeyer DD (1997b) Cytochrome c activation of CPP32-like proteolysis plays a critical role in a *Xenopus* cell-free apoptosis system. EMBO J 16:4639–4649

Koonin EV, Makarova KS, Rogozin IB, Davidovic L, Letellier MC, Pellegrini L (2003) The rhomboids: a nearly ubiquitous family of intramembrane serine proteases that probably evolved by multiple ancient horizontal gene transfers. Genome Biol 4:R19

Korsmeyer SJ (1992) Bcl-2 initiates a new category of oncogenes: regulators of cell death. Blood 80:879–886

Koshiba T, Detmer SA, Kaiser JT, Chen H, McCaffery JM, Chan DC (2004) Structural basis of mitochondrial tethering by mitofusin complexes. Science 305:858–862

Kroemer G, Galluzzi L, Brenner C (2007) Mitochondrial membrane permeabilization in cell death. Physiol Rev 87:99–163

Kuwana T, Mackey MR, Perkins G, Ellisman MH, Latterich M, Schneiter R, Green DR, Newmeyer DD (2002) Bid, Bax, and lipids cooperate to form supramolecular openings in the outer mitochondrial membrane. Cell 111:331–342

Labrousse AM, Zappaterra MD, Rube DA, Van der Bliek AM (1999) C. elegans dynamin-related protein DRP-1 controls severing of the mitochondrial outer membrane. Mol Cell 4:815–826

Lai Z, Ferry KV, Diamond MA, Wee KE, Kim YB, Ma J, Yang T, Benfield PA, Copeland RA, Auger KR (2001) Human mdm2 mediates multiple mono-ubiquitination of p53 by a mechanism requiring enzyme isomerization. J Biol Chem 276:31357–31367

Lee YJ, Jeong SY, Karbowski M, Smith CL, Youle RJ (2004) Roles of the mammalian mitochondrial fission and fusion mediators Fis1, Drp1, and Opa1 in apoptosis. Mol Biol Cell 15:5001–5011

Legros F, Lombes A, Frachon P, Rojo M (2002) Mitochondrial fusion in human cells is efficient, requires the inner membrane potential, and is mediated by mitofusins. Mol Biol Cell 13:4343–4354

Lei X, Chen Y, Du G, Yu W, Wang X, Qu H, Xia B, He H, Mao J, Zong W, Liao X, Mehrpour M, Hao X, Chen Q (2006) Gossypol induces Bax/Bak-independent activation of apoptosis and cytochrome c release via a conformational change in Bcl-2. FASEB J 20:2147–2149

Lemberg MK, Menendez J, Misik A, Garcia M, Koth CM, Freeman M (2005) Mechanism of intramembrane proteolysis investigated with purified rhomboid proteases. EMBO J 24:464–472

Lettre G, Hengartner MO (2006) Developmental apoptosis in C. elegans: a complex CEDnario. Nat Rev Mol Cell Biol 7:97–108

Leu JI, Dumont P, Hafey M, Murphy ME, George DL (2004) Mitochondrial p53 activates Bak and causes disruption of a Bak-Mcl1 complex. Nat Cell Biol 6:443–450

Leu JI, George DL (2007) Hepatic IGFBP1 is a prosurvival factor that binds to BAK, protects the liver from apoptosis, and antagonizes the proapoptotic actions of p53 at mitochondria. Genes Dev 21:3095–3109

Li H, Zhu H, Yuan J (1998) Cleavage of BID by caspase 8 mediates the mitochondrial damage in the Fas pathway of apoptosis. Cell 94:491–501

Li M, Luo J, Brooks CL, Gu W (2002) Acetylation of p53 inhibits its ubiquitination by Mdm2. J Biol Chem 277: 50607–50611

Liu X, Kim CN, Yang J, Jemmerson R, Wang X (1996) Induction of apoptotic program in cell-free extracts: requirement for dATP and cytochrome c. Cell 86:147–157

Luo X, Budihardjo I, Zou H, Slaughter C, Wang X (1998) Bid, a Bcl-2 interacting protein, mediates cytochrome c release from mitochondria in response to activation of cell surface death receptors. Cell 94:481–490

Lutkenhaus J (1998) Organelle division: from coli to chloroplasts. Curr Biol 8:R619–R621

Mahyar-Roemer M, Fritzsche C, Wagner S, Laue M, Roemer K (2004) Mitochondrial p53 levels parallel total p53 levels independent of stress response in human colorectal carcinoma and glioblastoma cells. Oncogene 23:6226–6236

Mai S, Klinkenberg M, Auburger G, Bereiter-Hahn J, Jendrach M (2010) Decreased expression of Drp1 and Fis1 mediates mitochondrial elongation in senescent cells and enhances resistance to oxidative stress through PINK1. J Cell Sci 123:917–926

Majewski N, Nogueira V, Bhaskar P, Coy PE, Skeen JE, Gottlob K, Chandel NS, Thompson CB, Robey RB, Hay N (2004) Hexokinase-mitochondria interaction mediated by Akt is required to inhibit apoptosis in the presence or absence of Bax and Bak. Mol Cell 16:819–830

Marchenko ND, Moll UM (2007) The role of ubiquitination in the direct mitochondrial death program of p53. Cell Cycle 6:1718–1723

Marchenko ND, Zaika A, Moll UM (2000) Death signal-induced localization of p53 protein to mitochondria. A potential role in apoptotic signaling. J Biol Chem 275:16202–16212

Martins LM, Iaccarino I, Tenev T, Gschmeissner S, Totty NF, Lemoine NR, Savopoulos J, Gray CW, Creasy CL, Dingwall C, Downward J (2002) The serine protease Omi/HtrA2 regulates apoptosis by binding XIAP through a reaper-like motif. J Biol Chem 277:439–444

Merino D, Giam M, Hughes PD, Siggs OM, Heger K, O'Reilly LA, Adams JM, Strasser A, Lee EF, Fairlie WD, Bouillet P (2009) The role of BH3-only protein Bim extends beyond inhibiting Bcl-2-like prosurvival proteins. J Cell Biol 186:355–362

Merkwirth C, Dargazanli S, Tatsuta T, Geimer S, Lower B, Wunderlich FT, Von Kleist-Retzow JC, Waisman A, Westermann B, Langer T (2008) Prohibitins control cell proliferation and apoptosis by regulating OPA1-dependent cristae morphogenesis in mitochondria. Genes Dev 22:476–488

Mihara M, Erster S, Zaika A, Petrenko O, Chittenden T, Pancoska P, Moll UM (2003) p53 has a direct apoptogenic role at the mitochondria. Mol Cell 11:577–590

Misaka T, Murate M, Fujimoto K, Kubo Y (2006) The dynamin-related mouse mitochondrial GTPase OPA1 alters the structure of the mitochondrial inner membrane when exogenously introduced into COS-7 cells. Neurosci Res 55:123–133

Miyashita T, Reed JC (1995) Tumor suppressor p53 is a direct transcriptional activator of the human *bax* gene. Cell 80:293–299

Mizuta T, Shimizu S, Matsuoka Y, Nakagawa T, Tsujimoto Y (2007) A Bax/Bak-independent mechanism of cytochrome c release. J Biol Chem 282:16623–16630

Moll UM, Zaika A (2001) Nuclear and mitochondrial apoptotic pathways of p53. FEBS Lett 493:65–69

Moll UM, Riou G, Levine AJ (1992) Two distinct mechanisms alter p53 in breast cancer: mutation and nuclear exclusion. Proc Natl Acad Sci USA 89:7262–7266

Moll UM, Laquaglia M, Benard J, Riou G (1995) Wild-type p53 protein undergoes cytoplasmic sequestration in undifferentiated neuroblastomas but not in differentiated tumors. Proc Natl Acad Sci USA 92:4407–4411

Morrow IC, Parton RG (2005) Flotillins and the PHB domain protein family: rafts, worms and anaesthetics. Traffic 6:725–740

Motz C, Martin H, Krimmer T, Rassow J (2002) Bcl-2 and porin follow different pathways of TOM-dependent insertion into the mitochondrial outer membrane. J Mol Biol 323:729–738

Muro I, Hay BA, Clem RJ (2002) The Drosophila DIAP1 protein is required to prevent accumulation of a continuously generated, processed form of the apical caspase DRONC. J Biol Chem 277:49644–49650

Nakamura N, Kimura Y, Tokuda M, Honda S, Hirose S (2006) MARCH-V is a novel mitofusin 2- and Drp1-binding protein able to change mitochondrial morphology. EMBO Rep 7:1019–1022

Nemajerova A, Erster S, Moll UM (2005) The post-translational phosphorylation and acetylation modification profile is not the determining factor in targeting endogenous stress-induced p53 to mitochondria. Cell Death Differ 12:197–200

Nguyen M, Branton PE, Walton PA, Oltvai ZN, Korsmeyer SJ, Shore GC (1994) Role of membrane anchor domain of Bcl-2 in suppression of apoptosis caused by E1B-defective adenovirus. J Biol Chem 269:16521–16524

Nijtmans LG, De Jong L, Artal Sanz M, Coates PJ, Berden JA, Back JW, Muijsers AO, Van der Spek H, Grivell LA (2000) Prohibitins act as a membrane-bound chaperone for the stabilization of mitochondrial proteins. EMBO J 19:2444–2451

Nikolaev AY, Li M, Puskas N, Qin J, Gu W (2003) Parc: a cytoplasmic anchor for p53. Cell 112:29–40

Oda E, Ohki R, Murasawa H, Nemoto J, Shibue T, Yamashita T, Tokino T, Taniguchi T, Tanaka N (2000) Noxa, a BH3-only member of the bcl-2 family and candidate mediator of p53-induced apoptosis. Science 288:1053–1058

Ohtsuka T, Ryu H, Minamishima YA, Macip S, Sagara J, Nakayama KI, Aaronson SA, Lee SW (2004) ASC is a Bax adaptor and regulates the p53-Bax mitochondrial apoptosis pathway. Nat Cell Biol 6:121–128

Okamoto K, Shaw JM (2005) Mitochondrial morphology and dynamics in yeast and multicellular eukaryotes. Annu Rev Genet 39:503–536

Olichon A, Emorine LJ, Descoins E, Pelloquin L, Brichese L, Gas N, Guillou E, Delettre C, Valette A, Hamel CP, Ducommun B, Lenaers G, Belenguer P (2002) The human dynamin-related protein OPA1 is anchored to the mitochondrial inner membrane facing the inter-membrane space. FEBS Lett 523:171–176

Olichon A, Baricault L, Gas N, Guillou E, Valette A, Belenguer P, Lenaers G (2003) Loss of OPA1 perturbates the mitochondrial inner membrane structure and integrity, leading to cytochrome c release and apoptosis. J Biol Chem 278:7743–7746

Olichon A, Landes T, Arnaune-Pelloquin L, Emorine LJ, Mils V, Guichet A, Delettre C, Hamel C, Amati-Bonneau P, Bonneau D, Reynier P, Lenaers G, Belenguer P (2007) Effects of OPA1 mutations on mitochondrial morphology and apoptosis: relevance to ADOA pathogenesis. J Cell Physiol 211:423–430

Olson MR, Holley CL, Gan EC, Colon-Ramos DA, Kaplan B, Kornbluth S (2003) A GH3-like domain in reaper is required for mitochondrial localization and induction of IAP degradation. J Biol Chem 278:44758–44768

Ott M, Norberg E, Walter KM, Schreiner P, Kemper C, Rapaport D, Zhivotovsky B, Orrenius S (2007) The mitochondrial TOM complex is required for tBid/Bax-induced cytochrome c release. J Biol Chem 282:27633–27639

Ott M, Norberg E, Zhivotovsky B, Orrenius S (2009) Mitochondrial targeting of tBid/Bax: a role for the TOM complex? Cell Death Differ 16:1075–1082

Park BS, Song YS, Yee SB, Lee BG, Seo SY, Park YC, Kim JM, Kim HM, Yoo YH (2005) Phospho-ser 15-p53 translocates into mitochondria and interacts with Bcl-2 and Bcl-xL in eugenol-induced apoptosis. Apoptosis 10:193–200

Park HH, Lo YC, Lin SC, Wang L, Yang JK, Wu H (2007) The death domain superfamily in intracellular signaling of apoptosis and inflammation. Annu Rev Immunol 25:561–586

Parone PA, James DI, da Cruz S, Mattenberger Y, Donze O, Barja F, Martinou JC (2006) Inhibiting the mitochondrial fission machinery does not prevent Bax/Bak-dependent apoptosis. Mol Cell Biol 26:7397–7408

Pellegrini L, Passer BJ, Canelles M, Lefterov I, Ganjei JK, Fowlkes BJ, Koonin EV, D'Adamio L (2001) PAMP and PARL, two novel putative metalloproteases interacting with the COOH-terminus of Presenilin-1 and -2. J Alzheimers Dis 3:181–190

Petit PX, Lecoeur H, Zorn E, Dauguet C, Mignotte B, Gougeon ML (1995) Alterations in mitochondrial structure and function are early events of dexamethasone-induced thymocyte apoptosis. J Cell Biol 130:157–167

Petit E, Oliver L, Vallette FM (2009) The mitochondrial outer membrane protein import machinery: a new player in apoptosis? Front Biosci 14:3563–3570

Petros AM, Gunasekera A, Xu N, Olejniczak ET, Fesik SW (2004) Defining the p53 DNA-binding domain/Bcl-x(L)-binding interface using NMR. FEBS Lett 559:171–174

Petros JA, Baumann AK, Ruiz-Pesini E, Amin MB, Sun CQ, Hall J, Lim S, Issa MM, Flanders WD, Hosseini SH, Marshall FF, Wallace DC (2005) mtDNA mutations increase tumorigenicity in prostate cancer. Proc Natl Acad Sci USA 102:719–724

Pietsch EC, Perchiniak E, Canutescu AA, Wang G, Dunbrack RL, Murphy ME (2008) Oligomerization of BAK by p53 utilizes conserved residues of the p53 DNA binding domain. J Biol Chem 283:21294–21304

Pitts KR, Yoon Y, Krueger EW, McNiven MA (1999) The dynamin-like protein DLP1 is essential for normal distribution and morphology of the endoplasmic reticulum and mitochondria in mammalian cells. Mol Biol Cell 10:4403–4417

Poole AC, Thomas RE, Andrews LA, McBride HM, Whitworth AJ, Pallanck LJ (2008) The PINK1/Parkin pathway regulates mitochondrial morphology. Proc Natl Acad Sci USA 105:1638–1643

Qin H, Yu T, Qing T, Liu Y, Zhao Y, Cai J, Li J, Song Z, Qu X, Zhou P, Wu J, Ding M, Deng H (2007) Regulation of apoptosis and differentiation by p53 in human embryonic stem cells. J Biol Chem 282:5842–5852

Quinn L, Coombe M, Mills K, Daish T, Colussi P, Kumar S, Richardson H (2003) Buffy, a Drosophila Bcl-2 protein, has anti-apoptotic and cell cycle inhibitory functions. EMBO J 22:3568–3579

Ross K, Rudel T, Kozjak-Pavlovic V (2009) TOM-independent complex formation of Bax and Bak in mammalian mitochondria during TNFalpha-induced apoptosis. Cell Death Differ 16:697–707

Sandu C, Ryoo HD, Steller H (2010) J Cell Biol 190:1039–1052

Schafer B, Quispe J, Choudhary V, Chipuk JE, Ajero TG, Du H, Schneiter R, Kuwana T (2009) Mitochondrial outer membrane proteins assist Bid in Bax-mediated lipidic pore formation. Mol Biol Cell 20:2276–2285

Schleiff E, Shore GC, Goping IS (1997) Human mitochondrial import receptor, Tom20p. Use of glutathione to reveal specific interactions between Tom20-glutathione S-transferase and mitochondrial precursor proteins. FEBS Lett 404:314–318

Schug ZT, Gottlieb E (2009) Cardiolipin acts as a mitochondrial signalling platform to launch apoptosis. Biochim Biophys Acta 1788:2022–2031

Scorrano L, Oakes SA, Opferman JT, Cheng EH, Sorcinelli MD, Pozzan T, Korsmeyer SJ (2003) BAX and BAK regulation of endoplasmic reticulum Ca2+: a control point for apoptosis. Science 300:135–139

Sesaki H, Jensen RE (2004) Ugo1p links the Fzo1p and Mgm1p GTPases for mitochondrial fusion. J Biol Chem 279:28298–28303

Sevrioukov EA, Burr J, Huang EW, Assi HH, Monserrate JP, Purves DC, Wu JN, Song EJ, Brachmann CB (2007) Drosophila Bcl-2 proteins participate in stress-induced apoptosis, but are not required for normal development. Genesis 45:184–193

Shaham S, Reddien PW, Davies B, Horvitz HR (1999) Mutational analysis of the Caenorhabditis elegans cell-death gene ced-3. Genetics 153:1655–1671

Shen Y, Shenk T (1994) Relief of p53-mediated transcriptional repression by the adenovirus E1B 19-kDa protein or the cellular Bcl-2 protein. Proc Natl Acad Sci USA 91:8940–8944

Sheridan C, Delivani P, Cullen SP, Martin SJ (2008) Bax- or Bak-induced mitochondrial fission can be uncoupled from cytochrome C release. Mol Cell 31:570–585

Shidara Y, Yamagata K, Kanamori T, Nakano K, Kwong JQ, Manfredi G, Oda H, Ohta S (2005) Positive contribution of pathogenic mutations in the mitochondrial genome to the promotion of cancer by prevention from apoptosis. Cancer Res 65:1655–1663

Smirnova E, Shurland DL, Ryazantsev SN, van der Bliek AM (1998) A human dynamin-related protein controls the distribution of mitochondria. J Cell Biol 143:351–358

Smirnova E, Griparic L, Shurland DL, van der Bliek AM (2001) Dynamin-related protein Drp1 is required for mitochondrial division in mammalian cells. Mol Biol Cell 12:2245–2256

Song Z, Chen H, Fiket M, Alexander C, Chan DC (2007) OPA1 processing controls mitochondrial fusion and is regulated by mRNA splicing, membrane potential, and Yme1L. J Cell Biol 178:749–755

Sot B, Freund SM, Fersht AR (2007) Comparative biophysical characterization of p53 with the pro-apoptotic BAK and the anti-apoptotic BCL-xL. J Biol Chem 282:29193–29200

Speidel D, Helmbold H, Deppert W (2006) Dissection of transcriptional and non-transcriptional p53 activities in the response to genotoxic stress. Oncogene 25:940–953

Steglich G, Neupert W, Langer T (1999) Prohibitins regulate membrane protein degradation by the m-AAA protease in mitochondria. Mol Cell Biol 19:3435–3442

Stennicke HR, Salvesen GS (2000) Caspases - controlling intracellular signals by protease zymogen activation. Biochim Biophys Acta 1477:299–306

Strom E, Sathe S, Komarov PG, Chernova OB, Pavlovska I, Shyshynova I, Bosykh DA, Burdelya LG, Macklis RM, Skaliter R, Komarova EA, Gudkov AV (2006) Small-molecule inhibitor of p53 binding to mitochondria protects mice from gamma radiation. Nat Chem Biol 2:474–479

Sugioka R, Shimizu S, Tsujimoto Y (2004) Fzo1, a protein involved in mitochondrial fusion, inhibits apoptosis. J Biol Chem 279:52726–52734

Suzuki Y, Imai Y, Nakayama H, Takahashi K, Takio K, Takahashi R (2001) A serine protease, HtrA2, is released from the mitochondria and interacts with XIAP, inducing cell death. Mol Cell 8:613–621

Sykes SM, Stanek TJ, Frank A, Murphy ME, McMahon SB (2009) Acetylation of the DNA binding domain regulates transcription-independent apoptosis by p53. J Biol Chem 284:20197–20205

Taguchi N, Ishihara N, Jofuku A, Oka T, Mihara K (2007) Mitotic phosphorylation of dynamin-related GTPase Drp1 participates in mitochondrial fission. J Biol Chem 282:11521–11529

Tan J, Zhuang L, Leong HS, Iyer NG, Liu ET, Yu Q (2005) Pharmacologic modulation of glycogen synthase kinase-3beta promotes p53-dependent apoptosis through a direct Bax-mediated mitochondrial pathway in colorectal cancer cells. Cancer Res 65:9012–9020

Tang X, Zhu Y, Han L, Kim AL, Kopelovich L, Bickers DR, Athar M (2007) CP-31398 restores mutant p53 tumor suppressor function and inhibits UVB-induced skin carcinogenesis in mice. J Clin Invest 117:3753–3764

Tang S, Le PK, Tse S, Wallace DC, Huang T (2009) Heterozygous mutation of Opa1 in Drosophila shortens lifespan mediated through increased reactive oxygen species production. PLoS One 4:e4492

Tomita Y, Marchenko N, Erster S, Nemajerova A, Dehner A, Klein C, Pan H, Kessler H, Pancoska P, Moll UM (2006) WT p53, but not tumor-derived mutants, bind to Bcl2 via the DNA binding domain and induce mitochondrial permeabilization. J Biol Chem 281:8600–8606

Tondera D, Grandemange S, Jourdain A, Karbowski M, Mattenberger Y, Herzig S, da Cruz S, Clerc P, Raschke I, Merkwirth C, Ehses S, Krause F, Chan DC, Alexander C, Bauer C, Youle R, Langer T, Martinou JC (2009) SLP-2 is required for stress-induced mitochondrial hyperfusion. EMBO J 28:1589–1600

van Loo G, van Gurp M, Depuydt B, Srinivasula SM, Rodriguez I, Alnemri ES, Gevaert K, Vandekerckhove J, Declercq W, Vandenabeele P (2002) The serine protease Omi/HtrA2 is released from mitochondria during apoptosis. Omi interacts with caspase-inhibitor XIAP and induces enhanced caspase activity. Cell Death Differ 9:20–26

Vayssiere JL, Petit PX, Risler Y, Mignotte B (1994) Commitment to apoptosis is associated with changes in mitochondrial biogenesis and activity in cell lines conditionally immortalized with simian virus 40. Proc Natl Acad Sci USA 91:11752–11756

Verhagen AM, Ekert PG, Pakusch M, Silke J, Connolly LM, Reid GE, Moritz RL, Simpson RJ, Vaux DL (2000) Identification of DIABLO, a mammalian protein that promotes apoptosis by binding to and antagonizing IAP proteins. Cell 102:43–53

Vousden KH, Lane DP (2007) p53 in health and disease. Nat Rev Mol Cell Biol 8:275–283

Wakabayashi J, Zhang Z, Wakabayashi N, Tamura Y, Fukaya M, Kensler TW, Iijima M, Sesaki H (2009) The dynamin-related GTPase Drp1 is required for embryonic and brain development in mice. J Cell Biol 186:805–816

Wang C, Youle RJ (2009) The role of mitochondria in apoptosis. Annu Rev Genet 43:95–118

Wasilewski M, Scorrano L (2009) The changing shape of mitochondrial apoptosis. Trends Endocrinol Metab 20:287–294

Westermann B (2008) Molecular machinery of mitochondrial fusion and fission. J Biol Chem 283:13501–13505

White K, Grether ME, Abrams JM, Young L, Farrell K, Steller H (1994) Genetic control of programmed cell death in *Drosophila*. Science 264:677–683

Wilson R, Goyal L, Ditzel M, Zachariou A, Baker DA, Agapite J, Steller H, Meier P (2002) The DIAP1 RING finger mediates ubiquitination of Dronc and is indispensable for regulating apoptosis. Nat Cell Biol 4:445–450

Wolozin B, Iwasaki K, Vito P, Ganjei JK, Lacana E, Sunderland T, Zhao B, Kusiak JW, Wasco W, D'Adamio L (1996) Participation of presenilin 2 in apoptosis: enhanced basal activity conferred by an Alzheimer mutation. Science 274:1710–1713

Xu D, Li Y, Arcaro M, Lackey M, Bergmann A (2005) The CARD-carrying caspase Dronc is essential for most, but not all, developmental cell death in Drosophila. Development 132:2125–2134

Yamaguchi R, Lartigue L, Perkins G, Scott RT, Dixit A, Kushnareva Y, Kuwana T, Ellisman MH, Newmeyer DD (2008) Opa1-mediated cristae opening is Bax/Bak and BH3 dependent, required for apoptosis, and independent of Bak oligomerization. Mol Cell 31:557–569

Yang J, Liu X, Bhalla K, Kim CN, Ibrado AM, Cai J, Peng TI, Jones DP, Wang X (1997) Prevention of apoptosis by Bcl-2: release of cytochrome c from mitochondria blocked. Science 275:1129–1132

Yin XM (2006) Bid, a BH3-only multi-functional molecule, is at the cross road of life and death. Gene 369:7–19

Yoo SJ, Huh JR, Muro I, Yu H, Wang L, Wang SL, Feldman RM, Clem RJ, Muller HA, Hay BA (2002) Hid, Rpr and Grim negatively regulate DIAP1 levels through distinct mechanisms. Nat Cell Biol 4:416–424

Yoon Y, McNiven MA (2001) Mitochondrial division: new partners in membrane pinching. Curr Biol 11:R67–R70

Yoon Y, Krueger EW, Oswald BJ, McNiven MA (2003) The mitochondrial protein hFis1 regulates mitochondrial fission in mammalian cells through an interaction with the dynamin-like protein DLP1. Mol Cell Biol 23:5409–5420

Yoshida Y, Izumi H, Torigoe T, Ishiguchi H, Itoh H, Kang D, Kohno K (2003) P53 physically interacts with mitochondrial transcription factor A and differentially regulates binding to damaged DNA. Cancer Res 63:3729–3734

Youle RJ, Strasser A (2008) The BCL-2 protein family: opposing activities that mediate cell death. Nat Rev Mol Cell Biol 9:47–59

Zamzami N, Marchetti P, Castedo M, Zanin C, Vayssière JL, Petit PX, Kroemer G (1995) Reduction in mitochondrial potential constitutes an early irreversible step of programmed lymphocyte death *in vivo*. J Exp Med 181:1661–1672

Zanna C, Ghelli A, Porcelli AM, Karbowski M, Youle RJ, Schimpf S, Wissinger B, Pinti M, Cossarizza A, Vidoni S, Valentino ML, Rugolo M, Carelli V (2008) OPA1 mutations associated with dominant optic atrophy impair oxidative phosphorylation and mitochondrial fusion. Brain 131:352–367

Zhang H, Kim JK, Edwards CA, Xu Z, Taichman R, Wang CY (2005) Clusterin inhibits apoptosis by interacting with activated Bax. Nat Cell Biol 7:909–915

Zhong LT, Sarafian T, Kane DJ, Charles AC, Mah SP, Edwards RH, Bredesen DE (1993) *bcl-2* inhibits death of central neural cells induced by multiple agents. Proc Natl Acad Sci USA 90:4533–4537

Zhu W, Cowie A, Wasfy GW, Penn LZ, Leber B, Andrews DW (1996) Bcl-2 mutants with restricted subcellular location reveal spatially distinct pathways for apoptosis in different cell types. EMBO J 15:4130–4141

Chapter 8
Inherited Mitochondrial Disorders

Josef Finsterer

Abstract Though inherited mitochondrial disorders (MIDs) are most well known for their syndromic forms, for which widely known acronyms (MELAS, MERRF, NARP, LHON etc.) have been coined, the vast majority of inherited MIDs presents in a non-syndromic form. Since MIDs are most frequently multisystem disorders already at onset or during the disease course, a MID should be suspected if there is a combination of neurological and non-neurological abnormalities. Neurological abnormalities occurring as a part of a MID include stroke-like episodes, epilepsy, migraine-like headache, movement disorders, cerebellar ataxia, visual impairment, encephalopathy, cognitive impairment, dementia, psychosis, hypopituitarism, aneurysms, or peripheral nervous system disease, such as myopathy, neuropathy, or neuronopathy. Non-neurological manifestations concern the ears, the endocrine organs, the heart, the gastrointestinal tract, the kidneys, the bone marrow, and the skin. Whenever there is an unexplained combination of neurological and non-neurological disease in a patient or kindred, a MID should be suspected and appropriate diagnostic measures initiated. Genetic testing should be guided by the phenotype, the biopsy findings, and the biochemical results.

Keywords Neuromuscular • Encephalomyopathy • Metabolic disease • Multisystem disease • Genetics • Mitochondrial DNA

8.1 Introduction

Inherited mitochondrial disorders (MIDs) can be classified as single-system or multisystem or as syndromic or non-syndromic conditions (Chinnery 2010; Chinnery and Turnbull 1999; DiMauro and Schon 2003; Finsterer et al. 2009; Leonard and Schapira 2000a, b; McFarland et al. 2010). Inherited MIDs may be caused by mutations in genes located in the mitochondrial DNA (mtDNA) or the nuclear DNA (nDNA) (Chinnery 2010; Leonard and Schapira 2000a, b; McFarland et al. 2010). MIDs may present at any age and are characterized by extensive phenotypic and genetic heterogeneity. Mutations in mtDNA genes impair the respiratory chain exclusively, whereas mutations in nDNA genes impair various mitochondrial molecules, structures, or pathways in addition to the respiratory

J. Finsterer, MD, Ph.D. (✉)
Danube University Krems, Postfach 20, 1180 Vienna, Austria, Europe
e-mail: fifigs1@yahoo.de

R. Scatena et al. (eds.), *Advances in Mitochondrial Medicine*, Advances in Experimental Medicine and Biology 942, DOI 10.1007/978-94-007-2869-1_8,

chain, such as the mtDNA-replication, beta-oxidation, the coenzyme-Q metabolism the pyruvat-dehydrogenation, the mitochondrial biogenesis, carrier-proteins, or pore-proteins. Since MIDs most frequently derive from respiratory chain dysfunction, this chapter will focus on MIDs directly or indirectly impairing the function of respiratory chain complexes (RCC) I-V including the oxidative phosphorylation (OXPHOS). The chapter will be divided into a description of syndromic and non-syndromic MIDs. Each mitochondrial syndromes will be presented in form of a vignette, following the structure trait of inheritance, clinical presentation, instrumental findings, onset of the manifestations, and pathogenesis. Since treatment of MIDs is largely symptomatic and supportive, it will not be covered in this review.

8.2 Syndromic MIDs

Syndromic MIDs will be classified into those predominantly due to mtDNA mutations, due to both mtDNA and nDNA mutations, and those predominantly due to nDNA mutations. MIDs predominantly due to mtDNA mutations will be further divided into those due to point mutations and those due to rearrangements, such as single deletions or duplications (Table 8.1). Syndromic MIDs predominantly due to nDNA mutations will be divided into those due to affection of RCC subunits, assembly factors of RCCs, the machinery responsible for the maintenance of the mtDNA, the coenzyme-Q metabolism, the machinery responsible for mitochondrial bioenergetics, and the lipid milieu (Table 8.1).

Table 8.1 Inherited syndromic MIDs due to predominantly mtDNA mutations or predominantly nDNA mutations

mtDNA mutations
  Point mutations
    tRNAs
      MELAS, MERRF, MIDD
    rRNA
      Aminoglycosid-induced deafness
    Protein-encoding
      LHON, NARP
    Deletions/duplications
      Pearson-syndrome, mtPEO, KSS
nDNA mutations affecting
  Subunits or assembly factors of RCCs
    Leigh-syndrome, Leigh-like syndrome, GRACILE syndrome
  Machinery for mtDNA maintenance
    Breakage syndromes (multiple deletions)
      adPEO, arPEO, MNGIE, ANS (SANDO, MIRAS), MEMSA, AHS, MCHS
    Depletion syndromes
      Myopathic MDD (myopathy), encephalomyopathic MDD (Leigh-syndrome, Leigh-like syndrome, IOSCA), encephalohepatic MDD
    Translation defects (protein synthesis machinery)
      PCH, LBSL, MLASA
  Coenzyme-Q metabolism
    Pure ataxia, pure myopathy, Leigh syndrome, cardio-facio-cutaneous syndrome
  Lipid milieu
    Barth syndrome
  Mitochondrial transport machinery
    DDS/Mohr-Tranebjaerg–syndrome, XLASA/A
  Mitochondrial biogenesis (fusion/fission)
    ADOA/ADOAD, CMT2A, DIDMOAD

8.2.1 Syndromic MIDs Resulting Predominantly from mtDNA Mutations

8.2.1.1 mtDNA Point Mutations

MIDs predominantly due to tRNA mutations

MELAS

MELAS (mitochondrial encephalomyopathy, lactacidosis, and stroke-like-episodes) syndrome is a maternally-inherited, multi-system disorder clinically presenting with stroke-like-episodes (SLEs), which usually occur before age 40 years and impair motor abilities, vision (cortical blindness), and cognition (mentation), tonic-clonic seizures, which frequently accompany SLEs, migraine-like headache, confusional state, dementia, psychosis, deafness, and recurrent vomiting (Goto et al. 1990). Short stature is common. Less common features include episodic coma, ophthalmoparesis, myoclonus, cerebellar ataxia, heart failure, hirsutism, gastrointestinal dysmotility, or renal insufficiency. Instrumental investigations include elevated lactate in the serum and CSF, elevated CSF-protein, optic atrophy, pigmentary retinopathy, diabetes, or intestinal pseudo-obstruction. MRI of the brain typically shows T2-hyperintense lesions, most frequently in an occipito-temporal distribution, which are also hyperintense on ADC and spread slowly during the weeks following the onset of a SLE. CT scans of the cerebrum may show uni- or bilateral basal ganglia calcifications. Nerve conduction studies and electromyography may show neuropathy or myopathy in up to one quarter of the cases. Muscle biopsy typically shows ragged-red fibers (RRF) or ragged-blue fibers (hyper-reactive succinate dehydrogenase (SDH) stain). RRF are typically positive for cytochrome-c-oxidase (COX), contrary to myoclonus epilepsy with RRF (MERRF) syndrome and Kearns-Sayre syndrome (KSS). Additionally, the number of mitochondria is increased in smooth muscle and endothelial cells of intramuscular blood vessels, best seen as strongly SDH-reactive blood vessels on SDH. Biochemical investigations of the muscle homogenate may show multiple partial defects, predominantly complex I or complex IV defects, or may be normal. Cardiologic examination may show cardiac conduction defects or cardiomyopathy. Onset is typically between age 2–10 years or occasionally in early adolescence. Early psychomotor development is usually normal. Frequent initial manifestations include seizures, headache, and vomiting.

In ~80% of the cases MELAS-syndrome is caused by the heteroplasmic transition m.3243A>G in the *tRNA(Leu(UUR))* gene (Goto et al. 1990). The second most frequent mtDNA mutation is the transition m.3271T>C occurring in ~8% of the patients. The third most frequent mutation is the transition m.3252A>G. Other mtDNA genes mutated in MELAS-syndrome include the *tRNA(Phe), tRNA(Val), tRNA(Lys), COXII, COXIII, ND1, ND5, ND6,* or *rRNA* gene. Though MELAS mutations are present in all tissues the heteroplasmy rate may vary between tissues. This may impede the detection of the mutation in blood lymphocytes why investigations of other tissues may be helpful in such cases. The genotype-phenotype correlation of the m.3243A>G mutation is weak, since it also causes maternally-inherited progressive external ophthalmoplegia (PEO), KSS, maternally inherited diabetes and deafness (MDD), Leigh-syndrome (LS), cluster headache, isolated myopathy, isolated cardiomyopathy, renal failure, or pancreatitis. In single cases polymerase-gamma (POLG1) mutations may cause MELAS (Deschauer et al. 2007). The phenotypic heterogeneity may be explained with the variable heteroplasmy rates and tissue distribution of the m.3243A>G mutation but not with the threshold level, which is assumed constant among individuals.

MERRF

MERRF syndrome is a maternally-inherited, multisystem disorder clinically characterized by myoclonus, generalized epilepsy, myopathy, neuropathy, cerebellar ataxia, deafness, short stature, or dementia

(Hirano and DiMauro 1996). Myocloni are often the initial manifestation. Occasionally, patients develop SLEs, spasticity, ophthalmoparesis, lipomatosis (Ekbom syndrome), or depression (Naini et al. 2005; Nishigaki et al. 2003). A rare phenotypic variant may be multiple systemic lipomatosis (MSL), which is accompanied by PEO, deafness, cerebellar ataxia, myopathy, and neuropathy (Naumann et al. 1997). Rare clinical manifestations include spasmodic dysphonia, myalgia, Parkinsonism, or sudden respiratory failure (van de Glind et al. 2007; Horvath et al. 2007; Peng et al. 2003; Wiedemann et al. 2008). Blood chemical investigations may show lactacidosis at rest, which increases after moderate exercise. The cerebrospinal fluid (CSF) protein may be mildly elevated. Cerebral imaging may show basal ganglia atrophy. Other instrumental investigations may reveal optic atrophy, pigmentary retinopathy, polyneuropathy, cardiomyopathy (histiocytoid cardiomyopathy), cardiac conduction abnormalities, including pre-excitation (Wolff-Parkinson-White syndrome or sudden cardiac death), or pancytopenia. EEG may show generalized spike-wave discharges or focal epileptiform discharges with background slowing. Cerebral imaging may reveal atrophy of the putamina, brainstem, or cerebellum, or basal ganglia calcification. Muscle biopsy typically shows RRF, SDH hyper-reactivity, and COX-negative RRF. The diagnosis is based on the four canonical features myoclonus, generalized epilepsy, ataxia, and RRF. Onset is usually in childhood after normal early development.

The most common mtDNA mutation causing MERRF-syndrome is the *tRNA(Lys)* transition m.8344A>G. It is responsible for the phenotype in >80% of the cases. Though the mutation can be found in all tissues, it may be detected only in skin fibroblasts, urinary epithelial cells, oral mucosa, hair follicles, or most reliably, muscle cells. The three transitions m.8356T>C, m.8361G>A, or m.8363G>A are responsible for about 10% of the MERRF cases. The remaining 10% of the MERRF cases may be due to the transitions m.611G>A in the *tRNA(Phe)* gene or m.15967G>A in the *tRNA(Pro)* gene (Mancuso et al. 2004). Although the genotype-phenotype correlation of the m.8344A>G mutation is tighter than that of other mtDNA mutations, it also causes phenotypes as different as LS, isolated myoclonus, familial lipomatosis, or isolated myopathy (Finsterer et al. 2009). Patients with the transition m.8356T>C may present as MELAS/MERRF overlap syndrome. MSL may not only be due to the m.8344A>G mutation but also due to multiple mtDNA deletions.

MIDD

MIDD (maternally inherited diabetes and deafness) is clinically characterized by the combination of inherited diabetes mellitus and hypoacusis following a maternal trait of inheritance (Van den Ouweland et al. 1995). Single patients may additionally present with seizures, migraine, short stature, mental retardation, stroke-like-episodes (Chen et al. 2004), or hypertrophic cardiomyopathy with or without heart failure (Nijveldt et al. 2004).

Genes mutated in MIDD include the *tRNA(Leu)* or *tRNA(Lys)* genes. The most frequently reported mutation causing MIDD is the transition m.3243A>G (Chen et al. 2004; Chinnery et al. 2000; Van den Ouweland et al. 1995). In single patients MIDD was due to large-scale mtDNA tandem duplications or deletions/duplications.

MIDs due to rRNA mutations

Aminoglycoside-induced deafness

Mitochondrial rRNA mutations are only rarely responsible for MIDs. One of these disorders is the aminoglycoside-induced deafness (Guan 2011). Aminoglycoside-induced deafness is clinically characterized by the occurrence of hearing loss during or after aminoglycoside treatment or by deterioration of pre-existing impaired hearing after antibiotic treatment with aminoglycosides (Rydzanicz et al. 2010).

Aminoglycoside-induced deafness is due to the point mutation m.1555A>G in the *12SrRNA* gene. The frequency of the mutation varies between different ethnia. The *12SrRNA* gene is not only a hot spot of aminoglycoside-induced hearing loss but also non-syndromic hearing loss. Homoplasmic mutations most frequently associated with non-syndromic hearing loss are the m.1555A>G and the m.1494C>T in a highly conserved region of the gene (Guan 2011). Putative other pathogenic variants include the substitutions m.669T>C, m.827A>G, or m.961 delT+C(ins) (Rydzanicz et al. 2010).

MIDs due to Protein-encoding Gene Mutations

LHON

LHON (Leber's hereditary optic neuropathy) follows a maternal trait of inheritance but in about 40% of the cases the family history is negative. LHON is clinically characterized by bilateral, acute or subacute loss of vision in young adults (Man et al. 2002). In about three quarters of the cases visual loss is unilateral at onset but becomes bilateral within 6 months. Males are four times more frequently affected than females. Occasionally, patients additionally develop postural tremor, Parkinsonism, or cardiomyopathy with cardiac conduction abnormalities (Man et al. 2002). Women may present with a phenotype mimicking multiple sclerosis (Kellar-Wood et al. 1994; Jansen et al. 1996; Bhatti and Newman 1999). Ophthalmologic investigations may show retinal ganglia degeneration or demyelination or optic nerve atrophy. Other abnormal instrumental findings include disc swelling, edema of the peripapillary nerve layer, retinal teleangiectasias, or increased vascular tortuosity. Also abnormal may be the fluorescin angiography, perimetry, visually-evoked potentials, or retinography (Sadun et al. 2006). Some patients develop polyneuropathy or myopathy (Nikoskelainen et al. 1995). In other studies affection of the myocardium and the cardiac conduction system have been reported (Nikoskelainen 1994). Onset is usually in the second or third decade. Until then affected individuals are entirely asymptomatic. More than 90% of the cases manifest by age 50 years. In females onset is usually a few years later than in males.

LHON is caused by ~20 different mtDNA mutations but three are most commonly found in all human populations, m.3460G>A (*ND1*, 60–80% of the cases), m.11778G>A (*ND4*, 0–50% of the cases (most common LHON-mutation)), and m.14484T>C (*ND6*, 0–65% of the cases), and considered as high-risk (primary LHON mutations) (Finsterer et al. 2009). The majority of the LHON mutations are homoplasmic. Only 10–15% of the mutations are heteroplasmic. The m.11778G>A mutation causes the most severe phenotype and the m.14484T>C mutation has the best long-term prognosis. The penetrance of LHON is ~50% in males and ~10% in females and varies within a single family. The most frequent secondary LHON mutations are the transitions m.4216T>C, m.13708G>A, and m.15257G>A (Howell et al. 1995). LHON may overlap with MELAS in case of the *ND1* mutations m.3376G>A and m.3697G>A (Blakely et al. 2005; Spruijt et al. 2007).

NARP

NARP (neurogenic weakness, ataxia, and retinitis pigmentosa) is a maternally-inherited, multisystem disease, clinically characterized by proximal neurogenic muscle weakness, ataxia, and visual impairment (Holt et al. 1990). Some patients may additionally present with short stature, ophthalmoplegia, learning difficulties, dementia, sleep apnea, or seizures (Santorelli et al. 1997). Instrumental findings include axonal sensorimotor polyneuropathy and cerebellar atrophy on MRI. Ophthalmologic investigations may show optic atrophy, salt and pepper retinopathy, bull's eye maculopathy, or retinitis pigmentosa with bone spicule formation (Ortiz et al. 1993). The electroretinogram may show predominantly cone dysfunction in some pedigrees and predominantly rod dysfunction in others (Chowers et al. 1999). EMG may be myopathic. Muscle biopsy may show myopathic alterations but no RRFs. ECG may show cardiac conduction defects. Onset is in early childhood with ataxia and learning difficulties (Thorburn and Rahman 2006). Patients may remain stable for years but experience episodic deterioration during infections.

NARP arises from the heteroplasmic transversion m.8993T>G or the transition m.8993T>C in the *ATP6* gene (Thorburn and Rahman 2006). If the heteroplasmy rate exceeds 95% the mutation manifests as maternally inherited LS (MILS). NARP and MILS may coexist within the same family. The mutation load may vary among different tissues and may increase or decrease with age. In some patients the mutation may be undetectable in blood lymphocytes and may be only detectable in hair follicles, urine sediment, skin fibroblasts or, most reliably, in the skeletal muscle.

8.2.1.2 Single Deletions or Duplications

KSS

KSS is a sporadic, severe MID clinically characterized by the invariant triad of PEO, pigmentary retinopathy, and onset <20 years. Frequent additional features include short stature, progressive cerebellar syndrome, limb weakness, cognitive impairment, or dysphagia due to cricopharyngeal achalasia. In single cases ataxia may even dominate the presentation (Zoccolella et al. 2006). Rare additional features include glaucoma, deafness, dementia, primary amenorrhea, or pyramidal signs (Riera et al. 2008; Zoccolella et al. 2006). Epilepsy and SLE are extremely rare. Instrumental investigations may show myopathy, endocrine dysfunction (growth hormone deficiency, diabetes, hypothyroidism, hypoparathyroidism, irregular menses) atrio-ventricular-block, increased CSF protein, or lactacidosis. Low light vision is compromised. Cerebral MRI may show cerebellar atrophy, supratentorial atrophy, or T2-hyperintensities in the deep gray matter nuclei, the cerebellar white matter, or the subcortical white matter (Hourani et al. 2006). KSS is associated with general choroid plexus failure (Spector and Johanson 2010). Muscle biopsy shows COX-negative RRF. Onset is per definition before age 20 years but usually in childhood. KSS is slowly progressive and patients die in early adulthood.

In >90% of the cases, KSS is due to sporadic, single large-scale mtDNA deletions ranging between 2 and 10 kb (common deletion) (Hourani et al. 2006). These deletions are often undetectable in blood lymphocytes, why other tissues, in particular muscle, are the preferred tissues for genetic testing. In some individuals duplications coexist with large-scale deletions (Poulton et al. 1998). The family history is usually negative for the disease. Rarely, the deletion is maternally transmitted. mtDNA deletions occur most likely during germline development in the mothers' oocytes or in the embryo during early embryogenesis. Deleted mtDNA from the blastocyst may enter all three germ layers causing KSS, may predominantly enter the hematopoietic lineage causing Pearson syndrome, or the muscle causing PEO (DiMauro and Schon 2003).

Pearson-Syndrome

Pearson-syndrome initially presents with tiredness and liability to infectious diseases (Lee et al. 2007). With progression of the disease patients additionally develop muscle weakness and hypotonia, tremor, ataxia, hepatopathy, renal insufficiency, or exocrine pancreas dysfunction (Lee et al. 2007; McShane et al. 1991). Instrumental investigations include pancytopenia, or sideroblastic anemia, and exocrine pancreas insufficiency. Some patients develop hepatopathy and metabolic acidosis. Muscle biopsy may show typical features of mitochondrial myopathy (McShane et al. 1991). Bone marrow biopsy may show vacuolization of marrow progenitor cells, including ringed sideroblasts or normoblasts with excessive deposition of iron within the mitochondria. Onset is in early infancy. Affected patients usually die in infancy from intractable infections, kachexia, stroke, or renal failure. Infants surviving into childhood develop features of KSS (Lee et al. 2007).

Pearson syndrome is due to rare sporadic single, large-scale mtDNA deletions or duplications, why the family history is usually negative for the disease (Lee et al. 2007; McShane et al. 1991).MtDNA deletions are usually more frequent in blood than in other tissues.

8.2.2 MIDs Resulting from mtDNA or nDNA Mutations

8.2.2.1 PEO

PEO follows an autosomal recessive, autosomal dominant (PEO plus) or maternal trait of inheritance, or may occur sporadically. Sporadic PEO is clinically characterized by bilateral ptosis and ophthalmoplegia and is frequently associated with weakness and exercise-intolerance. Occasionally, patients additionally present with ataxia or hearing loss. Instrumental investigations may reveal cataract, retinitis pigmentosa, or cardiomyopathy (Finsterer et al. 2009). Autosomal recessive and autosomal dominant PEO may additionally present with axonal neuropathy and sensory disturbances, dysarthria, seizures, migraine, Parkinsonism, ataxia, hearing loss, mental retardation, or hypogonadism (Luoma et al. 2004). Rarely, affected patients develop cardiomyopathy or gastrointestinal dysmotility. Instrumental investigations may show neuropathy, myopathy, or hepatopathy. Onset of Mendelian PEO is in adulthood.

Sporadic PEO is due to single large-scale mtDNA deletions, which may be detected only in the muscle. In less than 20% of the cases PEO is due to the common *tRNA(Lys)* mutation m.3243A>G. In single patients PEO arised from mutations in the *tRNA(Ala)* and *tRNA(Val)* genes (Hirano and DiMauro 2001). Mendelian PEO is due to heterozygous mutations in four different genes: *POLG1* encoding the catalytic subunit of the mtDNA-specific polymerase-gamma (Van Goethem et al. 2001); *PEO1* encoding the mtDNA helicase twinkle (Spelbrink et al. 2001); *SLC25A4* encoding the muscle-heart-specific mitochondrial adenine nucleotide translocator ANT1 (Kaukonen et al. 2000); or ECGF1 encoding the thymidine phosphorylase (see MNGIE). *POLG1* mutations are the most common cause of Mendelian PEO. *POLG1*-associated PEO is characterized by accumulation of multiple mtDNA deletions (breakage syndrome).

8.2.3 MIDs Predominantly Resulting from nDNA Mutations

8.2.3.1 MIDs Due to Mutations in Genes Encoding Respiratory Chain Subunits or Assembly Factors of RCCs

Leigh Syndrome

LS (Leigh syndrome), also termed subacute necrotizing encephalomyopathy, is clinically characterized by severe, developmental psychomotor delay, cerebellar ataxia, pyramidal signs, myoclonic or generalized tonic-clonic seizures, movement disorders including chorea, dystonia, respiratory abnormalities, ophthalmoparesis, or muscle weakness and hypotonia (floppy infant). Involvement of the brain stem may cause respiratory insufficiency (hyperventilation, irregular ventilation, hypoventilation, or apnea), dysphagia, recurrent vomiting, or abnormal thermoregulation (hypo/hyperthermia) (Rahman et al. 1996). Patients with MILS may additionally present with dysmorphism or SLEs. Lactate may be elevated in the serum and CSF. Cerebral MRI typically shows focal, symmetric lesions of the basal ganglia, thalamus, brainstem, cerebellum, or posterior columns of the spinal cord (Rossi et al. 2003). These lesions typically spread, contrary to Alpers-Huttenlocher disease (AHS), centrifugally from the brainstem and basal ganglia to the cortex. Histologically, these lesions show demyelination, gliosis, and vascular proliferation. Nerve conduction studies and electromyography may indicate myopathy or polyneuropathy. Muscle biopsy shows non-specific alterations (accumulation of intracytoplasmic lipid droplets) and RRF and COX-negative fibers are consistently absent, except for cases with MILS (Tsao et al. 2003). Biochemical investigations most commonly reveal RCCI or RCCIV defects, multiple RCC defects, or may be normal. About 10–20% of the cases with normal biochemical results of the muscle may have RCC defects in the myocardium, liver, skin fibroblasts, or white blood cells. Ophthalmologic investigations may show optic atrophy or retinitis pigmentosa. Cardiologic examination may reveal hypertrophic cardiomyopathy. Some patients may also develop hepatopathy or renal insufficiency (Tay et al. 2005). Onset is usually in early infancy between 3 and 12 months of age often following an infection. Patients usually die by age 2–3 years from respiratory or heart failure and only few survive into childhood or adulthood. The course is characterized by episodic deterioration and interspersed plateaus. Leigh-like syndrome is diagnosed if patients present with features strongly suggestive of LS but do not exactly fulfill the diagnostic criteria because of variable distribution (cortical) or character of the cerebral lesions or normal imaging or serum lactate.

LS is genetically heterogeneous. In 10–20% of the cases LS is due to the m.8993T>G or m.8993T>C mutation in the *ATP6* gene (NARP/MILS overlap) (Makino et al. 1998). In another 10–20% it is due to mutations in other mtDNA genes such as the *tRNA(Leu(UUA), tRNA(Lys), tRNA(Try), tRNA(Val), ND1, ND3, ND4, ND5, ND6,* or *COXIII*. More frequently, however, LS arises from an autosomal dominant, autosomal recessive, or X-linked defect, or occurs sporadically. Mendelian LS with RCCI deficiency may be due to mutations in genes encoding RCCI subunits *NDUFV1, NDUFS1, NDUFS2, NDUFS3, NDUFS4, NDUFS7, NDUFS8* (Finsterer 2008). Recently also mutations in the RCCI assembly factors *NDUFA12L, NDUFAF1, NDUFAF2,* or *C6ORF66. NDUFA12L* manifesting as leucencephalopathy have been described (Finsterer 2008). LS with RCCII defect may be due to *SDHA* mutations. LS with RCCIV defect arise from mutations in genes encoding COX assembly-factors such as *SCO1, SCO2, COX10,* or *COX15*. Mutations in the *SCO1, SCO2, COX10,* or *COX15* gene may be also associated with non-syndromic MIDs such as encephalopathy with cardiomyopathy (*SCO2, COX15*), nephropathy (*COX10*), or hepatopathy (*SCO1*). The French-Canadian Saguenay-Lac-Saint-Jean type of LS is due to mutations in the *LRPPRC* gene (Mootha et al. 2003). Only in two RCCV assembly genes pathogenic mutations have been identified so far. A mutation in the *ATP12* gene was associated with congenital lactacidosis and fatal infantile multisystem disease, involving brain, liver, heart, and muscle. *TMEM70* mutations caused isolated ATP-synthase deficiency and neonatal encephalo-cardiomyopathy. In case LS is X-linked or sporadic it is most frequently due to mutations in the E1-alpha-subunit of the pyruvate-dehydrogenase complex (*PDHA1* gene) (Lissens et al. 2000). Recently mutations in the *TACO1* gene encoding a translation factor of COXI has been reported to cause LS (Weraarpachai et al. 2009). All defects described in patients with LS affect the terminal oxidative metabolism and are likely to impair ATP-production.

Defects in mitochondrial translation are among the most common causes of mitochondrial disease, but the mechanisms that regulate mitochondrial translation remain largely unknown. In the yeast Saccharomyces cerevisiae, all mitochondrial mRNAs require specific translational activators, which recognize sequences in 5′ UTRs and mediate translation. As mammalian mitochondrial mRNAs do not have significant 5′ UTRs, alternate mechanisms must exist to promote translation. A recent study identified a specific defect in the synthesis of the mitochondrial DNA (mtDNA)-encoded COX I subunit in a pedigree segregating late-onset Leigh syndrome and cytochrome c oxidase (COX) deficiency. The authors mapped the defect to chromosome 17q by functional complementation and identified a homozygous single-base-pair insertion in CCDC44, encoding a member of a large family of hypothetical proteins containing a conserved DUF28 domain. CCDC44, renamed TACO1 for translational activator of COX I, shares a notable degree of structural similarity with bacterial homologues, and our findings suggest that it is one of a family of specific mammalian mitochondrial translational activators.

GRACILE

GRACILE (growth retardation, aminoaciduria, cholestasis, iron overload, lactacidosis, and early death) syndrome is a lethal infantile disorder in which fetal growth retardation, short stature, and hepato-encephalopathy are the dominant clinical findings (Morán et al. 2010). Cognitive functions are intact. Instrumental findings include aminoaciduria, cholestasis, iron overload, and lactacidosis. Biochemical investigations may reveal a RCCIII defect. Onset is in early childhood.

GRACILE syndrome is genetically due to mutations in a RCCIII assembly protein, known as *BCS1L*. *BCS1L* is an assembly factor that facilitates the insertion of the catalytic Rieske Fe-S subunit into RCCIII (Morán et al. 2010). *BCS1L* mutations disrupt the assembly of RCCIII. *BCS1L* mutations may also cause Bjornstad syndrome, characterized by sensorineural hearing loss and pili torti. The variable phenotypic expression of *BCS1L*mutations is attributed to the variable amount of reactive oxygen species resulting from these mutations (Hinson et al. 2007).

8.2.3.2 MIDs Due to Mutations in Genes Encoding Components of the mtDNA Maintenance Machinery

Breakage Syndromes

Breakage syndromes are characterized by multiple deletions and include MNGIE and the POLG1-related disorders. POLG1-related disorders include Mendelian PEO, the ataxia neuropathy spectrum (ANS), childhood myo-cerebro-hepathopathy spectrum (MCHS), myoclonic epilepsy, myopathy, and sensory ataxia (MEMSA), and AHS (Spinazzola and Zeviani 2007). ANS comprises the sensory ataxia, neuropathy, dysarthria, and ophthalmoplegia (SANDO) syndrome and the mitochondrial recessive ataxia syndrome (MIRAS) syndrome. Recently, also POLG1 mutations were made responsible for distal myopathy of the upper limbs (Giordano et al. 2010).

MNGIE

MNGIE (mitochondrial neuro-gastrointestinal encephalopathy) is a multisystem MID, which follows an autosomal recessive mode of inheritance. The clinical presentation is dominated by severe gastro-intestinal dysmotility associated with nausea, postprandial emesis, early satiety, dysphagia, gastro-intestinal reflux, episodic abdominal distensive pain, ascites, diarrhea, and kachexia (Debouverie et al. 1997; Hirano et al. 1994). Additional manifestations include short stature, PEO, dysphonia, dysarthria, neuropathy with sensory disturbances and distal weakness predominantly affecting the lower limbs, confusional state, and hypoacusis. The initial manifestation is gastrointestinal dysmotility in about two thirds of the cases, PEO in one fifth of the cases, and hypoacusis in about 10% of the cases (Teitelbaum et al. 2002). Carriers are not affected. Instrumental findings include hepato-spleno-megaly, steatosis hepatis, leucencephalopathy on MRI, mixed polyneuropathy, and myopathy with RRF and COX-negative muscle fibers. Highly variable findings include anemia, diverticulosis, autonomic nervous system dysfunction (arterial hypotension, sweating, bladder dysfunction), cardiomoypathy, increased CSF protein, and lactacidosis. Serum thymidine concentrations are increased >3 µmol/l and deoxyuridine concentrations >5 µmol/l (Martí et al. 2004). The thymidine phosphorylase activity in leucocytes is reduced to < 10% of normal (Nishino et al. 1999). Onset of the clinical manifestations is between the first and fifth decade, but in about two thirds of the cases onset is before age 20 years (Nishino et al. 2000). The prognosis is poor and most patients die between age 26–58 years (Nishino et al. 2000).

MNGIE is due to homozygous or compound homozygous mutations (missense mutations, splice-site mutations, microdeletions, insertions) in the *TYMP/ECGF1* gene. *TYMP* encodes the thymidine phosphorylase, which promotes the phosphorylation of thymidine to thymine and deoxyribose-phosphate. *TYMP* mutations result in systemic accumulation of thymidine and deoxyuridine, leading to deoxynucleotide pool imbalance and mtDNA instability. mtDNA instability results in mtDNA point mutations, multiple mtDNA deletions, or partial mtDNA depletion in the skeletal muscle (Nishigaki et al. 2004). mtDNA depletion or duplications may be found in any tissue by Southern blot or long-range PCR. *TYMP* mutations are detected by sequencing of the gene. Alternative splicing from splice-site mutations may be detected by reverse transcriptase PCR assay. A MNGIE-like phenotype due to *POLG1* mutations has been recently reported (van Goethem et al. 2001).

SANDO

SANDO follows an autosomal recessive trait of inheritance and is clinically characterized by the triad of cerebellar or sensory ataxia, dysarthria, and ophthalmoparesis (Fadic et al. 1997; Gago et al. 2006). Single patients may also present with dysphagia, muscle weakness, or neuropathy (Milone et al. 2008). Neuropathy may be motor, sensory, or mixed, and is severe enough to contribute to ataxia (sensory ataxia). Some patients may present with seizures. Up to one quarter of the patients develops muscle cramps. More rare manifestations include myoclonus, visual impairment, psychiatric abnormalities, headache, or hepatopathy (Wong et al. 2008; Tzoulis et al. 2006). Muscle biopsy may be normal or may show COX-negative fibers. Onset is usually in adulthood between age 16 and 40 years. Though SANDO shares features with AHS, it tends to be milder and more slowly progressive.

SANDO is due to *POLG1* mutations, which secondarily cause multiple mtDNA deletions (Gago et al. 2006; Milone et al. 2008). In single cases SANDO may be due to mutations in the *PEO1* gene (Hudson et al. 2005).

MIRAS

MIRAS (mitochondrial autosomal recessive ataxia syndrome) is characterized by cerebellar ataxia as the dominant phenotypic feature (Hakonen et al. 2008). In addition to ataxia affected patients present with polyneuropathy, dysarthria, mild cognitive impairment, involuntary movements, psychiatric abnormalities, and seizures (Hakonen et al. 2005). Biochemical investigations of the muscle homogenate may reveal reduced activity of RCCI and RCCIV. Onset of MIRAS is in juvenile age or early adulthood (Rantamäki et al. 2007).

MIRAS is caused by homozygous or compound heterozygous mutations in the *POLG1* gene, which secondarily cause multiple mtDNA deletions and to some extent also mtDNA depletion (Hakonen et al. 2008). Multiple mtDNA deletions are particularly present in the brain of these patients (Hakonen et al. 2008). In Northern Europe MIRAS should be considered as a first-line differential diagnosis of progressive ataxia since the carrier frequency in Finland and the number of patients in Norway are high (Hakonen et al. 2005).

MEMSA

Myoclonic epilepsy, myopathy, and sensory ataxia (MEMSA), formerly known as spinocerebellar ataxia with epilepsy (SCAE), is clinically characterized by myopathy, epilepsy and ataxia but without ophthalmoparesis. The phenotype resembles that of a spinocerebellar ataxia but additionally includes epilepsy (Galassi et al. 2008). Ataxia is usually followed by focal epilepsy, which generalizes with progression of the disease. Seizures may be so severe that they become refractory to conservative therapy including barbiturate anesthesia. Interictally, a progressive encephalopathy may develop. Single patients may additionally present with polyneuropathy, Parkinsonism, or depression. Myopathy is usually diffuse and manifests only as exercise intolerance. Onset is in early adulthood and the initial manifestation is most frequently cerebellar ataxia.

The syndrome is most frequently due to *POLG1* mutations, which secondarily cause multiple mtDNA deletions. Only in single cases mutations in the *PEO1* or *SLC25A4* genes have been described as causal (Galassi et al. 2008).

AHS

AHS (Alpers-Huttenlocher disease) is clinically characterized by severe, progressive encephalopathy with developmental delay and psychomotor regression, intractable epilepsy, headache, ataxia, neuropathy, hepatopathy, renal tubulopathy, fasting hypoglycemia, and early death (Gordon 2006; Naviaux and Nguyen 2005; Davidzon et al. 2006). Some patients additionally present with SLEs with cortical blindness (Gordon 2006). In half of the patients seizures are the initial clinical manifestation and may be focal, generalized, myoclonic, or may manifest as epilepsia partialis continua (Hakonen et al. 2005; Horvath et al. 2006; Naviaux and Nguyen 2005; Tzoulis et al. 2006). Another common initial manifestation is headache associated with visual sensations or visual auras (Hakonen et al. 2005; Tzoulis et al. 2006). Some patients develop Parkinsonism, which responds to L-DOPA (Luoma et al. 2004; Mancuso et al. 2004). Motor impairment may include weakness with hypotonia and spasticity predominantly of the lower limbs (Gordon 2006). There is cognitive impairment, which lastly evolves into dementia. More rare findings include retinitis pigmentosa and impaired hearing (Di Fonzo et al. 2003; Hakonen et al. 2005; Horvath et al. 2006). Liver enzymes and ultrasound investigations may indicate hepatopathy. CSF protein is usually normal or occasionally elevated. Nerve conduction studies may reveal polyneuropathy. Muscle biopsy usually shows COX-negative fibers (Kollberg et al. 2006). EEG may show slow, high-amplitude activity with small polyspikes or intermittent spike-wave activity (Worle et al. 1998). In case of epilepsia partialis continua the EEG may be normal, may show focal background slowing, or focal paroxysmal activity. Neuroimaging may show gliosis with progression of the disease, starting from the cortex (usually the occipital cortex) and progressing to the brainstem (contrary to LS). Neuropathological investigations may show cortical gliosis and subcortical neuronal loss, particularly in the thalamus (Kollberg et al. 2006). Onset is usually between 2 and 4 years but ranges from 1 month to 36 years. Psychomotor development is usually normal during the first few months.

AHS is most frequently due to mutations in the *POLG1* gene (Davidzon et al. 2005; Kollberg et al. 2006). It is the disorder with the most severe phenotype among the *POLG1*-related disorders. Recently, *PEO1* mutations have been described to cause a phenotype resembling that of AHS (Hakonen et al. 2007).

MCHS

The myo-cerebro-hepatopathy-spectrum (MCHS) disorders are clinically characterized by mitochondrial myopathy with hypotonia, lactacidosis and failure to thrive, developmental delay, dementia, and liver dysfunction (Wong et al. 2008). Additional features of MCHS disorders may be liver failure, renal tubular acidosis, pancreatitis, cyclic vomiting, or hearing loss. Seizures are no feature of the clinical presentation at least during the first few years. Onset of MCHS disorders is in the first few months up to three years. They are all due to POLG1 mutations and are thus part of the spectrum of POLG1 disorders (Wong et al. 2008).

Mitochondrial Depletion Disorders (MDDs)

MDDs are characterized by reduction of the mtDNA copy number, which is due to mutations in eight different genes (*DGUOK, MPV17, POLG1, RRM2B, SUCLA2, SUCLG1, TK2,* and *PEO1*). Their products are involved in mtDNA replication or regulation of the mitochondrial deoxy-ribo-nucleoside triphosphate (dNTP) pool. Genes most frequently mutated in MDDs are the *DGUOK* and the *POLG1* gene (18% each). Mutations in these genes may manifest in a single tissue (preferably muscle or liver), or in multiple tissues (heart, brain, kidney) (Ricci et al. 1992). All MDDs follow an autosomal recessive trait. mtDNA depletion may be confirmed by real-time quantitative PCR (qPCR) or by oligonucleotide array comparative genomic hybridization (oligo-aCGH).

Myopathic MDD

Myopathic MDD is clinically characterized by a pure myopathy. Myopathic MDD is most frequently due to mutations in the *TK2* gene (Saada et al. 2001). Mutations in this gene reduce the dNTP pool. *TK2* mutations are responsible for only approximately 20% of the cases. Urinary methylmalonic acid levels are normal.

Encephalo-Myopathic MDD

Encephalo-myopathic MDD is due to mutations in the *SUCLA2* gene, the *SUCLG1* gene, or the *RRM2B* gene. *SUCLA2* encodes the ß-subunit of the adenosine diphosphate-forming succinyl-CoA-ligase (Bourdon et al. 2007). Mutations in this gene manifest phenotypically as Leigh-like syndrome starting in early infancy with muscle hypotonia and myopathy preventing head and trunk control and ambulation. Later, patients develop progressive scoliosis, dystonia, athetosis, chorea, epilepsy (infantile spasms, generalized convulsions), hearing loss, and growth retardation. There may be moderate methyl-malonic-aciduria, lactacidosis, elevated CSF-lactate, increased C3-carnitine, or increased C4-dicarboxylic-carnitine. EMG may show enlarged motor units. Cerebral imaging may show atrophy, basal ganglia abnormalities, and delayed myelination. Muscle biopsy shows increased number of mitochondria and biochemical investigations RCCI, RCCIII, or RCCIV defects. Onset is between birth and 5 months. The disorder is lethal in early infancy. Mutations in the *SUCLG1* gene, encoding the alpha-subunit of the GDP-forming succinyl-CoA-ligase, manifest as fatal infantile lactacidosis, dysmorphism, or methyl-malonic-aciduria with muscle and liver mtDNA depletion. Muscle biopsy may reveal multiple RCC defects. The phenotype is indistinguishable from MDD due to *SUCLA2* mutations. mtDNA depletion may also derive from mutations in the p53-dependent ribonucleotide reductase (*RRM2B*) gene (Ostergaard et al. 2007). *RRM2B* encodes the p53-inducible subunit of the ribonucleotide reductase, which consists of a large catalytic subunit (R1) and a small R2 subunit, which is either maximally expressed during the S-phase or responsible for the DNA-repair and mtDNA-synthesis in non-proliferating cells. Ribonucleotide reductase is involved in the production of nucleotide precursors. *RRM2B* mutations manifest clinically as developmental delay, microcephaly, seizures, myopathy, muscle hypotonia, respiratory insufficiency, persistent lactacidosis, renal insufficiency with proximal tubulopathy, and diarrhea (Bourdon et al. 2007).

Hepato-Cerebral (Encephalo-Hepatic) MDD

Hepato-cerebral MDD is due to mutations in the *PEO1*, *POLG1*, *DGUOK*, or *MPV17* genes (Spinazzola and Zeviani 2007). Most frequently, hepato-cerebral MDD is due to *DGUOK* mutations (Sarzi et al. 2007). *DGUOK* mutations reduce the dNTP pool and either manifest as hepato-cerebral syndrome in neonates or as isolated hepatopathy (intrahepatic cholestasis, ascites, edema, hemorrhage) in infancy or childhood. The hepato-cerebral form manifests with developmental regression, typical rotatory nystagmus, which evolves into opsoclonus, and muscle hypotonia. Contrary to AHS, DGUOK-deficiency does not go along with seizures or abnormal cerebral imaging (Dimmock et al. 2008). Patients with isolated liver disease may also develop renal involvement. Liver enzymes and bilirubine are elevated. Morphology of liver mitochondria is abnormal on electron microscopy. Muscle biopsy may show subsarcolemmal accumulation of mitochondria, COX-negative RRF, and lipid droplets in RRFs (Mancuso et al. 2005). Biochemical investigations of the liver may show reduced RCCI,

RCCII, or RCCIV activity. Cause of death is usually hepatic failure. Mutations in *PEO1* impair mtDNA replication and cause an autosomal recessive AHS-like phenotype. Phenotypes of *POLG1* mutations, which cause mtDNA depletion, have been described above. *MPV17* encodes a protein of unknown function located at the inner mitochondrial membrane. *MPV17* mutations manifest as hepatic failure, hypoglycemia, muscle hypotonia, ataxia, dystonia, or polyneuropathy. Hepato-cerebral MDD from *MPV17* mutations is allelic to Navajo neuro-hepatopathy, clinically characterized by hepatopathy, severe sensory polyneuropathy, corneal anesthesia and scarring, acral mutilation, leucencephalopathy, failure to thrive, recurrent metabolic acidosis, and intercurrent infections (Spinazzola et al. 2006). In all hepato-cerebral MDDs urinary methylmalonic acid is normal.

IOSCA

IOSCA (infantile-onset spinocerebellar ataxia) is an autosomal recessive MID, which is clinically characterized by cerebellar ataxia, epilepsy, athetosis, muscle hypotonia, hypoacusis, PEO, sensory neuropathy, and hypogonadism (Lönnqvist et al. 1998; Nikali et al. 2005). Cerebral imaging may show progressive atrophy of the cerebellum, brainstem, or spinal cord (Nikali et al. 2005). Pathoanatomic studies confirm atrophy of the cerebellum, brainstem, and, most severely, spinal cord (Lönnqvist et al. 1998). Biochemical investigations may show deficiency of RCCI or RCCIV (Hakonen et al. 2008).

IOSCA is caused by mutations in the *PEO1* gene, which encodes the mitochondrial helicase twinkle (Hakonen et al. 2008). *PEO1* mutations secondarily cause mtDNA depletion in the brain and liver but also in other organs (Hakonen et al. 2008).

Translation Defects (Protein Synthesis Machinery)

Pontocerebellar Hypoplasia

Recently, a new autosomal recessive syndrome, pontocerebellar hypoplasia (PCH), comprising severe infantile encephalopathy associated with microcephaly, cerebral atrophy, thinning of the pons and gross atrophy and flattening of the cerebellar hemispheres, and multiple RCC defects has been described in three members of a consanguineous Sephardic Jewish family (Edvardson et al. 2007). Patients may manifest profound developmental delay with increased respiratory rate, poor feeding, edema of the hands and face, and transiently elevated blood and CSF-lactate (Rankin et al. 2010). Muscle biopsy may be normal including biochemical investigations or may show multiple RCC defects (Rankin et al. 2010). Meanwhile six subtypes have been described (Rankin et al. 2010). Onset of PCH is already prenatally.

Types 1 and 6 are due to missplicing intronic mutations in the *RARS2* gene encoding the mitochondrial tRNA(Arg) synthetase. *RARS2* mutations result in a marked reduction of the tRNA(Arg) transcript in fibroblasts. The CNS is assumed to be preferentially affected because of a tissue-specific vulnerability of the splicing machinery (Edvardson et al. 2007). Mutations in the transfer RNA splicing endonuclease subunit genes *TSEN54, TSEN2, TSEN34* were found to be associated with types 2 and 4 (Namavar et al. 2011). Mutations in the *TSEN54* gene manifest with a pathognomonic dragonfly-like cerebellar MRI-pattern, in which the cerebellar hemispheres are flat and severely reduced in size but the vermis is relatively spared (Namavar et al. 2011). *TSEN54* mutations additionally manifest with dyskinesia, dystonia, or generalized spasticity.

LBSL

Leucencephalopathy with brainstem and spinal cord involvement and lactacidosis (LBSL) is a recently described autosomal recessive syndromic MID clinically characterized by slowly progressive cerebellar ataxia, spasticity, and dorsal column dysfunction (Scheper et al. 2007). Some patients additionally develop mild cognitive impairment. There is a highly characteristic constellation of abnormalities on MRI (Scheper et al. 2007).

LBSL is caused by heterozygous mutations in the *DARS2* gene, which encodes the mitochondrial aspartyl-tRNA synthetase (Scheper et al. 2007). Homozygous *DARS2* mutations have not been reported and are assumed to be lethal (Isohanni et al. 2010). Though the activity of this enzyme is reduced in affected patients, the function of the respiratory chain is not impaired (Scheper et al. 2007). Multiple sclerosis, which is a differential of LBSL and MIDs in general (Bhatti and Newman 1999; Horvath et al. 2000; Jansen et al. 1996; Kellar-Wood et al. 1994), is not associated with DARS mutations (Isohanni et al. 2010).

MLASA

MLASA (myopathy, lactacidosis, and sideroblastic anemia) is a rare MID clinically characterized by the combination of sideroblastic anemia, mitochondrial myopathy, and lactacidosis (Fernandez-Vizarra et al. 2007; Patton et al. 2005; Scharfe et al. 2000; Zeharia et al. 2005). Additionally, patients may present with mental retardation or dysmorphic features, such as microcephaly, high palate, high filtrum, distichiasis, or micrognathia (Zeharia et al. 2005). Biochemical investigations may demonstrate reduced activity of RCCI-IV. Electron microscopy may show paracristalline inclusions or iron deposition in almost all mitochondria (Inbal et al. 1995).

MLASA is genetically heterogeneous and most frequently due to homozygous point mutations in the *PUS1* gene encoding the pseudouridine synthase I (Zeharia et al. 2005). Mutations in this gene result in the absence of any enzyme activity in cell lines of these patients (Patton et al. 2005) and in a complete lack of pseudouridylation at the corresponding sites in mitochondrial and cytoplasmic tRNAs. Meanwhile it has been shown that MLASA may be also due to mutations in the *YARS7* gene, which encodes the mitochondrial tyrosyl-tRNA synthetase (Riley et al. 2010).

8.2.3.3 Coenzyme-Q (CoQ)-Deficiency

CoQ-deficiency is a genetically and phenotypically heterogeneous group of MIDs, characterized by primary or secondary deficiency of CoQ. Phenotypically, primary CoQ-deficiency presents as a pure myopathy, as severe infantile neurologic syndrome with nephritis, as LS, or as pure ataxia (Montero et al. 2007). Among these four phenotypes, the ataxic variant is the most common dominated by cerebellar ataxia and cerebellar atrophy. Additionally, these patients may present with epilepsy, weakness, migraine, myoglobinuria, or developmental delay (Leshinsky-Silver et al. 2003). The second most frequent phenotype of primary CoQ-deficiency is characterized by a severe infantile multisystem MID with encephalomyopathy, recurrent myoglobinuria, and myopathy with RRF. CoQ-deficiency may also present as cardio-facio-cutaneous syndrome. Biochemically, there is deficiency of CoQ in muscle or fibroblasts (Montero et al. 2007). Defects of CoQ biosynthesis represent one of the few treatable mitochondrial diseases.

Primary CoQ-deficiency is due to mutations in genes encoding enzymes of the CoQ-biosynthesis, such as *COQ2* (nephropathy), *COQ4, COQ8 (ADCK3, CABC1), COQ9, PDSS1,* or *PDSS2* (Casarin et al. 2008; Mollet et al. 2008; Quinzii et al. 2008). Secondary CoQ-deficiency is due to mutations in genes not directly involved in the CoQ biosynthesis, which nonetheless cause secondary CoQ-deficiency. Genes mutated in secondary CoQ-deficiency include *APTX* (cerebellar ataxia*), ETFDH* (pure myopathy), or *BRAF, PTPN11, HRAS, KRAS, MEK1,* or *MEK2* (cardio-facio-cutaneous syndrome). In the majority of the cases, however, the causative mutation remains undetected. CoQ functions as a lipid-soluble component of virtually all cell membranes, transports electrons from RCCI and RCCII to RCCIII, and is essential for stabilizing RCCIII. Most cases with primary or secondary CoQ-deficiency respond favorably to CoQ-supplementation.

8.2.3.4 MIDs Due to Altered Lipid Milieu

Barth Syndrome

Barth syndrome is a rare, X-linked disorder, involving the heart, the skeletal muscles, and the hematologic system (Barth et al. 2004). Barth syndrome affects almost exclusively young males. Barth syndrome is clinically characterized by proportionate short stature and occasionally mild cognitive impairment. Congenital Barth syndrome additionally manifests with poor sucking, lethargy, hypotonia, and hypothermia. Single patients may experience ischemic, embolic stroke from noncompaction (hypertrabeculation) of the left ventricular apex and lateral wall (Ances et al. 2006). Instrumental investigations may demonstrate cardiomyopathy, which goes along with noncompaction in about half of the cases, cyclic neutropenia, low carnitine levels, increased urinary excretion of methyl-glutaconic acid, moderate hypocholesterolemia, and myopathy with mitochondrial abnormalities on muscle biopsy (Bleyl et al. 1997). Creatine-kinase may be mildly elevated in up to 15% of the patients (Spencer et al. 2006). Onset ranges from 1 to 49 years and peaks around puberty. Untreated boys die at infancy or early childhood from septicemia or cardiac failure (Bleyl et al. 1997). Mortality is highest in the first 4 years of life.

Barth syndrome is due to mutations in the G4.5 gene encoding taffazine (Bleyl et al. 1997). The gene product plays a crucial role in the mitochondrial cardiolipin metabolism (Osman et al. 2010). Cardiolipin itself is a dimeric phosphoglycerol-lipid predominantly present in mitochondrial membranes. Cardiolipin plays a pivotal role in the cellular energy metabolism, mitochondrial dynamics, and in the initiation of apoptotic pathways (Osman et al. 2010).

8.2.3.5 MIDs Due to Mutations in Genes Involved in the Mitochondrial Transport Machinery

Deafness Dystonia Syndrome (DDS, Mohr-Tranebjaerg-Syndrome (MTS))

MTS is a rare MID clinically characterized by early-onset postlingual sensorineural hearing loss, dystonia, cortical blindness, cataract, spasticity, dysphagia, and mental retardation (Tranebjaerg et al. 2000). Muscle biopsy is structurally and biochemically normal, but MRI and PET studies reveal hypometabolic areas in the right striatum and parietal cortex and atrophy of the occipital lobes.

MTS is due to mutations in the *DDP1* gene encoding the deafness-dystonia protein TIMM8a (Aguirre et al. 2008). Mutations in this gene affect the binding of Zn(2+) via the Cys(4) motif (Hofmann et al. 2002; Roesch et al. 2002). DDP1 mutations result in misfolding of the protein and consecutive inability of the protein to assemble with its cognate partner Tim13 to hetero-hexameric complexes. MTS may be also due to mutations in the ATG start codon of the *DDP1* gene leading to the absence of TIMM8a and marked reduction of Tim13 (Binder et al. 2003). In the allelic Jansen syndrome also a one-basepair deletion and a nonsense mutation have been described (Tranebjaerg et al. 2000). The phenotypic variability in MTS suggests the involvement of modifier factors influencing the phenotype (Aguirre et al. 2008).

X-Linked Sideroblastic Anemia with Ataxia (XLSA/A)

XLSA/A is a rare syndromic MID, characterized by mild sideroblastic anemia with hypochromia and microcytosis and cerebellar ataxia (Allikmets et al. 1999; Hellier et al. 2001; Pondarre et al. 2007). Cerebral imaging shows severe cerebellar atrophy. Only few cases have been reported so far.

XLSA/A is due to mutations in the mitochondrial *ATP-binding cassette transporter ABC7* gene (Pondarre et al. 2007; Maguire et al. 2001).

8.2.3.6 MIDs Due to Mutations in Genes Involved in the Mitochondrial Biogenesis (Fusion/Fission)

Autosomal Dominant Optic Atrophy and Deafness (ADOAD)

Autosomal dominant optic atrophy (ADOA) and deafness (ADOAD) is clinically characterized by ataxia, axonal, sensorimotor neuropathy, PEO, and myopathy (dominant optic atrophy "plus" syndrome) (Amati-Bonneau et al. 2008). Muscle biopsy may show mosaic COX-deficiency (Hudson et al. 2008). Biochemical investigations of the muscle may show defective ATP-production, similar to LHON, which is independent of the amount of multiple mtDNA deletions (Lodi et al. 2011).

The syndrome is due to mutations in the *OPA1* gene, encoding a dynamin-related GTPase, involved in mitochondrial fusion, fission, cristae organization, and apoptosis (Amati-Bonneau et al. 2008; Hudson et al. 2008; Liguori et al. 2008). Affected patients also harbor multiple mtDNA deletions, suggesting that *OPA1* is involved in mtDNA stability (Amati-Bonneau et al. 2008). *OPA1* appears to be generally responsible for mitochondrial quality control (Fuhrmann et al. 2010). At onset OPA1 mutations may manifest exclusively as isolated optic atrophy (ADOA) but during the disease course most patients develop ADOAD (Hudson et al. 2008).

CMT2A

MIDs may also manifest as one of the most common inherited neuropathies, CMT2A. CMT2A is a classical autosomal dominant axonal sensorimotor neuropathy characterized by earlier and more severe involvement of the lower extremities than the upper extremities, distal upper-extremity involvement as the neuropathy progresses, more prominent motor deficits than sensory deficits, and normal (>42 m/s) or only slightly decreased nerve conduction velocities. Postural tremor is common (Loiseau et al. 2007). The phenotype is characterized by degeneration of long peripheral axons, but the nature of this tissue selectivity remains unknown. Most affected individuals develop symptoms in the first or second decade. Although some individuals become dependent on crutches or a wheel-chair, most do not.

CMT2A is due to mutations in the mitofusin 2 (MFN2) gene. Mitofusins (MFN1, MFN2) are outer mitochondrial membrane proteins involved in regulating mitochondrial dynamics. There is increasing evidence that mitofusins play a key role in the regulation of the axonal transport of mitochondria. Importantly, both MFN1 and MFN2, interact with mammalian Miro (Miro1/Miro2) and Milton (OIP106/GRIF1) proteins, members of the molecular complex that links mitochondria to kinesin motors (Misko et al. 2010).

DIDMOAD (Diabetes Insipidus, Diabetes Mellitus, Optic Atrophy, and Deafness)

DIDMOAD or Wolfram syndrome (WFS) is a rare autosomal recessive neuro-degenerative disorder with juvenile onset (Medlej et al. 2004). The phenotype is characterized by diabetes and optic atrophy. Other less frequent features comprise psychiatric abnormalities, ataxia, urinary tract atony, joint contractures, cardiovascular and gastrointestinal autonomic neuropathy, hyper-gonadotropic hypogonadism, cardiac malformations, or pituitary dysfunction (Medlej et al. 2004). WFS is due to mutations in the *WFS1* gene encoding an endoplasmic reticulum membrane-embedded protein or due to mutations in the *CISD2* gene encoding a protein involved in mitochondrial integrity and aging (Ajlouni et al. 2002; Chen et al. 2010; Cryns et al. 2003). *WSF1* mutations secondarily cause single or multiple mtDNA deletions (Barrientos et al. 1996).

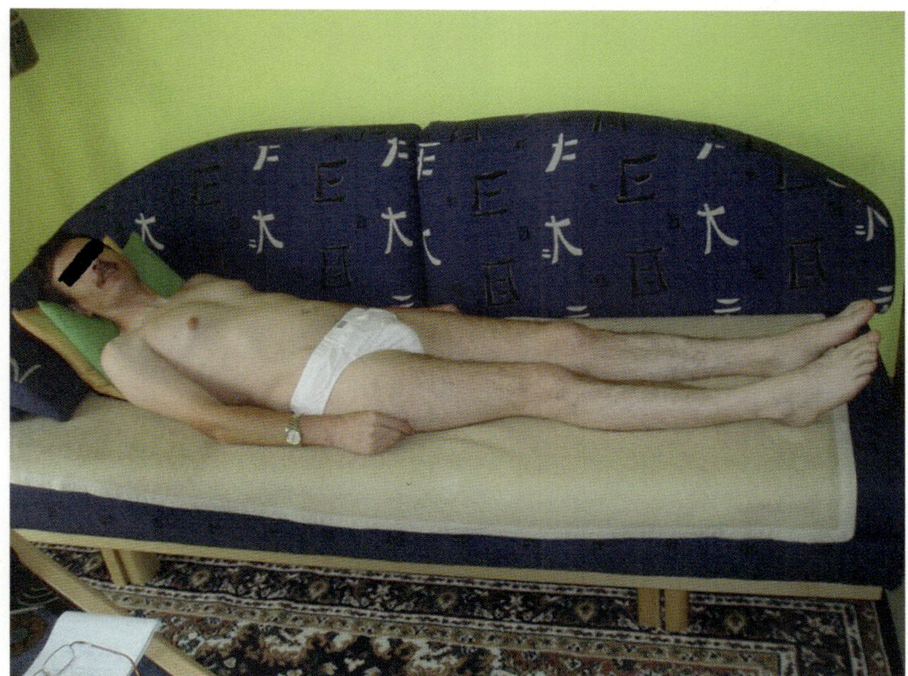

Fig. 8.1 Thirty-eight years-old patient with non-syndromic MID manifesting as epilepsy, stroke-like episodes, myopathy predominantly affecting the lower limbs, anarthria, and noncompaction of the left ventricular myocardium. The phenotype was due to the transition m.8381A>G

Non-syndromic MIDs

In the vast majority of the cases, MIDs typically exhibit wide genotypic and phenotypic heterogeneity. Due to the effects of tissue distribution, threshold effect and heteroplasmy a single mtDNA mutation may present with a broad spectrum of different clinical manifestations within a kindred or population. Because of the weak genotype-phenotype correlation of most mtDNA mutations, phenotypes of a specific mtDNA mutation are quite variable and patients display a cluster of clinical features, which either fall or mostly due not fall into a distinct clinical syndrome. Simultaneously, a distinct phenotype may be due to a number of different mutations, most well known in LS. Already in 2008 more than 40 mtDNA mutations and more than 20 mutated nDNA genes have been reported, which were associated with a LS phenotype (Finsterer 2008). Because of the complex genetic background and highly variable phenotypic expression it is frequently not possible to classify a certain phenotype as syndromic. In the majority of the MIDs, however, the phenotype does not neatly fit into one of the categories described above but represents a unique form within a continuum of phenotypic expression.

Though non-syndromic MIDs do not correspond to distinct phenotypes, they present with clusters of clinical manifestations. Non-syndromic MIDs may present as pure neurological problem, as pure non-neurological disease, or as both a neurological and non-neurological disorder. Pure neurological disorders include non-syndromic, fluctuating encephalopathies, encephalo-myopathies, or pure myopathies, classical mitochondrial myopathies, manifesting as exercise intolerance, easy fatigability, ptosis, ophthalmoparesis, bulbar weakness, limb weakness, axial weakness, or muscular respiratory insufficiency (Fig. 8.1). Pure cerebellar ataxia, epilepsy, spasticity, dystonia, migraine, cluster headache, or psychiatric abnormalities including confusional state, dementia, autism, or psychosis may be phenotypic expressions of an underlying mitochondrial defect. There may be also optic atrophy, pigmentary retinopathy, or pituitary

Fig. 8.2 Thirty-five years female with non-syndromic MID initially manifesting with intractable series of generalised seizures and epileptic states over 4 months. Biochemical investigations of the muscle homogenate revealed a RCCI defect. MRI of the cerebrum showed T2-hyperintense lesions in the thalamus and putamina bilaterally

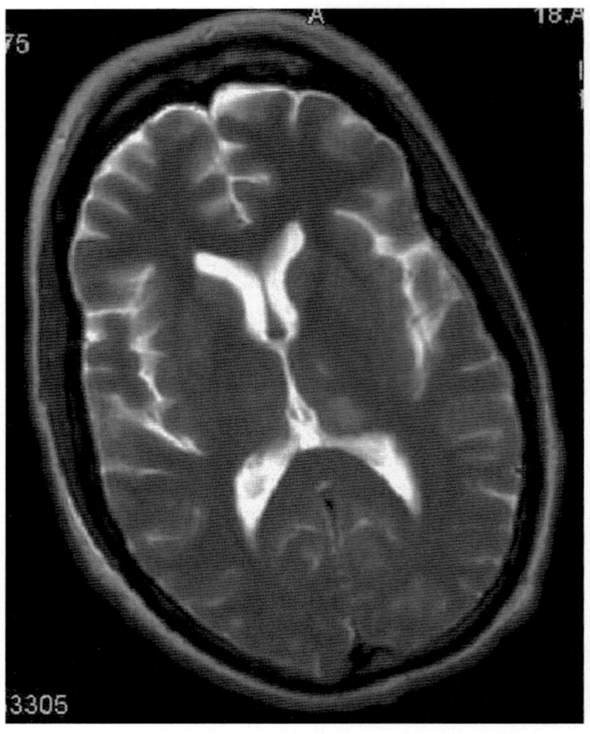

adenoma. Non-neurological manifestations of a non-syndromic MID include isolated cataract, hearing impairment, sicca syndrome, thyroid dysfunction, arrhythmias, cardiomyopathy, hepatopathy, liver cysts, pancreatitis, diabetes, vomiting, pseudoobstruction, diarrhea, renal insufficiency, renal cysts, dermatological disease, anemia, thrombocytopenia, thrombocytosis, or leucopenia. Even arteriopathy may be a non-neurological manifestation of a non-syndromic MID (Finsterer 2007). Frequently, there are also combinations of neurological and non-neurological manifestations such as hepato-encephalopathies or cardio-myo-encephalopathies. There are also indications that an increased number of pregnancy losses, the development of cysts in parenchymatous organs, and a tendency to develop aneurysms or diverticles represent manifestations of non-syndromic mitochondrial defects (Tay et al. 2006). Rarely, non-syndromic MID may manifest as vasculopathy resulting in arterial dissection or even rupture of an artery (Tay et al. 2006). If patients with an MID carry an increased risk to develop malignancy is so far unproven.

Because of the complexity and variable clinical presentation, a non-syndromic MID or syndromic MID in the early stages should be always suspected if there is isolated unexplained neurological disease, isolated unexplained non-neurological disease, or a combination of both. Suggestive of a MID are the presence of unexplained short stature, facial dysmorphism, a history of migraine, stroke-like episodes, seizures, cognitive decline, confusional state, psychosis, impaired hearing, impaired ocular motility, impaired vision, thyroid dysfunction, hypoparathyroidism, diabetes, hyponatriemia, hypogonadism, cardiomyopathy, cardiac conduction abnormalities, dry mouth and eyes, vomiting, gastrointestinal pseudoobstruction, diarrhea, hepatopathy, anemia, leucopenia, thrombocytopenia, thrombocytosis, renal insufficiency, renal cysts, myopathy, neuropathy, neuronopathy, or skin changes such as psoriasis. The suspicion of a non-syndromic MID is further supported if instrumental investigations additionally show recurrently elevated creatine-kinase, lactacidosis, reduced urine levels of aminoacids or organic acids, elevated lactate in the cerebro-spinal fluid, delayed visually-evoked potentials, or pigmentary retinopathy. Neuroimaging may show stroke-like lesions with cytotoxic or vasogenic edema, laminar cortical necrosis, basal ganglia necrosis, focal or diffuse white matter lesions, focal or diffuse atrophy, intra-cerebral calcifications, cysts, lacunas, microbleeds, cerebral hypoperfusion, intra-cerebral artery stenoses, intracranial dissection, aneurysms, or moyamoya syndrome (Fig. 8.2) (Finsterer 2009).

Table 8.2 Genes mutated in syndromic and non-syndromic MIDs

Mutated gene	Phenotype	Reference
mtDNA genes		
tRNA(Met)	tRNA misfolding	Jones et al. (2008)
tRNA(Trp)	Late-onset encephalopathy	Malfatti et al. (2010)
tRNA(Phe)	Psychosis, dementia, Parkinsonism	Young et al. (2010)
12SrRNA	Non-syndromic hearing loss	Pupo et al. (2008)
ATP6	Hereditary spastic paraplegia-like	Verny et al. (2011)
tDNA deletion	Endocrinopathy, deafness	Nicolino et al. (1997)
nDNA genes		
AIF	X-linked, encephalomyopathy, multiple RCC defects	Ghezzi et al. (2010)
C6orf66	Infantile encephalopathy	Saada et al. (2008)
C20orf7	Lethal neonatal MID	Sugiana et al. (2008)
DLP1	Microcephaly, optic atrophy, lactacidosis	Waterham et al. (2007)
EFG1	Infantile encephalopathy	Valente et al. (2007)
ETHE1	Retardation, diarrhea, acrocyanosis, petechiae	Barth et al. (2010)
FASTKD2	Developmental delay, epilepsy, atrophy, myopathy	Ghezzi et al. (2008)
FOXRED1	Infantile encephalopathy	Fassone et al. (2010)
GFER	Myopathy, cataract, multiple RCC defects	Di Fonzo et al. (2009)
GFM1	Leigh syndrome, hepatopathy, lactacidosis	Smits et al. (2011)
LIS1	Lissencephaly, mtDNA insertion	Millar et al. (2010)
MECP2	Rett syndrome	Condie et al. (2010)
MRPS16	Lactacidosis, dysmorphism, developmental delay	Miller et al. (2004)
NDUFS6	Neonatal lactacidosis in Caucasus Jews	Spiegel et al. (2009a)
NDUFV2	Parkinsonism	Nishioka et al. (2010)
NUBPL	RCCI deficiency	Calvo et al. (2010)
POLG2	adPEO	Ferraris et al. (2008)
POLG2	Ptosis, myopathy	Walter et al. (2010)
SCO1	Hepatopathy, severe encephalopathy	Valnot et al. (2000)
SLC25A3	Cardiomyopathy, lactacidosis	Mayr et al. (2007)
SLC25A19	Neuropathy, bilateral striatal necrosis, Amish microcephaly	Spiegel et al. (2009b)
SLC29A3	Scleroderma, hepatopathy, cardiac dysfunction	Morgan et al. (2010)
TRMU	Reversible hepatopathy	Zeharia et al. (2009)

Some of the mutated genes causing syndromic MIDs may also cause non-syndromic MIDs but are not mentioned in this list again

MR-spectroscopy may show intracerebral hypometabolism or lactacidosis. Muscle biopsy may show COX-positive or COX-negative RRF, COX-negative muscle fibers, SDH-hyper-reactivity, or increased number of or abnormally shaped or structured mitochondria. Most important for diagnosing non-syndromic MIDs is the biochemical investigation of the most severely affected tissue. It may reveal a single RCC defect, multiple RCC defects, or may be normal. Normal biochemical investigations, as well as normal muscle biopsy investigations do not exclude the presence of a MID.

Non-syndromic MIDs are best classified according to the mutated genes (Table 8.2). A number of genes has been reported during recent years of which mutations cause either syndromic or non-syndromic MIDs (m.1555A>G in *12SrRNA*) or only non-syndromic MIDs. Mutated genes, which cause only non-syndromic MIDs are listed in Table 8.2. Most recently, mutations in the *FOXRED1* gene, encoding a molecular chaperone responsible for the steady-state of RCCI, have been described (Fassone et al. 2010). Phenotypically, these mutations presented as infantile encephalopathy (Fassone et al. 2010). A non-.syndromic MID manifesting as developmental delay, cerebral atrophy, epilepsy, and myopathy with COX-deficiency was attributed to mutations in the *FASTKD2* gene, of which the product is involved in apoptosis. MIDs may also arise from mutations in the SLC29A3 gene encoding the mitochondrial and lysosomal nucleoside transporter hENT3 (Morgan et al. 2010). Phenotypically, these mutations express as scleroderma, hyperpigmentation, hypertrichosis, hepatomegaly, cardiac abnormalities, or musculoskeletal deformities, as pigmented hypertrichotic dermatosis with insulin-dependent diabetes syndrome, or as familial Rosai-Dorfman disease (short stature, familial histiocytosis, sinus histiocytosis with massive lymphadenopathy (SHML) (Kang et al. 2010). The number of mutated genes causing non-syndromic MIDs is further expanding and regular updates are required to meet and reflect the fast growing developments in the field.

8.3 Conclusion

The field of mitochondrial medicine is still expanding but the implications on the management of affected patients in health care systems is still poorly recognized and underestimated. Those involved in the management of these patients need to consider a MID whenever there is a progressive, multi-system disorder of unknown etiology. Diagnosing these conditions is challenging particularly in the early stages of the disease when there is often only a single organ affected. If the MID is not considered as a differential at this stage, these patients may be misdiagnosed and may become "fibromyalgia" patients, neurotic patients, or doctor shoppers during years until other manifestations arise and more clearly suggest the correct diagnosis. The diagnosis is facilitated when the clinical picture falls into one of the maternally-inherited or Mendelian syndromic forms. If the phenotype is complex or suggests a non-syndromic MID more comprehensive investigations are required. Since MIDs are increasingly recognized by physician involved in the management of MIDs their prevalence is mounting. The increasing prevalence of MIDs should urge the responsible political decision makers and managers of healthcare systems and those involved in the care of patients and education of students and physicians to establish specific units with multi-professional teams exclusively dedicated to the management of patients of this fastly growing field.

References

Aguirre LA, Pérez-Bas M, Villamar M, López-Ariztegui MA, Moreno-Pelayo MA, Moreno F, del Castillo I (2008) A Spanish sporadic case of deafness-dystonia (Mohr-Tranebjaerg) syndrome with a novel mutation in the gene encoding TIMM8a, a component of the mitochondrial protein translocase complexes. Neuromuscul Disord 18:979–981

Ajlouni K, Jarrah N, El-Khateeb M, El-Zaheri M, El Shanti H, Lidral A et al (2002) Wolfram syndrome: identification of a phenotypic and genotypic variant from Jordan. Am J Med Genet 115:61–65

Allikmets R, Raskind WH, Hutchinson A, Schueck ND, Dean M, Koeller DM (1999) Mutation of a putative mitochondrial iron transporter gene (ABC7) in X-linked sideroblastic anemia and ataxia (XLSA/A). Hum Mol Genet 8:743–749

Amati-Bonneau P, Valentino ML, Reynier P, Gallardo ME, Bornstein B, Boissière A et al (2008) OPA1 mutations induce mitochondrial DNA instability and optic atrophy 'plus' phenotypes. Brain 131:338–351

Ances BM, Sullivan J, Weigele JB, Hwang V, Messe SR, Kasner SE et al (2006) Stroke associated with Barth syndrome. J Child Neurol 21:805–807

Barrientos A, Casademont J, Saiz A, Cardellach F, Volpini V, Solans A et al (1996) Autosomal recessive Wolfram syndrome associated with an 8.5-kb mtDNA single deletion. Am J Hum Genet 58:963–970

Barth PG, Valianpour F, Bowen VM, Lam J, Duran M, Vaz FM et al (2004) X-linked cardioskeletal myopathy and neutropenia (Barth syndrome): an update. Am J Med Genet 126A:349–354

Barth M, Ottolenghi C, Hubert L, Chrétien D, Serre V, Gobin S, Romano S, Vassault A, Sefiani A, Ricquier D, Boddaert N, Brivet M, de Keyzer Y, Munnich A, Duran M, Rabier D, Valayannopoulos V, de Lonlay P (2010) Multiple sources of metabolic disturbance in ETHE1-related ethylmalonic encephalopathy. J Inherit Metab Dis (in press)

Bhatti MT, Newman NJ (1999) A multiple sclerosis-like illness in a man harboring the mtDNA 14484 mutation. J Neuroophthalmol 9:28–33

Binder J, Hofmann S, Kreisel S et al (2003) Clinical and molecular findings in a patient with a novel mutation in the deafness-dystonia peptide (DDP1) gene. Brain 126:1814–1820

Blakely EL, de Silva R, King A, Schwarzer V, Harrower T, Dawidek G, Turnbull DM, Taylor RW (2005) LHON/MELAS overlap syndrome associated with a mitochondrial MTND1 gene mutation. Eur J Hum Genet 13:623–627

Bleyl SB, Mumford BR, Brown-Harrison MC, Pagotto LT, Carey JC, Pysher TJ et al (1997) Xq28-linked noncompaction of the left ventricular myocardium: prenatal diagnosis and pathologic analysis of affected individuals. Am J Med Genet 72:257–265

Bourdon A, Minai L, Serre V, Jais JP, Sarzi E, Aubert S, Chrétien D, de Lonlay P, Paquis-Flucklinger V, Arakawa H, Nakamura Y, Munnich A, Rötig A (2007) Mutation of RRM2B, encoding p53-controlled ribonucleotide reductase (p53R2), causes severe mitochondrial DNA depletion. Nat Genet 39:776–780

Calvo SE, Tucker EJ, Compton AG, Kirby DM, Crawford G, Burtt NP, Rivas M, Guiducci C, Bruno DL, Goldberger OA, Redman MC, Wiltshire E, Wilson CJ, AltshulerD GSB, Daly MJ, Thorburn DR, Mootha VK (2010) High-throughput, pooledsequencing identifies mutations in NUBPL and FOXRED1 in human complex I deficiency. Nat Genet 42:851–858

Casarin A, Jimenez-Ortega JC, Trevisson E, Pertegato V, Doimo M, Ferrero-Gomez ML, Abbadi S, Artuch R, Quinzii C, Hirano M, Basso G, Ocaña CS, Navas P, Salviati L (2008) Functional characterization of human COQ4, a gene required for Coenzyme Q10 biosynthesis. Biochem Biophys Res Commun 372:35–39

Chen YN, Liou CW, Huang CC et al (2004) Maternally inherited diabetes and deafness (MIDD) syndrome: a clinical and molecular genetic study of a Taiwanese family. Chang Gung Med J 27:66–73

Chen YF, Wu CY, Kirby R, Kao CH, Tsai TF (2010) A role for the CISD2 gene in lifespan control and human disease. Ann N Y Acad Sci 1201:58–64

Chinnery PF (2010) Mitochondrial disorders overview, 2000 (updated 2010). In: Pagon RA, Bird TC, Dolan CR, Stephens K (eds) GeneReviews (Internet). University of Washington, Seattle WA, 1993-. Available from http://www.ncbi.nlm.nih.gov/bookshelf/br.fcgi?book=gene&part=mt-overview

Chinnery PF, Turnbull DM (1999) Mitochondrial DNA and disease. Lancet 354(suppl 1):17–21

Chinnery PF, Elliott C, Green GR et al (2000) The spectrum of hearing loss due to mitochondrial DNA defects. Brain 123:82–92

Chowers I, Lerman-Sagie T, Elpeleg ON, Shaag A, Merin S (1999) Cone and rod dysfunction in the NARP syndrome. Br J Ophthalmol 83:190–193

Condie J, Goldstein J, Wainwright MS (2010) Acquired microcephaly, regression of milestones, mitochondrial dysfunction, and episodic rigidity in a 46, XY male with a de novo MECP2 gene mutation. J Child Neurol 25:633–636

Cryns K, Sivakumaran TA, Van den Ouweland JM, Pennings RJ, Cremers CW, Flothmann K et al (2003) Mutational spectrum of the WFS1 gene in Wolfram syndrome, nonsyndromic hearing impairment, diabetes mellitus, and psychiatric disease. Hum Mutat 22:275–287

Davidzon G, Mancuso M, Ferraris S, Quinzii C, Hirano M, Peters HL et al (2005) POLG mutations and Alpers syndrome. Ann Neurol 57:921–923

Davidzon G, Greene P, Mancuso M, Klos KJ, Ahlskog JE, Hirano M, DiMauro S (2006) Early-onset familial parkinsonism due to POLG mutations. Ann Neurol 59:859–862

Debouverie M, Wagner M, Ducrocq X, Grignon Y, Mousson B, Weber M (1997) MNGIE syndrome in 2 siblings. Rev Neurol (Paris) 153:547–553

Deschauer M, Tennant S, Rokicka A, He L, Kraya T, Turnbull DM, Zierz S, Taylor RW (2007) MELAS associated with mutations in the POLG1 gene. Neurology 68:1741–1742

Di Fonzo A, Bordoni A, Crimi M, Sara G, Del Bo R, Bresolin N, Comi GP (2003) POLG mutations in sporadic mitochondrial disorders with multiple mtDNA deletions. Hum Mutat 22:498–499

Di Fonzo A, Ronchi D, Lodi T, Fassone E, Tigano M, Lamperti C, Corti S, Bordoni A, Fortunato F, Nizzardo M, Napoli L, Donadoni C, Salani S, Saladino F, Moggio M, Bresolin N, Ferrero I, Comi GP (2009) The mitochondrial disulfide relay system protein GFER is mutated in autosomal-recessive myopathy with cataract and combined respiratory-chain deficiency. Am J Hum Genet 84:594–604

DiMauro S, Schon EA (2003) Mitochondrial respiratory-chain diseases. N Engl J Med 348:2656–2668

Dimmock DP, Zhang Q, Dionisi-Vici C, Carrozzo R, Shieh J, Tang LY, Truong C, Schmitt E, Sifry-Platt M, Lucioli S, Santorelli FM, Ficicioglu CH, Rodriguez M, Wierenga K, Enns GM, Longo N, Lipson MH, Vallance H, Craigen WJ, Scaglia F, Wong LJ (2008) Clinical and molecular features of mitochondrial DNA depletion due to mutations in deoxyguanosine kinase. Hum Mutat 29:330–331

Edvardson S, Shaag A, Kolesnikova O, Gomori JM, Tarassov I, Einbinder T, Saada A, Elpeleg O (2007) Deleterious mutation in the mitochondrial arginyl-transfer RNA synthetase gene is associated with pontocerebellar hypoplasia. Am J Hum Genet 81:857–862

Fadic R, Russell JA, Vedanarayanan VV, Lehar M, Kuncl RW, Johns DR (1997) Sensory ataxic neuropathy as the presenting feature of a novel mitochondrial disease. Neurology 49:239–245

Fassone E, Duncan AJ, Taanman JW, Pagnamenta AT, Sadowski MI, Holand T, Qasim W, Rutland P, Calvo SE, Mootha VK, Bitner-Glindzicz M, Rahman S (2010) FOXRED1, encoding an FAD-dependent oxidoreductase complex-I-specific molecular chaperone, is mutated in infantile-onset mitochondrial encephalopathy. Hum Mol Genet 19:4837–4847

Fernandez-Vizarra E, Berardinelli A, Valente L, Tiranti V, Zeviani M (2007) Nonsense mutation in pseudouridylate synthase 1 (PUS1) in two brothers affected by myopathy, lactic acidosis and sideroblastic anaemia (MLASA). J Med Genet 44:173–180

Ferraris S, Clark S, Garelli E, Davidzon G, Moore SA, Kardon RH, Bienstock RJ, Longley MJ, Mancuso M, Gutiérrez Ríos P, Hirano M, Copeland WC, DiMauro S (2008) Progressive external ophthalmoplegia and vision and hearing loss in a patient with mutations in POLG2 and OPA1. Arch Neurol 65:125–131

Finsterer J (2007) Is atherosclerosis a mitochondrial disorder? VASA 36:229–240

Finsterer J (2008) Leigh and Leigh-like syndrome in children and adults. Pediatr Neurol 39:223–235

Finsterer J (2009) Central nervous system imaging in mitochondrial disorders. Can J Neurol Sci 36:143–153

Finsterer J, Harbo HF, Baets J, Van Broeckhoven C, Di Donato S, Fontaine B, De Jonghe P, Lossos A, Lynch T, Mariotti C, Schöls L, Spinazzola A, Szolnoki Z, Tabrizi SJ, Tallaksen CM, Zeviani M, Burgunder JM, Gasser T, European Federation of Neurological Sciences (2009) EFNS guidelines on the molecular diagnosis of mitochondrial disorders. Eur J Neurol 16:1255–1264

Fuhrmann N, Schimpf S, Kamenisch Y, Leo-Kottler B, Alexander C, Auburger G, Zrenner E, Wissinger B, Alavi MV (2010) Solving a 50 year mystery of a missing OPA1mutation: more insights from the first family diagnosed with autosomal dominantoptic atrophy. Mol Neurodegener 5:25

Gago MF, Rosas MJ, Guimarães J, Ferreira M, Vilarinho L, Castro L et al (2006) SANDO: two novel mutations in POLG1 gene. Neuromuscul Disord 16:507–509

Galassi G, Lamantea E, Invernizzi F, Tavani F, Pisano I, Ferrero I et al (2008) Additive effects of POLG1 and ANT1 mutations in a complex encephalomyopathy. Neuromuscul Disord 18:465–470

Ghezzi D, Saada A, D'Adamo P, Fernandez-Vizarra E, Gasparini P, Tiranti V, Elpeleg O, Zeviani M (2008) FASTKD2 nonsense mutation in an infantile mitochondrial encephalomyopathy associated with cytochrome c oxidase deficiency. Am J Hum Genet 83:415–423

Ghezzi D, Sevrioukova I, Invernizzi F, Lamperti C, Mora M, D'Adamo P, Novara F, Zuffardi O, Uziel G, Zeviani M (2010) Severe X-linked mitochondrial encephalomyopathy associated with a mutation in apoptosis-inducing factor. Am J Hum Genet 86:639–649

Giordano C, Pichiorri F, Blakely EL, Perli E, Orlandi M, Gallo P, Taylor RW, Inghilleri M, D'Amati G (2010) Isolated distalmyopathy of the upper limbs associated with mitochondrial DNA depletion and polymerase gamma mutations. Arch Neurol 67:1144–1146

Gordon N (2006) Alpers syndrome: progressive neuronal degeneration of children with liver disease. Dev Med Child Neurol 48:1001–1003

Goto Y, Nonaka I, Horai S (1990) A mutation in the tRNA(Leu)(UUR) gene associated with the MELAS subgroup of mitochondrial encephalomyopathies. Nature 348:651–653

Guan MX (2011) Mitochondrial DNA mutations associated with aminoglycoside ototoxicity. Mitochondrion 11(2): 237–245

Hakonen AH, Heiskanen S, Juvonen V, Lappalainen I, Luoma PT, Rantamaki M et al (2005) Mitochondrial DNA polymerase W748S mutation: a common cause of autosomal recessive ataxia with ancient European origin. Am J Hum Genet 77:430–441

Hakonen AH, Isohanni P, Paetau A, Herva R, Suomalainen A, Lönnqvist T (2007) Recessive Twinkle mutations in early onset encephalopathy with mtDNA depletion. Brain 130:3032–3040

Hakonen AH, Goffart S, Marjavaara S, Paetau A, Cooper H, Mattila K et al (2008) Infantile-onset spinocerebellar ataxia and mitochondrial recessive ataxia syndrome are associated with neuronal complex I defect and mtDNA depletion. Hum Mol Genet 17:3822–3835

Hellier KD, Hatchwell E, DuncombeAS KJ, Hammans SR (2001) X-linked sideroblastic anaemia with ataxia: another mitochondrial disease? J Neurol Neurosurg Psychiatry 70:65–69

Hinson JT, Fantin VR, Schönberger J, Breivik N, Siem G, McDonough B, Sharma P, Keogh I, Godinho R, Santos F, Esparza A, Nicolau Y, Selvaag E, Cohen BH, Hoppel CL, Tranebjaerg L, Eavey RD, Seidman JG, Seidman CE (2007) Missense mutations in theBCS1L gene as a cause of the Björnstad syndrome. N Engl J Med 356: 809–819

Hirano M, DiMauro S (1996) Clinical features of mitochondrial myopathies and encephalomyopathies. In: Lane RJM (ed) Handbook of muscle disease, vol 1. Marcel Dekker Inc, New York, pp 479–504

Hirano M, DiMauro S (2001) ANT1, Twinkle, POLG, and TP: new genes open our eyes to ophthalmoplegia. Neurology 57:2163–2165

Hirano M, Silvestri G, Blake DM, Lombes A, Minetti C, Bonilla E, Hays AP, Lovelace RE, Butler I, Bertorini TE (1994) Mitochondrial neurogastrointestinal encephalomyopathy (MNGIE): clinical, biochemical, and genetic features of an autosomal recessive mitochondrial disorder. Neurology 44:721–727

Hofmann S, Rothbauer U, Muhlenbein N et al (2002) The C66W mutation in the deafness dystonia peptide 1 (DDP1) affects the formation of functional DDP1/TIM13 complexes in the mitochondrial intermembrane space. J Biol Chem 277:23287–23293

Holt IJ, Harding AE, Petty RK, Morgan-Hughes JA (1990) A new mitochondrial disease associated with mitochondrial DNA heteroplasmy. Am J Hum Genet 46:428–433

Horvath R, Abicht A, Shoubridge EA, Karcagi V, Rozsa C, Komoly S, Lochmuller H (2000) Leber's hereditary optic neuropathy presenting as multiple sclerosis-like disease of the CNS. J Neurol 247:65–67

Horvath R, Hudson G, Ferrari G, Fütterer N, Ahola S, Lamantea E et al (2006) Phenotypic spectrum associated with mutations of the mitochondrial polymerase γ gene. Brain 129:1674–1684

Horvath R, Kley RA, Lochmuller H, Vorgerd M (2007) Parkinson syndrome, neuropathy, and myopathy caused by the mutation A8344G (MERRF) in tRNALys. Neurology 68:56–58

Hourani RG, Barada WM, Al-Kutoubi AM, Hourani MH (2006) Atypical MRI findings in Kearns-Sayre syndrome: T2 radial stripes. Neuropediatrics 37:110–113

Howell N, Kubacka I, Halvorson S, Howell B, McCullough DA, Mackey D (1995) Phylogenetic analysis of the mitochondrial genomes from Leber hereditary optic neuropathy pedigrees. Genetics 140:285–302

Hudson G, Deschauer M, Busse K, Zierz S, Chinnery PF (2005) Sensory ataxic neuropathy due to a novel C10Orf2 mutation with probable germline mosaicism. Neurology 64:371–373

Hudson G, Amati-Bonneau P, Blakely EL, Stewart JD, He L, Schaefer AM, Griffiths PG, Ahlqvist K, Suomalainen A, Reynier P, McFarland R, Turnbull DM, Chinnery PF, Taylor RW (2008) Mutation of OPA1 causes dominant optic atrophy with external ophthalmoplegia, ataxia, deafness and multiple mitochondrial DNA deletions: a novel disorder of mtDNA maintenance. Brain 131:329–337

Inbal A, Avissar N, Shaklai M, Kuritzky A, Schejter A, Ben-David E, Shanske S, Garty BZ (1995) Myopathy, lactic acidosis, and sideroblastic anemia: a new syndrome. Am J Med Genet 55:372–378

Isohanni P, Linnankivi T, Buzkova J, Lönnqvist T, Pihko H, Valanne L, Tienari PJ, Elovaara I, Pirttilä T, Reunanen M, Koivisto K, Marjavaara S, Suomalainen A (2010) DARS2 mutations in mitochondrial leucoencephalopathy and multiple sclerosis. J Med Genet 47:66–70

Jansen PH, van der Knaap MS, de Coo IF (1996) Leber's hereditary optic neuropathy with the 11 778 mtDNA mutation and white matter disease resembling multiple sclerosis: clinical, MRI and MRS findings. J Neurol Sci 135:176–180

Jones CN, Jones CI, Graham WD, Agris PF, Spremulli LL (2008) A disease-causing point mutation in human mitochondrial tRNAMet results in tRNA misfolding leading to defects in translational initiation and elongation. J Biol Chem 283:34445–34456

Kang N, Jun AH, Bhutia YD, Kannan N, Unadkat JD, Govindarajan R (2010) Human equilibrative nucleoside transporter-3 (hENT3) spectrum disorder mutations impair nucleoside transport, protein localization, and stability. J Biol Chem 285:28343–28352

Kaukonen J, Juselius JK, Tiranti V, Kyttala A, Zeviani M, Comi GP, Keranen S, Peltonen L, Suomalainen A (2000) Role of adenine nucleotide translocator 1 in mtDNA maintenance. Science 289:782–785

Kellar-Wood H, Robertson N, Govan GG, Compston DA, Harding AE (1994) Leber's hereditary optic neuropathy mitochondrial DNA mutations in multiple sclerosis. Ann Neurol 36:109–112

Kollberg G, Moslemi AR, Darin N, Nennesmo I, Bjarnadottir I, Uvebrant P et al (2006) POLG1 mutations associated with progressive encephalopathy in childhood. J Neuropathol Exp Neurol 65:758–768

Lee HF, Lee HJ, Chi CS, Tsai CR, Chang TK, Wang CJ (2007) The neurological evolution of Pearson syndrome: case report and literature review. Eur J Paediatr Neurol 11:208–214

Leonard JV, Schapira AVH (2000a) Mitochondrial respiratory chain disorders I: mitochondrial DNA defects. Lancet 355:299–304

Leonard JV, Schapira AVH (2000b) Mitochondrial respiratory chain disorders II: neurodegenerative disorders and nuclear gene defects. Lancet 355:389–394

Leshinsky-Silver E, Levine A, Nissenkorn A, Barash V, Perach M, Buzhaker E et al (2003) Neonatal liver failure and Leigh syndrome possibly due to CoQ-responsive OXPHOS deficiency. Mol Genet Metab 79:288–293

Liguori M, La Russa A, Manna I, Andreoli V, Caracciolo M, Spadafora P, Cittadella R, Quattrone A (2008) A phenotypic variation of dominant optic atrophy and deafness (ADOAD) due to a novel OPA1 mutation. J Neurol 255:127–129

Lissens W, De Meirleir L, Seneca S, Liebaers I, Brown GK, Brown RM, Ito M, Naito E, Kuroda Y, Kerr DS, Wexler ID, Patel MS, Robinson BH, Seyda A (2000) Mutations in the X-linked pyruvate dehydrogenase (E1) alpha subunit gene (PDHA1) in patients with a pyruvate dehydrogenase complex deficiency. Hum Mutat 15:209–219

Lodi R, Tonon C, Valentino ML, Manners D, Testa C, Malucelli E, La Morgia C, Barboni P, Carbonelli M, Schimpf S, Wissinger B, Zeviani M, Baruzzi A, Liguori R, Barbiroli B, Carelli V (2011) Defective mitochondrial adenosine triphosphate production in skeletal muscle from patients with dominant optic atrophy due to OPA1 mutations. Arch Neurol 68(1):67–73

Loiseau D, Chevrollier A, Verny C, Guillet V, Gueguen N, Pou de Crescenzo MA, Ferré M, Malinge MC, Guichet A, Nicolas G, Amati-Bonneau P, Malthièry Y, Bonneau D, Reynier P (2007) Mitochondrial coupling defect in Charcot-Marie-Tooth type 2A disease. Ann Neurol 61:315–323

Lönnqvist T, Paetau A, Nikali K, von Boguslawski K, Pihko H (1998) Infantile onset spinocerebellar ataxia with sensory neuropathy (IOSCA): neuropathological features. J Neurol Sci 161:57–65

Luoma P, Melberg A, Rinne JO, Kaukonen JA, Nupponen NN, Chalmers RM, Oldfors A, Rautakorpi I, Peltonen L, Majamaa K, Somer H, Suomalainen A (2004) Parkinsonism, premature menopause, and mitochondrial DNA polymerase gamma mutations: clinical and molecular genetic study. Lancet 364:875–882

Maguire A, Hellier K, Hammans S, May A (2001) X-linked cerebellar ataxia and sideroblastic anaemia associated with a missense mutation in the ABC7 gene predicting V411L. Br J Haematol 115:910–917

Makino M, Horai S, Goto Y, Nonaka I (1998) Confirmation that a T-to-C mutation at 9176 in mitochondrial DNA is an additional candidate mutation for Leigh's syndrome. Neuromuscl Disord 8:149–151

Malfatti E, Cardaioli E, Battisti C, Da Pozzo P, Malandrini A, Rufa A, Rocchi R, Federico A (2010) A novel point mutation in the mitochondrial tRNA((Trp)) gene produces late-onset encephalomyopathy, plus additional features. J Neurol Sci 297:105–108

Man PY, Turnbull DM, Chinnery PF (2002) Leber hereditary optic neuropathy. J Med Genet 39:162–169

Mancuso M, Filosto M, Mootha VK, Rocchi A, Pistolesi S, Murri L, DiMauro S, Siciliano G (2004) A novel mitochondrial tRNAPhe mutation causes MERRF syndrome. Neurology 62:2119–2121

Mancuso M, Ferraris S, Pancrudo J, Feigenbaum A, Raiman J, Christodoulou J, Thorburn DR, DiMauro S (2005) New DGK gene mutations in the hepatocerebral form of mitochondrial DNA depletion syndrome. Arch Neurol 62:745–747

Marti R, Spinazzola A, Nishino I, Andreu AL, Naini A, Tadesse S, Oliver JA, Hirano M (2002) Mitochondrial neurogastrointestinal encephalomyopathy and thymidine metabolism: results and hypotheses. Mitochondrion 2:143–147

Martí R, Spinazzola A, Tadesse S, Nishino I, Nishigaki Y, Hirano M (2004) Definitive diagnosis of mitochondrial neurogastrointestinal encephalomyopathy by biochemical assays. Clin Chem 50:120–124

Mayr JA, Merkel O, Kohlwein SD, Gebhardt BR, Böhles H, Fötschl U, Koch J, Jaksch M, Lochmüller H, Horváth R, Freisinger P, Sperl W (2007) Mitochondrial phosphate-carrier deficiency: a novel disorder of oxidative phosphorylation. Am J Hum Genet 80:478–484

McFarland R, Taylor RW, Turnbull DM (2010) A neurological perspective on mitochondrial disease. Lancet Neurol 9:829–840

McShane MA, Hammans SR, Sweeney M, Holt IJ, Beattie TJ, Brett EM et al (1991) Pearson syndrome and mitochondrial encephalomyopathy in a patient with a deletion of mtDNA. Am J Hum Genet 48:39–42

Medlej R, Wasson J, Baz P, Azar S, Salti I, Loiselet J et al (2004) Diabetes mellitus and optic atrophy: a study of Wolfram syndrome in the Lebanese population. J Clin Endocrinol Metab 89:1656–1661

Millar DS, Tysoe C, Lazarou LP, Pilz DT, Mohammed S, Anderson K, Chuzhanova N, Cooper DN, Butler R (2010) An isolated case of lissencephaly caused by the insertion of a mitochondrial genome-derived DNA sequence into the 5′ untranslated region of the PAFAH1B1 (LIS1) gene. Hum Genomics 4:384–393

Miller C, Saada A, Shaul N, Shabtai N, Ben-Shalom E, Shaag A, Hershkovitz E, Elpeleg O (2004) Defective mitochondrial translation caused by a ribosomal protein (MRPS16) mutation. Ann Neurol 56:734–738

Milone M, Brunetti-Pierri N, Tang LY, Kumar N, Mezei MM, Josephs K et al (2008) Sensory ataxic neuropathy with ophthalmoparesis caused by POLG mutations. Neuromuscl Disord 18:626–632

Misko A, Jiang S, Wegorzewska I, Milbrandt J, Baloh RH (2010) Mitofusin 2 is necessary for transport of axonal mitochondria and interacts with the Miro/Milton complex. J Neurosci 30:4232–4240

Mollet J, Delahodde A, Serre V et al (2008) CABC1 gene mutations cause ubiquinone deficiency with cerebellar ataxia and seizures. Am J Hum Genet 82:623–630

Montero R, Pineda M, Aracil A, Vilaseca MA, Briones P, Sánchez-Alcázar JA et al (2007) Clinical, biochemical and molecular aspects of cerebellar ataxia and Coenzyme Q10 deficiency. Cerebellum 6:118–122

Mootha VK, Lepage P, Miller K, Bunkenborg J, Reich M, Hjerrild M, Delmonte T, Villeneuve A, Sladek R, Xu F, Mitchell GA, Morin C, Mann M, Hudson TJ, Robinson B, Rioux JD, Lander ES (2003) Identification of a gene causing human cytochrome c oxidase deficiency by integrative genomics. Proc Natl Acad Sci U S A 100:605–610

Morán M, Marín-Buera L, Gil-Borlado MC, Rivera H, Blázquez A, Seneca S, Vázquez-López M, Arenas J, Martín MA, Ugalde C (2010) Cellular pathophysiologicalconsequences of BCS1L mutations in mitochondrial complex III enzyme deficiency. Hum Mutat 31:930–941

Morgan NV, Morris MR, Cangul H, Gleeson D, Straatman-Iwanowska A, Davies N, Keenan S, Pasha S, Rahman F, Gentle D, Vreeswijk MP, Devilee P, Knowles MA, Ceylaner S, Trembath RC, Dalence C, Kismet E, Köseo lu V, Rossbach HC, Gissen P, Tannahill D, Maher ER (2010) Mutations in SLC29A3, encoding an equilibrative nucleoside transporter ENT3, cause a familial histiocytosis syndrome (Faisalabad histiocytosis) and familial Rosai-Dorfman disease. PLoS Genet 6:e1000833

Naini AB, Lu J, Kaufmann P, Bernstein RA, Mancuso M, Bonilla E, Hirano M, DiMauro S (2005) Novel mitochondrial DNA ND5 mutation in a patient with clinical features of MELAS and MERRF. Arch Neurol 62:473–476

Namavar Y, Barth PG, Kasher PR, van Ruissen F, Brockmann K, Bernert G, Writzl K, Ventura K, Cheng EY, Ferriero DM, Basel-Vanagaite L, Eggens VR, Krägeloh-Mann I, De Meirleir L, King M, Graham JM Jr, von Moers A, Knoers N, Sztriha L, Korinthenberg R, Consortium P, Dobyns WB, Baas F, Poll-The BT (2011) Clinical, neuroradiological and genetic findings in pontocerebellar hypoplasia. Brain 134(1):143–156

Naumann M, Kiefer R, Toyka KV, Sommer C, Seibel P, Reichmann H (1997) Mitochondrial dysfunction with myoclonus epilepsy and ragged-red fibers point mutation in nerve, muscle, and adipose tissue of a patient with multiple symmetric lipomatosis. Muscle Nerve 20:833–839

Naviaux RK, Nguyen KV (2005) POLG mutations associated with Alpers syndrome and mitochondrial DNA depletion. Ann Neurol 58:491

Nicolino M, Ferlin T, Forest M, Godinot C, Carrier H, David M, Chatelain P, Mousson B (1997) Identification of a large-scale mitochondrial deoxyribonucleic acid deletion in endocrinopathies and deafness: report of two unrelated cases with diabetes mellitus and adrenal insufficiency, respectively. J Clin Endocrinol Metab 82:3063–3067

Nijveldt R, Serne EH, Sepers JM et al (2004) A man with diabetes and heart failure. Lancet 364:636

Nikali K, Suomalainen A, Saharinen J, Kuokkanen M, Spelbrink JN, Lönnqvist T et al (2005) Infantile onset spinocerebellar ataxia is caused by recessive mutations in mitochondrial proteins Twinkle and Twinky. Hum Mol Genet 14:2981–2990

Nikoskelainen EK (1994) Clinical picture of LHON. Clin Neurosci 2:115–120

Nikoskelainen EK, Marttila RJ, Huoponen K, Juvonen V, Lamminen T, Sonninen P, Savontaus ML (1995) Leber's "plus": neurological abnormalities in patients with Leber's hereditary optic neuropathy. J Neurol Neurosurg Psychiatry 59:160–164

Nishigaki Y, Tadesse S, Bonilla E, Shungu D, Hersh S, Keats BJ, Berlin CI, Goldberg MF, Vockley J, DiMauro S, Hirano M (2003) A novel mitochondrial tRNA(Leu(UUR)) mutation in a patient with features of MERRF and Kearns-Sayre syndrome. Neuromuscul Disord 13:334–340

Nishigaki Y, Marti R, Hirano M (2004) ND5 is a hot-spot for multiple atypical mitochondrial DNA deletions in mitochondrial neurogastrointestinal encephalomyopathy. Hum Mol Genet 13:91–101

Nishino I, Spinazzola A, Hirano M (1999) Thymidine phosphorylase gene mutations in MNGIE, a human mitochondrial disorder. Science 283:689–692

Nishino I, Spinazzola A, Papadimitriou A, Hammans S, Steiner I, Hahn CD, Connolly AM, Verloes A, Guimaraes J, Maillard I, Hamano H, Donati MA, Semrad CE, Russell JA, Andreu AL, Hadjigeorgiou GM, Vu TH, Tadesse S, Nygaard TG, Nonaka I, Hirano I, Bonilla E, Rowland LP, DiMauro S, Hirano M (2000) Mitochondrial neurogastrointestinal encephalomyopathy: an autosomal recessive disorder due to thymidine phosphorylase mutations. Ann Neurol 47:792–800

Nishioka K, Vilariño-Güell C, Cobb SA, Kachergus JM, Ross OA, Hentati E, Hentati F, Farrer MJ (2010) Genetic variation of the mitochondrial complex I subunit NDUFV2 and Parkinson disease. Parkinsonism Relat Disord 16(10):686–687

Ortiz RG, Newman NJ, Shoffner JM, Kaufman AE, Koontz DA, Wallace DC (1993) Variable retinal and neurologic manifestations in patients harboring the mitochondrial DNA 8993 mutation. Arch Ophthalmol 111:1525–1530

Osman C, Haag M, Wieland FT, Brügger B, Langer T (2010) A mitochondrial phosphatase required for cardiolipin biosynthesis: the PGP phosphatase Gep4. EMBO J 29:1976–1987

Ostergaard E, Christensen E, Kristensen E, Mogensen B, Duno M, Shoubridge EA, Wibrand F (2007) Deficiency of the alpha subunit of succinate-coenzyme A ligase causes fatal infantile lactic acidosis with mitochondrial DNA depletion. Am J Hum Genet 81:383–387

Patton JR, Bykhovskaya Y, Mengesha E, Bertolotto C, Fischel-Ghodsian N (2005) Mitochondrial myopathy and sideroblastic anemia (MLASA): missense mutation in the pseudouridine synthase 1 (PUS1) gene is associated with the loss of tRNA pseudouridylation. J Biol Chem 280:19823–19828

Peng Y, Crumley R, Ringman JM (2003) Spasmodic dysphonia in a patient with the A to G transition at nucleotide 8344 in mitochondrial DNA. Mov Disord 18:716–718

Pondarre C, Campagna DR, Antiochos B, Sikorski L, Mulhern H, Fleming MD (2007) Abcb7, the gene responsible for X-linked sideroblastic anemia with ataxia, is essential for hematopoiesis. Blood 109:3567–3569

Poulton J, Macaulay V, Marchington DR (1998) Mitochondrial genetics '98 is the bottleneck cracked? Am J Hum Genet 62:752–757

Pupo AC, Pirana S, Spinelli M, Lezirovitz K, Mingroni Netto RC, Macedo LS (2008) Study of a Brazilian family presenting non-syndromic hearing loss with mitochondrial inheritance. Braz J Otorhinolaryngol 74:786–789

Quinzii CM, López LC, Naini A, DiMauro S, Hirano M (2008) Human CoQ10 deficiencies. Biofactors 32:113–118

Rahman S, Blok RB, Dahl HH, Danks DM, Kirby DM, Chow CW, Christodoulou J, Thorburn DR (1996) Leigh syndrome: clinical features and biochemical and DNA abnormalities. Ann Neurol 39:343–351

Rankin J, Brown R, Dobyns WB, Harington J, Patel J, Quinn M, Brown G (2010) Pontocerebellar hypoplasia type 6: a British case with PEHO-like features. Am J Med Genet A 152A:2079–2084

Rantamäki M, Luoma P, Virta JJ, Rinne JO, Paetau A, Suomalainen A et al (2007) Do carriers of POLG mutation W748S have disease manifestations? Clin Genet 72:532–537

Ricci E, Moraes CT, Servidei S, Tonali P, Bonilla E, DiMauro S (1992) Disorders associated with depletion of mitochondrial DNA. Brain Pathol 2:141–147

Riera AR, Kaiser E, Levine P, Schapachnik E, Dubner S, Ferreira C et al (2008) Kearns-Sayre syndrome: electrovectorcardiographic evolution for left septal fascicular block of the his bundle. J Electrocardiol 41:675–678

Riley LG, Cooper S, Hickey P, Rudinger-Thirion J, McKenzie M, Compton A, Lim SC, Thorburn D, Ryan MT, Giegé R, Bahlo M, Christodoulou J (2010) Mutation of the mitochondrial tyrosyl-tRNA synthetase gene, YARS2, causes myopathy, lactic acidosis, and sideroblastic anemia–MLASA syndrome. Am J Hum Genet 87:52–59

Roesch K, Curran SP, Tranebjaerg L et al (2002) Human deafness dystonia syndrome is caused by a defect in assembly of the DDP1/TIMM8a-TIMM13 complex. Hum Mol Genet 11:477–486

Rossi A, Biancheri R, Bruno C, Di Rocco M, Calvi A, Pessagno A, Tortori-Donati P (2003) Leigh Syndrome with COX deficiency and SURF1 gene mutations: MR imaging findings. Am J Neuroradiol 24:1188–1191

Rydzanicz M, Wróbel M, Pollak A, Gawecki W, Brauze D, Kostrzewska-Poczekaj M, Wojsyk-Banaszak I, Lechowicz U, Mueller-Malesińska M, Ołdak M, Płoski R, Skarzy ski H, Szyfter K (2010) Mutation analysis of mitochondrial 12S rRNA gene in Polish patients with non-syndromic and aminoglycoside-induced hearing loss. Biochem Biophys Res Commun 395:116–121

Saada A, Shaag A, Mandel H, Nevo Y, Eriksson S, Elpeleg O (2001) Mutant mitochondrial thymidine kinase in mitochondrial DNA depletion myopathy. Nat Genet 29:342–344

Saada A, Edvardson S, Rapoport M, Shaag A, Amry K, Miller C, Lorberboum-Galski H, Elpeleg O (2008) C6ORF66 is an assembly factor of mitochondrial complex I. Am J Hum Genet 82:32–38

Sadun AA, Salomao SR, Berezovsky A, Sadun F, Denegri AM, Quiros PA, Chicani F, Ventura D, Barboni P, Sherman J, Sutter E, Belfort R Jr, Carelli V (2006) Subclinical carriers and conversions in Leber hereditary optic neuropathy: a prospective psychophysical study. Trans Am Ophthalmol Soc 104:51–61

Santorelli FM, Tanji K, Shanske S, DiMauro S (1997) Heterogeneous clinical presentation of the mtDNA NARP/T8993G mutation. Neurology 49:270–273

Sarzi E, Bourdon A, Chrétien D, Zarhrate M, Corcos J, Slama A, Cormier-Daire V, de Lonlay P, Munnich A, Rötig A (2007) Mitochondrial DNA depletion is a prevalent cause of multiple respiratory chain deficiency in childhood. J Pediatr 150:531–534

Scharfe C, Hauschild M, Klopstock T, Janssen AJ, Heidemann PH, Meitinger T, Jaksch M (2000) A novel mutation in the thiamine responsive megaloblastic anaemia gene SLC19A2 in a patient with deficiency of respiratory chain complex I. J Med Genet 37:669–673

Scheper GC, van der Klok T, van Andel RJ, van Berkel CG, Sissler M, Smet J et al (2007) Mitochondrial aspartyl-tRNA synthetase deficiency causes leukoencephalopathy with brain stem and spinal cord involvement and lactate elevation. Nat Genet 39:534–539

Smits P, Antonicka H, van Hasselt PM, Weraarpachai W, Haller W, Schreurs M, Venselaar H, Rodenburg RJ, Smeitink JA, van den Heuvel LP (2011) Mutation in subdomain G' of mitochondrial elongation factor G1 is associated with combined OXPHOSdeficiency in fibroblasts but not in muscle. Eur J Hum Genet 19(3):275–279

Spector R, Johanson CE (2010) Choroid plexus failure in the Kearns-Sayre syndrome. Cerebrospinal Fluid Res 7:14

Spelbrink JN, Li FY, Tiranti V, Nikali K, Yuan QP, Tariq M, Wanrooij S, Garrido N, Comi G, Morandi L, Santoro L, Toscano A, Fabrizi GM, Somer H, Croxen R, Beeson D, Poulton J, Suomalainen A, Jacobs HT, Zeviani M, Larsson C (2001) Human mitochondrial DNA deletions associated with mutations in the gene encoding Twinkle, a phage T7 gene 4-like protein localized in mitochondria. Nat Genet 28:223–231

Spencer CT, Bryant RM, Day J, Gonzalez IL, Colan SD, Thompson WR et al (2006) Cardiac and clinical phenotype in Barth syndrome. Pediatrics 118:e337–e346

Spiegel R, Shaag A, Mandel H, Reich D, Penyakov M, Hujeirat Y, Saada A, Elpeleg O, Shalev SA (2009a) Mutated NDUFS6 is the cause of fatal neonatal lactic acidemia in Caucasus Jews. Eur J Hum Genet 17:1200–1203

Spiegel R, Shaag A, Edvardson S, Mandel H, Stepensky P, Shalev SA, Horovitz Y, Pines O, Elpeleg O (2009b) SLC25A19 mutation as a cause of neuropathy and bilateral striatal necrosis. Ann Neurol 66:419–424

Spinazzola A, Zeviani M (2007) Disorders of nuclear-mitochondrial intergenomic communication. Biosci Rep 27:39–51

Spinazzola A, Viscomi C, Fernandez-Vizarra E, Carrara F, D'Adamo P, Calvo S, Marsano RM, Donnini C, Weiher H, Strisciuglio P, Parini R, Sarzi E, Chan A, DiMauro S, Rötig A, Gasparini P, Ferrero I, Mootha VK, Tiranti V, Zeviani M (2006) MPV17 encodes an inner mitochondrial membrane protein and is mutated in infantile hepatic mitochondrial DNA depletion. Nat Genet 38:570–575

Spruijt L, Smeets HJ, Hendrickx A, Bettink-Remeijer MW, Maat-Kievit A, Schoonderwoerd KC, Sluiter W, de Coo IF, Hintzen RQ (2007) A MELAS-associated ND1 mutation causing leber hereditary optic neuropathy and spastic dystonia. Arch Neurol 64:890–893

Sugiana C, Pagliarini DJ, McKenzie M, Kirby DM, Salemi R, Abu-Amero KK, Dahl HH, Hutchison WM, Vascotto KA, Smith SM, Newbold RF, Christodoulou J, Calvo S, Mootha VK, Ryan MT, Thorburn DR (2008) Mutation of C20orf7 disrupts complex I assembly and causes lethal neonatal mitochondrial disease. Am J Hum Genet 83:468–478

Tay SK, Sacconi S, Akman HO, Morales JF, Morales A, De Vivo DC, Shanske S, Bonilla E, DiMauro S (2005) Unusual clinical presentations in four cases of Leigh disease, Cytochrome C oxidase deficiency, and SURF1 gene mutations. J Child Neurol 20:670–674

Tay SH, Nordli DR Jr, Bonilla E, Null E, Monaco S, Hirano M, DiMauro S (2006) Aortic rupture in mitochondrial encephalopathy, lactic acidosis, and stroke-likeepisodes. Arch Neurol 63:281–283

Teitelbaum JE, Berde CB, Nurko S, Buonomo C, Perez-Atayde AR, Fox VL (2002) Diagnosis and management of MNGIE syndrome in children: case report and review of the literature. J Pediatr Gastroenterol Nutr 35:377–383

Thorburn DR, Rahman S (2006) Mitochondrial DNA-Associated Leigh Syndrome and NARP, 2003 (updated 2006). In: Pagon RA, Bird TC, Dolan CR, Stephens K (eds) GeneReviews (Internet). University of Washington, Seattle, WA, 1993-. Available from http://www.ncbi.nlm.nih.gov/bookshelf/br.fcgi?book=gene&part=narp

Tranebjaerg L, Elverland HH, Fagerheim T (2000) DFNA7. Adv Otorhinolaryngol 56:97–100

Tsao CY, Herman G, Boué DR et al (2003) Leigh disease with mitochondrial DNA A8344G mutation: case report and brief review. J Child Neurol 18:62–64

Tzoulis C, Engelsen BA, Telstad W, Aasly J, Zeviani M, Winterthun S, Ferrari G, Aarseth JH, Bindoff LA (2006) The spectrum of clinical disease caused by the A467T and W748S POLG mutations: a study of 26 cases. Brain 129:1685–1692

Valente L, Tiranti V, Marsano RM, Malfatti E, Fernandez-Vizarra E, Donnini C, Mereghetti P, De Gioia L, Burlina A, Castellan C, Comi GP, Savasta S, Ferrero I, Zeviani M (2007) Infantile encephalopathy and defective mitochondrial DNA translation in patients with mutations of mitochondrial elongation factors EFG1 and EFTu. Am J Hum Genet 80:44–58

Valnot I, Osmond S, Gigarel N, Mehaye B, Amiel J, Cormier-Daire V, Munnich A, Bonnefont JP, Rustin P, Rötig A (2000) Mutations of the SCO1 gene in mitochondrial cytochrome c oxidase deficiency with neonatal-onset hepatic failure and encephalopathy. Am J Hum Genet 67:1104–1109

van de Glind G, de Vries M, Rodenburg R, Hol F, Smeitink J, Morava E (2007) Resting muscle pain as the first clinical symptom in children carrying the MTTK A8344G mutation. Eur J Paediatr Neurol 11:243–246

Van den Ouweland JM, Lemkes HH, Gerbitz KD et al (1995) Maternally inherited diabetes and deafness (MIDD): a distinct subtype of diabetes associated with a mitochondrial tRNA(Leu)(UUR) gene point mutation. Muscle Nerve 3:S124–S130

Van Goethem G, Dermaut B, Löfgren A, Martin JJ, Van Broeckhoven C (2001) Mutation of POLG is associated with progressive external ophthalmoplegia characterized by mtDNA deletions. Nat Genet 28:211–212

Verny C, Guegen N, Desquiret V, Chevrollier A, Prundean A, Dubas F, Cassereau J, Ferre M, Amati-Bonneau P, Bonneau D, Reynier P, Procaccio V (2011) Hereditary spastic paraplegia-like disorder due to a mitochondrial ATP6 gene point mutation. Mitochondrion 11(1):70–75

Walter MC, Czermin B, Muller-Ziermann S, Bulst S, Stewart JD, Hudson G, Schneiderat P, Abicht A, Holinski-Feder E, Lochmüller H, Chinnery PF, Klopstock T, Horvath R (2010) Late-onset ptosis and myopathy in a patient with a heterozygous insertion in POLG2. J Neurol 257:1517–1523

Waterham HR, Koster J, van Roermund CW, Mooyer PA, Wanders RJ, Leonard JV (2007) A lethal defect of mitochondrial and peroxisomal fission. N Engl J Med 356:1736–1741

Weraarpachai W, Antonicka H, Sasarman F, Seeger J, Schrank B, Kolesar JE, Lochmüller H, Chevrette M, Kaufman BA, Horvath R, Shoubridge EA (2009) Mutation in TACO1, encoding a translational activator of COX I, results in cytochrome c oxidase deficiency and late-onset Leigh syndrome. Nat Genet 41:833–837

Wiedemann FR, Bartels C, Kirches E, Mawrin C, Wallesch CW (2008) Unusual presentations of patients with the mitochondrial MERRF mutation A8344G. Clin Neurol Neurosurg 110:859–863

Wong LJ, Naviaux RK, Brunetti-Pierri N, Zhang Q, Schmitt ES, Truong C, Milone M, Cohen BH, Wical B, Ganesh J, Basinger AA, Burton BK, Swoboda K, Gilbert DL, Vanderver A, Saneto RP, Maranda B, Arnold G, Abdenur JE, Waters PJ, Copeland WC (2008) Molecular and clinical genetics of mitochondrial diseases due to POLG mutations. Hum Mutat 29:E150–E172

Worle H, Kohler B, Schlote W, Winkler P, Bastanier CK (1998) Progressive cerebral degeneration of childhood with liver disease (Alpers-Huttenlocher disease) with cytochrome oxidase deficiency presenting with epilepsia partialis continua as the first clinical manifestation. Clin Neuropathol 17:63–68

Young TM, Blakely EL, Swalwell H, Carter JE, Kartsounis LD, O'Donovan DG, Turnbull DM, Taylor RW, de Silva RN (2010) Mitochondrial transfer RNA(Phe) mutation associated with a progressive neurodegenerative disorder characterized bypsychiatric disturbance, dementia, and akinesia-rigidity. Arch Neurol 67:1399–1402

Zeharia A, Fischel-Ghodsian N, Casas K, Bykhocskaya Y, Tamari H, Lev D, Mimouni M, Lerman-Sagie T (2005) Mitochondrial myopathy, sideroblastic anemia, and lactic acidosis: an autosomal recessive syndrome in Persian Jews caused by a mutation in the PUS1 gene. J Child Neurol 20:449–452

Zeharia A, Shaag A, Pappo O, Mager-Heckel AM, Saada A, Beinat M, Karicheva O, Mandel H, Ofek N, Segel R, Marom D, Rötig A, Tarassov I, Elpeleg O (2009) Acute infantile liver failure due to mutations in the TRMU gene. Am J Hum Genet 85:401–407

Zoccolella S, Torraco A, Amati A, Lamberti P, Serlenga L, Papa S et al (2006) Unusual clinical presentation of a patient carrying a novel single 1.8 kb deletion of mitochondrial DNA. Funct Neurol 21:39–41

Chapter 9
Role of Mitochondrial Function in Insulin Resistance

Myrte Brands, Arthur J. Verhoeven, and Mireille J. Serlie

Abstract The obesity pandemic increases the prevalence of type 2 diabetes (DM2).
DM2 develops when pancreatic β-cells fail and cannot compensate for the decrease in insulin sensitivity. How excessive caloric intake and weight gain cause insulin resistance has not completely been elucidated.

Skeletal muscle is responsible for a major part of insulin stimulated whole-body glucose disposal and, hence, plays an important role in the pathogenesis of insulin resistance.

It has been hypothesized that skeletal muscle mitochondrial dysfunction is involved in the accumulation of intramyocellular lipid metabolites leading to lipotoxicity and insulin resistance. However, findings on skeletal muscle mitochondrial function in relation to insulin resistance in human subjects are inconclusive. Differences in mitochondrial activity can be the result of several factors, including a reduced mitochondrial density, differences in insulin stimulated mitochondrial respiration, lower energy demand or reduced skeletal muscle perfusion, besides an intrinsic mitochondrial defect. The inconclusive results may be explained by the use of different techniques and study populations. Also, mitochondrial capacity is in far excess to meet energy requirements and therefore it may be questioned whether a reduced mitochondrial capacity limits mitochondrial fatty acid oxidation. Whether reduced mitochondrial function is causally related to insulin resistance or rather a consequence of the sedentary lifestyle remains to be elucidated.

Keywords Mitochondrial function • Oxidative phosphorylation • Obesity • Insulin resistance • Free fatty acids • Lipotoxicity

9.1 Introduction

The obesity pandemic is associated with an increase in the prevalence of type 2 diabetes mellitus (DM2). DM2 is characterized by insulin resistance and β-cell failure. Insulin sensitivity decreases during weight gain. This decrease in insulin sensitivity is accompanied by increased insulin secretion

M.J. Serlie (✉) • M. Brands
Department of Endocrinology and Metabolism, Academic Medical Center, F5-167, Meibergdreef 9,
1105 AZ, Amsterdam, The Netherlands
e-mail: M.J.Serlie@amc.uva.nl; M.Brands@amc.uva.nl

A.J. Verhoeven
Department of medical Biochemistry, Academic Medical Centre, Amsterdam, The Netherlands

R. Scatena et al. (eds.), *Advances in Mitochondrial Medicine*, Advances in Experimental
Medicine and Biology 942, DOI 10.1007/978-94-007-2869-1_9,
© Springer Science+Business Media B.V. 2012

to compensate for the insulin resistance. DM2 develops when β-cell function fails to further increase insulin secretion (Bergman 2007, 1489–501). The skeletal muscle is responsible for the major part (80%) of insulin-stimulated whole body glucose disposal, and hence plays an important role in the pathogenesis of insulin resistance (Boden 2002, 545–49; DeFronzo et al. 1985, 149–55). Insulin resistance precedes the onset of DM2. Therefore it is of great importance to gain more insight in the pathophysiology of insulin resistance.

Obese insulin resistant individuals are characterized by increased plasma free fatty acids (FFA) concentrations, an elevated basal rate of lipolysis and impaired suppression of lipolysis by insulin (Koutsari and Jensen 2006, 1643–50). Increased levels of FFA may directly mediate the development of insulin resistance since it was shown that plasma FFA concentration correlates with the degree of insulin resistance and experimental elevation of plasma FFA in young healthy individuals induces insulin resistance (Belfort et al. 2005, 1640–48). How increased FFA cause insulin resistance has not been completely elucidated. A growing body of evidence shows that nutrient overload causes accumulation of specific intramyocellular FFA metabolites. These metabolites interfere with the insulin signalling cascade and the glucose transporter GLUT 4 resulting in decreased insulin-mediated glucose uptake (Shulman 2000, 171–76).

Over the last decade it has been hypothesized that mitochondrial dysfunction is involved in the accumulation of these intramyocellular lipid metabolites leading to lipotoxicity and insulin resistance (Roden 2005, S111–S115). However not all studies report decreased mitochondrial capacity in relation to insulin resistance (Hancock et al. 2008, 7815–20; Holloway et al. 2007, E1782–E1789; Karakelides et al. 2010, 89–97; Nair et al. 2008, 1166–75; Toledo et al. 2008, 987–94; De Feyter et al. 2008, 643–53). This may be explained by the use of different techniques and study populations. In addition, insulin stimulates mitochondrial activity. This stimulation is decreased in obese individuals, and has been reported to be blunted in DM2 subjects (Asmann et al. 2006, 3309–19; Stump et al. 2003, 7996–8001). Therefore, decreased mitochondrial activity may not be an intrinsic mitochondrial defect but a functional defect related to an impaired insulin response. Furthermore, lower mitochondrial capacity in insulin resistant subjects could be a reflection of decreased mitochondrial content instead of an impaired mitochondrial function (Boushel et al. 2007, 790–96; Rabol et al. 2010, 857–63). A reduction in mitochondrial content may be caused by a decline in physical activity. Therefore decreased mitochondrial function could be more a consequence then a cause of the obese insulin-resistant state (Holloszy 2009, 463S–6S).

In this chapter we will summarize recent findings on mitochondrial function in DM2, obese and lean human subjects measured by different methods, and discuss whether impaired mitochondrial function is a cause or a consequence of obesity-induced insulin resistance.

9.1.1 Mitochondrial Function

Mitochondria are the energy producing organelles of the cell. All human cells, except the red blood cell, depend on the aerobe degradation of nutrients in the mitochondria for sufficient energy supply. A mitochondrion consists of a lipid bilayer of membranes: the inner and the outer mitochondrial membrane. The space between both layers is called the intermembrane space, the space surrounded by the inner membrane is called the matrix. The inner membrane is heavily folded into so-called cristae, possibly facilitating the coupling between the respiratory chain complexes (Wittig and Schagger 2009, 672–80).

In the matrix two important biochemical processes occur, i.e. (1) degradation of fatty acids (β-oxidation) and (2) oxidation of pyruvate and acetyl-coA in the tricarboxylic acid cycle (TCA cycle). These processes generate the energy-rich molecules NADH and FADH2.

The energy of these molecules is used by the electron transport chain located in the inner mitochondrial membrane to transport protons (H^+) into the intermembrane space. The proton gradient over the inner mitochondrial membrane is the driving force for the mitochondrial ATP production. When protons return to the matrix via the ATP-synthase complex (complex V), ADP is phosphorylated on the matrix side of complex V.

The ATP formed is transported over the inner mitochondrial membrane by the enzyme adenine nucleotide translocator (ANT). This enzyme exchanges cytosolic ADP for mitochondrial ATP. The rate of mitochondrial ATP production largely depends on the energy demand of the cell and the tightness of coupling of mitochondrial electron transport to ATP synthesis via the proton gradient across the inner mitochondrial membrane. Therefore mitochondrial function *in vivo* is defined as activity of the oxidative phosphorylation to produce ATP.

It should be noted that much of our knowledge on mitochondrial oxidative phosphorylation is derived from *in vitro* experiments with isolated mitochondria or isolated mitochondrial complexes, and that relative little information has become available on *in vivo* functioning of mitochondria.

Mitochondrial function is always the product of mitochondrial content and oxidative activity. Decreased mitochondrial function, i.e. mitochondrial dysfunction, can then be explained as an intrinsic abnormality in the respiratory chain or a decreased number of mitochondria, or both.

However, it is not always clear whether reported total mitochondrial function is corrected for differences in mitochondrial content. Furthermore, several other terms have been introduced; mitochondrial capacity, intrinsic mitochondrial function and basal mitochondrial function. Mitochondrial capacity means the capacity to upregulate mitochondrial activity under certain physiological conditions. Intrinsic mitochondrial function refers to the function of the isolated mitochondrion regardless of the regulating cellular processes. And basal function means mitochondrial function in the basal state, i.e. in a non-insulin stimulated condition. The use of these several terms in literature can be confusing.

In most studies relevant for this chapter, mitochondrial function has been measured *ex vivo* in permeabilized muscle fibers or isolated mitochondria purified from these muscle biopsies. Several techniques have been used to measure mitochondrial function.

9.2 Ex Vivo Mitochondrial Function

9.2.1 Functional Measurements

Ex vivo mitochondrial function can be measured by either oxygen consumption or ATP production. As stated above, mitochondrial ATP production depends on local energy demand. The advantage of *ex vivo* functional measurements is that mitochondrial function can be measured under specific and standardized substrate conditions. Therefore also energy demand by the addition of standardized ADP concentrations can be controlled. Furthermore, by addition of specific substrates, activity of the different complexes of the electron transport chain can be measured (Gnaiger 2009).

ATP production can be quantified in suspensions of isolated mitochondria using a bioluminescent technique that involves luciferin–luciferase ATP monitoring (Wibom et al. 2002, 139–51).

Mitochondrial ATP production measured using this latter technique in subjects with DM2 and non-diabetic obese subjects has been shown similar (Wibom et al. 2002, 139–51; Stump et al. 2003, 7996–8001; Asmann et al. 2006, 3309–19). Also in lean, insulin sensitive versus obese insulin resistant subjects matched for age no difference in mitochondrial ATP production has been found (Karakelides et al. 2010, 89–97).

Oxygen consumption can be measured in permeabilized muscle fibers or in isolated mitochondria by measuring the disappearance of oxygen using an oxygraph. Four different studies that measured mitochondrial function by oxygen consumption in DM2 subjects reported decreased oxidative respiration rates (Boushel et al. 2007, 790–96; Mogensen et al. 2007, 1592–99; Phielix et al. 2008; Rabol et al. 2010, 857–63).

In intact mitochondria (with a low permeability for protons) the amount of oxygen consumption accurately reflects the amount of ATP synthesis. However, mitochondria may also respire in the absence of ADP due to proton leak over the inner mitochondrial membrane. This is called uncoupled respiration. In rats the contribution of uncoupled respiration is significant and accounts for 16–31% of the resting metabolic rate (Rolfe and Brand 1996, C1380–C1389). In humans, the role of mitochondrial uncoupling is still unclear. It has been suggested that uncoupling is an additional process superimposed on the basic chemiosmotic model to control ATP synthesis (Boss et al. 2000, 143–56). Furthermore, mitochondrial uncoupling may serve to protect mitochondria against lipid-induced oxidative damage. It has been shown that in muscle expression of the mitochondrial uncoupling protein 3 (UCP3) is induced under high fat conditions (Schrauwen 2007, 33–41; Krook et al. 1998, 1528–31; Khalfallah et al. 2000, 25–31). This suggests that UCP3 is important in FFA-activated proton conductance, and might decrease the efficiency of oxidative phosphorylation when fatty acid supply does not match fatty acid oxidation and thereby preventing lipotoxicity. In pre-diabetic men UCP3 expression in muscle is reduced which suggests that lower expression of UCP3 might play a role in altered mitochondrial function and skeletal muscle insulin resistance (Schrauwen and Hesselink 2004, 1412–17). However, the exact physiological role of uncoupling proteins is human skeletal muscle has not been elucidated (Bao et al. 1998, 1935–40). The measurement of mitochondrial coupling can be established by either calculation of the P/O ratio or the respiratory control index. The relationship between ATP synthesis and oxygen consumption, the P/O ratio, can be measured by the addition of a known ADP concentration during the *ex vivo* measurement of mitochondrial oxygen consumption. The mean P/O ratio in isolated human quadriceps mitochondria is 3.0 (Tonkonogi and Sahlin 1997, 345–53). ATP production calculated from oxygen consumption and mitochondrial ATP synthesis as measured by the bioluminescent technique highly correlate (Tonkonogi and Sahlin 1997, 345–53). Another possibility to express the degree of coupling between oxygen consumption and ADP phosphorylation is the respiratory control index. This index compares respiration in the presence of ADP (state 3 respiration) and respiration after all the ADP has been phosphorylated (state 4 respiration). In subjects with DM2, state 4 respiration was not significantly different while state 3 respiration was decreased compared to obese controls (Mogensen et al. 2007, 1592–99). UCP3 expression in muscle was not different in this study suggesting no significant difference in uncoupled respiration between DM2 and obese individuals.

A third possibility to measure the amount of uncoupled respiration is to add a selective complex V inhibitor to the respiration medium. This abolishes ADP-stimulated respiration in intact mitochondria, while the remaining oxygen consumption reflects uncoupled respiration. Oligomycin and aurovertine are such phosphorylation inhibitors. Phielix et al. (2008) used this technique and reported that the uncoupled respiration in skeletal muscle of DM2 patients did not differ compared to BMI and age matched control subjects (Phielix et al. 2008), supporting the earlier observations by Mogensen et al. (2007, 1592–99).

ATP production, oxygen consumption, the respiratory control index and the mitochondrial P/O ratio depend not only on the degree of uncoupling, but also on the specific substrate(s) used in the experiment. Succinate for instance has a lower P/O ratio then substrates that deliver electrons to complex I. The use of physiological substrates is mandatory and optimization of the assay conditions is essential to prevent limitations (Gnaiger 2009; Rasmussen and Rasmussen 2000a, 37–44). Therefore to compare studies that measured *ex-vivo* mitochondrial function by these ex-vivo functional methods, one has to pay attention to differences in substrate fuelling.

In conclusion, direct measurement of *ex vivo* ATP synthesis as well as measurement of *ex vivo* oxygen consumption yields no significant differences in mitochondrial uncoupling while state 3 respiration seems to be reduced in DM2 subjects.

9.2.2 Mitochondrial Membrane Potential (MMP)

Mitochondrial function is driven by the proton motive force over the inner mitochondrial membrane which provides the energy for ATP synthesis. Numerous indicators have been used to monitor the membrane potential of mitochondria. These measurements are based on the distribution of a positively charged probe across the inner membrane that follows the Nernst equation (Scaduto and Grotyohann 1999, 469–77). In respiring mitochondria, such an indicator will be taken up by the mitochondria due to the negative potential inside.

Recently, fluorescent dyes have been developed for the measurement of the mitochondrial membrane potential instead of either electrodes or radioactive tracers (Scaduto and Grotyohann 1999, 469–77). This method provides a semiquantitative measurement of inner mitochondrial membrane potential and mitochondrial content in intact cells or tissue. However, this method generally only yields qualitative data and not a true estimation of the magnitude of the MMP.

We are not aware of any studies that used this method to compare insulin sensitive versus obese insulin resistant subjects. One study did, however, use this technique to measure the effect of a lipid infusion on mitochondrial function in healthy lean young men (Chavez et al. 2010, 422–29).

This study showed that a physiological increase in plasma FFA concentration during 6 h decreases the inner mitochondrial membrane potential, without altering gene expression, mitochondrial morphology, or content. Whether increased FFA indeed have a deleterious effect on mitochondrial function will be discussed below.

9.2.3 Measurement of Mitochondrial Enzymes

Mitochondrial function may also be studied by measuring the amount or activity of the enzymes involved in the respiratory chain complex. The electron transport chain (ETC) in the mitochondria consists of 5 large enzyme complexes. Each complex consists of at least 4 or more protein subunits.

The protein subunits from these complexes can be measured by immunoblotting. In overweight insulin resistant subjects the subunit protein levels in skeletal muscle were lower compared with the insulin sensitive group for each subunit measured. However, this was only statistically significant for complexes I and III (Heilbronn et al. 2007, 1467–73).

Also the enzyme activity of the different complexes can be measured. The assay for NADH oxidation by muscle mitochondria can be useful for an estimation of the activity of the entire electron transport chain and for estimation of the activity of complex I (Ritov et al. 2004, 27–38; Wibom et al. 2002, 139–51). A major challenge with the measurements of complex I and complex I + III activities is to sufficiently permeabilize the mitochondrial inner membrane to give NADH full access to its binding site at the matrix side of complex I without disrupting the integrity of the respiratory chain complexes (Rasmussen and Rasmussen 2000b, 473–80; Wibom et al. 2002, 139–51). Succinate oxidase represents mitochondria ETC activity from complexes II to IV. The enzyme-activity of NADH:O2 oxidoreductase and succinate oxidase in muscle mitochondria of DM2 patients and obese subjects compared with lean subjects has been reported to be decreased (Kelley et al. 2002, 2944–50; Ritov et al. 2005, 8–14).

Cytochrome C oxidase (COX, Complex IV) is the final electron acceptor of the mitochondrial respiratory chain. This enzyme complex catalyzes the four-electron reduction of O_2 to H_2O, while actively pumping protons from the matrix into the inter-membrane space. COX activity has been reported not to be statistically different between overweight and obese insulin resistant subjects matched for physical fitness and percentage body fat to insulin-sensitive subjects. Although, in the same study the expression of the mitochondrial encoded gene COX-1 was significantly decreased in the insulin resistant subjects (Heilbronn et al. 2007, 1467–73).

Other enzyme activities that are frequently measured regarding mitochondrial function are: creatine kinase (CK), citrate synthase (CS), succinate dehydrogenase (SDH) activity and beta-hydroxy-acyl-CoA dehydrogenase (HAD).

Activity of creatine kinase (CK) is measured as an index of muscle fiber content in biopsy samples (Kelley et al. 2002, 2944–50). Potential inclusion of connective tissue, fat, or blood could significantly affect the results of measurements of enzyme activity. Therefore, correction for CK activity instead of correction for mg wet muscle weight may be preferable (Kelley et al. 2002, 2944–50;Chi et al. 1983, C276–C287).

CS activity is a marker of nuclear expression of mitochondrial proteins, and hence a marker of mitochondrial content. However this measurement is not without limitations which will be discussed below. SDH activity is as an index for oxidative capacity. Skeletal muscle from obese and DM2 subjects had lower SDH activity than muscle from lean subjects. Furthermore lean individuals had a lower glycolytic-to-oxidative ratio. The latter was assessed by comparing the activity of the glycolytic enzyme α-GPDH to SDH activity (He et al. 2001, 817–23).

HAD is a mitochondrial enzyme that acts as an indicator of mitochondrial β-oxidation capacity. One of the first studies that measured oxidative enzyme activity in muscle of DM2 patients compared to obese normal-glycemic controls found a 30% reduction in CS activity but HAD was similar (Vondra et al. 1977, 527–29).

In conclusion, several studies found lower maximal activity of oxidative enzymes in skeletal muscle biopsies of DM2 and obese insulin resistant subjects compared to lean control subjects. Whether this relates to decreased mitochondrial capacity or mitochondrial function is not clear.

9.2.4 *Mitochondrial Morphology and Density*

The number, shape, and size of mitochondria are different for each cell type (Ogata and Yamasaki 1997, 214–23). Cells with high energy demand, like the skeletal muscle, contain up to 2,000 mitochondria while a platelet contains only 6–12 mitochondria.

Mitochondria are dynamic structures that constantly fuse and divide with other mitochondria.

Fusion serves to unify mitochondria. This enables mixing of compartments during cell development, energy dissipation, and regulation of the oxidative phosphorylation. Fission is required to promote transmission of the mitochondrial genome during mitochondrial replication and also participates in the distribution of the organelle throughout the cell (Civitarese and Ravussin 2008, 950–54). Furthermore, fission followed by selective fusion segregates dysfunctional mitochondria and permits their removal by autophagy. Fusion and fission events are strictly regulated and occur in pairs. Therefore, under most physiological conditions, mitochondrial shape and size remain relatively constant (Twig et al. 2008, 1092–97).

Electron microscopy (EM) allows quantification of mitochondrial density, size and shape.

It has been shown that mitochondrial size and total area are reduced in DM2 subjects and obese individuals compared to lean controls (Kelley et al. 2002, 2944–50). In addition, mitochondria in muscle from lean healthy volunteers have a more clearly defined internal membrane structure, including wider cristae, than those from obese and DM2 subjects (Kelley et al. 2002, 2944–50).

To conclude on impairment of mitochondrial function, the reduction in ETC activity has to be proportional greater than the decrease in mitochondrial content. Besides electron microscopy other measurements have been used to quantify mitochondrial content/density.

1. Mitochondrial-DNA (mt-DNA) content reflects the number of mitochondria (Puntschart et al. 1995, C619–C625). Mitochondrial proteins are encoded by nuclear genes, but 13 proteins that are critical in the electron transport chain are encoded in the mt-DNA. In trained athletes mt-DNA is 1.55 fold higher, but genomic DNA is not changed compared to sedentary men (Puntschart et al. 1995, C619–C625). In DM2 subjects mt-DNA content is similar to age, BMI and physical fitness matched non diabetic subjects (Phielix et al. 2008).
2. Citrate synthase is a nuclear encoded mitochondrial enzyme that is active in the mitochondrial matrix where it catalyses the first step of the Krebs cycle (Wang et al. 1999, 22–27).

    Citrate synthase activity and mt-DNA content in the vastus lateralis muscle from healthy subjects are positively correlated (Wang et al. 1999, 22–27). Endurance training increases citrate synthase activity, in parallel with mitochondrial content in healthy and DM2 subjects. However citrate synthase also increases following acute exercise (Tonkonogi et al. 1997, 435–36) or insulin stimulation (Stump et al. 2003, 7996–8001). These acute effects do not reflect changes in mitochondrial content. Therefore, measurement of mt-DNA is a more reliable marker as this is probably less sensitive to acute metabolic changes.
3. Cardiolipin is a specific lipid component of the inner mitochondrial membrane. Because its presence within this membrane is unique and in a relatively fixed ratio to protein and other lipids, determination of the amount of cardiolipin provides a quantitative assessment of the amount of inner mitochondrial membrane. Cardiolipin can be measured in small muscle biopsies from 10 to 20 mg wet weight (Ritov et al. 2006, 63–71). In a study of Toledo et al. cardiolipin, EM, and mt-DNA were used to measure mitochondrial content in 9 overweight/obese individuals before and after an intervention of weight loss by diet and exercise (7% weight loss within 16–20 weeks of intervention). After the intervention, mitochondrial density measured by EM increased while mitochondrial size did not differ. Cardiolipin increased together with an increase in ETC activity, measured as NADH oxireductase. Surprisingly however, mt-DNA did not increase (Toledo et al. 2008, 987–94).

In conclusion, the plasticity and number of mitochondria have an effect on mitochondrial function. Mitochondrial content can be measured reliably by different methods. However, EM is the only method to distinguish mitochondrial size from number. In obese insulin resistant DM2 subjects, it has been shown that the appearance of mitochondria differs from those in lean individuals. Whether this relates to disturbed function has to be elucidated in future studies.

9.2.5 *Mitochondrial Morphology and Density: Subsacrollemal vs Inter Myofibrillar Mitochondria*

The distribution of mitochondria within the skeletal muscle cell depends on local energy demand. It has been demonstrated that there are two different regions for mitochondrial localisation in the skeletal muscle. Sub-sarcolemmal (SS) mitochondria reside near the sarcolemma, and inter-myofibrillar (IMF) mitochondria are located between the myofibrils. The physiological role of these two mitochondrial populations may be different (Cogswell et al. 1993, C383–C389). IMF mitochondria supply energy for the muscle contractions, while SS mitochondria provide energy for membrane-related events including cell signalling, substrate and ion transport (Hood 2001, 1137–57).

Electron microscopy also allows analysis of mitochondrial distribution between the subsarcolemmal and intermyofibrillar space. Ritov et al. showed that in lean active subjects abundant subsarcolemmal mitochondria can be identified, while there is a striking decrease in obese and DM2 subjects. Although IMF mitochondria were also reduced, the deficit within the subsarcolemmal mitochondrial fraction in DM2 was greater. Furthermore, the reduction in electron transport chain activity in the subsarcolemmal mitochondrial fraction was nearly twofold greater than the reduction in mitochondria number compared to lean individuals, showing functional impairment of SS mitochondrial function (Ritov et al. 2005, 8–14). Compared to the obese individuals, IMF mitochondrial content and electron chain activity were similar, while ETC activity in SS mitochondria was significantly decreased in DM2.

It has been proposed that the observed preferential proliferation of subsarcolemmal vs. IMF mitochondria and the increase in intracellular lipid deposits during endurance training are two possible mechanisms by which muscle cells adapt to an increased use of fat as a fuel (Hoppeler et al. 1985, 320–27;Koves et al. 2005, C1074–C1082). This suggests that reduction in SS mitochondrial function may contribute to insulin resistance.

However, a 16-week physical activity intervention in 14 sedentary, obese men and women increased ETC activity in both SSM and IMF mitochondrial fractions by the same proportion (Menshikova et al. 2005, E818–E825).

Future research should focus on differences in the SS and IMF mitochondria between obese insulin resistant individuals and well matched controls (Holloway et al. 2009, 455S–62S).

9.2.6 Muscle Fiber Type

Human skeletal muscle consists of a mixed fiber type composition (Simoneau and Bouchard 1989, E567–E572). Mitochondrial shape and configuration are distinctive for each human skeletal muscle fiber type (Ogata and Yamasaki 1997, 214–23). Type 1 fibers, also known as red oxidative fibers, are slow in contraction time and have a high resistance to fatigue. Mitochondrial density in these fibers is high. Type 2 fibers, also known as white glycolytic fibers, are characterized by a short contraction time and a low resistance to fatigue. The mitochondria of this fiber type are more slender (Ogata and Yamasaki 1997, 214–23). Fast-twitch fibers are further divided into fast-twitch A (Type 2A) and fast-twitch B (Type 2B) fibers. Type 2A fibers are moderate resistant to fatigue, while type 2B two fibers are very sensitive to fatigue and therefore only used for short term activities. Mitochondrial density in type 2B fibers is low and they have a reduced oxidative enzyme activity.

The majority of the human studies assessed mitochondrial function in the vastus lateralis muscle. This muscle is known to be very homogenous with about 55% type I oxidative fibres and the content of connective tissue is modest (Tonkonogi and Sahlin 1997, 345–53).

Fiber type can be determined in small muscle biopsies by myosin staining. A study in 418 muscle biopsies obtained from vastus lateralis muscle of 270 healthy sedentary and 148 physically active Caucasian individuals of both sexes showed that there is a large inter-individual variation and gender difference in fiber type composition. On average, females have a slightly higher proportion of type 1 fibers, smaller fiber areas and a lower glycolytic capacity. The variability found in men and women was similar (Simoneau and Bouchard 1989, E567–E572). The determination of muscle fiber type is influenced by tissue sampling. Repeated measurements showed a 5–10% variation within the same muscle (Simoneau and Bouchard 1989, E567–E572).

Difference in fiber type composition may contribute to the lower mitochondrial content in subjects with DM2. Indeed, several studies found an increased proportion of type 2B and decreased proportion of type1 fibers in obese and DM2 subjects (Tanner et al. 2002, E1191–E1196; Oberbach et al. 2006, 895–900).

Although the different types of fiber cannot interconvert, training can cause selective hypertrophy of fibers based on the type of training. Also long term inactivity or immobilisation in former active subjects results in changes in muscle fiber type composition (Larsson and Ansved 1985, 714–22; Pette and

Staron 1997, 143–223). Differences in mitochondrial function between lean and obese subjects may therefore be related to a difference in fiber type composition caused by differences in physical activity and genetic predisposition. It has been shown that lean but insulin resistant first-degree relatives of DM2 patients are characterized by an increased number of type 2B muscle fibers (Nyholm et al. 1997, 1822–28). This may suggest that differences in fiber type composition are of primary genetic origin. He et al. (2001) showed that oxidative enzyme activity in muscle of DM2 and obese subjects is reduced within all fiber types compared to lean controls (He et al. 2001, 817–23). This result, however, can be influenced by the significant difference in age between the groups. During ageing there is a progressive decline in mitochondrial function (Menshikova et al. 2006, 534–40; Short et al. 2005, 5618–23).

Age related decline in mitochondrial function is probably neither related to adiposity nor insulin sensitivity. It has been shown that lean elderly physically active subjects display lower mitochondrial function while being equally insulin sensitive compared to lean young subjects (Karakelides et al. 2010, 89–97). The fact that men had a higher mitochondrial capacity, while women were more insulin sensitive, further dissociated the relation between insulin sensitivity and muscle mitochondrial function (Karakelides et al. 2010, 89–97).

In conclusion, differences in skeletal muscle fiber type may in part explain the differences in mitochondrial content and function described in obese insulin resistant DM2 subjects. A difference in fiber type composition can be of primary genetic origin or caused by selective physical training. Ageing causes a progressive decline in mitochondrial function.

9.2.7 Gene Expression

Mitochondria are inherited maternally, contain their own circular DNA and replicate them selves. However the majority of the mitochondrial proteins needed for ATP production and mitochondrial biogenesis are encoded in the nuclear genome (Hood 2001, 1137–57; Shoffner and Wallace 1992, 1179–86).

DNA microarrays can be used to identify changes in gene expression in human disease. Using this approach it was found that the expression of genes involved in the oxidative phosphorylation pathway were decreased in human muscle of DM2 patients (Mootha et al. 2003, 267–73; Sreekumar et al. 2002, 1913–20).

Peroxisome proliferator-activated receptor gamma coactivator 1-alpha (*PGC-1α*) is a very important transcription factor that regulates the activity of the oxidative phosphorylation pathway (Wu et al. 1999, 115–24). Expression of PGC-1α was found to be decreased by 36% in DM2 subjects and by 34% in non-diabetic subjects with a positive family history of DM2 (Patti et al. 2003, 8466–71).

More recent studies however, did not find changes in the expression of PGC-1α and other downstream PGC-1–regulated mitochondrial biosynthetic genes in DM2 offspring (Morino et al. 2005, 3587–93) and myotubes established from DM2 subjects (Frederiksen et al. 2008, 2068–77).

In conclusion, although the use of microarray's to identify changes in gene expression encoding mitochondrial proteins is of interest, controversial results have been published on lower expression of OXPHOS genes in obese insulin resistant subjects compared to controls.

9.3 In Vivo Measurement of Mitochondrial Function

9.3.1 Magnetic Resonance Spectroscopy (MRS)

The concentration and flux of intracellular metabolites can be measured non-invasively using nuclear magnetic resonance (NMR). Naturally-occurring isotopes of hydrogen (H), carbon (C) and phosphorus (P) are magnetically susceptible and detectable by nuclear magnetic resonance spectroscopy (Gadian and Radda 1981, 69–83; Shulman and Rothman 2001, 15–48).

Magnetic Resonance Spectroscopy (^{31}P-MRS) has been applied in two ways to assess mitochondrial ATP synthesis rates. In the magnetization saturation transfer method the unidirectional ATP synthesis rate is calculated from the fractional reduction of phosphate magnetization upon saturation of the γ-phosphate in ATP. Petersen et al. (2004) was the first to show an impaired ATP synthesis rate in skeletal muscle of insulin-resistant offspring of patients with DM2 using this method.

The same group developed a new method to also measure the TCA activity *in vivo*; during an intravenous infusion of [2-^{13}C]acetate, ^{13}C MRS was used to monitor the incorporation of the ^{13}C label into the muscle glutamate pool. Computer modelling of the enrichments of plasma [2-^{13}C]acetate and muscle [4-^{13}C]glutamate yielded the TCA cycle flux and provided a direct measure of muscle mitochondrial substrate oxidation rates (Befroy et al. 2007, 1376–81). Using this approach, it was shown that rates of muscle mitochondrial substrate oxidation were 30% lower in lean insulin resistant offspring compared with insulin-sensitive control subjects.

In DM2 subjects however, ATP synthesis measured by ^{31}P-MRS in the fasting state was 27% lower compared to lean young control subjects but did not differ compared to age and BMI matched controls (Szendroedi et al. 2007, e154). Moreover, the ATP saturation transfer method has been questioned as indicator of mitochondrial function due to the significant contribution of glycolytic ATP production (van den Broek et al. 2010, 1354–64).

Phosphocreatinine is an energy rich molecule that serves as a rapid energy source. In the first seconds of intense muscle exercise this energy is used to rapidly regenerate ATP.

During rest the muscle cell can quickly regenerate phosphocreatinine. This re-synthesis of phosphocreatine in human muscle after exercise is driven almost entirely by oxidative phosphorylation (Sahlin et al. 1997, C172–C178). Therefore the rate of phosphocreatine (PCr) recovery after exercise measured by ^{31}P MRS is an estimate of net oxidative ATP synthesis (Kemp et al. 1993, 66–72). Post-exercise PCr recovery half-time (PCrt1/2) using ^{31}P has been shown to be prolonged in DM2 patients when compared with BMI matched normoglycaemic control subjects (Schrauwen-Hinderling et al. 2007, 113–20; Phielix et al. 2008). However, when a more intense exercise protocol was used resulting in a larger PCr depletion, PCr recovery was not different between insulin-treated DM2 patients, subjects with early stage DM2 and sedentary, normal glycaemic BMI matched controls (De Feyter et al. 2008, 643–53).

The ATP-saturation transfer method measures the momentary flux of ATP-synthesis in the resting state, while PCr recovery measures mitochondrial capacity to produce extra ATP for recovery. This may explain the opposing findings.

In conclusion, *in vivo* measurement of ATP synthesis using NMR is a very promising method to measure mitochondrial function non-invasively. So far, it has been shown that ATP synthesis is reduced in insulin resistant offspring of DM2 patients but this has not convincingly been shown in obese insulin resistant or diabetic subjects and the results obtained may also have indicated a lower ATP demand in the insulin resistant group studied.

9.3.2 Oxygen Uptake

Indirect calorimetry using gas analysis is frequently used to measure indirect whole body resting energy expenditure and substrate oxidation (Frayn 1983, 628–34). Spiro-ergometry during the assessment of maximal exercise capacity yields rates of maximum whole body O_2 uptake (VO_2max). In subjects with normal cardiac and pulmonary function VO_2max is positively associated with mitochondrial content. Also the increase in mitochondrial volume upon endurance training is linearly correlated with the increase in VO_2max (Carter et al. 2001, 386–92; Hoppeler et al. 1985, 320–27). Therefore screening for VO_2max to match study participants has been used, especially because assessing physical fitness by questionnaires introduces more variation as the same quantity or quality of physical exercise may seem more or less strenuous to different individuals. VO_2max scores can improve with training and decrease with age, however the degree of trainability varies very widely and includes a significant genetic component: conditioning may double VO_2max in some individuals but will have only minimal effects in others (Bouchard et al. 1999, 1003–08).

A study in healthy young normal glucose tolerant men with either a first-degree relative (FDR) with DM2 ($n = 183$) or no family history of DM2 (control subjects, $n = 147$) showed that VO2 max was reduced in FDRs (40.5±0.6 vs. 45.2±0.9 ml O2/kg lean body mass respectively). This was despite identical physical activity scores (derived from a questionnaire) (Thamer et al. 2003, 2126–32). This might suggest that a family history of DM2 is associated with reduced maximal oxidative capacity, and is in agreement with the finding that mitochondrial content and ATP synthesis in FDR subjects is reduced.

Uptake of O2 by skeletal muscle can be used as an indirect estimate of mitochondrial function. This can be measured by assessment of arteriovenous differences in O_2 partial pressure and blood flow, or by kinetic analyses of dilution of $[^{15}O]O_2$, $[^{15}O]H_2O$ by position electron tomography (PET scan). Resting rates of oxygen consumption measured with the latter method were comparable between subjects with normal and high insulin sensitivity (Nuutila et al. 2000, 1084–91). No studies have been performed on insulin resistant subjects.

The muscle capillary network supplies oxygen to the mitochondria. Capillary hematocrit, erythrocyte spacing and oxygen saturation of myoglobin are critical variables that influence oxygen release from microvessels. During exercise good circulatory supply of oxygen and substrates (lactate, glucose and fatty acids) is important not to limit mitochondrial function. Differences in the microcirculation may therefore influence mitochondrial function. Under hyperinsulinemic conditions muscular perfusion is stimulated. In healthy humans, in response to hyperinsulinemia, both cardiac output and leg blood flow increased approximately 37% and 80% (p<0.01), respectively (Baron et al. 1993, 129–35). This insulin effect was blunted in obese insulin resistant humans (Baron et al. 1993, 129–35). This may hamper mitochondrial function.

In conclusion, maximal oxygen uptake is frequently used to match participants on physical activity. This seems to be more accurate than questionnaires. VO_2max correlates with mitochondrial content. Mitochondrial function measured by local oxygen uptake can be influenced by differences in the microcirculation which supplies oxygen and substrates to the myocyte. Changes in microcirculation may therefore have an independent effect on mitochondrial function and measurements of mitochondrial function.

9.4 Mitochondrial Dysfunction: Cause or Consequence of Insulin Resistance?

9.4.1 Direct Effect of Insulin on Mitochondrial Function

Insulin stimulates anabolic energy consuming processes, and hence stimulates mitochondrial ATP synthesis, both shown *in vivo* (Brehm et al. 2006, 136–40; Szendroedi et al. 2007, e154) and *in vitro* (Asmann et al. 2006, 3309–19; Stump et al. 2003, 7996–8001). In subjects with DM2, insulin-stimulated ATP synthesis was blunted during a hyperinsulinemic euglycemic clamp, while ATP synthesis increased by 11% in control subjects matched for age and BMI, and by 26% in young lean healthy subjects (Szendroedi et al. 2007, e154). The smaller increase in ATP synthesis in diabetic muscle in response to insulin can be the result of a lower rate of glucose transport into the insulin resistant muscles (Holloszy 2009, 463S–6S). To further study whether insulin stimulates mitochondrial function, Asmann et al. measured mitochondrial ATP production rate (MAPR) and expression of mitochondrial genes after 7 h of low dose and high dose insulin infusion. After the low-dose insulin infusion, muscle MAPR was not different between DM2 and non-diabetic subjects. Increasing insulin to postprandial levels by a 7-h high-dose insulin infusion showed a significant increase in MAPR only in non-diabetic subjects. This increase was associated with an increase in the expression of PGC-1, citrate synthase, and cytochrome c oxidase (Asmann et al. 2006, 3309–19). The latter finding suggests that insulin either directly or indirectly stimulates mitochondrial biogenesis. Indeed, in healthy individuals insulin stimulates mitochondrial protein turn-over, while in obese-insulin resistant subjects this stimulation is blunted (Guillet et al. 2009, 3044–50). In addition, in hyperglycaemic diabetic patients, a decrease in the expression of several key enzymes involved in mitochondrial energy metabolism was observed in skeletal muscle. This was reversed by insulin treatment and normalisation of blood glucose (Sreekumar et al. 2002, 1913–20).

In conclusion, these studies on insulin in relation to mitochondrial function indicate that differences in muscle mitochondrial function between DM2 patients and non-diabetic subjects may be related to an impaired insulin response.

9.4.2 *Impaired Function or Reduced Mitochondrial Content?*

Lower mitochondrial activity in DM2 and obesity suggests either a reduced mitochondrial function or reduced mitochondrial density in skeletal muscle. The latter is caused by either downregulation of mitochondrial biogenesis or by a difference in predominant fiber type.

Rabol et al. showed that mitochondrial content in skeletal muscle of DM2 subjects, compared to BMI matched controls, is reduced and that this reduction explains the lower total mitochondrial respiration rates. In skeletal muscle of the upper arm, mitochondrial function and content did not differ between these groups while mitochondrial respiration and content were significantly higher in leg muscle of the control subjects compared to DM2 subjects. This suggests that mitochondrial capacity is only reduced in muscles used for locomotor activity (Boushel et al. 2007, 790–96; Rabol et al. 2010, 857–63).

Differences in mitochondrial content between DM2 subjects and control subjects may be caused by a difference in physical activity. Endurance exercise-training results in an increase in mitochondrial content in skeletal muscles which are involved in exercise. A single bout of exercise or stimulation of muscle contractions induces a rapid increase in transcription of genes encoding proteins involved in mitochondrial biogenesis (Pilegaard et al. 2003, 851–58). Exercise physiologists recognised that a higher steady-state mitochondrial content can be reached upon a 6 week endurance training (Hood 2001, 1137–57). Trapolonsky et al. suggested that this increase in mitochondrial content is mainly an increase in the size of mitochondrial fragments (Tarnopolsky et al. 2007, R1271–R1278) while others showed increased number and size of mitochondria (Hoppeler et al. 1985, 320–27).

In the study of Kelley et al. mitochondrial oxidative enzyme activity was reduced in DM2 patients. However when the authors would have corrected for the reduction in CS activity, or the reduction in mitochondrial area found in the same study, the differences in oxidative capacity may have been less pronounced (Kelley et al. 2002, 2944–50).

Karakalides et al. measured MAPR in 24 obese and 24 lean participants matched for age and physical activity. It was shown that muscle mitochondrial function was neither related to adiposity nor to insulin sensitivity. Of interest, a higher mitochondrial ATP production capacity was noted in the men while the women were more insulin sensitive, demonstrating further dissociation between insulin sensitivity and muscle mitochondrial function (Karakelides et al. 2010, 89–97).

It is well known that exercise increases mitochondrial capacity. It has been shown that a 12 week endurance training program can restore mitochondrial function in DM2 to control levels, while the same training program had a less profound effect on the control subjects. Insulin sensitivity tended to improve in control subjects (rate of glucose disappearance (Rd) delta Rd 8% increase; P=0.08) and improved significantly in type 2 diabetic subjects (Meex et al. 2010, 572–79).

A combined intervention of weight loss and physical activity in previously sedentary obese adults increased skeletal muscle mitochondrial content and this was highly correlated with improvements in insulin sensitivity (Toledo et al. 2006, 3224–27; Toledo et al. 2008, 987–94). However, weight loss by dietary restriction improved insulin sensitivity to the same extent, while mitochondrial function was not altered (Toledo et al. 2008, 987–94).

Differences in mitochondrial content between lean and obese subjects may be related to a difference in fiber type composition caused by differences in physical activity and genetic predisposition (Oberbach et al. 2006, 895–900; Tanner et al. 2002, E1191–E1196).

In conclusion, mitochondrial function/capacity and content are highly associated with physical activity and fiber composition of skeletal muscle. Therefore, alterations in mitochondrial function in obese and DM2 subjects may be mainly related to differences in physical activity and fiber type.

9.4.3 *Is Mitochondrial Dysfunction an Inherited Defect?*

The development of DM2 is in part explained by genetic factors with a strong environmental influence. First-degree relatives (FDR) of DM2 patients have an approximately 40% lifetime risk of developing diabetes (Perseghin et al. 1997, 1001–09).

In 2004 Petersen et al. showed that mitochondrial function was decreased in FDR of DM2 patients by approximately 30%. This was associated with an increase in intramyocellular lipid and reduction in insulin sensitivity (Petersen et al. 2004, 664–71). It was suggested that insulin resistance in these young lean subjects was caused by an inherited defect in mitochondrial oxidative phosphorylation, resulting in a dysregulation of intramyocellular fatty acid metabolism. However by selecting only subjects with insulin resistance in the FDR-group, the insulin sensitive FDR were not studied. Therefore whether insulin-sensitive FDR have the same reduction in mitochondrial function in the presence of preserved insulin sensitivity is not known. Also, maybe this subgroup of FDR-subjects may represent another phenotype than the obese insulin resistant phenotype because rates of lipolysis and hepatic insulin sensitivity were normal in the insulin resistant FDR group while this is mostly disturbed in the obesity-induced insulin resistance phenotype.

In a study in 34 young sedentary men with ($n = 16$) or without ($n = 34$) a family history of DM2, insulin sensitivity and mitochondrial content were measured. It was found that insulin sensitivity measured as glucose uptake during a hyperinsulinemic euglycemic clamp was not different while mitochondrial content (measured as mt-DNA) was decreased in FDR (Ukropcova et al. 2007, 720–27). Mean VO_2 max was not significantly different in this study, while another study in 183 FDR versus 142 controls showed a significantly lower VO_2 max in FDR (Thamer et al. 2003, 2126–32).

Another study reported a 38% decrease in mitochondrial content in FDR of DM2 subjects (Morino et al. 2005, 3587–93). Differences in mitochondrial content may be related to difference in muscle fiber type, as it was shown that FDR of DM2 patients are characterized by an increased number of type 2B muscle fibers (Nyholm et al. 1997, 1822–28).

Controversial results have been published on lower expression of OXPHOS genes in FDR. Moreover, recent genome-wide association studies in DM2 subjects indicate that the hits are almost entirely for impaired beta-cell function instead of for insulin resistance (Florez 2008, 1100–10).

In conclusion, genetically determined decreased mitochondrial content as well as muscle fiber type may contribute to insulin resistance in FDR of DM2 patients. However, whether this can be translated to an obese insulin resistant individual without family history of DM2 is not known.

9.4.4 Nutrient Overload and Mitochondrial Dysfunction

In obese insulin resistant subjects, excess flow of fatty acids from adipose tissue to insulin sensitive organs like liver and skeletal muscle occurs. Over the last decade it has been hypothesized that this increased lipid availability could induce a mitochondrial defect which leads to impaired substrate oxidation and amplifies intramyocellular lipid accumulation. Several mechanisms have been postulated to explain how increased lipid availability could have a deleterious effect on mitochondrial function:

Firstly, increased supply of lipid substrate, in the absence of energy requiring processes (i.e., physical activity or anabolic processes), induces an imbalanced environment which encourage incomplete β-oxidation and intra-mitochondrial accumulation of acyl-CoAs. Their respective acylcarnitines and perhaps other as yet unidentified metabolites could contribute to mitochondrial dysfunction (Koves et al. 2008, 45–56).

Secondly, in cultured skeletal muscle cells it has been demonstrated that treatment with high concentrations of glucose or fatty acids induced mitochondrial damage via increased reactive oxygen species (ROS) production (Brownlee 2005, 1615–25; Costford et al. 2009, 2405–15).

Thirdly, obese individuals display elevated levels of muscle lipid peroxides (Russell et al. 2003, 104–06). Lipid peroxidation refers to the oxidative degradation of lipids. Free radicals "steal" electrons from the lipids in cell membranes, resulting in cell damage. This process proceeds by a free radical chain reaction mechanism (Schrauwen and Hesselink 2004, 1412–17).

Fourthly, increased concentration of cytosolic long-chain fatty acyl-CoA esters inhibits the mitochondrial adenine nucleotide translocator (Ciapaite et al. 2005, 944–51).

Finally, in healthy individuals prolonged lipid infusion for 48 h or 3 days of high fat feeding downregulates the transcription of genes involved in mitochondrial biogenesis (Richardson et al. 2005, 10290–97). These mechanistic data suggest that exposure to increased lipid availability has a detrimental effect on mitochondrial biogenesis and functioning.

Recently a few studies have been published on mitochondrial ATP synthesis in skeletal muscle during nutrient-induced insulin resistance. Brehm et al studied 10 healthy young men during a hyperinsulinemic euglycemic clamp with concomitant infusion of a lipid emulsion or control saline. *In vivo* ATP production was 30% lower during the lipid emulsion compared to the control saline infusion. During the saline infusion, ATP production increased during the 6 h of hyperinsulinemia by 30%. During the lipid infusion this increase was blunted. A recent study from our group showed that after 6 h of infusion of a lipid emulsion during a hyperinsulinemic euglycemic clamp *ex vivo* mitochondrial respiration was not different from the control situation, indicating decreased insulin signalling and decreased substrate uptake may be responsible for the decreased ATP production *in vivo* (Brands et al. 2011). However, short term elevation of plasma FFA by means of infusion of a lipid emulsion does not necessarily reflect or is representative for the chronic elevation of FFA in obese insulin resistant subjects. Studies in animals on the effect of prolonged lipid overload on mitochondrial function and insulin sensitivity show contradictory results.

In rats, a flaxseed/olive oil diet for 5 weeks, increased mitochondrial content in muscle and capacity of muscle to oxidize fat while insulin sensitivity significantly decreased (Hancock et al. 2008, 7815–20).

Bonnard et al. (2008) studied mice on a high fat high sugar (HFHS) diet for 16 weeks. After 4 weeks insulin resistance was already present whereas there was no change in mitochondrial function or content. After 16 weeks however both subsarcolemmal (31%, $P<0.05$) and IMF (41%, $P<0.01$) mitochondrial content in oxidative fibers were lower in the HFHS mice than in the control mice. Mitochondrial density measured by mtDNA and the expression of OXPHOS genes were also decreased. Respiration rates measured ex-vivo in permeabilized fibers were not altered after 4 weeks, but after 16 weeks a significant decrease in oxidative capacity was observed. Electron microscopy showed structural abnormalities: a number of mitochondria appeared swollen, with fewer cristae, and the inner and/or outer membranes were sometimes disrupted in the muscle of HFHS mice at 16 weeks. These results suggest that an alteration in mitochondrial function is a consequence of a hypercaloric diet and develops after alterations in insulin sensitivity occur (Bonnard et al. 2008, 789–800).

In has been hypothesized that disruption of the balance between fission and fusion can be an important etiologic factor in mitochondrial alterations found in diabetic subjects (Civitarese and Ravussin 2008, 950–54).

Mfn2 (mitofusin 2), a mitochondrial membrane protein that participates in mitochondrial fusion in mammalian cells, is induced during myogenesis and contributes to the maintenance and operation of the mitochondrial network (Bach et al. 2003, 17190–97). In the study of Bonnard expression of Mfn was significantly decreased in the HFHS group (Bonnard et al. 2008, 789–800).

At the moment there are no studies available that studied mitochondrial function during prolonged hyper caloric or high fat intake in humans. So far many studies compared obese insulin resistant individuals or DM2 patients to a selected control group. One study has shown the morphological alterations in obese insulin resistant individuals (Kelley et al. 2002, 2944–50). These morphological alterations improve after physical training (Toledo et al. 2006, 3224–27).

A common finding is that skeletal muscle of insulin resistant subjects has 30% decreased mitochondrial content. The capacity of skeletal muscle to up regulate mitochondrial activity is high. In healthy men, muscle oxygen uptake during strenuous exercise increases 150 fold, measured by femoral arterial-venous differences (Andersen and Saltin 1985, 233–49). Because the capacity of muscle to oxidize substrate is so far in excess of what is needed to supply the energy needs of resting muscle, it is questionable whether a 30% decrease in mitochondrial content has a significant effect on the ability of resting muscle to oxidize fat (Holloszy 2009, 463S–6S).

Increased storage of metabolites of fatty acids is associated with reduced insulin sensitivity. In obese insulin resistant subject intramyocellular lipid (IMCL) is increased and whole body fatty acid oxidation is decreased compared to lean individuals (Berggren et al. 2008, E726–E732). In difference with trained individuals the distribution of the lipid droplets is more central (Malenfant et al. 2001, 1316–21). Exercise endurance training increases mitochondrial capacity and IMCL, but also the proportion of IMCL in physical contact with mitochondria (Tarnopolsky et al. 2007, R1271–R1278). It is conceivable that close proximity between IMCL and mitochondria improves substrate flux from storage to metabolic use and reduces toxic metabolic by-products which may interfere with insulin signalling. Interestingly, the lower ability to oxidize fat persisted after massive weight loss, but improved after exercise in obese and extreme obese individuals (Berggren et al. 2008, E726–E732). This indicates again that reduction in mitochondrial function and fatty acid oxidation can be related to inactivity in the obese insulin resistant state.

9.5 Conclusion

Many different methods have been used to measure mitochondrial function. Methodological differences between studies make it difficult to conclude whether reduced mitochondrial capacity is associated with the insulin resistant state. The sensitivity of ex-vivo mitochondrial analysis is affected by processing of the muscle biopsy. To keep these influences as little as possible it's preferable to measure mitochondrial function in fresh permeabilized muscle fibers instead of isolated mitochondria or frozen biopsies (Szendroedi and Roden 2008, 2155–67).

The advantage of the ex-vivo functional measurement of mitochondrial capacity is that mitochondrial function can be measured under similar substrate conditions in all participants. Furthermore it allows studying intrinsic mitochondrial capacity of the different ETC complexes

(Gnaiger 2009). However ex-vivo mitochondrial function does not necessarily reflect metabolic mitochondrial activity *in vivo*.

Nuclear magnetic resonance makes it possible to non-invasively measure ATP synthesis in-vivo. In addition, in combination with labelled isotopes the activity of the TCA cycle can be assessed. Future research in which in-vivo and ex-vivo experiments will be combined, will give more insight in the role of mitochondrial function in relation to insulin sensitivity.

Differences in mitochondrial function can be the result of several factors, including a reduced mitochondrial density, differences in insulin stimulation, lower energy demand and, lower muscle blood perfusion, but also a true mitochondrial dysfunction (i.e. lower mitochondrial respiratory capacity per mitochondrion). To compare study results one should always be aware of the conditions under which mitochondrial function is measured and which groups are compared. This makes it difficult to make a simplified table with an overview of all the studies on mitochondrial function in human subjects.

A common finding in studies is that mitochondrial content is decreased in obese insulin resistant subjects. This may be related to differences in fiber type composition and lower physical activity. Exercise improves mitochondrial function and insulin sensitivity in insulin resistant subjects, while insulin sensitivity can also be improved solely by weight reduction. Moreover young obese and elderly obese individuals have preserved mitochondrial function while having lower insulin sensitivity compared to age matched lean controls. The age related decline in mitochondrial function could not be related to decrease in insulin sensitivity. This dissociates mitochondrial function and insulin resistance and indicates that reduction in mitochondrial function is probably a consequence of the sedentary life style.

It is unlikely that decreased mitochondrial function causes decreased fat oxidation capacity in the resting state leading to intracellular lipid accumulation. Moreover high caloric intake in combination with low physical inactivity causes lipid/energy storage and progression to obesity and diabetes. Whether prolonged overload of fat causes mitochondrial damage and therefore decreased function is not clear. From animal studies we can conclude that during nutrient overload insulin resistance develops far before the onset of mitochondrial alterations.

In FDR of DM2 patients, decreased mitochondrial content may be of primary genetic origin.

In combination with a high fat diet and low physical activity; this may favour lipid/energy storage and progression to obesity and diabetes at an earlier stage.

References

Andersen P, Saltin B (1985) Maximal perfusion of skeletal muscle in man. J Physiol 366:233–249

Asmann YW et al (2006) Skeletal muscle mitochondrial functions, mitochondrial DNA copy numbers, and gene transcript profiles in type 2 diabetic and nondiabetic subjects at equal levels of low or high insulin and euglycemia. Diabetes 55(12):3309–3319

Bach D et al (2003) Mitofusin-2 determines mitochondrial network architecture and mitochondrial metabolism. A novel regulatory mechanism altered in obesity. J Biol Chem 278(19):17190–17197

Bao S et al (1998) Expression of mRNAs encoding uncoupling proteins in human skeletal muscle: effects of obesity and diabetes. Diabetes 47(12):1935–1940

Baron AD et al (1993) Skeletal muscle blood flow. A possible link between insulin resistance and blood pressure. Hypertension 21(2):129–135

Befroy DE et al (2007) Impaired mitochondrial substrate oxidation in muscle of insulin-resistant offspring of type 2 diabetic patients. Diabetes 56(5):1376–1381

Belfort R et al (2005) Dose-response effect of elevated plasma free fatty acid on insulin signaling. Diabetes 54(6):1640–1648

Berggren JR et al (2008) Skeletal muscle lipid oxidation and obesity: influence of weight loss and exercise. Am J Physiol Endocrinol Metab 294(4):E726–E732

Bergman RN (2007) Orchestration of glucose homeostasis: from a small acorn to the California oak. Diabetes 56(6):1489–1501

Boden G (2002) Interaction between free fatty acids and glucose metabolism. Curr Opin Clin Nutr Metab Care 5(5):545–549

Bonnard C et al (2008) Mitochondrial dysfunction results from oxidative stress in the skeletal muscle of diet-induced insulin-resistant mice. J Clin Invest 118(2):789–800

Boss O, Hagen T, Lowell BB (2000) Uncoupling proteins 2 and 3: potential regulators of mitochondrial energy metabolism. Diabetes 49(2):143–156

Bouchard C et al (1999) Familial aggregation of VO(2max) response to exercise training: results from the HERITAGE Family Study. J Appl Physiol 87(3):1003–1008

Boushel R et al (2007) Patients with type 2 diabetes have normal mitochondrial function in skeletal muscle. Diabetologia 50(4):790–796

Brands M et al (2011) Short-term increase of plasma free fatty acids does not interfere with intrinsic mitochondrial function in healthy young men. Metabolism 60(10):1398–1405

Brehm A et al (2006) Increased lipid availability impairs insulin-stimulated ATP synthesis in human skeletal muscle. Diabetes 55(1):136–140

Brownlee M (2005) The pathobiology of diabetic complications: a unifying mechanism. Diabetes 54(6):1615–1625

Carter SL et al (2001) Changes in skeletal muscle in males and females following endurance training. Can J Physiol Pharmacol 79(5):386–392

Chavez AO et al (2010) Effect of short-term free Fatty acids elevation on mitochondrial function in skeletal muscle of healthy individuals. J Clin Endocrinol Metab 95(1):422–429

Chi MM et al (1983) Effects of detraining on enzymes of energy metabolism in individual human muscle fibers. Am J Physiol 244(3):C276–C287

Ciapaite J et al (2005) Modular kinetic analysis of the adenine nucleotide translocator-mediated effects of palmitoyl-CoA on the oxidative phosphorylation in isolated rat liver mitochondria. Diabetes 54(4):944–951

Civitarese AE, Ravussin E (2008) Mitochondrial energetics and insulin resistance. Endocrinology 149(3):950–954

Cogswell AM, Cogswell AM, Stevens RJ, Hood DA (1993) Properties of skeletal muscle mitochondria isolated from subsarcolemmal and intermyofibrillar regions. Am J Physiol 264(2 Pt 1):C383–C389

Costford SR et al (2009) Increased susceptibility to oxidative damage in post-diabetic human myotubes. Diabetologia 52(11):2405–2415

De Feyter HM et al (2008) Early or advanced stage type 2 diabetes is not accompanied by in vivo skeletal muscle mitochondrial dysfunction. Eur J Endocrinol 158(5):643–653

DeFronzo RA et al (1985) Effects of insulin on peripheral and splanchnic glucose metabolism in noninsulin-dependent (type II) diabetes mellitus. J Clin Invest 76(1):149–155

Florez JC (2008) Newly identified loci highlight beta cell dysfunction as a key cause of type 2 diabetes: where are the insulin resistance genes? Diabetologia 51(7):1100–1110

Frayn KN (1983) Calculation of substrate oxidation rates in vivo from gaseous exchange. J Appl Physiol 55(2):628–634

Frederiksen CM et al (2008) Transcriptional profiling of myotubes from patients with type 2 diabetes: no evidence for a primary defect in oxidative phosphorylation genes. Diabetologia 51(11):2068–2077

Gadian DG, Radda GK (1981) NMR studies of tissue metabolism. Annu Rev Biochem 50:69–83

Gnaiger E (2009) Capacity of oxidative phosphorylation in human skeletal muscle. New perspectives of mitochondrial physiology. Int J Biochem Cell Biol 41(10):1837–1845

Guillet C et al (2009) Changes in basal and insulin and amino acid response of whole body and skeletal muscle proteins in obese men. J Clin Endocrinol Metab 94(8):3044–3050

Hancock CR et al (2008) High-fat diets cause insulin resistance despite an increase in muscle mitochondria. Proc Natl Acad Sci USA 105(22):7815–7820

He J, Watkins S, Kelley DE (2001) Skeletal muscle lipid content and oxidative enzyme activity in relation to muscle fiber type in type 2 diabetes and obesity. Diabetes 50(4):817–823

Heilbronn LK et al (2007) Markers of mitochondrial biogenesis and metabolism are lower in overweight and obese insulin-resistant subjects. J Clin Endocrinol Metab 92(4):1467–1473

Holloszy JO (2009) Skeletal muscle "mitochondrial deficiency" does not mediate insulin resistance. Am J Clin Nutr 89(1):463S–466S

Holloway GP et al (2007) Skeletal muscle mitochondrial FAT/CD36 content and palmitate oxidation are not decreased in obese women. Am J Physiol Endocrinol Metab 292(6):E1782–E1789

Holloway GP, Bonen A, Spriet LL (2009) Regulation of skeletal muscle mitochondrial fatty acid metabolism in lean and obese individuals. Am J Clin Nutr 89(1):455S–462S

Hood DA (2001) Invited Review: contractile activity-induced mitochondrial biogenesis in skeletal muscle. J Appl Physiol 90(3):1137–1157

Hoppeler H et al (1985) Endurance training in humans: aerobic capacity and structure of skeletal muscle. J Appl Physiol 59(2):320–327

Karakelides H et al (2010) Age, obesity, and sex effects on insulin sensitivity and skeletal muscle mitochondrial function. Diabetes 59(1):89–97

Kelley DE et al (2002) Dysfunction of mitochondria in human skeletal muscle in type 2 diabetes. Diabetes 51(10):2944–2950

Kemp GJ, Taylor DJ, Radda GK (1993) Control of phosphocreatine resynthesis during recovery from exercise in human skeletal muscle. NMR Biomed 6(1):66–72

Khalfallah Y et al (2000) Regulation of uncoupling protein-2 and uncoupling protein-3 mRNA expression during lipid infusion in human skeletal muscle and subcutaneous adipose tissue. Diabetes 49(1):25–31

Koutsari C, Jensen MD (2006) Thematic review series: patient-oriented research. Free fatty acid metabolism in human obesity. J Lipid Res 47(8):1643–1650

Koves TR et al (2005) Subsarcolemmal and intermyofibrillar mitochondria play distinct roles in regulating skeletal muscle fatty acid metabolism. Am J Physiol Cell Physiol 288(5):C1074–C1082

Koves TR et al (2008) Mitochondrial overload and incomplete fatty acid oxidation contribute to skeletal muscle insulin resistance. Cell Metab 7(1):45–56

Krook A et al (1998) Uncoupling protein 3 is reduced in skeletal muscle of NIDDM patients. Diabetes 47(9):1528–1531

Larsson L, Ansved T (1985) Effects of long-term physical training and detraining on enzyme histochemical and functional skeletal muscle characteristic in man. Muscle Nerve 8(8):714–722

Malenfant P et al (2001) Fat content in individual muscle fibers of lean and obese subjects. Int J Obes Relat Metab Disord 25(9):1316–1321

Meex RC et al (2010) Restoration of muscle mitochondrial function and metabolic flexibility in type 2 diabetes by exercise training is paralleled by increased myocellular fat storage and improved insulin sensitivity. Diabetes 59(3):572–579

Menshikova EV et al (2005) Effects of weight loss and physical activity on skeletal muscle mitochondrial function in obesity. Am J Physiol Endocrinol Metab 288(4):E818–E825

Menshikova EV et al (2006) Effects of exercise on mitochondrial content and function in aging human skeletal muscle. J Gerontol A Biol Sci Med Sci 61(6):534–540

Mogensen M et al (2007) Mitochondrial respiration is decreased in skeletal muscle of patients with type 2 diabetes. Diabetes 56(6):1592–1599

Mootha VK et al (2003) PGC-1alpha-responsive genes involved in oxidative phosphorylation are coordinately down-regulated in human diabetes. Nat Genet 34(3):267–273

Morino K et al (2005) Reduced mitochondrial density and increased IRS-1 serine phosphorylation in muscle of insulin-resistant offspring of type 2 diabetic parents. J Clin Invest 115(12):3587–3593

Nair KS et al (2008) Asian Indians have enhanced skeletal muscle mitochondrial capacity to produce ATP in association with severe insulin resistance. Diabetes 57(5):1166–1175

Nuutila P et al (2000) Enhanced stimulation of glucose uptake by insulin increases exercise-stimulated glucose uptake in skeletal muscle in humans: studies using [15O]O2, [15O]H2O, [18F]fluoro-deoxy-glucose, and positron emission tomography. Diabetes 49(7):1084–1091

Nyholm B et al (1997) Evidence of an increased number of type IIb muscle fibers in insulin-resistant first-degree relatives of patients with NIDDM. Diabetes 46(11):1822–1828

Oberbach A et al (2006) Altered fiber distribution and fiber-specific glycolytic and oxidative enzyme activity in skeletal muscle of patients with type 2 diabetes. Diabetes Care 29(4):895–900

Ogata T, Yamasaki Y (1997) Ultra-high-resolution scanning electron microscopy of mitochondria and sarcoplasmic reticulum arrangement in human red, white, and intermediate muscle fibers. Anat Rec 248(2):214–223

Patti ME et al (2003) Coordinated reduction of genes of oxidative metabolism in humans with insulin resistance and diabetes: potential role of PGC1 and NRF1. Proc Natl Acad Sci USA 100(14):8466–8471

Perseghin G et al (1997) Metabolic defects in lean nondiabetic offspring of NIDDM parents: a cross-sectional study. Diabetes 46(6):1001–1009

Petersen KF et al (2004) Impaired mitochondrial activity in the insulin-resistant offspring of patients with type 2 diabetes. N Engl J Med 350(7):664–671

Pette D, Staron RS (1997) Mammalian skeletal muscle fiber type transitions. Int Rev Cytol 170:143–223

Phielix E et al (2008) Lower intrinsic ADP-stimulated mitochondrial respiration underlies in vivo mitochondrial dysfunction in muscle of male type 2 diabetic patients. Diabetes 57(11):2943–2949

Pilegaard H, Saltin B, Neufer PD (2003) Exercise induces transient transcriptional activation of the PGC-1alpha gene in human skeletal muscle. J Physiol 546(Pt 3):851–858

Puntschart A et al (1995) mRNAs of enzymes involved in energy metabolism and mtDNA are increased in endurance-trained athletes. Am J Physiol 269(3 Pt 1):C619–C625

Rabol R et al (2010) Regional anatomic differences in skeletal muscle mitochondrial respiration in type 2 diabetes and obesity. J Clin Endocrinol Metab 95(2):857–863

Rasmussen UF, Rasmussen HN (2000a) Human quadriceps muscle mitochondria: a functional characterization. Mol Cell Biochem 208(1-2):37–44

Rasmussen UF, Rasmussen HN (2000b) Human skeletal muscle mitochondrial capacity. Acta Physiol Scand 168(4):473–480

Richardson DK et al (2005) Lipid infusion decreases the expression of nuclear encoded mitochondrial genes and increases the expression of extracellular matrix genes in human skeletal muscle. J Biol Chem 280(11):10290–10297

Ritov VB, Menshikova EV, Kelley DE (2004) High-performance liquid chromatography-based methods of enzymatic analysis: electron transport chain activity in mitochondria from human skeletal muscle. Anal Biochem 333(1):27–38

Ritov VB et al (2005) Deficiency of subsarcolemmal mitochondria in obesity and type 2 diabetes. Diabetes 54(1):8–14

Ritov VB, Menshikova EV, Kelley DE (2006) Analysis of cardiolipin in human muscle biopsy. J Chromatogr B Analyt Technol Biomed Life Sci 831(1-2):63–71

Roden M (2005) Muscle triglycerides and mitochondrial function: possible mechanisms for the development of type 2 diabetes. Int J Obes (Lond) 29(S111)

Rolfe DF, Brand MD (1996) Contribution of mitochondrial proton leak to skeletal muscle respiration and to standard metabolic rate. Am J Physiol 271(4 Pt 1):C1380–C1389

Russell AP et al (2003) Lipid peroxidation in skeletal muscle of obese as compared to endurance-trained humans: a case of good vs. bad lipids? FEBS Lett 551(1–3):104–106

Sahlin K, Sahlin K et al (1997) Phosphocreatine content in single fibers of human muscle after sustained submaximal exercise. Am J Physiol 273(1 Pt 1):C172–C178

Scaduto RC Jr, Grotyohann LW (1999) Measurement of mitochondrial membrane potential using fluorescent rhodamine derivatives. Biophys J 76(1 Pt 1):469–477

Schrauwen P (2007) High-fat diet, muscular lipotoxicity and insulin resistance. Proc Nutr Soc 66(1):33–41

Schrauwen P, Hesselink MK (2004) Oxidative capacity, lipotoxicity, and mitochondrial damage in type 2 diabetes. Diabetes 53(6):1412–1417

Schrauwen-Hinderling VB et al (2007) Impaired in vivo mitochondrial function but similar intramyocellular lipid content in patients with type 2 diabetes mellitus and BMI-matched control subjects. Diabetologia 50(1):113–120

Shoffner JM, Wallace DC (1992) Mitochondrial genetics: principles and practice. Am J Hum Genet 51(6):1179–1186

Short KR et al (2005) Decline in skeletal muscle mitochondrial function with aging in humans. Proc Natl Acad Sci USA 102(15):5618–5623

Shulman GI (2000) Cellular mechanisms of insulin resistance. J Clin Invest 106(2):171–176

Shulman RG, Rothman DL (2001) 13C NMR of intermediary metabolism: implications for systemic physiology. Annu Rev Physiol 63:15–48

Simoneau JA, Bouchard C (1989) Human variation in skeletal muscle fiber-type proportion and enzyme activities. Am J Physiol 257(4 Pt 1):E567–E572

Sreekumar R et al (2002) Gene expression profile in skeletal muscle of type 2 diabetes and the effect of insulin treatment. Diabetes 51(6):1913–1920

Stump CS et al (2003) Effect of insulin on human skeletal muscle mitochondrial ATP production, protein synthesis, and mRNA transcripts. Proc Natl Acad Sci USA 100(13):7996–8001

Szendroedi J, Roden M (2008) Mitochondrial fitness and insulin sensitivity in humans. Diabetologia 51(12):2155–2167

Szendroedi J et al (2007) Muscle mitochondrial ATP synthesis and glucose transport/phosphorylation in type 2 diabetes. PLoS Med 4(5):e154

Tanner CJ et al (2002) Muscle fiber type is associated with obesity and weight loss. Am J Physiol Endocrinol Metab 282(6):E1191–E1196

Tarnopolsky MA et al (2007) Influence of endurance exercise training and sex on intramyocellular lipid and mitochondrial ultrastructure, substrate use, and mitochondrial enzyme activity. Am J Physiol Regul Integr Comp Physiol 292(3):R1271–R1278

Thamer C et al (2003) Reduced skeletal muscle oxygen uptake and reduced beta-cell function: two early abnormalities in normal glucose-tolerant offspring of patients with type 2 diabetes. Diabetes Care 26(7):2126–2132

Toledo FG, Watkins S, Kelley DE (2006) Changes induced by physical activity and weight loss in the morphology of intermyofibrillar mitochondria in obese men and women. J Clin Endocrinol Metab 91(8):3224–3227

Toledo FG et al (2008) Mitochondrial capacity in skeletal muscle is not stimulated by weight loss despite increases in insulin action and decreases in intramyocellular lipid content. Diabetes 57(4):987–994

Tonkonogi M, Sahlin K (1997) Rate of oxidative phosphorylation in isolated mitochondria from human skeletal muscle: effect of training status. Acta Physiol Scand 161(3):345–353

Tonkonogi M, Harris B, Sahlin K (1997) Increased activity of citrate synthase in human skeletal muscle after a single bout of prolonged exercise. Acta Physiol Scand 161(3):435–436

Twig G, Hyde B, Shirihai OS (2008) Mitochondrial fusion, fission and autophagy as a quality control axis: the bioenergetic view. Biochim Biophys Acta 1777(9):1092–1097

Ukropcova B et al (2007) Family history of diabetes links impaired substrate switching and reduced mitochondrial content in skeletal muscle. Diabetes 56(3):720–727

van den Broek NM et al (2010) Increased mitochondrial content rescues in vivo muscle oxidative capacity in long-term high-fat-diet-fed rats. FASEB J 24(5):1354–1364

Vondra K et al (1977) Enzyme activities in quadriceps femoris muscle of obese diabetic male patients. Diabetologia 13(5):527–529

Wang H et al (1999) Relationships between muscle mitochondrial DNA content, mitochondrial enzyme activity and oxidative capacity in man: alterations with disease. Eur J Appl Physiol Occup Physiol 80(1):22–27

Wibom R, Hagenfeldt L, von Dobeln U (2002) Measurement of ATP production and respiratory chain enzyme activities in mitochondria isolated from small muscle biopsy samples. Anal Biochem 311(2):139–151

Wittig I, Schagger H (2009) Supramolecular organization of ATP synthase and respiratory chain in mitochondrial membranes. Biochim Biophys Acta 1787(6):672–680

Wu Z et al (1999) Mechanisms controlling mitochondrial biogenesis and respiration through the thermogenic coactivator PGC-1. Cell 98(1):115–124

Chapter 10
Mitochondria and Diabetes. An Intriguing Pathogenetic Role

Philip Newsholme, Celine Gaudel, and Maurico Krause

Abstract Mitochondria play a key role in energy metabolism and ATP production in many tissues, including skeletal muscle, cardiac muscle, brain and liver. Inherent disorders of mitochondria such as mDNA deletions cause major disruption of metabolism and can result in severe disease phenotypes. However, the incidence of such mDNA based disorders is extremely rare and cannot account for the dramatic rise in human metabolic diseases, which are characterised by defects in energy metabolism. Mitochondrial dysfunction characterized by reduced ATP generation and reduced mitochondrial number in skeletal muscle or reduced ATP generation and mitochondrial stimulus-secretion coupling in the pancreatic beta cell has been implicated in the pathology of chronic metabolic disease associated with type 2 diabetes mellitus and also with aging. Additionally the generation of ROS from mitochondria and other cellular sources may interfere in insulin signaling in muscle, contributing to insulin resistance. Reduced mitochondrial oxidative capacity coupled with increased ROS generation underlies the accumulation of intramuscular fat, insulin resistance and muscle dysfunction in aging. We will review the molecular basis for optimal mitochondrial function or mechanisms of dysfunction and correlate with pathology of identified diseases and aging.

Keywords Insulin resistance and diabetes • Mitochondrial DNA • Mitochondrial dysfunction • Muscle dysfunction in aging • Reactive Oxygen Species (ROS)

10.1 Introduction

Mitochondria are abundant where efficient biological energy generation is required, such as skeletal and cardiac muscle and brain. The primary role of mitochondria is to convert the products of carbohydrate, protein, and fat metabolism to CO_2 and water, using key enzymes of the TCA cycle to generate

P. Newsholme (✉) • C. Gaudel
UCD School of Biomolecular and Biomedical Science and UCD Institute of Sport and Health,
UCD Dublin, Belfield Dublin 4, Ireland
e-mail: philip.newsholme@ucd.ie

School of Biochemical Sciences, Building 308 Room 122, GPO Box U1987, Curtin University, Perth,
Western Australia 6845

M. Krause
UCD School of Biomolecular and Biomedical Science and UCD Institute of Sport and Health,
UCD Dublin, Belfield Dublin 4, Ireland

Biomedical Research Group (BMRG), Department of Science,
Institute of Technology Tallaght, Dublin 24, Ireland

R. Scatena et al. (eds.), *Advances in Mitochondrial Medicine*, Advances in Experimental
Medicine and Biology 942, DOI 10.1007/978-94-007-2869-1_10,
© Springer Science+Business Media B.V. 2012

NADH and $FADH_2$ and of the electron transport chain including; NADH dehydrogenase (Complex I), succinate dehydrogenase (Complex II), cytochrome bc_1 (Complex III), and cytochrome c oxidase (Complex IV). During reactions specific to the electron transport chain, protons (H^+) are pumped from the matrix to the space between the inner and outer membranes, establishing a proton gradient. Protons moving down this gradient drive the synthesis of ATP by the enzyme ATP synthase (Complex V). The coupling of substrate oxidation with ATP formation in the mitochondria is called oxidative phosphorylation and is central to energy generation in a variety of tissues and organs. Dysfunction of these mitochondrial complexes may also play an important role in the pathogenesis of some chronic diseases. However, it is not clear whether mitochondria responsible for, or victims of, metabolic dysregulation. In this chapter, we will present and review data supporting the hypothesis that mitochondrial dysfunction underlies the metabolic abnormalities associated with type 2 diabetes and aging.

10.2 Overview of Mitochondrial Oxidative Phosphorylation

Mitochondria generate cellular energy through TCA cycle activity and the associated electron transport chain of the inner membrane. The reducing equivalents [NADH and $FADH_2$] that are produced from the TCA cycle are reoxidized via a process that involves transfer of electrons through the electron transport chain (ETC) and associated translocation of protons across the mitochondrial inner membrane, creating the transmembrane electrochemical gradient (estimated as 150–200 mV negative to the cytosol). This gradient provides the electrochemical potential to make ATP from ADP and P_i, driven by proton movement back through the ATP synthase complex. Under normal conditions, the proton gradient is also diminished by H^+ 'leak' to the matrix. The 'leak' occurs either via non-protein membrane pores, protein/lipid interfaces (H^+ leak), or by proton channels known as uncoupling proteins (UCPs) (Fig. 10.1).

However, mitochondria can generate significant ROS (reactive oxygen species) and reactive nitrogen species because of unavoidable oxidative phosphorylation chemistry. Superoxide anions (O_2^-) are a byproduct of single electron reduction of ubiquinone. Furthermore, these anions are the major contributors to other reactive species inside mitochondrion (Evans et al. 2002), for example, the reaction of O_2^- with nitric oxide produces peroxynitrite. Superoxide anions, peroxynitrite, and other reactive species are very powerful chemical oxidants (Evans et al. 2002; Turrens 2003).

The electron transport chain dependent movement of protons across the inner mitochondrial membrane establishes an electrochemical gradient of which mitochondrial membrane potential ($\Delta\psi_m$) is an important component. An increase in $\Delta\psi_m$ will result in elevated ATP production but reduced electron transport capability thus leading to increased ROS production (Korshunov et al. 1997). Uncoupling agents (for example, UCPs) reduce the proton gradient across the mitochondrial inner membrane and decrease $\Delta\psi_m$, causing decreased ATP and ROS production but increased ADP concentration. Between 0.2% and 2% of oxygen taken up by cells is converted into ROS (Harper et al. 2004).

Cells require antioxidant systems to neutralize ROS. For example, O_2^- are enzymatically converted to hydrogen peroxide by a manganese-superoxide dismutase (MnSOD) within mitochondria. Hydrogen peroxide can then be rapidly removed by the mitochondrial enzyme glutathione (GSH) peroxidase. The inner mitochondrial membrane also contains vitamin E, which is a powerful antioxidant as it can accept unpaired electrons to produce a stable product. A further antioxidant enzyme, catalase, is the major hydrogen peroxide detoxifying enzyme found exclusively in peroxisomes (Evans et al. 2002) (Fig. 10.2).

However, while cells have a number of antioxidant mechanisms available, it is still possible for ROS to evade antioxidant defense mechanisms, resulting in a slow accumulation of chronic damage. Both the mitochondrion and nucleus contain a variety of DNA repair enzymes to correct oxidant induced modifications (Evans et al. 2002, 2004) but damage most likely occurs when the endogenous

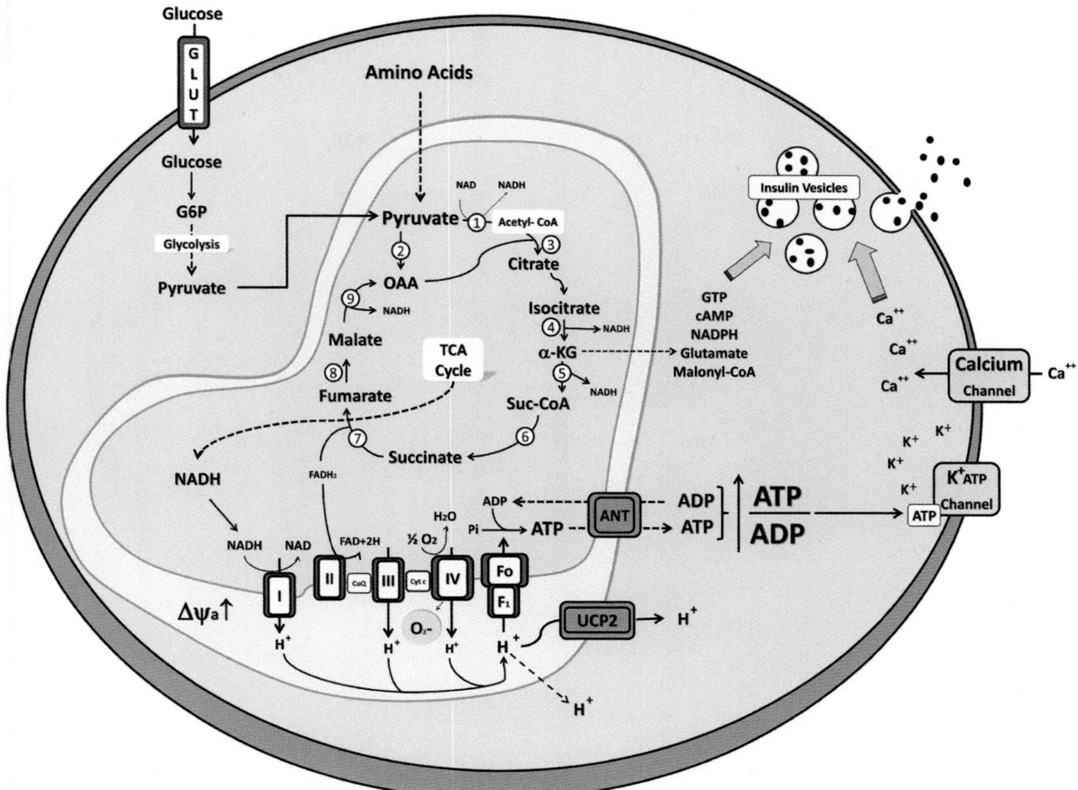

Fig. 10.1 *General view of the mitochondrial metabolism in pancreatic β-cells.* Products of carbohydrate, protein, and fat metabolism can be converted to CO_2 and water by the mitochondria, using key enzymes of TCA cycle and the electron transport chain; NADH dehydrogenase (Complex I), succinate dehydrogenase (Complex II), cytochrome bc_1 (Complex III), and cytochrome c oxidase (Complex IV). During these reactions, protons (H^+) are pumped from the matrix to the space between the inner and outer membranes, establishing a proton gradient. Protons diffusing back along this gradient drive the synthesis of ATP by the enzyme ATP synthase (Complex V). Mitochondria generate cellular energy through TCA cycle activity and the associated electron transport chain of the inner membrane. The reducing equivalents [NADPH and $FADH_2$] produced from the TCA cycle are reoxidized via a process that involves transfer of electrons through the electron transport chain (ETC) and associated translocation of protons across the mitochondrial inner membrane, creating the transmembrane electrochemical gradient which is used to provide the electrochemical potential to make ATP through the ATP synthase complex. In the case of β-cells, the increased ATP/ADP ratio leads to the closure of the K_{ATP}^+ channels leading to membrane depolarization followed by calcium influx that, together with other co-factors (such as glutamate, NADPH, Malonyl-CoA, cAMP, GTP) induces the translocation and exocytosis of the insulin vesicles. Under normal conditions, the proton gradient formed across the mitochondrial inner membrane can be diminished by $H+$leak to the matrix via non-protein membrane pores or by proton channels known as uncoupling proteins (UCPs). Since superoxide anions ($O2^-$) are a byproduct of single electron reduction of ubiquinone, mitochondria can also generate significant ROS by the unavoidable oxidative phosphorylation chemistry. UCPs reduce the proton gradient across the mitochondrial inner membrane and decrease $\Delta\psi m$, causing decreased ATP and ROS production but increased ADP concentration. ① Pyruvate Dehydrogenase, ② Pyruvate carboxylase, ③ Citrate synthase, ④ Isocitrate dehydrogenase, ⑤ α-ketoglutarate dehydrogenase ⑥ Succinate thiokinase ⑦ Succinate dehydrogenase, ⑧ Fumarase, ⑨ Malate dehydrogenase, *ANT* adenine nucleotide translocator

antioxidant network and repair systems are overwhelmed (Hutter et al. 2007; Maiese et al. 2007; Rachek et al. 2007). However, it is essential to repair oxidant induced damage to DNA or mutations may result in impaired transcription. Damaged mitochondria may be removed by autophagy, but many aspects of this process are obscure (Evans et al. 2004). However, it is known that mitochondrial biogenesis is regulated by some specific transcriptional activators and co-activators as well as by

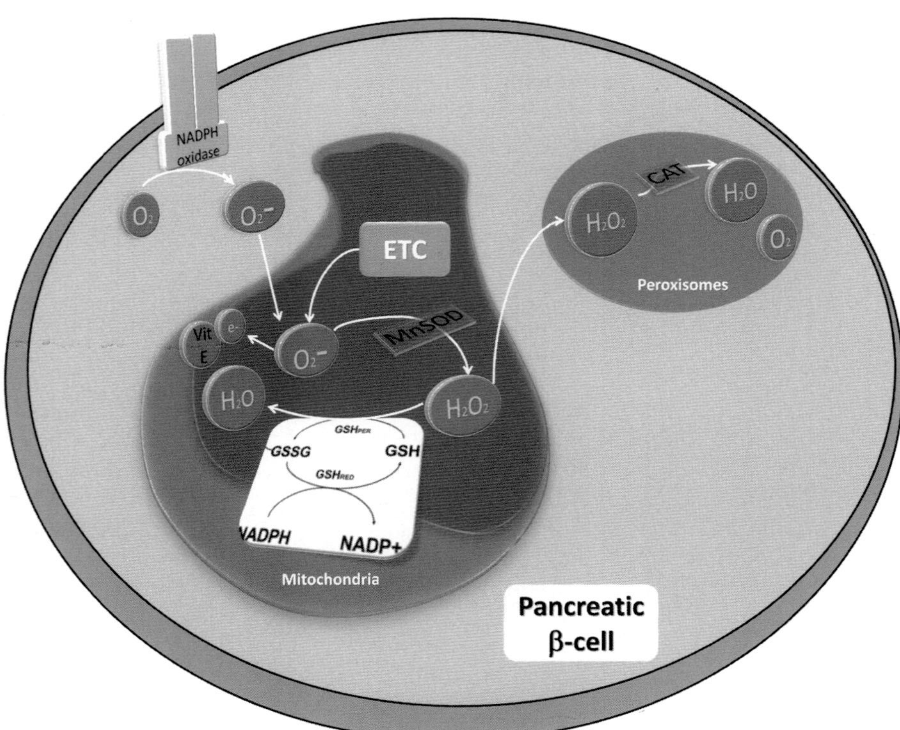

Fig. 10.2 *Superoxide production and the major antioxidant mechanisms in pancreatic β-cells.* Superoxide anions can be synthesized by the activation of the membrane NADPH oxidase and also in normal conditions by the electron transport chain. An increased mitochondrial membrane potential ($\Delta\psi m$) can result in elevated ATP production but reduced electron transport capability thus leading to increased ROS production. The excess of superoxide anions are enzymatically converted to hydrogen peroxide by a manganese-superoxide dismutase (MnSOD) within mitochondria. Hydrogen peroxide can then be rapidly removed by the mitochondrial enzyme glutathione (GSH) peroxidase, which uses glutathione as the electron donor forming glutathione disulphide (GSSG). Glutathione can be resynthesized by the action of the enzyme glutathione reductase (using NADPH as substrate). The inner mitochondrial membrane also contains vitamin E, which is a powerful antioxidant as it can accept unpaired electrons to produce a stable product. Also, catalase is the major hydrogen peroxide detoxifying enzyme found exclusively in peroxisomes

hormones (Goffart and Wiesner 2003). Any imbalance in these processes will lead to cell dysfunction and possibly death resulting in oxidative stress-related diseases. However, the molecular and biochemical mechanisms that link oxidative stress-related processes and diseases remain elusive.

10.3   ROS and Insulin Resistance

Excessive levels of reactive oxygen species not only directly damage cells by oxidizing DNA, protein, and lipids, but indirectly damage cells by activating a variety of stress-sensitive intracellular signalling pathways such as NF-kB, p38 MAPK, JNK/SAPK, hexosamine, and others. Activation of these pathways results in the increased expression of numerous gene products that may cause cellular damage and play a major role in the etiology of the late complications of diabetes. In addition, recent data *in vitro* and *in vivo* suggest that activation of the same or similar stress pathways results in insulin resistance and impaired insulin secretion (Newsholme et al. 2007). Accordingly, it has been proposed the existence of a link among the hyperglycemia- and FFA-induced increases in ROS and oxidative stress, activation of stress-sensitive pathways and the eventual development of not only the late complications of diabetes but also insulin resistance and beta-cell dysfunction (Newsholme et al. 2007). Although our understanding of how hyperglycemia induced oxidative stress ultimately leads to tissue damage has advanced considerably in recent years (Rolo and Palmeira 2006; Vincent et al. 2005), effective therapeutic strategies to prevent or delay the development of this damage remain limited.

The involvement of 'non-damaging' levels ROS in signal transduction is now firmly accepted and examples include roles in cell growth or programmed cell death (apoptosis) (Burdon 1995; Irani 2000; Irani et al. 1997), kinase activation (Lo et al. 1996; Lu et al. 1993), immune responses (Valko et al. 2007), cell calcium signaling (Bedard and Krause 2007) and gene expression (Schoonbroodt and Piette 2000). For example, increased inducible nitric oxide synthase (iNOS) expression in response to redox-dependent transcription factor NFκB activation is a specific example of ROS regulated gene expression. Vascular tone and inhibition of platelet adhesion is regulated by a nitric oxide and hydrogen peroxide dependent activation of guanylate cyclase. Angiotensin II, Thrombin, PDGF (platelet-derived growth factor) and TNF-α (tumor necrosis factor-α) are known to increase ROS production in vascular smooth muscle cells through activation of an isoform of the NOX family NADPH oxidase.

However, since expression levels of antioxidant enzymes such as catalase, and glutathione peroxidase are very low in beta-cells compared to other tissues (Lenzen et al. 1996; Tiedge et al. 1997), beta-cells are thought as targets for oxidative stress-mediated tissue damage (Evans et al. 2002; Maechler et al. 1999; Robertson et al. 2003; Tanaka et al. 2002). Thus it is likely that inflammatory cytokine or saturated fatty acid production of ROS and subsequent oxidative stress is involved in beta-cell deterioration in type 2 diabetes. Whether the source of ROS in the beta cell is mainly mitochondrial or membrane associated NADPH oxidase is open to debate, but the authors have recently published evidence in favour of a key role for NADPH oxidase (Michalska et al. 2010).

There is strong evidence for oxidative stress dependent changes in intracellular signalling, resulting in chronic inflammation and insulin resistance *in vivo* as reported by others (Brownlee 2005; Fridlyand and Philipson 2005; Katakam et al. 2005). While mitochondrial ROS generation may be important for regulation of mitochondrial UCP activity and thus cellular energy metabolism (see below) the NADPH oxidase associated ROS may *specifically* alter parameters of signal transduction, insulin secretion, insulin action and cell proliferation or cell death. From a mechanistic perspective, an increase in reactive molecules can trigger the activation of stress-sensitive serine/threonine kinase signalling pathways such as JNK, NF-kB, p38 MAPK (and others) that in turn phosphorylate multiple targets, including the insulin receptor and IRS proteins. Increased serine phosphorylation of IRS reduces its ability to undergo tyrosine phosphorylation and may accelerate the degradation of IRS-1, offering a plausible explanation for the molecular basis of oxidative stress-induced insulin resistance. There are convincing data to support an important role for the activation of JNK, IKK, PKC, and perhaps other stress and inflammation-activated kinases in the pathogenesis of oxidative stress-induced insulin resistance, and suggest that they might be attractive pharmacological targets to increase insulin sensitivity. The use of antioxidants and pharmacological inhibitors in suppressing the chronic activation of these pathways is consistent with this idea. Moreover, identification of the molecular basis and sites of action for the protection afforded by a variety of antioxidants against oxidative stress-induced damage might lead to the discovery of additional pharmacological targets for novel therapies to prevent, reverse, or delay the onset of oxidative stress-induced insulin resistance.

Despite considerable advances in technology to measure parameters of human mitochondrial function, we are still unable to determine whether impaired function occurs because of alterations in the function of individual mitochondria, a reduction in mitochondrial density (number and/or size of normally functioning mitochondria), differences in O_2 delivery to the mitochondria, or decreased cellular energy demand (Szendroedi and Roden 2008). However, mitochondrial dysfunction is associated with the pathogenesis of insulin resistance related to type 2 diabetes. Using isolated mitochondria from muscle biopsy tissue of insulin-resistant individuals, reduced levels of mRNA for mitochondrial genes (Patti et al. 2003; Heilbronn et al. 2007; Mootha et al. 2003; Morino et al. 2005), decreased mtDNA (Ritov et al. 2005; Boushel et al. 2007), lower protein expression of respiratory chain subunits (Heilbronn et al. 2007), reduced oxidative enzyme activities and decreased mitochondrial size and density (Heilbronn et al. 2007; Kelley et al. 2002; Morino et al. 2005; Ritov et al. 2005) have been reported. Impaired basal and insulin-stimulated mitochondrial metabolism *in vivo* was also demonstrated in patients with type-2 diabetes (Schrauwen-Hinderling et al. 2007) and first-degree relatives of type-2 diabetes patients (Petersen et al. 2004; Befroy et al. 2007). Therefore it is generally well accepted that muscle mitochondrial capacity to produce ATP is reduced in type-2 diabetes patients and insulin-resistant offspring. What remains to be determined is whether this is a result of mitochondrial dysfunction or is secondary to the diabetic or insulin-resistant state.

10.4 Pancreatic Beta Cell Mitochondrial Function

In the pancreatic beta cell the end product of glycolysis, pyruvate, is metabolised by either pyruvate dehydrogenase (PDH; the glucose oxidation pathway) or pyruvate carboxylase (PC; the anaplerosis/ cataplerosis pathway) to acetyl-CoA or oxaloacetate, respectively, resulting in enhanced mitochondrial tricarboxycylic acid (TCA) cycle activity. Among the enzymes responsible for glucose metabolism, glucokinase (GK), PC, and PDH appear to play particularly important regulatory roles in the insulin-secretory pathway. Beta cell PC activity is high even though the cell does not participate in gluconeogenesis, which suggests this enzyme exerts anaplerotic functions. Note that beta cells lack phosphoenolpyruvate carboxykinase (an essential enzyme for gluconeogenesis, converting oxaloacetate to phosphoenol pyruvate). A recent study has highlighted that siRNA targeted to PC resulted in a reduction of insulin secretion from INS-1 cells (Xu et al. 2008), consistent with the observation that PC activity may be reduced in type 2 diabetes (MacDonald et al. 1996). Conversely, overexpression of PC in INS-1 cells resulted in increased insulin release (Xu et al. 2008), again supporting an important role for this enzyme in the maintenance of glucose stimulated insulin secretion (GSIS).

Transfer of electrons from TCA cycle to the mitochondrial electron transport chain is mediated by NADH and $FADH_2$ formation, resulting in ATP generation. The increase in intracellular ATP to ADP ratio leads to the characteristic closure of K_{ATP} channels, membrane depolarization, opening of voltage-gated Ca^{2+} channels, and rapid rise in intracellular Ca^{2+} concentration, leading to mobilization and ultimately fusion of insulin-containing granules with the plasma membrane and insulin release. The primary actions of glucose are mediated by potentiation of ATP concentration by enhanced TCA cycle substrate (oxidative and anaplerotic) supply. Generation of other additive factors derived from glucose metabolism might also be promoted by mitochondrial Ca^{2+} elevation.

Pyruvate may be converted in the beta cell to both acetyl-CoA and oxaloacetate, as discussed above. A number of possibilities for mitochondrial metabolism of pyruvate exist: (i) generation of CO_2 via TCA cycle activity; (ii) export from the mitochondria as glutamate (due to 2-oxoglutarate conversion to glutamate via transamination or glutamate dehydrogenase activity); (iii) export from the mitochondria as malate to be converted back to pyruvate by $NADP^+$ dependent malic enzyme; and (iv) export from the mitochondria as citrate to be acted on by ATP citrate lyase and subsequently acetyl CoA carboxylase to form malonyl-CoA which is an inhibitor of carnitine palmitoyl transferase-1 and thus an inhibitor of fatty acid oxidation (malonyl-CoA can subsequently be used for fatty acid synthesis via the action of fatty acid synthase).

One of these pathways, the so-called pyruvate-malate cycle, predicts a role for malate in insulin secretion via generation of the stimulus-secretion coupling factor NADPH (Jensen et al. 2008). Flow of the cycle requires oxaloacetate derived from pyruvate (via PC) to be converted to malate via a reversal of the malate dehydrogenase reaction, consuming NADH and generating NAD^+ in the mitochondrial matrix. Following this, malate is exported to the cytosol, converted to pyruvate via $NADP^+$ dependent malate dehydrogenase, generating NADPH. Glucose stimulation of beta cells or isolated rodent islet cells increases malate levels and while it is theoretically possible for the malate-pyruvate cycle to operate in the pancreatic beta cell (recently reviewed Jensen et al. 2008) concerns have been raised as to the activity and impact of this cycle under physiologic conditions.

Normal TCA cycle activity ensures the malate $\rightarrow$ oxaloacetate direction of flux, thus generating NADH in the mitochondrial matrix. In addition, malate $\rightarrow$ oxaloacetate conversion forms part of the malate-aspartate shuttle, which has a high activity in the beta cell, and is essential for transfer of cytosolic NADH to the mitochondrial matrix (for review Bender et al. 2006b). In beta cells, reducing equivalents may be transported to the mitochondrial matrix by either the glycerol-phosphate or the malate-aspartate shuttle (Eto et al. 1999). Inhibition of the malate-aspartate shuttle by amino-oxyacetate (which acts on transamination reactions and inhibits cytosolic NADH reoxidation) has been demonstrated to attenuate the secretory response to nutrients, thus highlighting the dominance of this latter shuttle in the beta cell. Most recently Aralar1, a mitochondrial aspartate-glutamate carrier which is an integral component in the malate-aspartate shuttle, has been demonstrated to play an important role in glucose-induced insulin secretion, as its deletion in INS-1 cells leads to a complete loss of malate-aspartate shuttle activity in mitochondria, and to a 25% decrease of insulin release in response to glucose (Marmol et al. 2009).

As described above, one key constituent of the malate-aspartate NADH shuttle is the mitochondrial aspartate-glutamate transporter, with its two Ca^{2+}-sensitive isoforms, Citrin and Aralar1, expressed in excitatory tissue. However, Aralar1 is the dominant aspartate-glutamate transporter isoform expressed in beta cells. Adenoviral-mediated overexpression of Aralar1 in INS-1E beta cells and rat pancreatic islets enhanced glucose-evoked NAD(P)H generation, electron transport chain activity, and mitochondrial ATP formation, and Aralar1 was demonstrated to exert its effect on insulin secretion upstream of the TCA cycle (Rubi et al. 2004). Indeed, the capacity of the aspartate-glutamate transporter appeared to limit NADH shuttle activity and subsequent mitochondrial metabolism. Thus, it is highly *improbable* that a malate-pyruvate cycle is active and important to insulin secretion, if the malate-aspartate shuttle is indeed an active component of stimulus-secretion coupling.

An alternative pyruvate cycling pathway has been proposed, where generation of citrate from condensation of oxaloacetate (OAA) and acetyl-CoA occurs in the TCA cycle, followed by export of citrate from the mitochondria via the citrate-isocitrate carrier, cleavage of citrate by ATP citrate lyase to OAA and acetyl-CoA, and recycling to pyruvate via a cytosolic malate dehydrogenase and $NADP^+$-dependent malic enzyme (Jensen et al. 2008). In this proposed cycle, OAA to malate formation occurs in the cytosol, similar to the malate-aspartate shuttle. Acetyl-CoA can also serve a substrate for acetyl-CoA carboxylase, leading to formation of long-chain acyl-CoA accumulation in the cytosol via malonyl-CoA. In beta cells, glucose stimulation increases malonyl-CoA levels before insulin release and addition of long-chain acyl-CoA results in a stimulation of insulin secretion.

While current research is exploring the capacity of each of the above mitochondrial pathways, shuttles and cycles in the beta cell, relatively little is known about their impairment in type-2 diabetes. It is highly probable that impairment of metabolic stimulus-secretion coupling at multiple sites does occur in the beta cell leading to impaired insulin secretion, hyperglycaemia and type 2 diabetes.

10.5 Mitochondrial DNA Mutations and Type 2 Diabetes

Type 2 diabetes is the most common metabolic disease in the world, but the primary mechanism(s) leading to the development of the disease is still unknown. Insulin resistance plays an early role in the pathogenesis of the disease, eventually leading to defects in insulin secretion by pancreatic beta-cells and progression to hyperglycemia. As full mitochondrial function is required to achieve normal glucose-stimulated insulin secretion from pancreatic beta-cells, both dysfunction of the mitochondrial oxidative pathway and/or defects in mitochondrial DNA (mtDNA) can be involved in the development of type 2 diabetes.

Deletions occurring in mtDNA cause the formation of mutant mtDNA and lead to the development of the most widely recognised mitochondrial diseases, such as Kearns-Sayre syndrome and Pearson syndrome. These neuromuscular disorders result in severe impairment in muscle coordination, cardiac and respiratory functions, and even lead to death, usually in infancy or early childhood. These conditions are rare, but ask the question of the possible contribution of mutations in mtDNA to a more common disease such as type 2 diabetes.

A number of studies have described reduced levels of mRNA for mitochondrial genes (Patti et al. 2003; Heilbronn et al. 2007; Mootha et al. 2003; Morino et al. 2005), decreased mtDNA (Ritov et al. 2005; Boushel et al. 2007) and lower protein expression of respiratory chain subunits (Heilbronn et al. 2007) in mitochondria isolated from muscle biopsy of insulin-resistant individuals. Moreover mitochondrial mutations are known to be present in 2% of T2DM patients (particularly in regions affecting the replication and transcription process), and several mtDNA polymorphisms have been observed, particularly in the NADH and cytochrome c oxidase genes, two important components of the respiratory chain. A non-silent polymorphism of the mitochondrial coding region of the *ND1* gene (a subunit of the NADH dehydrogenase enzyme) has been reported in a large ($n = 245$) group of non-diabetic Pima Indians, a population highly susceptible to developing T2DM (Jackman et al. 2008). More precisely, a single-nucleotide polymorphism leading to a change from isoleucine to valine at amino acid 81 (site 3,457) is associated with a significantly lower resting metabolic rate (RMR), meaning that this ND1 polymorphism could alter respiratory capacity, electron transport or the proton gradient across the inner mitochondrial membrane. However, further investigation into the functional mitochondrial consequences in a small sub-sample of this group revealed no detrimental effect of the ND1 polymorphism on the functional capacity of isolated skeletal muscle mitochondria, indicating that the observed association between a lower RMR and the ND1 polymorphism was not related to mitochondrial function (Jackman et al. 2008). Mitochondrial deletions and myopathies can result in major metabolic disruption but it is still not clear whether less significant mitochondrial mutations can cause mitochondrial and thus cellular dysfunction.

Mutations occurring at levels other than mitochondrial DNA can also result in mitochondrial dysfunction and T2DM. One example is the mitochondrial inner membrane protein known as uncoupling protein 2 (UCP2). When activated, this membrane protein allows protons to move across the inner membrane into the matrix, uncoupling glucose oxidative metabolism from ATP production (Vina et al. 2009). Because it decreases the amount of ATP generated from metabolic fuels, UCP2 negatively regulates glucose-stimulated insulin secretion. Indeed it has been demonstrated that overexpression of UCP2 in cultured pancreatic beta-cells decreased glucose-stimulated insulin secretion (Chan et al. 2001), while targeted inactivation of the UCP2 gene in mice had the opposite effect (Zhang et al. 2001).

10.6 Mitochondrial Dysfunction and Mutations Associated with Aging

Aging is commonly described as a progressive decline in the condition and function of an organism, including important changes in the body composition associated with a progressive decrease in physiologic activity and an increased susceptibility to diseases (Troen 2003). Among these diseases, type 2 diabetes appears to be the most common chronic metabolic disease in the elderly. A recent study comparing healthy young and elderly people has shown that the elderly group developed insulin resistance, mostly evident in the skeletal muscle. Insulin resistance is the result of an age-associated reduction in both mitochondrial oxidative and phosphorylation activity and number (Petersen et al. 2003). Aging has also been associated with accumulation of mutations in control sites for mitochondrial replication (Michikawa et al. 1999). Many other studies also support the idea that a decline in mitochondrial oxidative and ATP generating activity may have an important role in the decline in muscle function in aging (Petersen et al. 2003; Short et al. 2005; Barazzoni et al. 2000; Menshikova et al. 2006; Rooyackers et al. 1996; Muller-Hocker et al. 1992; Trounce et al. 1989; Tonkonogi et al. 2003; Conley et al. 2000). The decrease of the number of cardiac muscle mitochondria appears to be also important in the aging process as the level of old rat mitochondrial proteins were lower than in the heart of young animals, suggesting mitochondriogenesis is impaired with aging (Vina et al. 2009). In humans, the maximal ATP production rate in muscle appears to decline by 8% per decade (Short et al. 2005), due to a combination of reduced mitochondrial content and a functional alteration of the existing mitochondria.

However, dysfunction is not the unique mitochondrial defect associated with aging. In the early 1980s the mitochondrial theory of aging was first published, postulating that during a lifetime a progressive accumulation of somatic mutations in mtDNA occurs, leading to an inevitable decline in mitochondrial function (Miquel et al. 1980). In neurones from patients with Parkinson's disease it has been shown an age-related high level of accumulation of mtDNA deletions compared with the age-matched controls (Bender et al. 2006a; Kraytsberg et al. 2006). In skeletal muscle from Rhesus monkeys, the number of cytochrome c oxidase deficient fibres strongly increases with age and high levels of mtDNA deletions have been found in the areas of cytochrome c oxidase deficiency (Lee et al. 1993). The same observation has been made in skeletal muscle from aging rats (Herbst et al. 2007) correlating sarcopenia to mtDNA mutations. Moreover, animal models of aging have been used to study this accumulation of mtDNA mutations during the aging process and also link it to type 2 diabetes. Indeed, by disrupting the nuclear gene encoding mitochondrial transcription factor A (TFAM) specifically in pancreatic beta-cells to reduce mtDNA expression, Silva et al. observed altered mitochondrial membrane potential, impaired insulin signalling, reduced insulin secretion and an age-associated beta-cell loss (Silva et al. 2000). Therefore it is possible that both mitochondrial oxidative dysfunction and mtDNA mutations play a role in the aging process associated with the development of type 2 diabetes.

10.7 Conclusion

In conclusion, a number of underlying mechanisms responsible for impaired mitochondrial function in metabolic disorders such as insulin resistance and type 2 diabetes have been described while others remain to be discovered. Prospective clinical trials investigating mitochondrial function in various ethnic populations (at rest and during exercise) and the impact on muscle metabolism and development of insulin resistance and type 2 diabetes need to be conducted to delineate the complex interplay between these variables. Reductions in pancreatic beta cell insulin secretion and correlation with beta cell mitochondrial dysfunction including aspects of impaired metabolic stimulus-secretion coupling, needs further exploration in the context of reduced insulin action and muscle dysfunction associated with type 2 diabetes and aging (Fig. 10.3).

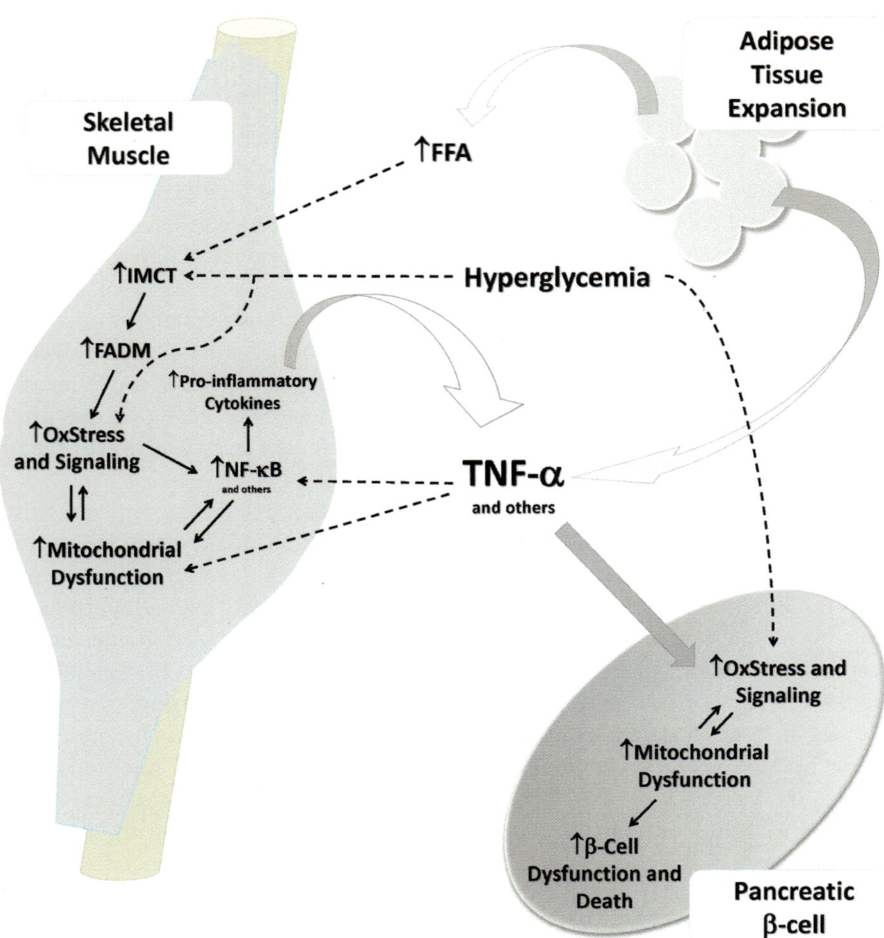

Fig. 10.3 *Possible mechanisms involved in mitochondrial/cell dysfunction in Type 2 diabetes mellitus.* Adipose tissue expansion increases the levels of free fatty acids (FFA), which together with the hyperglycemia increase the synthesis and accumulation of intramyocellular triglycerides (IMCT). Sedentary behaviour and aging are related with a decreased mobilization of the IMCT's resulting in an increased synthesis of toxic fatty-acid-delivered metabolites (FADM). These metabolites causes a elevation in production of ROS and RNS, resulting in oxidative stress, mitochondrial dysfunction and the activation of stress signals such as NF-κB followed by the increased production and release of pro-inflammatory cytokines (TNF-α and others). TNF-α is one of the major molecules that induces insulin resistance in skeletal muscle cells. This cytokine can also induce activation of stress signals in pancreatic β-cells, leading to mitochondrial dysfunction that culminates in cell dysfunction and death

References

Barazzoni R, Short KR, Nair KS (2000) Effects of aging on mitochondrial DNA copy number and cytochrome c oxidase gene expression in rat skeletal muscle, liver, and heart. J Biol Chem 275:3343–3347

Bedard K, Krause KH (2007) The NOX family of ROS-generating NADPH oxidases: physiology and pathophysiology. Physiol Rev 87:245–313

Befroy DE, Petersen KF, Dufour S, Mason GF, de Graaf RA, Rothman DL, Shulman GI (2007) Impaired mitochondrial substrate oxidation in muscle of insulin-resistant offspring of type 2 diabetic patients. Diabetes 56:1376–1381

Bender A, Krishnan KJ, Morris CM, Taylor GA, Reeve AK, Perry RH, Jaros E, Hersheson JS, Betts J, Klopstock T, Taylor RW, Turnbull DM (2006a) High levels of mitochondrial DNA deletions in substantia nigra neurons in aging and Parkinson disease. Nat Genet 38:515–517

Bender K, Newsholme P, Brennan L, Maechler P (2006b) The importance of redox shuttles to pancreatic beta-cell energy metabolism and function. Biochem Soc Trans 34:811–814

Boushel R, Gnaiger E, Schjerling P, Skovbro M, Kraunsoe R, Dela F (2007) Patients with type 2 diabetes have normal mitochondrial function in skeletal muscle. Diabetologia 50:790–796

Brownlee M (2005) The pathobiology of diabetic complications: a unifying mechanism. Diabetes 54:1615–1625

Burdon RH (1995) Superoxide and hydrogen peroxide in relation to mammalian cell proliferation. Free Radic Biol Med 18:775–794

Chan CB, de Leo D, Joseph JW, McQuaid TS, Ha XF, Xu F, Tsushima RG, Pennefather PS, Salapatek AM, Wheeler MB (2001) Increased uncoupling protein-2 levels in beta-cells are associated with impaired glucose-stimulated insulin secretion: mechanism of action. Diabetes 50:1302–1310

Conley KE, Jubrias SA, Esselman PC (2000) Oxidative capacity and ageing in human muscle. J Physiol 526(Pt 1):203–210

Eto K, Tsubamoto Y, Terauchi Y, Sugiyama T, Kishimoto T, Takahashi N, Yamauchi N, Kubota N, Murayama S, Aizawa T, Akanuma Y, Aizawa S, Kasai H, Yazaki Y, Kadowaki T (1999) Role of NADH shuttle system in glucose-induced activation of mitochondrial metabolism and insulin secretion. Science 283:981–985

Evans JL, Goldfine ID, Maddux BA, Grodsky GM (2002) Oxidative stress and stress-activated signaling pathways: a unifying hypothesis of type 2 diabetes. Endocr Rev 23:599–622

Evans MD, Dizdaroglu M, Cooke MS (2004) Oxidative DNA damage and disease: induction, repair and significance. Mutat Res 567:1–61

Fridlyand LE, Philipson LH (2005) Oxidative reactive species in cell injury: mechanisms in diabetes mellitus and therapeutic approaches. Ann N Y Acad Sci 1066:136–151

Goffart S, Wiesner RJ (2003) Regulation and co-ordination of nuclear gene expression during mitochondrial biogenesis. Exp Physiol 88:33–40

Harper ME, Bevilacqua L, Hagopian K, Weindruch R, Ramsey JJ (2004) Ageing, oxidative stress, and mitochondrial uncoupling. Acta Physiol Scand 182:321–331

Heilbronn LK, Gan SK, Turner N, Campbell LV, Chisholm DJ (2007) Markers of mitochondrial biogenesis and metabolism are lower in overweight and obese insulin-resistant subjects. J Clin Endocrinol Metab 92:1467–1473

Herbst A, Pak JW, McKenzie D, Bua E, Bassiouni M, Aiken JM (2007) Accumulation of mitochondrial DNA deletion mutations in aged muscle fibers: evidence for a causal role in muscle fiber loss. J Gerontol A Biol Sci Med Sci 62:235–245

Hutter E, Skovbro M, Lener B, Prats C, Rabol R, Dela F, Jansen-Durr P (2007) Oxidative stress and mitochondrial impairment can be separated from lipofuscin accumulation in aged human skeletal muscle. Aging Cell 6:245–256

Irani K (2000) Oxidant signaling in vascular cell growth, death, and survival: a review of the roles of reactive oxygen species in smooth muscle and endothelial cell mitogenic and apoptotic signaling. Circ Res 87:179–183

Irani K, Xia Y, Zweier JL, Sollott SJ, Der CJ, Fearon ER, Sundaresan M, Finkel T, Goldschmidt-Clermont PJ (1997) Mitogenic signaling mediated by oxidants in Ras-transformed fibroblasts. Science 275:1649–1652

Jackman MR, Ravussin E, Rowe MJ, Pratley R, Milner MR, Willis WT (2008) Effect of a polymorphism in the ND1 mitochondrial gene on human skeletal muscle mitochondrial function. Obesity (Silver Spring) 16:363–368

Jensen MV, Joseph JW, Ronnebaum SM, Burgess SC, Sherry AD, Newgard CB (2008) Metabolic cycling in control of glucose-stimulated insulin secretion. Am J Physiol Endocrinol Metab 295:E1287–E1297

Katakam AK, Chipitsyna G, Gong Q, Vancha AR, Gabbeta J, Arafat HA (2005) Streptozotocin (STZ) mediates acute upregulation of serum and pancreatic osteopontin (OPN): a novel islet-protective effect of OPN through inhibition of STZ-induced nitric oxide production. J Endocrinol 187:237–247

Kelley DE, He J, Menshikova EV, Ritov VB (2002) Dysfunction of mitochondria in human skeletal muscle in type 2 diabetes. Diabetes 51:2944–2950

Korshunov SS, Skulachev VP, Starkov AA (1997) High protonic potential actuates a mechanism of production of reactive oxygen species in mitochondria. FEBS Lett 416:15–18

Kraytsberg Y, Kudryavtseva E, McKee AC, Geula C, Kowall NW, Khrapko K (2006) Mitochondrial DNA deletions are abundant and cause functional impairment in aged human substantia nigra neurons. Nat Genet 38:518–520

Lee CM, Chung SS, Kaczkowski JM, Weindruch R, Aiken JM (1993) Multiple mitochondrial DNA deletions associated with age in skeletal muscle of rhesus monkeys. J Gerontol 48:B201–B205

Lenzen S, Drinkgern J, Tiedge M (1996) Low antioxidant enzyme gene expression in pancreatic islets compared with various other mouse tissues. Free Radic Biol Med 20:463–466

Lo YY, Wong JM, Cruz TF (1996) Reactive oxygen species mediate cytokine activation of c-Jun NH2-terminal kinases. J Biol Chem 271:15703–15707

Lu D, Maulik N, Moraru II, Kreutzer DL, Das DK (1993) Molecular adaptation of vascular endothelial cells to oxidative stress. Am J Physiol 264:C715–C722

Macdonald MJ, Tang J, Polonsky KS (1996) Low mitochondrial glycerol phosphate dehydrogenase and pyruvate carboxylase in pancreatic islets of Zucker diabetic fatty rats. Diabetes 45:1626–1630

Maechler P, Jornot L, Wollheim CB (1999) Hydrogen peroxide alters mitochondrial activation and insulin secretion in pancreatic beta cells. J Biol Chem 274:27905–27913

Maiese K, Morhan SD, Chong ZZ (2007) Oxidative stress biology and cell injury during type 1 and type 2 diabetes mellitus. Curr Neurovasc Res 4:63–71

Marmol P, Pardo B, Wiederkehr A, del Arco A, Wollheim CB, Satrustegui J (2009) Requirement for aralar and its Ca2+-binding sites in Ca2+ signal transduction in mitochondria from INS-1 clonal beta-cells. J Biol Chem 284:515–524

Menshikova EV, Ritov VB, Fairfull L, Ferrell RE, Kelley DE, Goodpaster BH (2006) Effects of exercise on mitochondrial content and function in aging human skeletal muscle. J Gerontol A Biol Sci Med Sci 61:534–540

Michalska M, Wolf G, Walther R, Newsholme P (2010) The effects of pharmacologic inhibition of NADPH oxidase or iNOS on pro-inflammatory cytokine, palmitic acid or H2O2 -induced mouse islet or clonal pancreatic beta cell dysfunction. Biosci Rep. doi:10.1042/BSR20090138

Michikawa Y, Mazzucchelli F, Bresolin N, Scarlato G, Attardi G (1999) Aging-dependent large accumulation of point mutations in the human mtDNA control region for replication. Science 286:774–779

Miquel J, Economos AC, Fleming J, Johnson JE Jr (1980) Mitochondrial role in cell aging. Exp Gerontol 15:575–591

Mootha VK, Lindgren CM, Eriksson KF, Subramanian A, Sihag S, Lehar J, Puigserver P, Carlsson E, Ridderstrale M, Laurila E, Houstis N, Daly MJ, Patterson N, Mesirov JP, Golub TR, Tamayo P, Spiegelman B, Lander ES, Hirschhorn JN, Altshuler D, Groop LC (2003) PGC-1alpha-responsive genes involved in oxidative phosphorylation are coordinately downregulated in human diabetes. Nat Genet 34:267–273

Morino K, Petersen KF, Dufour S, Befroy D, Frattini J, Shatzkes N, Neschen S, White MF, Bilz S, Sono S, Pypaert M, Shulman GI (2005) Reduced mitochondrial density and increased IRS-1 serine phosphorylation in muscle of insulin-resistant offspring of type 2 diabetic parents. J Clin Invest 115:3587–3593

Muller-Hocker J, Schneiderbanger K, Stefani FH, Kadenbach B (1992) Progressive loss of cytochrome c oxidase in the human extraocular muscles in ageing–a cytochemical-immunohistochemical study. Mutat Res 275:115–124

Newsholme P, Haber EP, Hirabara SM, Rebelato ELO, Procopio J, Morgan D, Oliveira-Emilio HC, Carpinelli AR, Curi R (2007) Diabetes associated cell stress and dysfunction – Role of mitochondrial and non-mitochondrial ROS production and activity. J Physiol 583:9–24

Patti ME, Butte AJ, Crunkhorn S, Cusi K, Berria R, Kashyap S, Miyazaki Y, Kohane I, Costello M, Saccone R, Landaker EJ, Goldfine AB, Mun E, Defronzo R, Finlayson J, Kahn CR, Mandarino LJ (2003) Coordinated reduction of genes of oxidative metabolism in humans with insulin resistance and diabetes: potential role of PGC1 and NRF1. Proc Natl Acad Sci USA 100:8466–8471

Petersen KF, Befroy D, Dufour S, Dziura J, Ariyan C, Rothman DL, Dipietro L, Cline GW, Shulman GI (2003) Mitochondrial dysfunction in the elderly: possible role in insulin resistance. Science 300:1140–1142

Petersen KF, Dufour S, Befroy D, Garcia R, Shulman GI (2004) Impaired mitochondrial activity in the insulin-resistant offspring of patients with type 2 diabetes. N Engl J Med 350:664–671

Rachek LI, Musiyenko SI, Ledoux SP, Wilson GL (2007) Palmitate induced mitochondrial deoxyribonucleic acid damage and apoptosis in l6 rat skeletal muscle cells. Endocrinology 148:293–299

Ritov VB, Menshikova EV, He J, Ferrell RE, Goodpaster BH, Kelley DE (2005) Deficiency of subsarcolemmal mitochondria in obesity and type 2 diabetes. Diabetes 54:8–14

Robertson RP, Harmon J, Tran PO, Tanaka Y, Takahashi H (2003) Glucose toxicity in beta-cells: type 2 diabetes, good radicals gone bad, and the glutathione connection. Diabetes 52:581–587

Rolo AP, Palmeira CM (2006) Diabetes and mitochondrial function: role of hyperglycemia and oxidative stress. Toxicol Appl Pharmacol 212:167–178

Rooyackers OE, Adey DB, Ades PA, Nair KS (1996) Effect of age on in vivo rates of mitochondrial protein synthesis in human skeletal muscle. Proc Natl Acad Sci USA 93:15364–15369

Rubi B, del Arco A, Bartley C, Satrustegui J, Maechler P (2004) The malate-aspartate NADH shuttle member Aralar1 determines glucose metabolic fate, mitochondrial activity, and insulin secretion in beta cells. J Biol Chem 279:55659–55666

Schoonbroodt S, Piette J (2000) Oxidative stress interference with the nuclear factor-kappa B activation pathways. Biochem Pharmacol 60:1075–1083

Schrauwen-Hinderling VB, Kooi ME, Hesselink MK, Jeneson JA, Backes WH, van Echteld CJ, van Engelshoven JM, Mensink M, Schrauwen P (2007) Impaired in vivo mitochondrial function but similar intramyocellular lipid content in patients with type 2 diabetes mellitus and BMI-matched control subjects. Diabetologia 50:113–120

Short KR, Bigelow ML, Kahl J, Singh R, Coenen-Schimke J, Raghavakaimal S, Nair KS (2005) Decline in skeletal muscle mitochondrial function with aging in humans. Proc Natl Acad Sci USA 102:5618–5623

Silva JP, Kohler M, Graff C, Oldfors A, Magnuson MA, Berggren PO, Larsson NG (2000) Impaired insulin secretion and beta-cell loss in tissue-specific knockout mice with mitochondrial diabetes. Nat Genet 26:336–340

Szendroedi J, Roden M (2008) Mitochondrial fitness and insulin sensitivity in humans. Diabetologia 51:2155–2167

Tanaka Y, Tran PO, Harmon J, Robertson RP (2002) A role for glutathione peroxidase in protecting pancreatic beta cells against oxidative stress in a model of glucose toxicity. Proc Natl Acad Sci USA 99:12363–12368

Tiedge M, Lortz S, Drinkgern J, Lenzen S (1997) Relation between antioxidant enzyme gene expression and antioxidative defense status of insulin-producing cells. Diabetes 46:1733–1742

Tonkonogi M, Fernstrom M, Walsh B, Ji LL, Rooyackers O, Hammarqvist F, Wernerman J, Sahlin K (2003) Reduced oxidative power but unchanged antioxidative capacity in skeletal muscle from aged humans. Pflugers Arch 446:261–269
Troen BR (2003) The biology of aging. Mt Sinai J Med 70:3–22
Trounce I, Byrne E, Marzuki S (1989) Decline in skeletal muscle mitochondrial respiratory chain function: possible factor in ageing. Lancet 1:637–639
Turrens JF (2003) Mitochondrial formation of reactive oxygen species. J Physiol 552:335–344
Valko M, Leibfritz D, Moncol J, Cronin MT, Mazur M, Telser J (2007) Free radicals and antioxidants in normal physiological functions and human disease. Int J Biochem Cell Biol 39:44–84
Vina J, Gomez-Cabrera MC, Borras C, Froio T, Sanchis-Gomar F, Martinez-Bello VE, Pallardo FV (2009) Mitochondrial biogenesis in exercise and in ageing. Adv Drug Deliv Rev 61:1369–1374
Vincent AM, Stevens MJ, Backus C, McLean LL, Feldman EL (2005) Cell culture modeling to test therapies against hyperglycemia-mediated oxidative stress and injury. Antioxid Redox Signal 7:1494–1506
Xu J, Han J, Long YS, Epstein PN, Liu YQ (2008) The role of pyruvate carboxylase in insulin secretion and proliferation in rat pancreatic beta cells. Diabetologia 51:2022–2030
Zhang CY, Baffy G, Perret P, Krauss S, Peroni O, Grujic D, Hagen T, Vidal-Puig AJ, Boss O, Kim YB, Zheng XX, Wheeler MB, Shulman GI, Chan CB, Lowell BB (2001) Uncoupling protein-2 negatively regulates insulin secretion and is a major link between obesity, beta cell dysfunction, and type 2 diabetes. Cell 105:745–755

Chapter 11
Mitochondria and Heart Disease

Elinor J. Griffiths

Abstract Mitochondria play a key role in the normal functioning of the heart, and in the pathogenesis and development of various types of heart disease. Physiologically, mitochondrial ATP supply needs to be matched to the often sudden changes in ATP demand of the heart, and this is mediated to a large extent by the mitochondrial Ca^{2+} transport pathways allowing elevation of mitochondrial $[Ca^{2+}]$ ($[Ca^{2+}]_m$). In turn this activates dehydrogenase enzymes to increase NADH and hence ATP supply. Pathologically, $[Ca^{2+}]_m$ is also important in generation of reactive oxygen species, and in opening of the mitochondrial permeability transition pore (MPTP); factors involved in both ischaemia-reperfusion injury and in heart failure. The MPTP has proved a promising target for protective strategies, with inhibitors widely used to show cardioprotection in experimental, and very recently human, studies. Similarly mitochondrially-targeted antioxidants have proved protective in various animal models of disease and await clinical trials. The mitochondrial Ca^{2+} transport pathways, although in theory promising therapeutic targets, cannot yet be targeted in human studies due to non-specific effects of drugs used experimentally to inhibit them. Finally, specific mitochondrial cardiomyopathies due to mutations in mtDNA have been identified, usually in a gene for a tRNA, which, although rare, are almost always very severe once the mutation has exceeded its threshold.

Keywords Ischaemia • Ischemia • Reperfusion • Cardiomyopathy • Hypertrophy • Congenital heart disease • Heart failure • Calcium • Permeability transition pore • Mitochondrial DNA • Calcium uniporter • Cyclosporine A

Abbreviations

mCU	Mitochondrial calcium uniporter
mNCX	Mitochondrial sodium calcium exchanger
MPTP	Mitochondrial permeability transition pore
ROS	Reactive oxygen species
RuR	Ruthenium red

E.J. Griffiths (✉)
Bristol Heart Institute and Department of Biochemistry, University of Bristol, Bristol, UK

Department of Biochemistry, School of Medical Sciences, University Walk, Bristol BS8 1TD, UK
e-mail: Elinor.Griffiths@bristol.ac.uk

R. Scatena et al. (eds.), *Advances in Mitochondrial Medicine*, Advances in Experimental Medicine and Biology 942, DOI 10.1007/978-94-007-2869-1_11,
© Springer Science+Business Media B.V. 2012

11.1 Introduction: Heart Diseases and Mitochondria

Mitochondria provide over 90% of the ATP required for the heart to function normally (Harris and Das 1991). The heart also has to have a way of increasing ATP supply rapidly upon increases in demand, such as occurs during increased workload or adrenergic stimulation. To give and idea of how quickly this has to happen, in a canine heart the entire ATP pool is turned over in 1 min under normal conditions, and in about 10 s under conditions of high workload (Khouri et al. 1965; Balaban 2009; Katz et al. 1989). Oxygen is not rate limiting for ATP synthesis until below about 20 μM (McCormack et al. 1990), a level much lower than that occurring physiologically. Pathologically, however, O_2 levels can decrease for a variety of reasons, leading to partial or total ischaemia, which will then impair ATP synthesis. This occurs when arteries become narrowed during atherosclerosis, either causing angina or a heart attack, in the case of unstable plaques that rupture and block the artery completely. Ischaemia also occurs during cardiac surgery when the aorta is cross-clamped, the heart stopped and the body placed on a heart-lung bypass machine. Reperfusion of the heart is obviously necessary but paradoxically can cause further damage. Clinically reperfusion damage can therefore occur during cardiac surgery, spontaneously following a myocardial infarction (MI), and in patients undergoing thrombolysis or angioplasty for treatment of MI.

Mitochondria, in particular mitochondrial Ca^{2+} overload and oxygen free radical formation, are associated with the transition from reversible to irreversible damage following ischaemia: The discovery that the mitochondrial permeability transition pore (MPTP) plays a key role in the development of reperfusion injury has opened the way for protective strategies targeted at the pore – these are discussed below. Similarly the oxidative stress cause by reactive oxygen species (ROS) has been shown to contribute to the pathogenesis of both reperfusion injury and lately to the development of heart failure; free radical scavengers have been used experimentally to prevent such damage, and recently scavengers targeted specifically at the mitochondria have been designed that afford better protection; see Sect. 11.3.1.

Some specific cardiomyopathies arising from defects in mitochondrial DNA (mtDNA) have been identified, and these will be highlighted below. However, there are a myriad of other diseases arising from defects in mtDNA that affect the nervous system and muscular tissue. This chapter will not deal with these non heart-specific defects, which are covered in the chapter on inherited diseases (see Chap. 8 by Finsterer). Neither will I cover congenital heart disease arising from defects in cardiac structure or function during development since these are not specifically mitochondrial; for reviews see Bruneau (2008), Nemer (2008).

11.2 The Central Role of Mitochondria in Cardiac Ischaemia/Reperfusion Injury

11.2.1 Regulation of ATP Supply and Demand in the Heart

Normal mitochondrial physiology including oxidative phosphorylation is covered in Chap. 1 (by Papa) of this volume and has been reviewed recently (Balaban 2009; Denton 2009; Griffiths 2009). However, I will discuss the parts relevant to understanding the role of mitochondria in heart disease, particularly the mitochondrial Ca^{2+} transport pathways.

Oxygen acts as the final electron acceptor in the respiratory chain; as oxygen becomes limiting, electron carriers can no longer be re-oxidised, resulting in a build up of NAD(P)H and $FADH_2$ generated by dehydrogenases in the citric acid cycle. This has been measured using autofluorescence at the relevant wavelength in both whole hearts and isolated myocytes (Katz et al. 1987; Heineman and

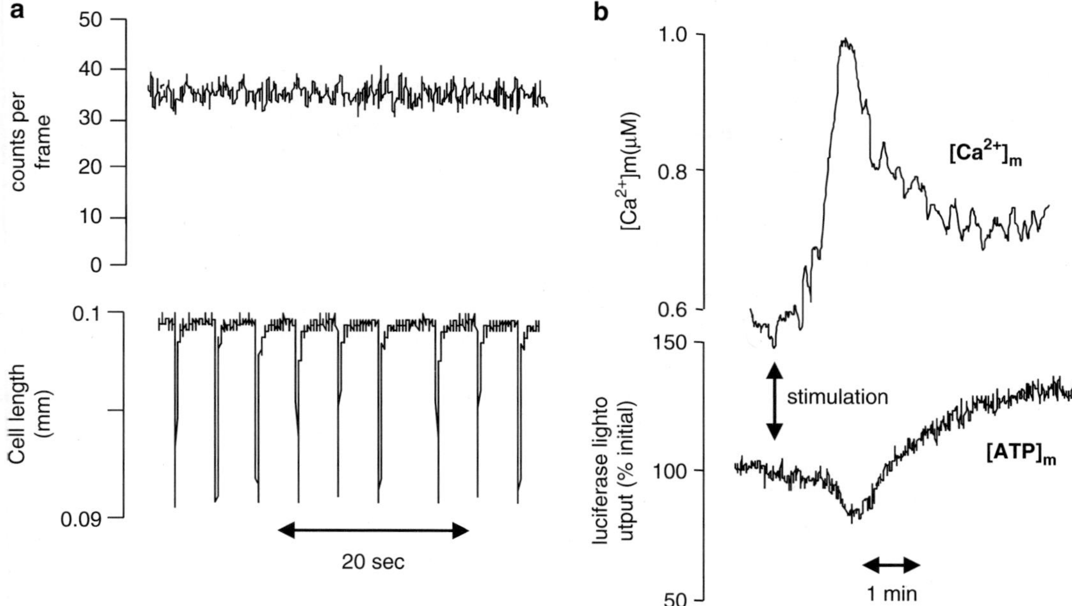

Fig. 11.1 *ATP and mitochondrial [Ca²⁺] levels in beating cardiomyocytes.* (**a**) $[ATP]_m$ was measured using targeted luciferase in synchronously beating adult cardiomyocytes stimulated to contract at 0.2 Hz. Parallel cell length measurements were taken from a single cell to highlight the lack of change in $[ATP]_m$ during a single contraction, (**b**) $[Ca^{2+}]_m$ and $[ATP]_m$ were measured using targeted aequorin and luciferase, respectively, in parallel experiments on small populations of cells stimulated to contract at 2 Hz from rest in presence of isoproterenol. In this figure the average $[Ca^{2+}]_m$ is shown – see text for discussion (Figure based on work of the author data first published in Bell et al. 2006)

Balaban 1993; White and Wittenberg 1993; Griffiths et al. 1997). The importance of ensuring adequate O_2 supply for maintaining supply-demand balance was illustrated when initial studies on whole hearts found an increase in the NAD(P)H/NAD(P)⁺ ratio fluorescence upon increased workload – however, this was subsequently found to be due to inadequate perfusion of the hearts; in vivo and in well-oxygenated hearts, there was no such increase (Katz et al. 1987; Heineman and Balaban 1993).

Thus there has to be a mechanism of ensuring that ATP supply is matched exactly to demand, and early studies in isolated mitochondria found that the ADP/ATP ratio was the main regulator of ATP production (Chance and Williams 1956). However later studies in beating hearts found that the ratio did not change in well-oxygenated hearts even during large increases in workload (Katz et al. 1989; Neely et al. 1972). In support of this, we found recently, using targeted luciferase, that ATP levels in beating cardiomyocytes were remarkably constant in both cytosolic and mitochondrial compartments (Bell et al. 2006); and see Fig. 11.1. The discovery by Denton and McCormack that Ca²⁺ could activate the mitochondrial dehydrogenases – pyruvate dehydrogenase (PDH), oxoglutarate dehydrogenase (OGDH) and isocitrate dehydrogenase (ICDH) – in the physiological range lead them to propose a parallel activation model where an increase in intramitochondrial free $[Ca^{2+}]$ ($[Ca^{2+}]_m$) activated the dehydrogenases to increase NADH and hence ATP production (McCormack et al. 1990; Denton 2009); see Fig. 11.2. The observation that ATP levels do not change on a beat to beat basis, or under conditions of increases workload in the heart imply that $[Ca^{2+}]_m$ plays the key role under physiological conditions in the heart. However, Balaban has argued that, given the importance of ensuring a rapid response system of ATP synthesis in the myocardium, more than one mechanism is likely to operate to coordinate ATP supply and demand (Balaban 2009). This can be seen under conditions where the heart was stimulated to beat rapidly from rest when there is an initial drop in ATP before it recovers, the timecourse of which correlates with the time taken for mitochondria to take up Ca²⁺ (Fig. 11.2).

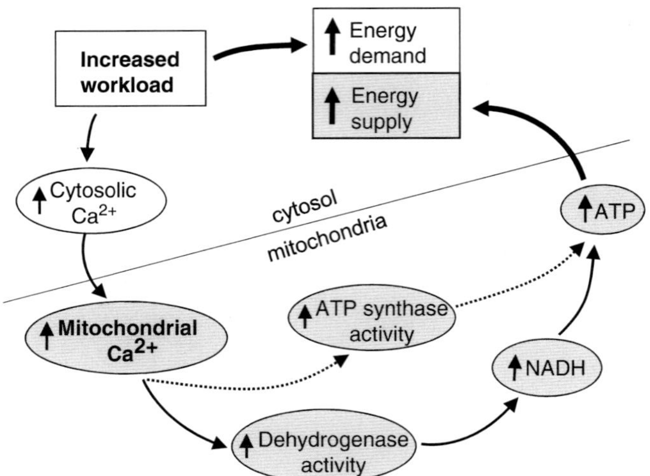

Fig. 11.2 *Parallel activation model of dehydrogenase activation by mitochondrial [Ca²⁺].* Increases in cytosolic Ca²⁺ resulting form increases in heart workload or adrenergic stimulation are relayed to the mitochondrial matrix via the mitochondrial Ca²⁺ uniporter (mCU). $[Ca^{2+}]_m$ activates dehydrogenase of the citric acid cycle and possibly the ATP synthase to increase ATP supply in line with the increased demand. See text for further details

Role of Ca²⁺ in regulating mitochondrial function is discussed in more detail in Chap. 3 (by Brini), and in recent reviews (Griffiths 2009; Maack and O'Rourke 2007; Dedkova and Blatter 2008). Briefly, mitochondrial Ca²⁺ uptake occurs by a uniporter (mCU), and efflux via a sodium calcium exchanger (mNCX); a summary of the mitochondrial pathways for Ca²⁺ transport together with known inhibitors is shown in Fig. 11.3. Studies using isolated mitochondria found that the kinetics of the channels indicated they were too slow to play any role in intracellular Ca²⁺ signalling during excitation-contraction (EC) coupling of the heart (reviewed in Nicholls and Crompton 1980; Gunter and Pfeiffer 1990) and it was predicted that net Ca²⁺ influx would occur only when external [Ca²⁺] rose above about 500 nM (Nicholls and Crompton 1980; Gunter and Pfeiffer 1990), much higher than the resting cytosolic free [Ca²⁺] ($[Ca^{2+}]_c$) of 100–200 nM. However, evidence from non-cardiac and more recently cardiac cells has revealed that the mCU is located in close proximity to the sarcoplasmic reticular (SR) Ca²⁺ release channel, at least in some subcellular populations of mitochondria, and therefore is exposed to a much higher but very localised $[Ca^{2+}]_c$ than previously thought (Griffiths 2009; Maack and O'Rourke 2007; Dedkova and Blatter 2008). It therefore may change on a rapid timescale and be able to modulate EC coupling.

The Ca²⁺-induced mitochondrial permeability transition pore (MPTP), first described as an increase in inner membrane permeability in 1976 (Hunter et al. 1976), can act as a Ca²⁺ efflux mechanism but is not specific for Ca²⁺, allowing transport of small molecules with a molecular weight of less than about 1.5 kDa. The MPTP also requires additional factors such as adenine nucleotide depletion, oxidative stress and elevated phosphate; this makes a physiological role for the MPTP unlikely but these conditions are exactly those that occur during ischaemia/reperfusion injury; this is discussed further below.

11.2.2 Mitochondrial Dysfunction and Ca²⁺ Transport During Ischaemia and Reperfusion

Whether the result of gradual or sudden ischaemia, mitochondrial ATP production will become progressively less as oxygen levels and substrate supply decrease. The ionic changes that result from reduced ATP supply are summarised in Fig. 11.3, and reviewed in Suleiman et al. (2001), Murphy and

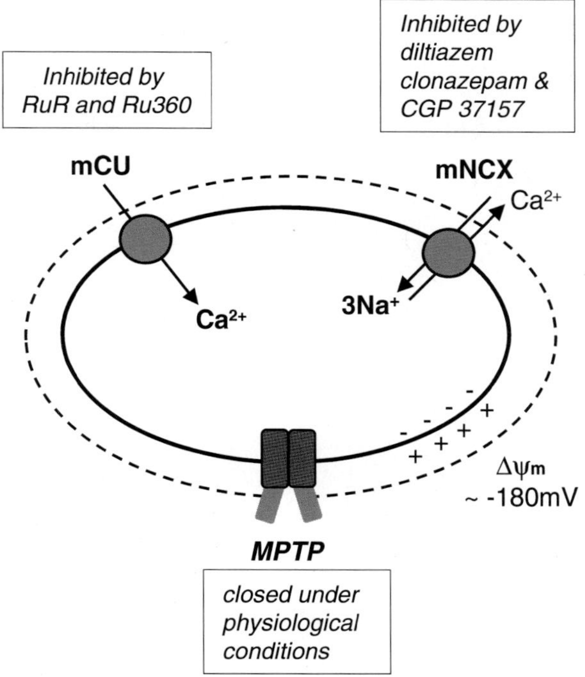

Fig. 11.3 *Ca²⁺ transport pathways of mitochondria. mCU* Calcium uniporter, *mNCX* mitochondrial sodium calcium exchanger, *MPTP* mitochondrial permeability transition pore, *RuR* ruthenium red. $\Delta\psi_m$ – mitochondrial membrane potential, approximately −180 mV in actively respiring mitochondria (inside negative). *Solid oval* depicts the inner membrane and *dashed oval* the permeable outer membrane. The MPTP is probably closed under physiological conditions but when open can act as an efflux pathway for Ca²⁺; is also permeable to other small molecules of less than about 1,500 Da. The MPTP is shown here as consisting of both inner and outer membrane proteins; see text for a discussion of pore components

Steenbergen (2008a). The reduced ATP levels lead to failure of the Na⁺/K⁺-ATPase, Na⁺ loading (Haigney et al. 1994), and subsequently Ca²⁺ loading via reversal of the Na⁺/Ca²⁺ exchanger (Silverman and Stern 1994), and build up of lactic acid causes intracellular acidosis. The ionic changes occurring during ischaemia/reperfusion and the role of mitochondria are summarised in Fig. 11.4 and reviewed in Suleiman et al. (2001), Murphy and Steenbergen (2008b). In isolated myocytes, $[Ca^{2+}]_m$ only increased following ATP depletion-dependent rigor contracture. Reperfusion of hearts or myocytes before rigor-contracture causes reversible damage "stunning", but usually recovery with time. Whether or not cardio-myocytes recovered from hypoxia depended on the level of $[Ca^{2+}]_m$ achieved at the end of the hypoxic period: cells having $[Ca^{2+}]_m$ greater than about 250–300 nM invariably hypercontracted upon reperfusion (Miyata et al. 1992; Griffiths et al. 1998). Similar increases have been observed in mitochondria isolated from whole hearts following ischaemia/reperfusion – $[Ca^{2+}]_m$ rose from pre-hypoxic values of 160–360 and 570 nM after 50 and 80 min of hypoxia, respectively (Allen et al. 1993). But a much greater increase in $[Ca^{2+}]_m$ occurs upon reperfusion (Delcamp et al. 1998; Chacon et al. 1994), for example in whole hearts following 80 min hypoxia, reperfusion led to a 10-fold increase in $[Ca^{2+}]_m$ (Allen et al. 1993). Although normally mitochondria have the capacity to take up huge amounts of Ca²⁺ (Nicholls and Crompton 1980; Gunter and Pfeiffer 1990) and thus could potentially remove toxic levels of Ca²⁺ from the cytosol, such accumulation of Ca²⁺ can eventually damage mitochondria both by competing for ATP production and more importantly by inducing the mitochondrial permeability transition pore (MPTP). Other factors upon reperfusion also lower the threshold of $[Ca^{2+}]_m$ needed for the MPTP to open; for example low adenine nucleotides, free radical generation, and return to normal pH. Hence the MPTP can open at values of $[Ca^{2+}]_m$ that may not be much higher than physiological.

But it should be remembered that limited (rather than excessive) Ca²⁺ uptake by mitochondria on reperfusion has the capacity to be protective: for example, by activation of PDH. Increased glucose

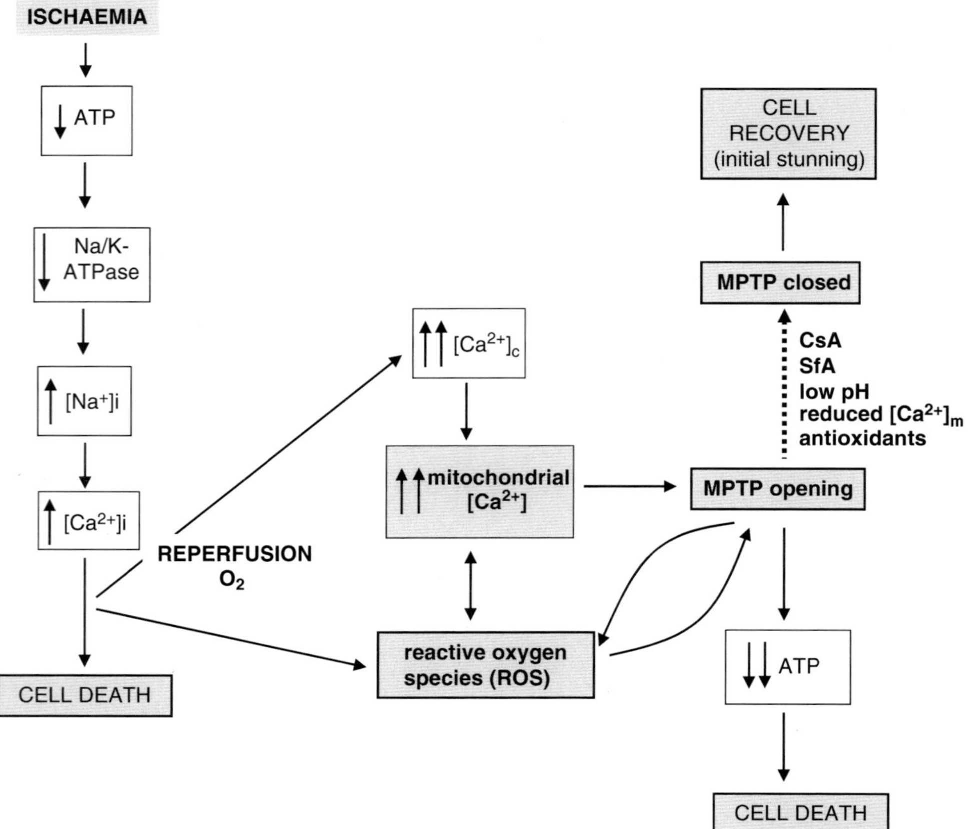

Fig. 11.4 *Ionic changes during ischaemia and reperfusion injury showing central role of mitochondrial [Ca²⁺] and the MPTP. Ischaemia* leads to an inhibition of oxidative phosphorylation, the resulting decrease in ATP causes ion channel dysfunction, leading to increases in $[Na^+]_i$, $[Ca^{2+}]_c$ and $[Ca^{2+}]_m$. Of ischaemia is of short duration, the cell can recovery as the changes will not be severe enough to cause opening of the MPTP, although stunning (reversible injury) may occur. However, following prolonged ischaemia, the increase in $[Ca^{2+}]_m$, reactive oxygen species and low ATP levels cause opening of the MPTP. ATP levels can then not recover and ROS production is exacerbated, leading to cell death. Agents that either prevent the increase in $[Ca^{2+}]_m$, inhibit pore components (SfA and CsA), or inhibit the pore indirectly (low pH and free radical scavengers), will allow the pore to close, or prevent opening, shifting the balance towards cell recovery. See text for further discussion

oxidation on reperfusion improves recovery of the heart, and drugs like ranolazine, which increase PDH activity, can improve post-ischaemic recovery (Clarke et al. 1993). So in designing protective strategies, it is a matter of getting the balance right between beneficial versus harmful effects of mitochondrial Ca^{2+} uptake. The situation is further complicated by the fact that many other factors on reperfusion affect this balance.

Although several studies had reported an increase in $[Ca^{2+}]_m$ during hypoxia (see above), the mechanism of entry of the Ca^{2+} was either not discussed, or assumed to be the mCU. But mitochondrial membrane potential ($\Delta\Psi_m$) depolarises during hypoxia (Di Lisa et al. 1995), and this would be expected to inhibit Ca^{2+} uptake through the mCU. However, we found that the increase in myocyte $[Ca^{2+}]_m$ during hypoxia could *not* be prevented by RuR (at concentrations of RuR, 20 μM, that could inhibit $[Ca^{2+}]_m$ increases in response to a cytosolic Ca^{2+} load) but instead the $[Ca^{2+}]_m$ increase could be prevented by clonazepam, an inhibitor of mNCX. By contrast, upon reoxygenation, RuR once again inhibited Ca^{2+} uptake, whilst clonazepam inhibited efflux (Griffiths et al. 1998). This allowed us to propose the following model: during hypoxia Ca^{2+} entry into mitochondria occurs via mNCX, and the mCU is largely inactive. Upon reoxygenation, however, the transporters regain their normal directionality.

We have provided further evidence that entry of Ca^{2+} during hypoxia occurs via mNCX by showing, using a model of simulated hypoxia, that the process is Na^+-dependent (Griffiths 1999). And a reversal of the mNCX under conditions of metabolic inhibition was also found in a study on cultured renal epithelial cells, supporting our hypothesis (Smets et al. 2004).

11.2.3 The Mitochondrial Permeability Transition Pore

It has been known for many years that Ca^{2+}-induced mitochondrial dysfunction during ischaemia is associated with the transition from reversible to irreversible cell damage; see above and Bush et al. (1980), Sordahl and Stewart (1980), Fleckenstein et al. (1983): Mitochondria accumulate deposits of calcium phosphate, become swollen, and eventually rupture. This sequence of events, whereby mitochondrial Ca^{2+} uptake leads to mitochondrial dysfunction and prevents oxidative phosphorylation was later found to be due to Ca^{2+}-induced opening of the MPTP. The MPTP plays a key role in cell death by both necrosis and apoptosis, and has been discussed in recent reviews (Hajnóczky et al. 2006; Rasola and Bernardi 2007; Roy and Hajnóczky 2008; Leung and Halestrap 2008; Pinton et al. 2008). In absence of specific inhibitors of mitochondrial Ca^{2+} uptake that can be used on reperfusion, which, as mentioned above, may not be ideal since some Ca^{2+} would be needed to activated mitochondrial dehydrogenases, the discovery of relatively specific inhibitors of the MPTP have provided firstly a useful tool for investigation of the role of the MPTP, and secondly as therapies for ischaemia/reperfusion damage.

However, the exact components of the MPTP are still not known; for a number of years the MPTP was generally thought to consist of the outer membrane voltage-dependent anion channel (VDAC), the inner membrane adenine nucleotide translocase (ANT) and the matrix protein cyclophilin D (CyP-D). Studies on transgenic mice confirmed the role of CyP-D as having a critical regulatory role in pore-opening (Baines et al. 2005), but have shown that neither the ANT (Kokoszka et al. 2004) nor VDAC (Baines et al. 2007) are essential components of the pore, though they may also play a regulatory role; the composition and regulation of the pore are discussed fully in recent reviews (Di Lisa and Bernardi 2006; Halestrap 2009; Javadov et al. 2009). The latest and more compelling evidence indicates that the inner membrane phosphate carrier (PiC) rather than the ANT is likely to be a pore component (Leung et al. 2008), and a working model has been proposed by Halestrap (2009). There is a suggestion that there is no single protein responsible for pore formation, but rather it is due to aggregation of misfolded proteins, or proteins damaged by oxidative stress (He and Lemasters 2002). However, the specific properties of the pore; Ca^{2+} activation, inhibition by CsA, and modulation by activators and inhibitors of the ANT or PiC make this unlikely (Halestrap 2009).

11.2.4 Mitochondria as a Target for Cardioprotection During Ischaemia and Reperfusion

11.2.4.1 Studies Using Inhibitors of Mitochondrial Ca^{2+} Transport

Ruthenium red (RuR) has been shown to protect hearts or myocytes from reperfusion/reoxygenation damage at concentrations ranging from 0.1 to 6 μM (Peng et al. 1980; Leperre et al. 1995; Miyamae et al. 1996; Grover et al. 1990; Benzi and Lerch 1992; Figueredo et al. 1991; Park et al. 1990; Carry et al. 1989; Stone et al. 1989). However, at these concentrations RuR can also inhibit Ca^{2+} channels of the SR and myocyte contraction (Griffiths 2000), whereas much higher levels are required to inhibit mitochondria Ca^{2+} uptake in myocytes (Griffiths et al. 1998). It therefore seems more likely that the protective effects were due to an energy sparing effect as a result of reducing $[Ca^{2+}]_c$ (Benzi and Lerch 1992). Unfortunately at higher concentrations RuR has non-specific damaging effects on hearts, making it unsuitable to accurately assess the contribution of mitochondrial Ca^{2+} uptake to reperfusion-induced damage.

Ru360 is a more specific inhibitor of the mCU, although there are problems with permeability in isolated myocytes (Bell et al. 2006; Robert et al. 2001). It has, however, been reported to protect whole hearts against ischaemia/reperfusion injury: pre-treatment of isolated rat hearts with 10 μM Ru360 provided protection against reperfusion injury, as determined from infarct size and enzyme release (Zhang et al. 2006). But in another study lower concentrations of Ru360 were required: recovery of rat hearts from ischaemia was optimal between 0.25–1 μM Ru360 and declined at higher concentrations (de Jesus et al. 2005). $[Ca^{2+}]_m$ (as measured following isolation of mitochondria at the end of the perfusion protocol) was also decreased in Ru360 treated hearts (de Jesus et al. 2005).

With regard to inhibitors of the mNCX, diltiazem can protect hearts from ischaemia/reperfusion damage, but this has mainly been attributed to its effects on sarcolemmal L-type Ca^{2+}-channels (Winniford et al. 1985) or Na^+ channels (Takeo et al. 2004); both of which would indirectly preserve mitochondrial integrity. Clonazepam cannot be used in whole hearts as it appears to inhibit contractility by a non-myocyte effect (Griffiths, unpublished observation), even though it was protective and prevented the ischaemia-induced increase in $[Ca^{2+}]_m$ in isolated myocytes (Griffiths et al. 1998; Sharikabad et al. 2004), as discussed above. There have been no reports of the effects of CGP37157 in whole hearts; it has been used to inhibit Ca^{2+} entry in isolated myocytes (Maack et al. 2006), although there can be problems with solubilising the compound (Griffiths et al. 1997); it has not been used in any models of ischaemia/reperfusion injury.

Intracellular acidification, such as occurs during ischaemia, can also decrease the rate of Ca^{2+} uptake, probably as a consequence of reduced $\Delta\Psi_m$ (Gursahani and Schaefer 2004). Maintaining an acid pH upon reperfusion is known to delay intracellular Ca^{2+} accumulation and protect against reperfusion injury (Panagiotopoulos et al. 1990), and additionally inhibits opening of the MPTP (Halestrap 1991).

11.2.4.2 Inhibitors of the Permeability Transition Pore

A non-specific pore in the mitochondrial inner membrane that allowed permeability of molecules up to 1.5 kDa was first identified in the 1970s by Haworth and Hunter (Hunter and Haworth 1979a, b; Haworth and Hunter 1979). Crompton then determined that the MPTP was being regulated by Ca^{2+} and oxidative stress (Crompton et al. 1987), and realised its implications for myocardial reperfusion injury (Crompton and Costi 1990). The discovery that opening of the MPTP could be inhibited by cyclosporine A (Crompton et al. 1988) suggested a possible protective strategy, and Crompton subsequently showed that cyclosporine A (CsA), a potent inhibitor of the pore in isolated mitochondria, was protective in a myocyte model of hypoxia/reoxygenation (Nazareth et al. 1991). We found CsA to be cardioprotective in a perfused rat heart model of IR injury (Griffiths and Halestrap 1993), and further that the MPTP opened only upon reperfusion, not during ischaemia (Griffiths and Halestrap 1995); see Fig. 11.4. Opening occurred during the first 5 min of reperfusion (Kerr et al. 1999), and giving CsA on reperfusion was also protective (Hausenloy et al. 2003). Cyclosporine A is an immunosuppressant commonly used in transplant operations. However its effect on the MPTP is by an entirely separate mechanism – it inhibits the peptidyl-prolyl cis-trans isomerase activity of CyP-D, an effect that greatly decreases the sensitivity of the pore to Ca^{2+}, although the inhibition by CsA can be overcome at high enough Ca^{2+}. We found that analogues of CsA that inhibit the MPTP but are not immunosuppressive are still cardioprotective (Griffiths and Halestrap 1993), indicating it is the mitochondrial effect that is important. Other inhibitors of the pore have subsequently been found to be cardioprotective, such as sanglifehrin A (SfA), which also acts on CyP-D, Debio-025(Gomez et al. 2007), pyruvate (a free radical scavenger and which maintains low pH), propofol (an anaesthetic and free radical scavenger), and low pH – more information on these compounds is given in recent reviews (Di Lisa and Bernardi 2006; Halestrap and Pasdois 2009).

It has nevertheless taken some time for these findings to be translated to a clinical setting: in a pilot trial patients presenting with acute ST-elevation following myocardial infarction (STEMI) were given CsA or control saline before undergoing PCI, and administering CsA at the time of reperfusion was associated with a smaller infarct (Piot et al. 2008). Another study investigated the effect of a single dose of CsA administered at the time of reperfusion following MI on LV remodelling and function 5 days and 6 months following the MI; there was a reduction in infarct size at 6 months follow up in the CsA-group (Mewton et al. 2010). Both studies are promising but require a further large scale trial.

11.2.4.3   Ischaemic Pre- and Post-conditioning

Ischaemic preconditioning is a protective strategy that has been widely used experimentally, where short periods of ischaemia protect against a prolonged period. Various end-effectors and mediators of the pathway have been proposed, including different signalling pathways and kinases, plus the mitochondrial ATP-sensitive K^+ (mK_{ATP}) channels (reviewed in Hausenloy and Yellon 2007; Ardehali and O'Rourke 2005; Lawrence et al. 2001). Ischaemic postconditioning (IPost) is another protective strategy that may be more clinically relevant (Hausenloy and Yellon 2007), since the short ischaemia episodes are applied following reperfusion. A full discussion of these pathways is beyond the scope of this review, but IPC is associated with a reduction in MPTP opening (Javadov et al. 2003), and so is relevant here. Several studies have now found IPC to be associated with a reduced $[Ca^{2+}]_m$ (Wang et al. 2001; Crestanello et al. 2000; Murata et al. 2001; Hausenloy et al. 2004a; Smart et al. 2006), which may then lead to a reduction in MPTP opening (reviewed in Halestrap et al. 2007). IPC and IPost both cause suppression of MPTP opening upon reperfusion (Javadov et al. 2003; Hausenloy et al. 2004b; Argaud et al. 2005).

As mentioned above, mice deficient in CyP-D are resistant to pore opening, and have smaller infarcts in response to IR injury (Baines et al. 2005; Nakagawa et al. 2005; Lim et al. 2007). However, the CyP-D deficient mice could not be further protected by IPC, IPost, or pharmacological agents such as bradykinin (that mimics IPC), CsA or SfA (Lim et al. 2007), confirming the MPTP as essential in the cardioprotection afforded by either type of conditioning, and proposing it as an end-effector of the two pathways (Lim et al. 2007). The mechanism of this protection is not known, though various signalling pathways have been proposed, including involvement of Akt, GSK-3 and PKC -see review (Hausenloy and Yellon 2007). However, it appears unlikely that these act directly to phosphorylate mitochondrial proteins, but rather by reducing oxidative stress (Clarke et al. 2008). There is also evidence that transient opening of the MPTP may act as the trigger for IPC, since including CsA or SfA during the preconditioning ischaemia reduced the infarct-limiting effects of IPC (Hausenloy et al. 2004a).

Despite all the experimental studies showing protective effects of pre and post-conditioning, their translation to the clinical setting has been disappointing (Ludman et al. 2010). IPC (Murry et al. 1986) is clearly limited by the fact that it has to be applied before ischaemia, but IPost (Zhao et al. 2003) seems more promising. Clinically, IPost has been used by inflating/deflating an angioplasty balloon following insertion of a stent in the affected artery; reported to reduce infarct size at 6 months and improve function after 1 year (Thibault et al. 2008).

11.3   Mitochondria and Heart Failure

11.3.1   Role of Reactive Oxygen Species (ROS)

Heart failure is a major cause of morbidity and mortality in developed countries (Cleland et al. 2001), and an increasing problem in aging populations (Tsutsui et al. 2008). It can result from a variety of causes, such hypertension or coronary artery disease, progressing from compensated hypertrophy through to failure, or result from inherited or acquired valvular disease or cardiomyopathy. A link between mitochondrial dysfunction and heart failure was observed as early as 1962 using a guinea-pig model of heart failure induced by aortic banding, where a reduced oxidative phosphorylation capacity of mitochondria was observed. Although the authors could not prove a causal relationship, they suggested that mitochondria played a critical role in the development of the disease (Schwartz and Lee 1962).

Heart failure progresses by cardiac remodelling, where the myocytes enlarge, often preceded by compensated hypertrophy, followed by deterioration in pump function. Many experimental and clinical studies have now shown that the remodelling proceeds by myocyte loss via apoptosis – reviewed in van Empel et al. (2005). The role of mitochondria in apoptosis is well known, and covered by Chap. 7 in this volume (Mignotte). However, the role of oxidative stress induced by the generation of reactive oxygen species (ROS) in the pathogenesis of heart failure appears is also becoming increasingly well accepted (Tsutsui et al. 2008); these damaging species can causes deleterious effects on DNA (mitochondrial and nuclear), protein and cell structure, as well as acting as signalling molecules in their own right that contribute towards the development of the remodelling process, in hypertrophy and heart failure (Tsutsui et al. 2008; Seddon et al. 2007).

Mitochondria are a major source of ROS in the heart since the respiratory chain generates the superoxide anion, O_2^-, as part of normal respiration, and this can then trigger formation of other ROS (Murphy 2009). Mitochondria are more susceptible to ROS damage than nuclear DNA since they have poor DNA repair mechanisms and no protective histones; additionally O_2^- generated by the respiratory chain is not easily membrane permeable so may become trapped within the mitochondriua (Tsutsui et al. 2009). The mutation rate of mtDNA is more than ten times that of nuclear DNA (Chen et al. 2006). Increased O_2^- production by mitochondria was found in a canine model of heart failure (Ide et al. 2000), and markers of ROS generation in blood of patients with heart failure (Mallat et al. 1998). However ROS from other sources may also play a role, such as xanthine oxidase, NADPH oxidase, or uncoupled nitric oxide synthase in either myocytes or endothelial cells in the heart (Seddon et al. 2007). mtDNA encodes essential subunits of respiratory chain proteins (see below), and so damage to a mitochondrial gene can rapidly lead to deleterious effects on the whole cell. Recently, mitochondrially-targeted antioxidants have been produced, to try and effectively combat ROS-induced diseases (James et al. 2005; Murphy and Smith 2007). MitoQ$_{10}$ is a ubiquinol antioxidant with a triphenylphosphonium lipophilic tail that accumulates several 100-fold in mitochondria because of their highly negative membrane potential (James et al. 2005). In experimental studies, mostly on rat models of heart disease so far, MitoQ$_{10}$ has been shown to be beneficial in protecting against ischaemia/reperfusion damage (Adlam et al. 2005), hypertension and hypertrophy (Graham et al. 2009), and sepsis-induced cardiac dysfunction (Supinski et al. 2009). However, MitoQ$_{10}$ did not completely prevent hypertension, indicating that mitochondrial ROS production is not the only contributing factor (Graham et al. 2009).

The heart has various antioxidant defence mechanisms; these do not appear to be downregulated in heart failure, rather it is the increase in ROS production that overwhelms the anti-oxidant capacity (Tsutsui et al. 2008). Mitochondria contain several enzymes that detoxify ROS: manganese superoxide dismutase (Mn-SOD) converts O_2^- to H_2O_2, and glutathione peroxidase and peroxiredoxins convert H_2O_2 to water (Murphy 2009). So as well as adding exogenous anti-oxidants, strategies that upregulate the endogenous defence pathways are candidates for the prevention or treatment of heart failure. One such enzyme is glutathione peroxidase, present in both cytosol and mitochondria, which scavenges H_2O_2 and prevents formation of hydroxyl radicals: overexpression of this enzyme in mice prevented the development of heart failure following myocardial infarction (Shiomi et al. 2004). Using a similar model in rats, dietary supplementation with vitamin E also protected against cardiac dysfunction leading to heart failure; this was associated with increased activities of catalase and glutathione peroxidase (Hill et al. 2005). Knocking out Mn-SOD in mitochondria similarly leads to dilated cardiomyopathy in mice, which die within 10 days of birth (Li et al. 1995). The role of oxidative stress in the heart is covered in more detail by recent reviews (Tsutsui et al. 2008; Seddon et al. 2007) and in Chap. 5 of this volume (by Lenaz).

Pacing induced heart failure is a common model of human dilated cardiomyopathy (Moe and Armstrong 1999), and is associated with defects in mitochondrial function such as reduced respiratory chain activity and beta-oxidation, and depletion of high energy phosphates (Marin-Garcia et al. 2001). A time course study in this model revealed parallel increases in markers of oxidative stress, apoptosis, and respiratory chain dysfunction (Marin-Garcia et al. 2009). Defects in complexes I, III and V were found in the left ventricle whereas in the left atrium only complex V was deficient, and markers of apoptosis were also found in both left ventricle and atrium (Marin-Garcia et al. 2009). However, there were no differences in the level of citrate synthase (a common marker of mitochondrial content), complex II or complex IV, indicating that the changes were specific for certain enzymes only, and not due simply to an overall decrease in mitochondrial content – rather there were selective changes in both nuclear-encoded and mitochondrial-encoded components of the respiratory chain. Thus it is clear that mitochondrial dysfunction occurs in heart failure and that mitochondrially generated ROS contribute to the development of the disease.

11.3.2 *Mitochondrial [Ca²⁺] and Heart Failure*

In a rabbit model of heart failure, mitochondrial Ca^{2+} uptake was unchanged during the early stages of hypertrophy, but this was followed by a decrease in Ca^{2+} uptake as the disease progressed (Sordahl et al. 1973). There was a parallel initial increase in respiratory chain activity in hypertrophy but which decreased on progression to failure (Sordahl et al. 1973); this decline in respiration fits with a lower $[Ca^{2+}]_m$, although that was not directly shown in this study. In myocytes isolated from hearts of cardiomyopathic hamsters that develop heart failure, there was a reduction in PDH activity, and also a reduced $[Ca^{2+}]_m$ in response to rapid electrical stimulation compared with control hearts (Di Lisa et al. 1993). This seemed likely due to a reduction in the systolic Ca^{2+} transient, leading to reduced $[Ca^{2+}]_m$ and failure to activate PDH. The hearts also exhibited reduced developed pressure and adenine nucleotide content (Wikman-Coffelt et al. 1986). Mitochondria isolated from the hearts also showed a reduced Ca^{2+} uptake (Lin et al. 2007) and this was associated with a lower $\Delta\psi_m$ and reduced activities of complexes I and IV. It is possible but untested that inhibiting the mNCX in these hearts would be beneficial in restoring $[Ca^{2+}]_m$ and activating PDH.

Recent work from O'Rourke's group has shown that dysregulation of Na^+ homeostasis in heart failure may be a primary cause of mitochondrial dysfunction (Maack et al. 2006; Liu and O'Rourke 2008): in a guinea-pig model of heart failure (induced by aortic constriction), intracellular $[Na^+]$ was 16 mM compared with 5 mM in control cells (Liu and O'Rourke 2008). Rapid pacing of the cells induced a decrease in NAD(P)H fluorescence, an indirect indicator of respiratory chain activity, whereas this was maintained in controls. An inhibitor of mNCX, CGP 37157, was able to prevent the decrease in NADH in the failing myocytes. It is thus likely to restore ATP levels in the failing hearts: earlier work showed that the mNCX is capable of regulating $[Ca^{2+}]_m$ and dehydrogenase activity since adding Na^+ to isolated mitochondria shifts the activation curves for PDH and OGDH by Ca^{2+} to the right (Denton et al. 1980).

$[Ca^{2+}]_m$ may also play a role in regulating levels of oxidative stress: In the model of guinea-pig heart failure used above, increased workload resulted in a transient oxidation of NAD(P)H, but which was re-reduced as $[Ca^{2+}]_m$ increased (Kohlhaas et al. 2010). Concomitant with this was a rise in H_2O_2, measured using the fluorescent indicator CMH_2-DCF-DA. The ROS production was enhanced in the presence of Ru360 to block mitochondrial Ca^{2+} uptake, or when Ca^{2+}-eflux was accelerated using increased $[Na^+]_i$. Myocytes from failing hearts showed elevated basal ROS production by the mitochondria, and this was prevented by inhibiting mNCX (Kohlhaas et al. 2010). The transient oxidation of NAD(P)H was closely associated with an increase in mitochondrial H_2O_2 formation. The authors argue that since NAD(P)H levels correlate positively with the glutathione redox state but inversely with ROS formation (Aon et al. 2007), prevention of recovery of NAD(P)H by the reduced $[Ca^{2+}]_m$ is the underlying cause of the observed increase in ROS in these myocytes. They suggest therefore that mitochondrial Ca^{2+} uptake is not just important for balancing energy supply with demand, but also for the ability of the mitochondria to scavenge free radicals by maintaining the redox state of the matrix (Kohlhaas et al. 2010).

However, the benzodiazepine inhibitors of the mNCX like clonazepam and diltiazem cannot be used in the whole heart as specific antagonists of mitochondrial Ca^{2+} efflux, because of their effects on coronary vessels (diltiazem, for example, is used to reduce high blood pressure). Design of more specific inhibitors of the mNCX may be of benefit in states where ATP synthesis is impaired, such as in heart failure, since maintaining $[Ca^{2+}]_m$ at higher levels could in turn increase ATP production, and also reduce ROS formation by mitochondria (Kohlhaas et al. 2010). There is some precedent for the idea that inhibiting the mNCX can enhance [ATP]: in pancreatic islets CGP37157 increased oxidative phosphorylation, and potentiated glucose-stimulated insulin release (Lee et al. 2003), prompting the authors to suggest it as a novel insulin secretagogue.

## 11.4	Mitochondria and Inherited Cardiomyopathies

### 11.4.1	Mitochondrial DNA and Disease

Mitochondrial DNA (mtDNA) is circular, double stranded, and encodes 13 subunits of oxidative phosphorylation, (in complexes I, III, IV and V), 2 rRNA subunits and 22 tRNA's; this is covered in detail in Chap. 2 of this volume (by Bai) and reviewed in (Tuppen et al. 2010). Mutations in mtDNA lead to diseases that predominantly affect the nervous system, skeletal and cardiac muscle. Defects in mitochondrial proteins, whether nuclear or mitochondrially encoded, can cause cardiomyopathy but also myopathy and neuropathy – this is not surprising and has been known for many years – for more information see reviews (Li et al. 1995; Naviaux 2000; Fosslien 2003). Although cardiac defects often form a part of the "mitochondrial disease", I will restrict this section to specific cardiomyopathies arising from mitochondrial defects – other diseases of mitochondria are the subject of another chapter in this issue (Chap. 8 by Finsterer).

### 11.4.2	Mitochondrial Cardiomyopathies

Cardiomyopathies are diseases that cause cardiac dysfunction such as heart failure, arrhythmia, and sudden death; they represent a major cause of morbidity and mortality in both children and adults (Hughes and McKenna 2005). Types of cardiomopathy include dilated cardiomyopathy (DCM) and hypertrophic cardiomyopathy (HCM) (Hughes and McKenna 2005). DCM is the most common cause of heart failure, affecting 40 people out of every 100,000 (Towbin and Bowles 2002). About 50% of individuals die within 5 years of diagnosis, either from pump failure or sudden death, although the situation us improving with development of new drugs. Although the aetiology is not always known, about 30–40% of cases of DCM have the familial form, with autosomal dominant inheritance the main form of inheritance. DCM and HCM can be cause by defects in contractile and structural proteins, for example in HCM most mutations are small (single point or small deletions/insertions) in genes for β-myosin heavy chain, cardiac troponin T or I, and myosin binding protien C (Marian et al. 2001). HCM is also a main cause of sudden death in young and apparently healthy individuals and athletes (Towbin and Bowles 2002).

Mitochondrial inheritance of cardiomyopathy like all mitochondrial diseases is complicated (Goldstein et al. 1999): inheritance is by the maternal line, since mitochondria in the embryo derive almost entirely from oocyte mitochondria. However, manifestation of a disease varies due to heteroplasmy – the presence of different populations of mitochondrial DNA within the same cell. The offspring may inherit all, none, or intermediate amounts of the damaged mitochondrial genome from the mother. The disease may therefore not become apparent until the mutated mtDNA reaches a certain amount – the threshold effect (Chen et al. 2006).

mtDNA diseases that only affect the heart are rare and often fatal, but specific cardiomyopathies have been reported (Goldstein et al. 1999). More than 50 point mutations have now been identified that lead to diseases with cardiomyopathy; these are usually within genes for tRNA, and affect multiple systems since more than one mitochondrial protein is affected. Large deletions of mtDNA are present in patients with Kearns-Sayre syndrome, who also have a cardiac conduction block (rather than cardiomyopathy) (Goldstein et al. 1999).

An example of a point mutation causing disease occurred in two families with hypertrophic cardiomyopathy where clinical abnormalities were confined to the heart: an A to G transition in the tRNA^{Ile} gene caused severely depressed respiratory chain enzyme activity (in complexes I and IV) (Terasaki et al. 2001). All family members had hypertrophy, some had or went on to develop LV dilation and failure; there were two childhood deaths, one heart transplant recipient and another family member awaiting one. Another study on an infant with cardiomyopathy found a mutation (C to T) in the mitochondrial tRNA^{Leu} gene that lead to partial deficiencies of complexes I and IV (Goldstein et al. 1999) Although the same mutation could be detected in mother and siblings, they were asymptomatic, despite having up to 74% of the mutant genomes, whereas mitochondria from the infant with the cardiomyopathy contained 100% of the abnormal gene. The infant died aged 6 months following cardiac failure, and microscopic examination on autopsy revealed major abnormalities confined to the heart – hypertrophic cardiomyopathy; enlarged mitochondria but abnormal cristae – "whorls" (Goldstein et al. 1999).

Another patient with congestive heart failure showed a novel point mutation in the gene for mitochondrial tRNA^{Lys} (Terasaki et al. 2001). In a biopsy taken from the left ventricular wall during an operation, electron microscopy showed that the failing tissue contained giant mitochondria surrounded by numerous smaller mitochondria, which had concentric circular cristae (Kanzaki et al. 2010). The giant mitochondria had possibly occurred via fusion of several mitochondria, possible in an attempt to compensate for the reduced function. By contrast normal tissue contained continuous rows of uniform mitochondria with the classical cristae appearance.

As well as mutations in mtDNA genes themselves, defective transcription can also have severe consequences: mitochondrial transcription factor (TFAM) is a nuclear-encoded transcription factor that binds to mitochondrial DNA. Cardiac-specific knockout of TFAM in mice caused dilated cardiomyopathy in addition to reduced mitochondrial copy number (Wang et al. 1999). Conversely, overexpressing TFAM in mice prevented the decline in mitochondrial copy number and attenuated heart failure following myocardial infarction (Ikeuchi et al. 2005). The restored respiratory chain activity could then reduce ROS production and the increases in mitochondrial copy number also maintained ATP synthesis (Tsutsui et al. 2009).

Mutations in nuclear DNA can also cause mitochondrial cardiomyopathies resulting from severe enzyme defects, since most proteins in mitochondria are encoded by the nuclear genome. Deficiencies in cytochrome c oxidase caused infantile hypertrophic cardiomyopathy (Servidei et al. 1994), and cardiomyopathy is the most common cause of death in infants with complex I deficiency associated with severe lactic acidosis (Goldstein et al. 1999). A cardiomyopathy was also seen in two patients with ATPase deficiency (Holme et al. 1992). Diseases associated with defects in nuclear-encoded mitochondrial proteins, including those involved in fatty acid synthesis or citric acid cycle enzymes are discussed more fully in Chap. 8 (by Finsterer).

There is an X-linked cardiomyopathy, Barth syndrome, which affects mitochondrial function: Barth syndrome is caused by a defect in the cardiolipin transacylase enzyme, tafazzin. Cardiolipin is a phospholipid characteristic of the mitochondrial inner membrane and synthesised in mitochondria but then remodeled to produce cardiolipin rich in unsaturated fatty acids, particularly linoleic acid (Hauff and

Hatch 2006; Claypool et al. 2008). Mitochondria have membrane protein contents much higher than those of other membranes (Claypool et al. 2008), and optimal cardiolipin content is essential for correct function and organisation of many mitochondrial enzymes, including those of the respiratory chain, the ATP synthase and adenine nucleotide translocase. Various mutations in the tafazzin gene have been described (Hauff and Hatch 2006), and lead to a reduced cardiolipin content of mitochondria, more saturated fatty acids in the cardiolipin, and an accumulation of monolysocardiolpin. Patients all show alterations in mitochondrial structure, and depressed oxidative phospgorylation (Claypool et al. 2008). Infants have LV dysfunction and dilation, and can succumb to sudden death although most survive infancy (Towbin and Bowles 2002).

There are also inherited diseases that cause electrophysiological disturbances in the heart, causing arrhythmias, long QT syndrome, and Brugada syndrome amongst others (Marcus 2000). However, although mitochondria, in particular mitochondrial Ca^{2+} signalling, is becoming increasingly recognised as being capable of modulation EC coupling in the heart, few of the mitochondria ion transporters have been characterised, and there are as yet no known mutations in mitochondrial proteins that lead directly to arrhythmias.

11.5   Conclusions

It is clear that mitochondria play a major role in both normal and pathological heart function, either as a primary cause or in the development of heart disease. Very recently clinical trials utilising probes acting on mitochondria have begun: CsA, which acts on the MPTP, and the mitochondrially-targeted antioxidants. Particularly promising are strategies like CsA and IPost that can be used at the point of reperfusion.

Thus these carefully targeted strategies should give better clinical outcomes, than for example, generally antioxidants that may not reach the main site of ROS production, the mitochondria, effectively. It is essential to continue our basic research in this area: the MPTP was a curious phenomenon observed initially in isolated mitochondria, but it is now generally agreed to be a critical mediator of reperfusion injury, and targeted as the end-effector of various protective strategies. However, basic science findings need to be shaped by the constraints and practicalities of clinical applications, hence despite the numerous studies on IPC, it has proved limited as a clinical tool.

Finally, design of specifically targeted drugs against the MPTP or mitochondrial Ca^{2+} transport pathways have I believe, tremendous potential, but first these elusive proteins need to be fully identified and characterised. There may also be as yet unidentified cardiomyopathies due to inheritance of abnormal genes for these proteins.

References

Adlam VJ, Harrison JC, Porteous CM, James AM, Smith RA, Murphy MP et al (2005) Targeting an antioxidant to mitochondria decreases cardiac ischemia-reperfusion injury. FASEB J 19(9):1088–1095

Allen SP, Darley-Usmar VM, McCormack JG, Stone D (1993) Changes in mitochondrial matrix free calcium in perfused rat hearts subjected to hypoxia-reoxygenation. J Mol Cell Cardiol 25(8):949–958

Aon MA, Cortassa S, Maack C, O'Rourke B (2007) Sequential opening of mitochondrial ion channels as a function of glutathione redox thiol status. J Biol Chem 282(30):21889–21900

Ardehali H, O'Rourke B (2005) Mitochondrial K(ATP) channels in cell survival and death. J Mol Cell Cardiol 39(1):7–16

Argaud L, Gateau-Roesch O, Raisky O, Loufouat J, Robert D, Ovize M (2005) Postconditioning inhibits mitochondrial permeability transition. Circulation 111(2):194–197

Baines CP, Kaiser RA, Purcell NH, Blair NS, Osinska H, Hambleton MA et al (2005) Loss of cyclophilin D reveals a critical role for mitochondrial permeability transition in cell death. Nature 434(7033):658–662

Baines CP, Kaiser RA, Sheiko T, Craigen WJ, Molkentin JD (2007) Voltage-dependent anion channels are dispensable for mitochondrial-dependent cell death. Nat Cell Biol 9(5):550–555

Balaban RS (2009) The role of Ca(2+) signaling in the coordination of mitochondrial ATP production with cardiac work. Biochim Biophys Acta 1787(11):1334–1341

Bell CJ, Bright NA, Rutter GA, Griffiths EJ (2006) ATP regulation in adult rat cardiomyocytes: time-resolved decoding of rapid mitochondrial calcium spiking imaged with targeted photoproteins. J Biol Chem 281(38):28058–28067

Benzi RH, Lerch R (1992) Dissociation between contractile function and oxidative metabolism in postischemic myocardium. Attenuation by ruthenium red administered during reperfusion. Circ Res 71(3):567–576

Bruneau BG (2008) The developmental genetics of congenital heart disease. Nature 451(7181):943–948

Bush LR, Shlafer M, Haack DW, Lucchesi BR (1980) Time-dependent changes in canine cardiac mitochondrial function and ultrastructure resulting from coronary occlusion and reperfusion. Basic Res Cardiol 75(4):555–571

Carry MM, Mrak RE, Murphy ML, Peng CF, Straub KD, Fody EP (1989) Reperfusion injury in ischemic myocardium: protective effects of ruthenium red and of nitroprusside. Am J Cardiovasc Pathol 2(4):335–344

Chacon E, Reece JM, Nieminen AL, Zahrebelski G, Herman B, Lemasters JJ (1994) Distribution of electrical potential, pH, free Ca2+, and volume inside cultured adult rabbit cardiac myocytes during chemical hypoxia: a multiparameter digitized confocal microscopic study. Biophys J 66(4):942–952

Chance B, Williams GR (1956) Respiratory enzymes in oxidative phosphorylation. VI. The effects of adenosine diphosphate on azide-treated mitochondria. J Biol Chem 221(1):477–489

Chen J, Hattori Y, Nakajima K, Eizawa T, Ehara T, Koyama M et al (2006) Mitochondrial complex I activity is significantly decreased in a patient with maternally inherited type 2 diabetes mellitus and hypertrophic cardiomyopathy associated with mitochondrial DNA C3310T mutation: a cybrid study. Diabetes Res Clin Pract 74(2):148–153

Clarke B, Spedding M, Patmore L, McCormack JG (1993) Protective effects of ranolazine in guinea-pig hearts during low-flow ischaemia and their association with increases in active pyruvate dehydrogenase. Br J Pharmacol 109(3):748–750

Clarke SJ, Khaliulin I, Das M, Parker JE, Heesom KJ, Halestrap AP (2008) Inhibition of mitochondrial permeability transition pore opening by ischemic preconditioning is probably mediated by reduction of oxidative stress rather than mitochondrial protein phosphorylation. Circ Res 102(9):1082–1090

Claypool SM, Boontheung P, McCaffery JM, Loo JA, Koehler CM (2008) The cardiolipin transacylase, tafazzin, associates with two distinct respiratory components providing insight into Barth syndrome. Mol Biol Cell 19(12):5143–5155

Cleland JG, Khand A, Clark A (2001) The heart failure epidemic: exactly how big is it? Eur Heart J 22(8):623–626

Crestanello JA, Doliba NM, Babsky AM, Doliba NM, Niibori K, Osbakken MD et al (2000) Opening of potassium channels protects mitochondrial function from calcium overload. J Surg Res 94(2):116–123

Crompton M, Costi A (1990) A heart mitochondrial Ca2(+)-dependent pore of possible relevance to re-perfusion-induced injury. Evidence that ADP facilitates pore interconversion between the closed and open states. Biochem J 266(1):33–39

Crompton M, Costi A, Hayat L (1987) Evidence for the presence of a reversible Ca2+-dependent pore activated by oxidative stress in heart mitochondria. Biochem J 245(3):915–918

Crompton M, Ellinger H, Costi A (1988) Inhibition by cyclosporin A of a Ca2+-dependent pore in heart mitochondria activated by inorganic phosphate and oxidative stress. Biochem J 255(1):357–360

de Jesus GRG, Guerrero-Hernandez A, Guerrero-Serna G, Rodriguez-Zavala JS, Zazueta C (2005) Inhibition of the mitochondrial calcium uniporter by the oxo-bridged dinuclear ruthenium amine complex (Ru360) prevents from irreversible injury in postischemic rat heart. FEBS J 272(13):3477–3488

Dedkova EN, Blatter LA (2008) Mitochondrial Ca2+ and the heart. Cell Calcium 44(1):77–91

Delcamp TJ, Dales C, Ralenkotter L, Cole PS, Hadley RW (1998) Intramitochondrial [Ca2+] and membrane potential in ventricular myocytes exposed to anoxia-reoxygenation. Am J Physiol 275(2 Pt 2):H484–H494

Denton RM (2009) Regulation of mitochondrial dehydrogenases by calcium ions. Biochim Biophys Acta 1787(11):1309–1316

Denton RM, McCormack JG, Edgell NJ (1980) Role of calcium ions in the regulation of intramitochondrial metabolism. Effects of Na+, Mg2+ and ruthenium red on the Ca2+-stimulated oxidation of oxoglutarate and on pyruvate dehydrogenase activity in intact rat heart mitochondria. Biochem J 190(1):107–117

Di Lisa F, Bernardi P (2006) Mitochondria and ischemia-reperfusion injury of the heart: fixing a hole. Cardiovasc Res 70(2):191–199

Di Lisa F, Fan CZ, Gambassi G, Hogue BA, Kudryashova I, Hansford RG (1993) Altered pyruvate dehydrogenase control and mitochondrial free Ca2+ in hearts of cardiomyopathic hamsters. Am J Physiol 264(6 Pt 2):H2188–H2197

Di Lisa F, Blank PS, Colonna R, Gambassi G, Silverman HS, Stern MD et al (1995) Mitochondrial membrane potential in single living adult rat cardiac myocytes exposed to anoxia or metabolic inhibition. J Physiol 486(Pt 1):1–13

Figueredo VM, Dresdner KP Jr, Wolney AC, Keller AM (1991) Postischaemic reperfusion injury in the isolated rat heart: effect of ruthenium red. Cardiovasc Res 25(4):337–342

Fleckenstein A, Frey M, Fleckenstein-Grun G (1983) Consequences of uncontrolled calcium entry and its prevention with calcium antagonists. Eur Heart J 4(Suppl H):43–50

Fosslien E (2003) Review: mitochondrial medicine–cardiomyopathy caused by defective oxidative phosphorylation. Ann Clin Lab Sci 33(4):371–395

Goldstein JD, Shanske S, Bruno C, Perszyk AA (1999) Maternally inherited mitochondrial cardiomyopathy associated with a C-to-T transition at nucleotide 3303 of mitochondrial DNA in the tRNA(Leu(UUR)) gene. Pediatr Dev Pathol 2(1):78–85

Gomez L, Thibault H, Gharib A, Dumont JM, Vuagniaux G, Scalfaro P et al (2007) Inhibition of mitochondrial permeability transition improves functional recovery and reduces mortality following acute myocardial infarction in mice. Am J Physiol Heart Circ Physiol 293(3):H1654–H1661

Graham D, Huynh NN, Hamilton CA, Beattie E, Smith RA, Cocheme HM et al (2009) Mitochondria-targeted antioxidant MitoQ10 improves endothelial function and attenuates cardiac hypertrophy. Hypertension 54(2):322–328

Griffiths EJ (1999) Reversal of mitochondrial Na/Ca exchange during metabolic inhibition in rat cardiomyocytes. FEBS Lett 453(3):400–404

Griffiths EJ (2000) Use of ruthenium red as an inhibitor of mitochondrial Ca(2+) uptake in single rat cardiomyocytes. FEBS Lett 486(3):257–260

Griffiths EJ (2009) Mitochondrial calcium transport in the heart: physiological and pathological roles. J Mol Cell Cardiol 46(6):789–803

Griffiths EJ, Halestrap AP (1993) Protection by Cyclosporin A of ischemia/reperfusion-induced damage in isolated rat hearts. J Mol Cell Cardiol 25(12):1461–1469

Griffiths EJ, Halestrap AP (1995) Mitochondrial non-specific pores remain closed during cardiac ischaemia, but open upon reperfusion. Biochem J 307(Pt 1):93–98

Griffiths EJ, Wei SK, Haigney MC, Ocampo CJ, Stern MD, Silverman HS (1997) Inhibition of mitochondrial calcium efflux by clonazepam in intact single rat cardiomyocytes and effects on NADH production. Cell Calcium 21(4):321–329

Griffiths EJ, Ocampo CJ, Savage JS, Rutter GA, Hansford RG, Stern MD et al (1998) Mitochondrial calcium transporting pathways during hypoxia and reoxygenation in single rat cardiomyocytes. Cardiovasc Res 39(2):423–433

Grover GJ, Dzwonczyk S, Sleph PG (1990) Ruthenium red improves postischemic contractile function in isolated rat hearts. J Cardiovasc Pharmacol 16(5):783–789

Gunter TE, Pfeiffer DR (1990) Mechanisms by which mitochondria transport calcium. Am J Physiol 258(5 Pt 1): C755–C786

Gursahani HI, Schaefer S (2004) Acidification reduces mitochondrial calcium uptake in rat cardiac mitochondria. Am J Physiol Heart Circ Physiol 287(6):H2659–H2665

Haigney MC, Lakatta EG, Stern MD, Silverman HS (1994) Sodium channel blockade reduces hypoxic sodium loading and sodium-dependent calcium loading. Circulation 90(1):391–399

Hajnóczky G, Csordás G, Das S, Garcia-Perez C, Saotome M, Sinha Roy S et al (2006) Mitochondrial calcium signalling and cell death: approaches for assessing the role of mitochondrial Ca^{2+} uptake in apoptosis. Cell Calcium 40(5-6): 553–560

Halestrap AP (1991) Calcium-dependent opening of a non-specific pore in the mitochondrial inner membrane is inhibited at pH values below 7. Implications for the protective effect of low pH against chemical and hypoxic cell damage. Biochem J 278(Pt 3):715–719

Halestrap AP (2009) What is the mitochondrial permeability transition pore? J Mol Cell Cardiol 46(6):821–831

Halestrap AP, Pasdois P (2009) The role of the mitochondrial permeability transition pore in heart disease. Biochim Biophys Acta 1787(11):1402–1415

Halestrap AP, Clarke SJ, Khaliulin I (2007) The role of mitochondria in protection of the heart by preconditioning. Biochim Biophys Acta – Bioenergetics 1767(8):1007–1031

Harris DA, Das AM (1991) Control of mitochondrial ATP synthesis in the heart. Biochem J 280(Pt 3):561–573

Hauff KD, Hatch GM (2006) Cardiolipin metabolism and Barth syndrome. Prog Lipid Res 45(2):91–101

Hausenloy DJ, Yellon DM (2007) Preconditioning and postconditioning: united at reperfusion. Pharmacol Ther 116(2): 173–191

Hausenloy DJ, Duchen MR, Yellon DM (2003) Inhibiting mitochondrial permeability transition pore opening at reperfusion protects against ischaemia-reperfusion injury. Cardiovasc Res 60(3):617–625

Hausenloy D, Wynne A, Duchen M, Yellon D (2004a) Transient mitochondrial permeability transition pore opening mediates preconditioning-induced protection. Circulation 109(14):1714–1717

Hausenloy DJ, Yellon DM, Mani-Babu S, Duchen MR (2004b) Preconditioning protects by inhibiting the mitochondrial permeability transition. Am J Physiol Heart Circ Physiol 287(2):H841–H849

Haworth RA, Hunter DR (1979) The Ca2+-induced membrane transition in mitochondria. II. Nature of the Ca2+ trigger site. Arch Biochem Biophys 195(2):460–467

He L, Lemasters JJ (2002) Regulated and unregulated mitochondrial permeability transition pores: a new paradigm of pore structure and function? FEBS Lett 512(1–3):1–7

Heineman FW, Balaban RS (1993) Effects of afterload and heart rate on NAD(P)H redox state in the isolated rabbit heart. Am J Physiol Heart Circ Physiol 264(2):H433–H440

Hill MF, Palace VP, Kaur K, Kumar D, Khaper N, Singal PK (2005) Reduction in oxidative stress and modulation of heart failure subsequent to myocardial infarction in rats. Exp Clin Cardiol 10(3):146–153

Holme E, Greter J, Jacobson CE, Larsson NG, Lindstedt S, Nilsson KO et al (1992) Mitochondrial ATP-synthase deficiency in a child with 3-methylglutaconic aciduria. Pediatr Res 32(6):731–735

Hughes SE, McKenna WJ (2005) New insights into the pathology of inherited cardiomyopathy. Heart 91(2):257–264

Hunter DR, Haworth RA (1979a) The Ca2+-induced membrane transition in mitochondria. I. The protective mechanisms. Arch Biochem Biophys 195(2):453–459

Hunter DR, Haworth RA (1979b) The Ca2+-induced membrane transition in mitochondria. III. Transitional Ca2+ release. Arch Biochem Biophys 195(2):468–477

Hunter DR, Haworth RA, Southard JH (1976) Relationship between configuration, function, and permeability in calcium-treated mitochondria. J Biol Chem 251(16):5069–5077

Ide T, Tsutsui H, Kinugawa S, Suematsu N, Hayashidani S, Ichikawa K et al (2000) Direct evidence for increased hydroxyl radicals originating from superoxide in the failing myocardium. Circ Res 86(2):152–157

Ikeuchi M, Matsusaka H, Kang D, Matsushima S, Ide T, Kubota T et al (2005) Overexpression of mitochondrial transcription factor a ameliorates mitochondrial deficiencies and cardiac failure after myocardial infarction. Circulation 112(5):683–690

James AM, Cocheme HM, Smith RA, Murphy MP (2005) Interactions of mitochondria-targeted and untargeted ubiquinones with the mitochondrial respiratory chain and reactive oxygen species. Implications for the use of exogenous ubiquinones as therapies and experimental tools. J Biol Chem 280(22):21295–21312

Javadov SA, Clarke S, Das M, Griffiths EJ, Lim KH, Halestrap AP (2003) Ischaemic preconditioning inhibits opening of mitochondrial permeability transition pores in the reperfused rat heart. J Physiol 549(Pt 2):513–524

Javadov S, Karmazyn M, Escobales N (2009) Mitochondrial permeability transition pore opening as a promising therapeutic target in cardiac diseases. J Pharmacol Exp Ther 330(3):670–678

Kanzaki Y, Terasaki F, Okabe M, Otsuka K, Katashima T, Fujita S et al (2010) Giant mitochondria in the myocardium of a patient with mitochondrial cardiomyopathy: transmission and 3-dimensional scanning electron microscopy. Circulation 121(6):831–832

Katz LA, Koretsky AP, Balaban RS (1987) Respiratory control in the glucose perfused heart. A 31P NMR and NADH fluorescence study. FEBS Lett 221(2):270–276

Katz LA, Swain JA, Portman MA, Balaban RS (1989) Relation between phosphate metabolites and oxygen consumption of heart in vivo. Am J Physiol 256(1 Pt 2):H265–H274

Kerr PM, Suleiman MS, Halestrap AP (1999) Reversal of permeability transition during recovery of hearts from ischemia and its enhancement by pyruvate. Am J Physiol 276(2 Pt 2):H496–H502

Khouri EM, Gregg DE, Rayford CR (1965) Effect of exercise on cardiac output, left coronary flow and myocardial metabolism in the unanesthetized dog. Circ Res 17(5):427–437

Kohlhaas M, Liu T, Knopp A, Zeller T, Ong MF, Bohm M et al (2010) Elevated cytosolic Na+ increases mitochondrial formation of reactive oxygen species in failing cardiac myocytes. Circulation 121(14):1606–1613

Kokoszka JE, Waymire KG, Levy SE, Sligh JE, Cai J, Jones DP et al (2004) The ADP/ATP translocator is not essential for the mitochondrial permeability transition pore. Nature 427(6973):461–465

Lawrence CL, Billups B, Rodrigo GC, Standen NB (2001) The KATP channel opener diazoxide protects cardiac myocytes during metabolic inhibition without causing mitochondrial depolarization or flavoprotein oxidation. Br J Pharmacol 134(3):535–542

Lee B, Miles PD, Vargas L, Luan P, Glasco S, Kushnareva Y et al (2003) Inhibition of mitochondrial Na+-Ca2+ exchanger increases mitochondrial metabolism and potentiates glucose-stimulated insulin secretion in rat pancreatic islets. Diabetes 52(4):965–973

Leperre A, Millart H, Prevost A, Trenque T, Kantelip JP, Keppler BK (1995) Compared effects of ruthenium red and cis [Ru(NH3)4Cl2]Cl on the isolated ischaemic-reperfused rat heart. Fundam Clin Pharmacol 9(6):545–553

Leung AW, Halestrap AP (2008) Recent progress in elucidating the molecular mechanism of the mitochondrial permeability transition pore. Biochim Biophys Acta 1777(7–8):946–952

Leung AW, Varanyuwatana P, Halestrap AP (2008) The mitochondrial phosphate carrier interacts with cyclophilin D and may play a key role in the permeability transition. J Biol Chem 283(39):26312–26323

Li Y, Huang TT, Carlson EJ, Melov S, Ursell PC, Olson JL et al (1995) Dilated cardiomyopathy and neonatal lethality in mutant mice lacking manganese superoxide dismutase. Nat Genet 11(4):376–381

Lim SY, Davidson SM, Hausenloy DJ, Yellon DM (2007) Preconditioning and postconditioning: the essential role of the mitochondrial permeability transition pore. Cardiovasc Res 75(3):530–535

Lin L, Sharma VK, Sheu SS (2007) Mechanisms of reduced mitochondrial Ca2+ accumulation in failing hamster heart. Pflugers Arch 454(3):395–402

Liu T, O'Rourke B (2008) Enhancing mitochondrial Ca2+ uptake in myocytes from failing hearts restores energy supply and demand matching. Circ Res 103(3):279–288

Ludman AJ, Yellon DM, Hausenloy DJ (2010) Cardiac preconditioning for ischaemia: lost in translation. Dis Model Mech 3(1–2):35–38

Maack C, O'Rourke B (2007) Excitation-contraction coupling and mitochondrial energetics. Basic Res Cardiol 102(5):369–392

Maack C, Cortassa S, Aon MA, Ganesan AN, Liu T, O'Rourke B (2006) Elevated cytosolic Na+ decreases mitochondrial Ca^{2+} uptake during excitation-contraction coupling and impairs energetic adaptation in cardiac myocytes. Circ Res 99(2):172–182

Mallat Z, Philip I, Lebret M, Chatel D, Maclouf J, Tedgui A (1998) Elevated levels of 8-iso-prostaglandin F2alpha in pericardial fluid of patients with heart failure: a potential role for in vivo oxidant stress in ventricular dilatation and progression to heart failure. Circulation 97(16):1536–1539

Marcus FI (2000) Electrocardiographic features of inherited diseases that predispose to the development of cardiac arrhythmias, long QT syndrome, arrhythmogenic right ventricular cardiomyopathy/dysplasia, and Brugada syndrome. J Electrocardiol 33(Suppl):1–10

Marian AJ, Salek L, Lutucuta S (2001) Molecular genetics and pathogenesis of hypertrophic cardiomyopathy. Minerva Med 92(6):435–451

Marin-Garcia J, Goldenthal MJ, Moe GW (2001) Abnormal cardiac and skeletal muscle mitochondrial function in pacing-induced cardiac failure. Cardiovasc Res 52(1):103–110

Marin-Garcia J, Goldenthal MJ, Damle S, Pi Y, Moe GW (2009) Regional distribution of mitochondrial dysfunction and apoptotic remodeling in pacing-induced heart failure. J Card Fail 15(8):700–708

McCormack JG, Halestrap AP, Denton RM (1990) Role of calcium ions in regulation of mammalian intramitochondrial metabolism. Physiol Rev 70(2):391–425

Mewton N, Croisille P, Gahide G, Rioufol G, Bonnefoy E, Sanchez I et al (2010) Effect of cyclosporine on left ventricular remodeling after reperfused myocardial infarction. J Am Coll Cardiol 55(12):1200–1205

Miyamae M, Camacho SA, Weiner MW, Figueredo VM (1996) Attenuation of postischemic reperfusion injury is related to prevention of [Ca2+]m overload in rat hearts. Am J Physiol Heart Circ Physiol 271(5):H2145–H2153

Miyata H, Lakatta EG, Stern MD, Silverman HS (1992) Relation of mitochondrial and cytosolic free calcium to cardiac myocyte recovery after exposure to anoxia. Circ Res 71(3):605–613

Moe GW, Armstrong P (1999) Pacing-induced heart failure: a model to study the mechanism of disease progression and novel therapy in heart failure. Cardiovasc Res 42(3):591–599

Murata M, Akao M, O'Rourke B, Marban E (2001) Mitochondrial ATP-sensitive potassium channels attenuate matrix Ca^{2+} overload during simulated ischemia and reperfusion: possible mechanism of cardioprotection. Circ Res 89(10):891–898

Murphy MP (2009) How mitochondria produce reactive oxygen species. Biochem J 417(1):1–13

Murphy MP, Smith RA (2007) Targeting antioxidants to mitochondria by conjugation to lipophilic cations. Annu Rev Pharmacol Toxicol 47:629–656

Murphy E, Steenbergen C (2008a) Ion transport and energetics during cell death and protection. Physiology (Bethesda) 23:115–123

Murphy E, Steenbergen C (2008b) Mechanisms underlying acute protection from cardiac ischemia-reperfusion injury. Physiol Rev 88(2):581–609

Murry CE, Jennings RB, Reimer KA (1986) Preconditioning with ischemia: a delay of lethal cell injury in ischemic myocardium. Circulation 74(5):1124–1136

Nakagawa T, Shimizu S, Watanabe T, Yamaguchi O, Otsu K, Yamagata H et al (2005) Cyclophilin D-dependent mitochondrial permeability transition regulates some necrotic but not apoptotic cell death. Nature 434(7033):652–658

Naviaux RK (2000) Mitochondrial DNA disorders. Eur J Pediatr 159(Suppl 3):S219–S226

Nazareth W, Yafei N, Crompton M (1991) Inhibition of anoxia-induced injury in heart myocytes by cyclosporin A. J Mol Cell Cardiol 23(12):1351–1354

Neely JR, Denton RM, England PJ, Randle PJ (1972) The effects of increased heart work on the tricarboxylate cycle and its interactions with glycolysis in the perfused rat heart. Biochem J 128(1):147–159

Nemer M (2008) Genetic insights into normal and abnormal heart development. Cardiovasc Pathol 17(1):48–54

Nicholls DG, Crompton M (1980) Mitochondrial calcium transport. FEBS Lett 111(2):261–268

Panagiotopoulos S, Daly MJ, Nayler WG (1990) Effect of acidosis and alkalosis on postischemic Ca gain in isolated rat heart. Am J Physiol Heart Circ Physiol 258(3):H821–H828

Park Y, Bowles DK, Kehrer JP (1990) Protection against hypoxic injury in isolated-perfused rat heart by ruthenium red. J Pharmacol Exp Ther 253(2):628–635

Peng CF, Kane JJ, Straub KD, Murphy ML (1980) Improvement of mitochondrial energy production in ischemic myocardium by in vivo infusion of ruthenium red. J Cardiovasc Pharmacol 2(1):45–54

Pinton P, Giorgi C, Siviero R, Zecchini E, Rizzuto R (2008) Calcium and apoptosis: ER-mitochondria Ca2+ transfer in the control of apoptosis. Oncogene 27(50):6407–6418

Piot C, Croisille P, Staat P, Thibault H, Rioufol G, Mewton N et al (2008) Effect of cyclosporine on reperfusion injury in acute myocardial infarction. N Engl J Med 359(5):473–481

Rasola A, Bernardi P (2007) The mitochondrial permeability transition pore and its involvement in cell death and in disease pathogenesis. Apoptosis 12(5):815–833

Robert V, Gurlini P, Tosello V, Nagai T, Miyawaki A, Di Lisa F et al (2001) Beat-to-beat oscillations of mitochondrial [Ca^{2+}] in cardiac cells. EMBO J 20(17):4998–5007

Roy SS, Hajnóczky G (2008) Calcium, mitochondria and apoptosis studied by fluorescence measurements. Methods 46(3):213–223

Schwartz A, Lee KS (1962) Study of heart mitochondria and glycolytic metabolism in experimentally induced cardiac failure. Circ Res 10:321–332

Seddon M, Looi YH, Shah AM (2007) Oxidative stress and redox signalling in cardiac hypertrophy and heart failure. Heart 93(8):903–907

Servidei S, Bertini E, DiMauro S (1994) Hereditary metabolic cardiomyopathies. Adv Pediatr 41:1–32

Sharikabad MN, Ostbye KM, Brors O (2004) Effect of hydrogen peroxide on reoxygenation-induced Ca2+ accumulation in rat cardiomyocytes. Free Radic Biol Med 37(4):531–538

Shiomi T, Tsutsui H, Matsusaka H, Murakami K, Hayashidani S, Ikeuchi M et al (2004) Overexpression of glutathione peroxidase prevents left ventricular remodeling and failure after myocardial infarction in mice. Circulation 109(4): 544–549

Silverman HS, Stern MD (1994) Ionic basis of ischaemic cardiac injury: insights from cellular studies. Cardiovasc Res 28(5):581–597

Smart N, Mojet MH, Latchman DS, Marber MS, Duchen MR, Heads RJ (2006) IL-6 induces PI 3-kinase and nitric oxide-dependent protection and preserves mitochondrial function in cardiomyocytes. Cardiovasc Res 69(1):164–177

Smets I, Caplanusi A, Despa S, Molnar Z, Radu M, vandeVen M et al (2004) Ca2+ uptake in mitochondria occurs via the reverse action of the Na+/Ca2+ exchanger in metabolically inhibited MDCK cells. Am J Physiol Renal Physiol 286(4):F784–F794

Sordahl LA, Stewart ML (1980) Mechanism(s) of altered mitochondrial calcium transport in acutely ischemic canine hearts. Circ Res 47(6):814–820

Sordahl LA, McCollum WB, Wood WG, Schwartz A (1973) Mitochondria and sarcoplasmic reticulum function in cardiac hypertrophy and failure. Am J Physiol 224(3):497–502

Stone D, Darley-Usmar V, Smith DR, O'Leary V (1989) Hypoxia-reoxygenation induced increase in cellular Ca2+ in myocytes and perfused hearts: the role of mitochondria. J Mol Cell Cardiol 21(10):963–973

Suleiman MS, Halestrap AP, Griffiths EJ (2001) Mitochondria: a target for myocardial protection. Pharmacol Ther 89(1):29–46

Supinski GS, Murphy MP, Callahan LA (2009) MitoQ administration prevents endotoxin-induced cardiac dysfunction. Am J Physiol Regul Integr Comp Physiol 297(4):R1095–R1102

Takeo S, Tanonaka K, Iwai T, Motegi K, Hirota Y (2004) Preservation of mitochondrial function during ischemia as a possible mechanism for cardioprotection of diltiazem against ischemia/reperfusion injury. Biochem Pharmacol 67(3):565–574

Terasaki F, Tanaka M, Kawamura K, Kanzaki Y, Okabe M, Hayashi T et al (2001) A case of cardiomyopathy showing progression from the hypertrophic to the dilated form: association of Mt8348A–>G mutation in the mitochondrial tRNA(Lys) gene with severe ultrastructural alterations of mitochondria in cardiomyocytes. Jpn Circ J 65(7):691–694

Thibault H, Piot C, Staat P, Bontemps L, Sportouch C, Rioufol G et al (2008) Long-term benefit of postconditioning. Circulation 117(8):1037–1044

Towbin JA, Bowles NE (2002) The failing heart. Nature 415(6868):227–233

Tsutsui H, Kinugawa S, Matsushima S (2008) Oxidative stress and mitochondrial DNA damage in heart failure. Circ J 72(Suppl A):A31–A37

Tsutsui H, Kinugawa S, Matsushima S (2009) Mitochondrial oxidative stress and dysfunction in myocardial remodelling. Cardiovasc Res 81(3):449–456

Tuppen HA, Blakely EL, Turnbull DM, Taylor RW (2010) Mitochondrial DNA mutations and human disease. Biochim Biophys Acta 1797(2):113–128

van Empel VP, Bertrand AT, Hofstra L, Crijns HJ, Doevendans PA, De Windt LJ (2005) Myocyte apoptosis in heart failure. Cardiovasc Res 67(1):21–29

Wang J, Wilhelmsson H, Graff C, Li H, Oldfors A, Rustin P et al (1999) Dilated cardiomyopathy and atrioventricular conduction blocks induced by heart-specific inactivation of mitochondrial DNA gene expression. Nat Genet 21(1): 133–137

Wang L, Cherednichenko G, Hernandez L, Halow J, Camacho SA, Figueredo V et al (2001) Preconditioning limits mitochondrial Ca2+ during ischemia in rat hearts: role of KATP channels. Am J Physiol Heart Circ Physiol 280(5):H2321–H2328

White RL, Wittenberg BA (1993) NADH fluorescence of isolated ventricular myocytes: effects of pacing, myoglobin, and oxygen supply. Biophys J 65(1):196–204

Wikman-Coffelt J, Sievers R, Parmley WW, Jasmin G (1986) Cardiomyopathic and healthy acidotic hamster hearts: mitochondrial activity may regulate cardiac performance. Cardiovasc Res 20(7):471–481

Winniford MD, Willerson JT, Hillis LD (1985) Calcium antagonists for acute ischemic heart disease. Am J Cardiol 55(3):116B–124B

Zhang SZ, Gao Q, Cao CM, Bruce IC, Xia Q (2006) Involvement of the mitochondrial calcium uniporter in cardioprotection by ischemic preconditioning. Life Sci 78(7):738–745

Zhao ZQ, Corvera JS, Halkos ME, Kerendi F, Wang NP, Guyton RA et al (2003) Inhibition of myocardial injury by ischemic postconditioning during reperfusion: comparison with ischemic preconditioning. Am J Physiol Heart Circ Physiol 285(2):H579–H588

Chapter 12
Mitochondria in Neurodegeneration

Lezi E and Russell H. Swerdlow

Abstract Many neurodegenerative diseases demonstrate abnormal mitochondrial morphology and biochemical dysfunction. Alterations are often systemic rather than brain-limited. Mitochondrial dysfunction may arise as a consequence of abnormal mitochondrial DNA, mutated nuclear proteins that interact directly or indirectly with mitochondria, or through unknown causes. In most cases it is unclear where mitochondria sit in relation to the overall disease cascades that ultimately causes neuronal dysfunction and death, and there is still controversy regarding the question of whether mitochondrial dysfunction is a necessary step in neurodegeneration. In this chapter we highlight and catalogue mitochondrial perturbations in some of the major neurodegenerative diseases including Alzheimer's disease (AD), Parkinson's disease (PD), amyotrophic lateral sclerosis (ALS), and Huntington's disease (HD). We consider data that suggest mitochondria may be critically involved in neurodegenerative disease neurodegeneration cascades.

Keywords Cybrid • Mitochondria • Mitochondrial DNA • Neurodegenerative disease

12.1 The Quintessential Neurodegenerative Diseases

Neurodegenerative diseases are characterized by gradually progressive, selective loss of anatomically or physiologically related neuronal systems. The clinical syndromes associated with particular neuro-anatomical patterns of cell dysfunction and loss are typically categorized by whether they initially affect cognition, movement, strength, coordination, sensation, vision, or autonomic control. Prototypical examples include AD, PD, ALS, and HD. HD is strictly an autosomal dominant disorder. With AD, PD, and ALS most cases are age-related and show sporadic epidemiology, although rare Mendelian variants do occur. As life expectancy continues to advance in developed countries the incidence of these disorders increases and will continue to do so.

Mitochondrial dysfunction is a common theme in these diseases. Mitochondria are known to play a central role in many cell functions including ATP generation, intracellular Ca^{2+} homeostasis, reactive

Lezi E • R.H. Swerdlow, MD (✉)
Departments of Neurology, Molecular and Integrative Physiology, University of Kansas
School of Medicine, MSN 2012, Landon Center on Aging, 3901 Rainbow Blvd,
Kansas City, KS 66209, USA
e-mail: le2@kumc.edu; rswerdlow@kumc.edu

R. Scatena et al. (eds.), *Advances in Mitochondrial Medicine*, Advances in Experimental
Medicine and Biology 942, DOI 10.1007/978-94-007-2869-1_12,
© Springer Science+Business Media B.V. 2012

oxygen species (ROS) formation, and apoptosis. Neurons are particularly dependent on mitochondria because of their high energy demands. It seems reasonable to hypothesize neurons are relatively intolerant of mitochondrial dysfunction. This assumption is supported by the fact that maternally inherited diseases with known homoplasmic or near-homoplasmic mitochondrial DNA (mtDNA) mutations tend to affect the central nervous system and muscle, the body's two most aerobic tissues.

12.2   Alzheimer's Disease

AD is the most common neurodegenerative disease and the most frequent cause of dementia. By far the greatest risk factor for AD is ageing, and approximately one in ten persons over 65 and nearly half of those over 85 have AD (Antuono and Beyer 1999). With such high prevalence rates among the oldest old it is difficult to not consider AD pathology from outside the context of aging itself (Swerdlow 2007a).

AD can be divided into early versus late onset forms as well as sporadic and autosomal-dominant variants. Autosomal dominant AD represents the minority of AD cases and typically presents before the age of 65. It is caused by mutations in genes encoding for either the amyloid precursor protein (APP), presenilin 1 (PS1), or presenilin 2 (PS2), and these mutations appear to alter processing of APP towards the 42 amino acid beta amyloid (Aβ) derivative (Scheuner et al. 1996). Aβ is the major constituent of amyloid plaques observed in particular brain regions of AD patients, including neocortex, hippocampus, and other subcortical regions essential for cognitive function. In 1992 the "amyloid cascade hypothesis" was proposed (Hardy and Higgins 1992). This hypothesis states altered processing of APP or changes in Aβ stability result in a chronic imbalance between Aβ production and clearance. Gradual accumulation of aggregated Aβ initiates a complex, multistep process that includes gliosis, inflammatory changes, neuritic/synaptic change, neurofibrillary tangles, reductions in neurotransmitters, and finally neurodegeneration and neuronal cell death.

However, it is not quite clear how Aβ might induce neurodegeneration. One possible mechanism is that Aβ interferes with mitochondrial function. When maintained in the presence of Aβ, isolated mitochondria show diminished respiratory capacity in general, and specifically inhibition of several key enzymes including cytochrome oxidase, α-ketoglutarate dehydrogenase, and pyruvate dehydrogenase (Pereira et al. 1998; Canevari et al. 1999; Casley et al. 2002). Brief exposure of cultured rat hippocampal neurons to sub-lethal Aβ concentrations resulted in rapid and severe impairment of mitochondrial transport without inducing apparent cell death (Rui et al. 2006). At concentrations insufficient to kill cells, Aβ appears to induce an increase in mitochondrial DNA (mtDNA) levels and reduces the number of normal appearing mitochondria (Diana et al. 2008). Cells depleted of endogenous mtDNA (ρ0) cells, which lack functional electron transport chains (ETC), are impervious to Aβ (Cardoso et al. 2001). A further study reports a positive correlation between levels of soluble Aβ and hydrogen peroxide in brain mitochondria isolated from APP transgenic mice (Manczak et al. 2006), which supports the view that mutant APP or soluble Aβ impairs mitochondrial metabolism. Physical associations between mitochondria and APP as well as between mitochondria and Aβ have been reported in transgenic mice (Manczak et al. 2006). Aβ binds to a mitochondrial protein called Aβ-binding alcohol dehydrogenase (ABAD), and it has been demonstrated that blocking the interaction of Aβ and ABAD can suppress Aβ-induced apoptosis and free-radical generation in neurons (Lustbader et al. 2004). These physical associations have also been supported by human AD studies (Lustbader et al. 2004; Anandatheerthavarada et al. 2003; Crouch et al. 2005; Caspersen et al. 2005; Devi et al. 2006). Physical associations between PS1 and mitochondria are also reported (Hansson et al. 2004).

Besides functional changes, extensive literature indicates mitochondrial structural dynamics are also altered in AD patients. Quantitative ultrastructural morphometric analysis shows that compared to age-matched control group brains AD brains contain a significantly lower percentage of normal

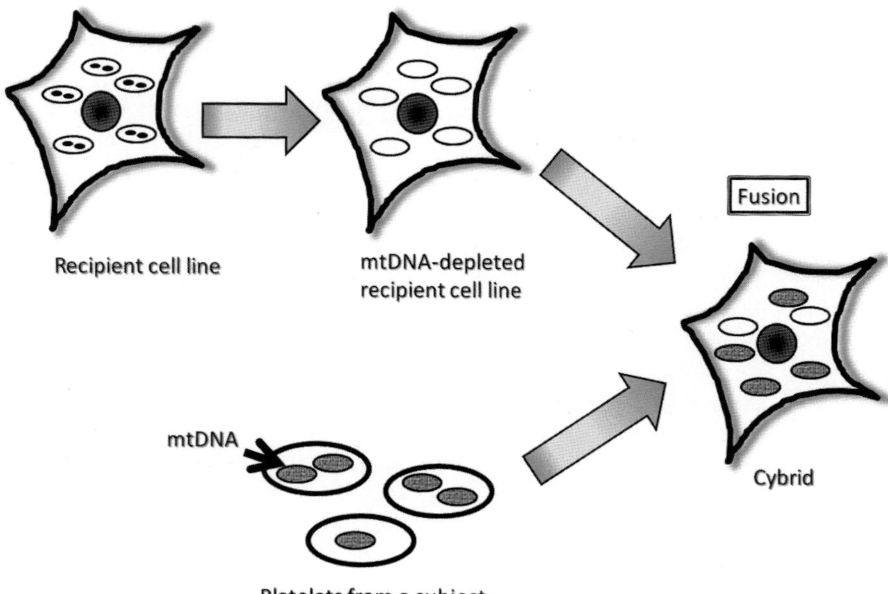

Fig. 12.1 *The cybrid technique.* The *black circles* represent nuclei in parental cells. The *ovals* represent mitochondria. The *black dots within the ovals* represent mitochondrial DNA

mitochondria (de la Monte et al. 2000) and a significantly higher percentage of mitochondria with broken cristae (Hirai et al. 2001). Also, in fibroblasts from sporadic AD patients mitochondria are longer, with two or more mitochondria often joined together, while those of age-matched normal human fibroblasts are much shorter and appear sausage-shaped or rounded (Wang et al. 2008a). Similar morphological changes are also found in neurons over-expressing wild-type APP. APP over-expressing cells actually show mitochondria with heterogeneous morphologies; approximately 50% of cells contain fragmented, punctiform mitochondria and the mitochondria in some cells show elongated, net-like structures (Wang et al. 2008b).

It is known that the activities of several mitochondrial enzymes including complex IV (cytochrome c oxidase; COX), pyruvate dehydrogenase complex, and α-ketoglutarate dehydrogenase complex are reduced in AD (Swerdlow and Kish 2002). COX is the last enzyme in the respiratory ETC of mitochondria and receives electrons from cytochrome c. It contains several metal prosthetic sites and 13 protein subunits of which ten are encoded by nuclear and three by mtDNA genes. In 1990, deficient COX activity was found in platelets of AD patients. A similar finding was made in AD brains in 1992 (Parker et al. 1990a; Kish et al. 1992). Subsequently, the finding of reduced COX activity in AD patients has been replicated in platelets (Parker et al. 1994; Bosetti et al. 2002; Cardoso et al. 2004a), fibroblasts (Curti et al. 1997), focal brain regions (Bosetti et al. 2002), and large parts of the brain (Mutisya et al. 1994; Wong-Riley et al. 1997). These reports indicate mitochondrial dysfunction occurs in AD and that AD mitochondrial dysfunction is systemic rather than brain-limited.

COX reduction has also been reported at all stages of the disease, including mild cognitive impairment (MCI) (Swerdlow and Kish 2002; Valla et al. 2006). APP transgenic mice also develop early signs of mitochondrial perturbation; expression of mitochondrial genes is altered when these mice are only 2 months old, which precedes by months the appearance of cognitive signs (Manczak et al. 2006).

Cytoplasmic hybrid (cybrid) studies suggest mtDNA is at least partly responsible for the reduced activity of COX in AD patients (Swerdlow et al. 1997). A diagram that provides an overview of the cybrid technique is shown in Fig. 12.1. When platelet mtDNA from AD patients is expressed within neuronal cell lines grown in culture (cytoplasmic hybrid cell lines, or cybrids), the resulting cells continue to manifest reduced COX activity and this specific biochemical defect persists over time in the cybrid lines (Swerdlow et al. 1997; Swerdlow 2007b). It also has been observed that AD cybrid cell lines containing AD subject mitochondria/mtDNA overproduce free radicals, accumulate Aβ, and have decreased ATP levels (Swerdlow 2007b; Khan et al. 2000; Cardoso et al. 2004b). Since three of the 13 COX subunits are encoded by mtDNA, this phenomenon suggests mtDNA differs between AD patients and control subjects, and indirectly supports the view that mtDNA contributes to the AD-associated COX activity reduction.

It remains unclear how mtDNA from AD subjects specifically differs from that of control subjects. Several studies show oxidative modification of both nuclear DNA and mtDNA are increased in AD brains (Gabbita et al. 1998; Mecocci et al. 1994; Wang et al. 2005). Levels of 8-hydroxy-2-deoxyguanosine (8-OHdG) are widely considered to reflect levels of oxidative stress (Valavanidis et al. 2009), and mtDNA 8-OHdG is increased in AD patient cortical brain regions (Mecocci et al. 1994). It is known that mtDNA with large mtDNA deletions (including a 4,977 base-pair deletion that involves mtDNA cytochrome oxidase subunit genes) preferentially accumulates in human AD brains compared to control aged brain (Corral-Debrinski et al. 1994; Hamblet and Castora 1997) and the frequency of point mutations are also higher in several brain regions including parietal gyrus, hippocampus, and cerebellum of AD subjects (Chang et al. 2000). Although AD mtDNA sequences contain a higher number of substitutions in tRNA genes, without a corresponding biochemical analysis it is hard to know whether these mtDNA mutations constitute a major etiological factor in sporadic AD (Elson et al. 2006).

Mitochondrial genes contain frequent polymorphic variations, and mtDNA gene products function in the context of nuclear-encoded proteins that also contain polymorphic variations. It is possible that polymorphism-defined ETC subunit combinations do not function identically. If so, this could explain why epidemiologic associations between mtDNA polymorphisms and AD risk are difficult to establish (Swerdlow and Kish 2002).

Although clear mtDNA features contributing to the pathogenesis of AD are still not known, the possibility that maternal mitochondrial inheritance may influence disease risk and pathology has been considered. While several studies actually conclude there is no evidence of a maternal effect in AD, or even that there is predominant paternal transmission (Ehrenkrantz et al. 1999; Payami and Hoffbuhr 1993), other epidemiological studies find maternal inheritance strongly influences AD risk (Duara et al. 1993; Edland et al. 1996). Among AD patients with one affected parent, the ratio of mothers to fathers affected is 3:1; for cases in which affected proband relations include one affected parent and at least sibling, the mother to father ratio increases to 9:1 (Edland et al. 1996). Recently, a genetic study indentified new possible regions of linkage on chromosome 10 and 12 only among families with maternal transmission of late-onset AD (Bassett et al. 2002). Brain imaging techniques also provide evidence of maternal transmission of AD risk. Positron emission tomography (PET) imaging, when using 2-[^{18}F] fluoro-2-deoxy-D-glucose (FDG) as the tracer, can be used to determine the cerebral metabolic rate of glucose (CMR$_{glc}$). It has been demonstrated that in AD patients, CMR$_{glc}$ is reduced in several neuroanatomic areas including the parietotemporal, posterior cingulate, and to a smaller extent frontal cortex and medial temporal lobe regions (Mosconi 2005). These reductions occur years before AD symptom onset. One FDG-PET study reported that cognitively intact subjects (aged from 46 to 80) with AD mothers but not AD fathers had AD-like patterns of CMR$_{glc}$ reduction even after accounting for other possible AD risk factors (Mosconi et al. 2007, 2009).

The amyloid cascade hypothesis, which assumes AD is always a primary amyloidosis, has dominated thinking in the AD research field for decades but other etiologic hypotheses have been formulated. The "mitochondrial cascade hypothesis" was proposed in 2004 (Swerdlow and Khan 2004). In the mitochondrial cascade hypothesis, mitochondria sit at the apex of AD histopathology and neurodegeneration. It assumes AD mitochondrial dysfunction drives amyloidosis, tau phosphorylation, and cell cycle re-entry (Swerdlow and Khan 2009; Swerdlow 2007c). As mentioned above, since AD mitochondrial dysfunction is systemic altered mitochondrial function in AD cannot simply represent a consequence of neurodegeneration. Although many investigators believe that mitochondrial dysfunction is a downstream event in the development of AD and may play a minor role in the disease, the results of several studies including cell culture and transgenic mouse studies support that brain mitochondrial bioenergetic defects (such as oxidative damage, COX activity, oxygen consumption, and H_2O_2 production) precedes or drives Aβ production/deposition and plaque formation (Khan et al. 2000; Manczak et al. 2006; Prat#ico et al. 2001; Yao et al. 2009). The mitochondrial cascade hypothesis also takes aging phenomena into account. It postulates inheritance determines mitochondrial baseline function and durability, which in turn influences how mitochondria change with age. It is presumed more durable mitochondria adequately function for more decades than less durable mitochondria. When mitochondrial change reaches a threshold and bioenergetic homeostasis can no longer be maintained, AD histopathology and symptoms may ensue (Swerdlow 2007c).

In summary, mounting evidence indicates altered mitochondrial function associates with AD. If mitochondrial dysfunction is critical for the initiation and progression of AD, the susceptibility of mitochondria to environmental and genetic risk factors should play a role in the development of AD and mitochondria need to be considered in late-onset, sporadic AD prevention and treatment development efforts.

12.3 Parkinson's Disease

PD is the most common neurodegenerative movement disorder. It affects ~1% of the population above the age of 60 (Abou-Sleiman et al. 2006) and 1–3% of those over 80 years of age (Tanner and Goldman 1996). PD is clinically characterized by rigidity, resting tremor, bradykinesia and postural instability. The key symptoms and signs arise from a preferential loss of dopaminergic neurons of the substantia nigra pars compacta, although early neurodegeneration also occurs in other discrete brainstem and basal forebrain nuclei. Another hallmark is that surviving nigral neurons may contain Lewy bodies, intracytoplasmic inclusions that are mainly composed of fibrillar α-synuclein protein (Spillantini et al. 1997). The presence of nigral Lewy Bodies establishes the histological diagnosis of PD.

Like AD, PD is clinically partitioned into early versus late onset variants and Mendelian versus non-Mendelian forms. With advancing age the percentage of cases caused by Mendelian gene mutations declines. Most PD (~90%) is sporadic and does not show Mendelian inheritance (Trimmer and Bennett 2009).

Mitochondrial dysfunction has long been implicated in the pathogenesis of PD. Evidence first emerged in the 1980s that drug abusers developed an acute and irreversible parkinsonian syndrome after using 1-methyl-4-phenyl-1,2,3,6-tetrahydropyridine (MPTP). The active metabolite of MPTP, 1-methyl-4-phenylpyridinium (MPP$^+$), is transported intracellularly by the dopamine transporter (DAT). Perhaps because of DAT uptake it accumulates in dopaminergic neurons and inhibits complex I (Nicklas et al. 1985). MPP$^+$-induced complex I inhibition further leads to increased free radical production/oxidative stress, decreased ATP production, increased intracellular calcium concentration, excitotoxicity, nitric oxide-related cellular damage, and ultimately the death of dopaminergic neurons (Beal 1998; Hantraye et al. 1996; Mizuno et al. 1988; Ng et al. 1996; Sheehan et al. 1997; Smith et al. 1994; Ali et al. 1994). MPTP has been extensively used for PD cell culture and animal modeling.

In 1989, several groups reported that complex I activity was reduced in the substantia nigra, platelets, and skeletal muscle of patients with idiopathic PD (Parker et al. 1989; Schapira et al. 1989; Bindoff et al. 1989). Since then altered complex I activity was also reported in fibroblasts and frontal cortex (Mytilineou et al. 1994; Parker et al. 2008). It has been hypothesized that this PD systemic complex I activity reduction may be a consequence of exposure to exogenous inhibitors, systemic endogenous production of an inhibitory factor, or mtDNA-encoding of complex I subunits

Table 12.1 Interactions between mitochondria and proteins encoded by genes that are mutated in Mendelian Parkinson's Disease

Locus	Gene product	Inheritance & comments	Direct or indirect interaction with mitochondria
PARK1/4	α-Synuclein	AD	Mutant α-synuclein sensitizes neurons to oxidative stress and damage.
PARK2	Parkin	AR, most common cause of recessive juvenile PD	Parkin mutations lead to increased oxidative stress and in turn mitochondrial dysfunction can affect parkin function.
PARK6	PINK1	AR, second most common cause of recessive juvenile PD	A mitochondria-localized kinase; its deficiency sensitizes mitochondria to rotenone and induces degeneration of dopaminergic neurons.
PARK7	DJ-1	AR	A possible redox sensor; binds to mitochondrial complex I and maintain its activity.
PARK8	LRRK2	AD, most common cause of dominant PD	Associates with the outer mitochondrial membrane and can bind parkin.
PARK13	OMI/HTRA2	AD?[a]	A mitochondrial protease; acts downstream of PINK1; loss of HtrA2 results in the accumulation of unfolded proteins in the mitochondria and increased production of ROS.

AD autosomal dominant, *AR* autosomal recessive
[a]Not uniformly accepted

(Swerdlow 2000). Data supporting all of these possibilities are published. For example, the complex I inhibitor rotenone has been used to model PD in rats. Rats administered rotenone develop a PD-like syndrome characterized by loss of substantia nigra neurons and the formation of α-synuclein-rich inclusion bodies (Betarbet et al. 2000; Cannon et al. 2009).

Several nuclear gene mutations associated with autosomal dominant and recessive forms of Mendelian PD have also been identified (Table 12.1). Examples of such genes are α-synuclein, Parkin, phosphate and tensin homologue-induced kinase 1 (PINK1), DJ1, leucine-rich repeat kinase 2 (LRRK2), and Htr A serine peptidase 2 (HTRA2). Genetically modified organisms based on knock-out, over-expression, or mutant versions of these genes have since been generated for purposes of PD animal modeling. Interestingly, many of these nuclear genes also implicate a role for mitochondria in PD pathogenesis.

In transgenic mice over-expressing α-synuclein, mitochondrial function is impaired, oxidative stress increases, and in the face of complex I inhibitors the threshold for nigral degeneration is reduced (Song et al. 2004). In another study of mice that over-express mutant α-synuclein, α–synuclein immunostaining suggested this protein directly affects mitochondria (Martin et al. 2006).

Parkin, a ubiquitin ligase, is believed to protect neuron mitochondria (Palacino et al. 2004). It has been reported in *drosophila* and mouse models that parkin deficiency or mutations lead to increased oxidative stress and mitochondrial impairment (Palacino et al. 2004; Pesah et al. 2004). It is important to note that mitochondrial dysfunction and oxidative stress also affect parkin function and exacerbate the consequences of parkin mutations (Chung et al. 2004).

PINK1, a mitochondria-localized kinase, appears to protect against cell death (Silvestri et al. 2005). This protective effect is abrogated by PD-related mutations that disable its kinase function (Petit et al. 2005). PINK deficiency increases the sensitivity of mitochondria to rotenone and induces degeneration of dopaminergic neurons in *drosophila* (Yang et al. 2006). These reports and others provide strong evidence that mitochondrial dysfunction plays an important role in the pathogenesis of Mendelian PD, and are consistent with an important role for mitochondrial function in sporadic PD.

As mentioned above, reduced complex I activity is a systemic event in PD. Complex I is a large multimeric enzyme containing 46 known protein subunits. At least seven of these subunits are encoded by genes on mtDNA. Because mtDNA makes such an important contribution to the structure and function of complex I and mtDNA abnormalities can produce sporadic disease, in 1989 it was hypothesized that mtDNA alteration might constitute a key risk factor for the development of idiopathic PD (Parker et al. 1989). An early study found levels of the common mtDNA deletion were increased in PD brains, but this study did not use age-matched controls (Ikebe et al. 1990). Other studies using DNA isolated from brain homogenates found that relative to age-matched controls, mtDNA deletions were not increased (Schapira et al. 1990; Lestienne et al. 1991). More recently it was shown that mtDNA deletion burdens increase with advancing age and are further increased in nigral neurons from PD subjects (Bender et al. 2006; Kraytsberg et al. 2006).

Multiple groups have used the cybrid technique to show transfer of mitochondria and mtDNA from sporadic PD subject platelets produces cell lines with persistently reduced complex I activity (Swerdlow et al. 1996a; Gu et al. 1998; Esteves et al. 2008, 2010). PD cybrid cell lines also have increased reactive oxygen species production, reduced mitochondrial calcium storage, less ATP production, depolarized mitochondria, and higher caspase 3 activity. PD cybrid cell lines generate Lewy body-like inclusions without the need for exogenous protein expression or toxin-mediated inhibition of mitochondrial or proteasomal function (Trimmer et al. 2004). Mitochondrial respiration and pathways influenced by aerobic metabolism are also altered in PD cybrid cell lines. A recent study reported PD cybrid mitochondria have an increased proton leak and decreased respiratory reserve capacity. In these cybrid cell lines levels of the transcriptional co-activator PGC1-α, which coordinates mitochondrial biogenesis, were reduced (Esteves et al. 2010).

Although the actual mtDNA alterations that account for these findings are still unknown, these results strongly suggest mtDNA contributes to reduced complex I activity in sporadic PD. This mtDNA contribution could derive from inherited or somatic mtDNA mutations. Several lines of investigation support a role for mtDNA inheritance. Epidemiologic studies suggest for non-Mendelian cases who nevertheless have a PD-affected parent, the affected parent is more likely to be the mother (Wooten et al. 1997; Swerdlow et al. 2001). Mitochondrial haplogroup and polymorphism association studies demonstrate mtDNA variations alter PD risk as well (Swerdlow 2000; van der Walt et al. 2003). The systemic nature of the PD complex I defect, in conjunction with the fact that expression of PD subject platelet mtDNA probably accounts for the results of PD cybrid studies, also suggests mtDNA inheritance is more likely to play a key role than somatic mutation acquisition (Swerdlow 2009).

As discussed above, the use of PD tissues and a number of experimental PD models has contributed to our recognition and understanding of how mitochondria are important to PD pathogenesis. *In vivo* human studies also contribute to this knowledge base. Proton and phosphorus magnetic resonance spectroscopy (^{1}H and ^{31}P MRS) are powerful, noninvasive techniques that facilitate quantitative *in vivo* measurements of metabolism pathway intermediates. ^{31}P MRS allows quantitative measurements of high energy phosphates such as adenosine triphosphate and phosphocreatine, and can be used to provide an indication of brain energy stores (Henchcliffe et al. 2008). One study using these techniques found high-energy phosphates were reduced in the putamen and midbrain of both early and advanced PD patient groups (Hattingen et al. 2009).

Most would agree mitochondria play an important role in PD pathogenesis. Abundant evidence supports this view. Although identifying the actual mtDNA features that associate with sporadic PD warrants further investigation, at this point targeting mitochondrial function in PD treatment development efforts is well-justified.

12.4   Amyotrophic Lateral Sclerosis

ALS is a neurodegenerative disease that primarily affects strength. It is characterized by upper and lower motor neuron degeneration. Weakness and muscle atrophy usually begin asymmetrically and distally in a single limb, spreads within the neuro-axis to involve contiguous muscle groups innervated by nearby motor neurons, and eventually also affects more rostral motor neurons. Approximately 10% of ALS cases are familial and the rest are sporadic. Similar to AD and PD, the incidence of ALS increases with increasing age, and the older the age of onset the less likely Mendelian inheritance is responsible. Among familial cases, the most common mutations occur in the copper-zinc superoxide dismutase (SOD1) gene on chromosome 21. SOD1 mutations account for about 20% of the familial cases and 2% of all cases. More recently, mutations in two RNA processing proteins, TDP-43 and FUS/TLW (Kabashi et al. 2008; Sreedharan et al. 2008; Vance et al. 2009; Kwiatkowski et al. 2009), have also been found in kindreds with familial ALS variants.

Mitochondrial alterations have been described in sporadic ALS as well as in models of familial ALS. Mitochondrial morphological changes, such as bizarre giant mitochondria and spiny or stubby mitochondria, are found at greater than normal frequencies (Hirano et al. 1984; Masui et al. 1985; Nakano et al. 1987). Abnormal mitochondria accumulate in the axon hillock and initial segment of axons (Sasaki and Iwata 1996). Changes are observed in both neural and non-neural tissues (Swerdlow et al. 2000). Changes in mitochondrial electron transport chain activities have been noted by several groups using biopsies from patients with ALS and animal models of ALS. While the overall results of many different studies support the overall view that mitochondria and mitochondrial function are altered in ALS, particular results from these studies are not homogeneous. In one study, complex I activity was increased in postmortem brain tissue from a patient with familial ALS (Bowling et al. 1993). Reduced complex IV activity was shown in patients with sporadic ALS (Fujita et al. 1996). Complex I and II-III deficiencies were observed in patients with familial ALS due to SOD1 mutations and also in an SOD1 transgenic mouse model (Browne et al. 1998).

When the cybrid technique was used to study the function of mitochondria obtained from ALS subject platelets, ALS cybrids produced on a neuroblastoma nuclear background showed a significant reduction in complex I activity and non-significant trends towards reduced complex III and IV activities (Swerdlow et al. 1996b, 1998). In another study that used spinal cord tissue from patients with ALS, it was reported that activity of citrate synthase, which is often used as a marker of mitochondrial mass, was significantly lower than it was in control subjects. Along with the decreased activities of respiratory chain complexes I + III, II + III, and IV this paper reported, low citrate synthase activity suggests there is a loss of mitochondria from spinal cords of ALS patients (Wiedemann et al. 2002).

Cell ROS levels may increase when mitochondrial respiration is impaired, although ROS itself may impair mitochondrial function (Bacman et al. 2006). There is certainly abundant evidence that indicates oxidative stress in increased in ALS. In sporadic ALS cases both lipid and protein oxidation are enhanced in spinal cord motor neurons and glia (Shibata et al. 2001). Also, the percentage of oxidized CoQ10 in sporadic ALS subject cerebrospinal fluid exceeds that of age-matched controls and positively correlates with illness duration (Murata et al. 2008). Markers of immune system activation are significantly elevated in ALS postmortem CNS tissue (Simpson et al. 2004), and increased blood ROS and lactate production levels suggests a close relationship between mitochondrial function and oxidative stress in ALS (Siciliano et al. 2002). Some propose oxidation-induced DNA damage contributes to sporadic ALS pathogenesis (Murata et al. 2008).

As to whether alterations in mtDNA are associated with ALS, diminished levels of mtDNA were observed in skeletal muscle of patients with sporadic ALS (Vielhaber et al. 2000). Mitochondrial DNA haplogroups also appear to influence ALS risk (Mancuso et al. 2004). Other studies suggest levels of the 4,977-base pair mtDNA common deletion are elevated in sporadic ALS (Ro et al. 2003; Dhaliwal and Grewal 2000). Since correlation does not establish causality, though, further investigation is needed to determine whether mtDNA somatic mutations play a causal role in sporadic ALS or are merely a byproduct of upstream events.

Most ALS laboratory modeling is accomplished using transgenic rodents that express an ALS-associated SOD1 mutation. The SOD1 gene was the first gene recognized to cause autosomal dominant ALS, and more than 100 different mutations have been mapped to it (Bacman et al. 2006). SOD1 protein functions as a ubiquitous antioxidant enzyme that catalyzes the dismutation of superoxide radicals to hydrogen peroxide, which can be converted to molecular oxygen by additional antioxidant enzymes such as catalase and glutathione peroxidase. It localizes predominantly to the cytoplasm, but both wild type and mutant SOD1 protein have been found in the intermembrane space, matrix and outer membrane of mitochondria of ALS-affected tissues (Higgins et al. 2002; Velde et al. 2008; Vijayvergiya et al. 2005; Liu et al. 2004). It is postulated that mutant SOD1 accumulates and aggregates in the outer mitochondrial membrane, that this impairs mitochondrial protein import, and disrupting mitochondrial protein import perturbs mitochondrial function (Liu et al. 2004).

Extensive mitochondrial fragmentation occurs in cell models of mutant SOD1 overexpression (Raimondi et al. 2006; Menzies et al. 2002). Mitochondrial vacuolation is another abnormal morphologic feature characteristic of SOD1 ALS models. This is seen in spinal motor neurons from these mice, and it occurs in conjunction with expansion of the intermembrane space and the mitochondrial outer membrane (Higgins et al. 2003). A transient explosive increase in vacuoles is observed in mutant SOD1-expressing transgenic mice just prior to motor neuron demise (Kong and Xu 1998), which suggests mitochondrial dysfunction may trigger ALS cell death cascades.

SOD1-induced mitochondrial membrane damage discharges the mitochondrial membrane potential, impairs mitochondrial respiration, and reduces the ability of mitochondria to buffer cytosolic calcium (Borthwick et al. 1999; Jung et al. 2002; Carri et al. 1997). In SOD1 mice these changes precede the onset of motor signs (Damiano et al. 2006).

Substantial evidence suggests mitochondrial dysfunction plays a crucial role in ALS motor neuron degeneration. Where mitochondrial dysfunction sits in the ALS pathologic cascade is unclear and where mitochondria sit in the degeneration hierarchy of Mendelian and sporadic ALS variants may differ. In the Mendelian forms mitochondrial dysfunction certainly must occur downstream of the causative mutation, but even in Mendelian ALS mitochondrial dysfunction may play a fairly upstream role. In sporadic ALS it is possible that mitochondrial dysfunction occupies the apex of the ALS pathology pyramid, but this remains unproven (Beal 1995).

12.5 Huntington's Disease

HD is a degenerative movement disorder clinically characterized by choreiform movements, psychiatric disturbances, and dementia. Symptoms may develop in childhood or young adulthood but usually manifest in middle age. Clinical changes reflect neuron dysfunction and loss that preferentially affects GABAergic medium spiny striatal neurons (Vonsattel and DiFiglia 1998). The disease becomes less neuroanatomically specific during later stages as it extends to other brain regions. HD is strictly an autosomal dominant disorder and it is caused by a CAG triplet repeat expansion (>35 CAGs) in the first exon of the Huntingtin (HTT) gene on chromosome 4 (Huntington's Disease Collaborative Research Group 1993).

Impaired cell energy production and metabolism in HD were recognized before the responsible gene mutation was identified. Energy metabolism-related deficits were predicted in the early 1980s following observations of excessive weight loss and deficient brain FDG uptake on PET (Sanberg et al. 1981; Kuhl et al. 1982). In the early 1990s proton nuclear magnetic resonance spectroscopy further revealed increased lactate in the cortex and basal ganglia of HD subjects (Jenkins et al. 1993).

Several electron transport chain enzyme activities are deficient in HD tissues. Complex II, III and IV activities are significantly reduced in HD subject brains (Gu et al. 1996; Browne et al. 1997). Additional data suggest the complex II defect is particularly relevant to the demise of neuron populations affected in HD (Benchoua et al. 2006). Complex II inhibitors have successfully been used to model HD; systemic administration of the complex II inhibitors 3-nitropropionic acid and malonate to rodents and primates recreates an HD-like pattern of neurodegeneration and an HD-consistent behavioral phenotype (Beal et al. 1993; Brouillet et al. 1995). Surprisingly, though, for two non-brain tissues (platelets and muscle) complex I activity is reduced but complex II, III, and IV activities are not (Arenas et al. 1998; Parker et al. 1990b).

Since HTT polyglutamine repeat expansion is the primary cause of HD, the question arises as to how and why mitochondrial dysfunction arises in HD. This could conceivably result from direct or indirect effects that HTT may have on mitochondria. Another question that requires consideration is whether mitochondrial dysfunction plays an important intermediary role in HD dysfunction and neurodegeneration cascades. These questions have been studied using transgenic mice that express all or part of the mutant huntingtin gene, but despite considerable efforts decisive conclusions remain elusive.

Available data do indicate polyglutamine-expanded HTT directly associates with mitochondria. A study of mice expressing a 72 glutamine-long expansion found brain mitochondria had lower mitochondrial membrane potentials and depolarized at lower calcium exposures than did mitochondria from control mouse brains. These biochemical defects preceded the onset of structural and behavioral abnormalities by months (Panov et al. 2002). This study further found that when normal mitochondria were incubated with a fusion protein containing an abnormally long polyglutamine repeat, the mitochondria developed calcium handling deficits consistent with those seen in human HD subject tissues and HD transgenic animal models. A different study also found mitochondria from HD transgenic mice were overly sensitive to calcium-induced mitochondria permeability transitions. This phenomena was also observed in normal mitochondria exposed to mutant HTT (Choo et al. 2004).

Other data indicate mutant HTT may indirectly influence mitochondrial function by altering mitochondria-relevant transcription events. HTT appears to interact with several transcription factors, including p53, CREB-binding protein, Sp1, and PGC1-α (Bae et al. 2005; Sugars and Rubinsztein 2003; Weydt et al. 2006; Cui et al. 2006). p53 is a tumor suppressor protein that also regulates genes involved in mitochondrial function and oxidative stress. A recent study reported mutant HTT binds p53, upregulates nuclear p53 levels and transcriptional activity, and through these effects causes mitochondrial membrane depolarization. p53 suppression prevented mitochondrial depolarization and HTT-induced cytotoxicity (Bae et al. 2005). PGC-1α is a transcription coactivator that regulates mitochondrial biogenesis and metabolic pathways relevant to cell bioenergetics. PGC-1α knock-out mice have an HD-like phenotype (Lin et al. 2004), and reduced expression of PGC-1α target genes is seen in HD patient and HD transgenic mouse striatum (Weydt et al. 2006). Crossing PGC-1α knock-out mice with HD transgenic mice exacerbates striatal neurodegeneration and motor abnormalities, while lentivirus-mediated delivery of PGC-1α to the striatum is neuroprotective in HD transgenic mice (Cui et al. 2006).

Resveratrol, an activator of the sirtuin Sir2 homolog 1 (SIRT1) may also protect against mutant HTT-induced metabolic dysfunction (Parker et al. 2005). SIRT1 deacetylates and activates PGC-1α (Nemoto et al. 2005; Rodgers et al. 2005). PGC-1α activation is under consideration for its potential as an HD therapeutic target.

12.6 Conclusions

Depicting the hierarchical cascades that drive and mediate neuron dysfunction and death in neurodegenerative diseases is extremely complex (Fig. 12.2). Identifying individual pathologies is easier than defining how they interact. Strong evidence acquired over decades shows mitochondrial abnormalities

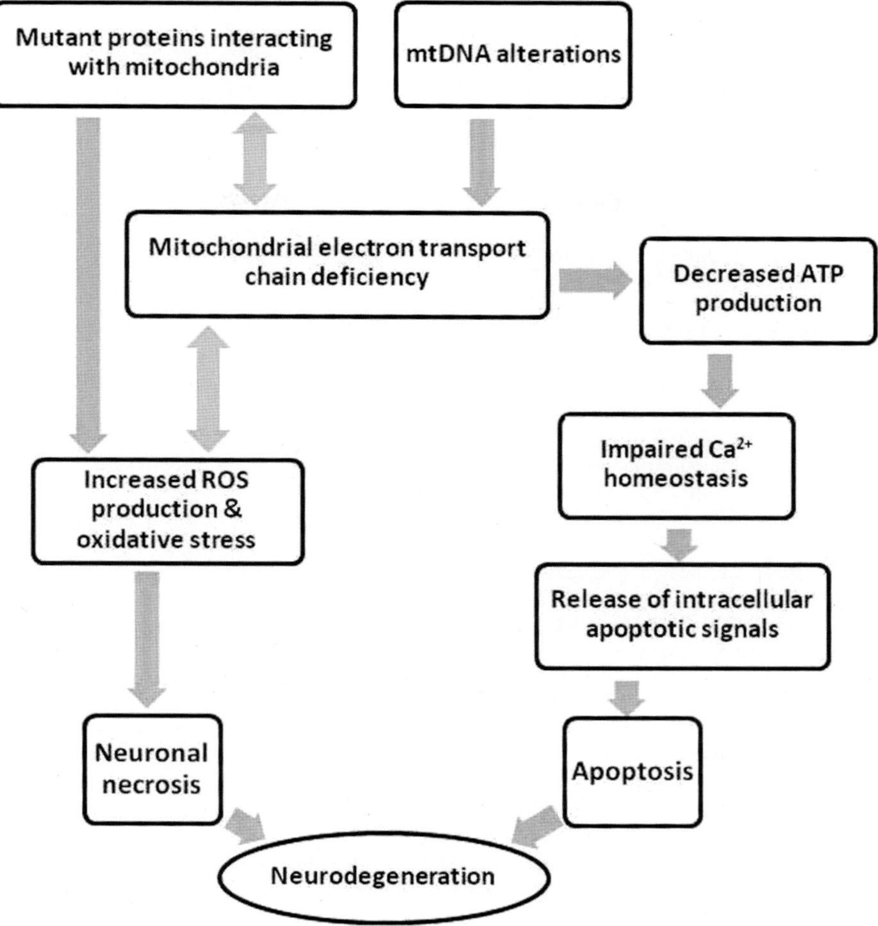

Fig. 12.2 Attempt to summarize relationships between mitochondria and other characteristic neurodegeneration features

occur in persons with various neurodegenerative diseases, and further shows distinct mitochondrial abnormalities are characteristic of particular disorders. This is the case for very rare neurodegenerative diseases and also for very common age-related disorders such as AD and PD. It has been considered for some time that mitochondria might play a quite upstream role in sporadic neurodegenerations. It is now also known that a remarkable number of proteins that cause neurodegeneration in their mutant forms interact with mitochondria or affect mitochondrial function. It is important that studies of the mitochondria-neurodegeneration nexus continue for many reasons. Such studies could yield insights into and treatments for diseases that devastate millions of people.

References

Abou-Sleiman PM, Muqit MMK, Wood NW (2006) Expanding insights of mitochondrial dysfunction in Parkinson's disease. Nat Rev Neurosci 7(3):207–219

Ali SF, David SN, Newport GD, Cadet JL, Slikker W Jr (1994) MPTP-induced oxidative stress and neurotoxicity are age-dependent: evidence from measures of reactive oxygen species and striatal dopamine levels. Synapse 18:27–34

Anandatheerthavarada HK, Biswas G, Robin M-A, Avadhani NG (2003) Mitochondrial targeting and a novel transmembrane arrest of Alzheimer's amyloid precursor protein impairs mitochondrial function in neuronal cells. J Cell Biol 161(1):41–54

Antuono P, Beyer J (1999) The burden of dementia. A medical and research perspective. Theor Med Bioethics 20(1):3–13

Arenas J, Campos Y, Ribacoba R, Martin MA, Rubio JC, Ablanedo P, Cabello A (1998) Complex I defect in muscle from patients with Huntington's disease. Ann Neurol 43:397–400

Bacman SR, Bradley WG, Moraes CT (2006) Mitochondrial involvement in amyotrophic lateral sclerosis: trigger or target? Mol Neurobiol 33(2):113–131

Bae BI, Xu H, Igarashi S, Fujimuro M, Agrawal N, Taya Y, Hayward SD, Moran TH, Montell C, Ross CA, Snyder SH, Sawa A (2005) p53 mediates cellular dysfunction and behavioral abnormalities in Huntington's disease. Neuron 47:29–41

Bassett SS, Avramopoulos D, Fallin D (2002) Evidence for parent of origin effect in late-onset Alzheimer disease. Am J Med Genet B Neuropsychiatr Genet 114(6):679–686

Beal MF (1995) Aging, energy, and oxidative stress in neurodegenerative diseases. Ann Neurol 38(3):357–366

Beal MF (1998) Excitotoxicity and nitric oxide in Parkinson's disease pathogenesis. Ann Neurol 44:S110–S114

Beal MF, Brouillet E, Jenkins BG, Ferrante RJ, Kowall NW, Miller JM, Storey E, Srivastava R, Rosen BR, Hyman BT (1993) Neurochemical and histologic characterization of striatal excitotoxic lesions produced by the mitochondrial toxin 3-nitropropionic acid. J Neurosci 13(10):4181–4192

Benchoua A, Trioulier Y, Zala D, Gaillard MC, Lefort N, Dufour N, Saudou F, Elalouf JM, Hirsch E, Hantraye P, Déglon N, Brouillet E (2006) Involvement of mitochondrial complex II defects in neuronal death produced by N-terminus fragment of mutated huntingtin. Mol Biol Cell 17(4):1652–1663

Bender A, Krishnan KJ, Morris CM, Taylor GA, Reeve AK, Perry RH, Jaros E, Hersheson JS, Betts J, Klopstock T, Taylor RW, Turnbull DM (2006) High levels of mitochondrial DNA deletions in substantia nigra neurons in aging and Parkinson disease. Nat Genet 38(5):515–517

Betarbet R, Sherer TB, Mackenzie G, Garcia-Osuna M, Panov AV, Greenamyre JT (2000) Chronic systemic pesticide exposure reproduces features of Parkinson's disease. Nat Neurosci 3(12):1301–1306

Bindoff LA, Birch-Machin M, Cartlidge NEF, Parker WD, Turnbull DM (1989) Mitochondrial function in Parkinson's disease. Lancet 2(8653):49

Borthwick GM, Johnson MA, Ince PG, Shaw PJ, Turnbull DM (1999) Mitochondrial enzyme activity in amyotrophic lateral sclerosis: implications for the role of mitochondria in neuronal cell death. Ann Neurol 46:787–790

Bosetti F, Brizzi F, Barogi S, Mancuso M, Siciliano G, Tendi EA, Murri L, Rapoport SI, Solaini G (2002) Cytochrome c oxidase and mitochondrial F1F0-ATPase (ATP synthase) activities in platelets and brain from patients with Alzheimer's disease. Neurobiol Aging 23(3):371–376

Bowling AC, Schulz JB, Brown RH, Beal MF (1993) Superoxide dismutase activity, oxidative damage, and mitochondrial energy metabolism in familial and sporadic amyotrophic lateral sclerosis. J Neurochem 61(6):2322–2325

Brouillet E, Hantraye P, Ferrante RJ, Dolan R, Leroy-Willig A, Kowall NW, Beal MF (1995) Chronic mitochondrial energy impairment produces selective striatal degeneration and abnormal choreiform movements in primates. Proc Natl Acad Sci USA 92:7105–7109

Browne SE, Bowling AC, Macgarvey U, Baik MJ, Berger SC, Muqit MM, Bird ED, Beal MF (1997) Oxidative damage and metabolic dysfunction in Huntington's disease: selective vulnerability of the basal ganglia. Ann Neurol 41(5):646–653

Browne SE, Bowling AC, Baik MJ, Gurney M, Brown RH, Beal MF (1998) Metabolic dysfunction in familial, but not sporadic, amyotrophic lateral sclerosis. J Neurochem 71:281–287

Canevari L, Clark JB, Bates TE (1999) β-Amyloid fragment 25–35 selectively decreases complex IV activity in isolated mitochondria. FEBS Lett 457(1):131–134

Cannon JR, Tapias V, Na HM, Honick AS, Drolet RE, Greenamyre JT (2009) A highly reproducible rotenone model of Parkinson's disease. Neurobiol Dis 34(2):279–290

Cardoso SM, Santos S, Swerdlow RH, Oliveira CR (2001) Functional mitochondria are required for amyloid beta-mediated neurotoxicity. FASEB J 15(8):1439–1441

Cardoso SM, Proença MT, Santos S, Santana I, Oliveira CR (2004a) Cytochrome c oxidase is decreased in Alzheimer's disease platelets. Neurobiol Aging 25(1):105–110

Cardoso SM, Santana I, Swerdlow RH, Oliveira CR (2004b) Mitochondria dysfunction of Alzheimer's disease cybrids enhances Abeta toxicity. J Neurochem 89(6):1417–1426

Carri MT, Ferri A, Battistoni A, Famhy L, Gabbianelli R, Poccia F, Rotilio G (1997) Expression of a Cu, Zn superoxide dismutase typical of familial amyotrophic lateral sclerosis induces mitochondrial alteration and increase of cytosolic Ca2+ concentration in transfected neuroblastoma SH-SY5Y cells. FEBS Lett 414(2):365–368

Casley CS, Canevari L, Land JM, Clark JB, Sharpe MA (2002) β-Amyloid inhibits integrated mitochondrial respiration and key enzyme activities. J Neurochem 80(1):91–100

Caspersen C, Wang N, Yao J, Sosunov A, Chen X, Lustbader JW, Xu HW, Stern D, Mckhann G, Yan SD (2005) Mitochondrial Abeta: a potential focal point for neuronal metabolic dysfunction in Alzheimer's disease. FASEB J 19(14):2040–2041

Chang S-W, Zhang D, Chungb HD, Zassenhaus HP (2000) The frequency of point mutations in mitochondrial DNA is elevated in the Alzheimer's brain. Biochem Biophys Res Commun 273(1):203–208

Choo YS, Johnson GV, Macdonald M, Detloff PJ, Lesort M (2004) Mutant huntingtin directly increases susceptibility of mitochondria to the calcium-induced permeability transition and cytochrome c release. Hum Mol Genet 13(14):1407–1420

Chung KKK, Thomas B, Li X, Pletnikova O, Troncoso JC, Marsh L, Dawson VL, Dawson TM (2004) S-nitrosylation of parkin regulates ubiquitination and compromises parkin's protective function. Science 304(5675):1328–1331

Corral-Debrinski M, Horton T, Lott MT, Shoffner JM, Mckee AC, Beal MF, Graham BH, Wallace DC (1994) Marked changes in mitochondrial DNA deletion levels in Alzheimer brains. Genomics 23:471–476

Crouch PJ, Blake R, Duce JA, Ciccotosto GD, Li Q-X, Barnham KJ, Curtain CC, Cherny RA, Cappai R, Dyrks T, Masters CL, Trounce IA (2005) Copper-dependent inhibition of human cytochrome c oxidase by a dimeric conformer of amyloid-beta1-42. J Neurosci 25(3):672–679

Cui L, Jeong H, Borovecki F, Parkhurst CN, Tanese N, Krainc D (2006) Transcriptional repression of PGC-1alpha by mutant huntingtin leads to mitochondrial dysfunction and neurodegeneration. Cell 127(1):59–69

Curti D, Rognoni F, Gasparini L, Cattaneo A, Paolillo M, Racchi M, Zani L, Bianchetti A, Trabucchi M, Bergamaschi S, Govoni S (1997) Oxidative metabolism in cultured fibroblasts derived from sporadic Alzheimer's disease (AD) patients. Neurosci Lett 236(1):13–16

Damiano M, Starkov AA, Petri S, Kipiani K, Kiaei M, Mattiazzi M, Beal MF, Manfredi G (2006) Neural mitochondrial Ca2+ capacity impairment precedes the onset of motor symptoms in G93A Cu/Zn-superoxide dismutase mutant mice. J Neurochem 96(5):1349–1361

De La Monte SM, Luong T, Neely TR, Robinson D, Wands JR (2000) Mitochondrial DNA damage as a mechanism of cell loss in Alzheimer's disease. Lab Invest 80(8):1323–1335

Devi L, Prabhu BM, Galati DF, Avadhani NG, Anandatheerthavarada HK (2006) Accumulation of amyloid precursor protein in the mitochondrial import channels of human Alzheimer's disease brain is associated with mitochondrial dysfunction. J Neurosci 26(35):9057–9068

Dhaliwal GK, Grewal RP (2000) Mitochondrial DNA deletion mutation levels are elevated in ALS brains. Neuroreport 11(11):2507–2509

Diana A, Simic G, Sinforiani E, Orru N, Pichiri G, Bono G (2008) Mitochondria morphology and DNA content upon sublethal exposure to beta-amyloid(1-42) peptide. Coll Antropol 32(Suppl 1):51–58

Duara R, Lopez-Alberola RF, Barker WW, Loewenstein DA, Zatinsky M, Eisdorfer CE, Weinberg GB (1993) A comparison of familial and sporadic Alzheimer's disease. Neurology 43:1377–1384

Edland SD, Silverman JM, Peskind ER, Tsuang D, Wijsman E, Morns JC (1996) Increased risk of dementia in mothers of Alzheimer's disease cases: evidence for maternal inheritance. Neurology 47:254–256

Ehrenkrantz D, Silverman JM, Smith CJ, Birstein S, Marin D, Mohs RC, Davis KL (1999) Genetic epidemiological study of maternal and paternal transmission of Alzheimer's disease. Am J Med Genet B Neuropsychiatr Genet 88:378–382

Elson JL, Herrnstadt C, Preston G, Thal L, Morris CM, Edwardson JA, Beal MF, Turnbull DM, Howell N (2006) Does the mitochondrial genome play a role in the etiology of Alzheimer's disease? Hum Genet 119:241–254

Esteves ARF, Domingues F, Ferreira IL, Januário C, Swerdlow RH, Oliveira CR, Cardoso SM (2008) Mitochondrial function in Parkinson's disease cybrids containing an nt2 neuron-like nuclear background. Mitochondrion 8(3):219–228

Esteves AR, Lu J, Rodova M, Onyango I, Lezi E, Dubinsky R, Lyons KE, Pahwa R, Burns JM, Cardoso SM, Swerdlow RH (2010) Mitochondrial respiration and respiration associated proteins in cell lines created through Parkinson's subject mitochondrial transfer. J Neurochem 113(3):674–682

Fujita K, Yamauchi M, Shibayama K, Ando M, Honda M, Nagata Y (1996) Decreased cytochrome c oxidase activity but unchanged superoxide dismutase and glutathione peroxidase activities in the spinal cords of patients with amyotrophic lateral sclerosis. J Neurosci Res 45:276–281

Gabbita SP, Lovell MA, Markesbery WR (1998) Increased nuclear DNA oxidation in the brain in Alzheimer's disease. J Neurochem 71:2034–2040

Gu M, Gash MT, Mann VM, Javoy-Agid F, Cooper JM, Schapira AH (1996) Mitochondrial defect in Huntington's disease caudate nucleus. Ann Neurol 39:385–389

Gu M, Cooper JM, Taanman JW, Schapira AHV (1998) Mitochondrial DNA transmission of the mitochondrial defect in Parkinson's disease. Ann Neurol 44:177–186

Hambleta NS, Castora FJ (1997) Elevated levels of the Kearns-Sayre syndrome mitochondrial DNA deletion in temporal cortex of Alzheimer's patients. Mutat Res 379:253–262

Hansson CA, Frykman S, Farmery MR, Tjernberg LO, Nilsberth C, Pursglove SE, Ito A, Winblad B, Cowburn RF, Thyberg J, Ankarcrona M (2004) Nicastrin, presenilin, APH-1, and PEN-2 form active gamma-secretase complexes in mitochondria. J Biol Chem 279:51654–51660

Hantraye P, Brouillet E, Ferrante R, Palfi S, Dolan R, Matthews RT, Beal MF (1996) Inhibition of neuronal nitric oxide synthase prevents MPTP-induced parkinsonism in baboons. Nat Med 2:1017–1021

Hardy JA, Higgins GA (1992) Alzheimer's disease: the amyloid cascade hypothesis. Science 256:184–185

Hattingen E, Magerkurth J, Pilatus U, Mozer A, Seifried C, Steinmetz H, Zanella F, Hilker R (2009) Phosphorus and proton magnetic resonance spectroscopy demonstrates mitochondrial dysfunction in early and advanced Parkinson's disease. Brain 132:3285–3297

Henchcliffe C, Shungu DC, Mao X, Huang C, Nirenberg MJ, Jenkins BG, Beal MF (2008) Multinuclear magnetic resonance spectroscopy for in vivo assessment of mitochondrial dysfunction in Parkinson's disease. Ann N Y Acad Sci 1147:206–220

Higgins CMJ, Jung C, Ding H, Xu Z (2002) Mutant Cu, Zn superoxide dismutase that causes motoneuron degeneration is present in mitochondria in the CNS. J Neurosci 22:RC215

Higgins CM, Jung C, Xu Z (2003) ALS-associated mutant SOD1G93A causes mitochondrial vacuolation by expansion of the intermembrane space and by involvement of SOD1 aggregation and peroxisomes. BMC Neurosci 4:16

Hirai K, Aliev G, Nunomura A, Fujioka H, Russell RL, Atwood CS, Johnson AB, Kress Y, Vinters HV, Tabaton M, Shimohama S, Cash AD, Siedlak SL, Harris PLR, Jones PK, Petersen RB, Perry G, Smith MA (2001) Mitochondrial abnormalities in Alzheimer's disease. J Neurosci 21:3017–3023

Hirano A, Donnenfeld H, Sasaki S, Nakano I (1984) Fine structural observations of neuroWlamentous changes in amyotrophic lateral sclerosis. J Neuropathol Exp Neurol 43:461–470

Huntington's Disease Collaborative Research Group (1993) A novel gene containing a trinucleotide repeat that is expanded and unstable on Huntington's disease chromosomes. Cell 72:971–983

Ikebe S, Tanaka M, Ohno K, Sato W, Hattori K, Kondo T, Mizuno Y, Ozawa T (1990) Increase of deleted mitochondrial DNA in the striatum in Parkinson's disease and senescence. Biochem Biophys Res Commun 170:1044–1048

Jenkins BG, Koroshetz WJ, Beal MF, Rosen BR (1993) Evidence for impairment of energy metabolism in vivo in Huntington's disease using localized 1 H NMR spectroscopy. Neurology 43:2689–2695

Jung C, Higgins CMJ, Xu Z (2002) A quantitative histochemical assay for activities of mitochondrial electron transport chain complexes in mouse spinal cord sections. J Neurosci Methods 114:165–172

Kabashi E, Valdmanis PN, Dion P, Spiegelman D, Mcconkey BJ, Vande Velde C, Bouchard JP, Lacomblez L, Pochigaeva K, Salachas F, Pradat PF, Camu W, Meininger V, Dupre N, Rouleau GA (2008) TARDBP mutations in individuals with sporadic and familial amyotrophic lateral sclerosis. Nat Genet 40:572–574

Khan SM, Cassarino DS, Abramova NN, Keeney PM, Borland MK, Trimmer PA, Krebs CT, Bennett JC, Parks JK, Swerdlow RH, Parker WD, Bennett JP (2000) Alzheimer's disease cybrids replicate beta-amyloid abnormalities through cell death pathways. Ann Neurol 48:148–155

Kish SJ, Bergeron C, Rajput A, Dozic S, Mastrogiacomo F, Chang LJ, Wilson JM, Distefano LM, Nobrega JN (1992) Brain cytochrome oxidase in Alzheimer's disease. J Neurochem 59:776–779

Kong J, Xu Z (1998) Massive mitochondrial degeneration in motor neurons triggers the onset of amyotrophic lateral sclerosis in mice expressing a mutant SOD1. J Neurosci 18:3241–3250

Kraytsberg Y, Kudryavtseva E, Mckee AC, Geula C, Kowall NW, Khrapko K (2006) Mitochondrial DNA deletions are abundant and cause functional impairment in aged human substantia nigra neurons. Nat Genet 38:518–520

Kuhl DE, Phelps ME, Markham CH, Metter EJ, Riege WH, Winter J (1982) Cerebral metabolism and atrophy in Huntington's disease determined by 18FDG and computed tomographic scan. Ann Neurol 12:425–434

Kwiatkowski TJ, Bosco DA, Leclerc AL, Tamrazian E, Vanderburg CR, Russ C, Davis A, Gilchrist J, Kasarskis EJ, Munsat T, Valdmanis P, Rouleau GA, Hosler BA, Cortelli P, De Jong PJ, Yoshinaga Y, Haines JL, Pericak-Vance MA, Yan J, Ticozzi N, Siddique T, Mckenna-Yasek D, Sapp PC, Horvitz HR, Landers JE, Brown RH (2009) Mutations in the FUS/TLS gene on chromosome 16 cause familial amyotrophic lateral sclerosis. Science 323:1205–1208

Lestienne P, Nelson I, Riederer P, Reichmann H, Jellinger K (1991) Mitochondrial DNA in postmortem brain from patients with Parkinson's disease. J Neurochem 56:1819

Lin J, Wu PH, Tarr PT, Lindenberg KS, St-Pierre J, Zhang CY, Mootha VK, Jäger S, Vianna CR, Reznick RM, Cui L, Manieri M, Donovan MX, Wu Z, Cooper MP, Fan MC, Rohas LM, Zavacki AM, Cinti S, Shulman GI, Lowell BB, Krainc D, Spiegelman BM (2004) Defects in adaptive energy metabolism with CNS-linked hyperactivity in PGC-1alpha null mice. Cell 119:121–135

Liu J, Lillo C, Jonsson PA, Velde CV, Ward CM, Miller TM, Subramaniam JR, Rothstein JD, Marklund S, Andersen PM, Brännström T, Gredal O, Wong PC, Williams DS, Cleveland DW (2004) Toxicity of familial ALS-linked SOD1 mutants from selective recruitment to spinal mitochondria. Neuron 43:5–17

Lustbader JW, Cirilli M, Lin C, Xu HW, Takuma K, Wang N, Caspersen C, Chen X, Pollak S, Chaney M, Trinchese F, Liu S, Gunn-Moore F, Lue L-F, Walker DG, Kuppusamy P, Zewier ZL, Arancio O, Stern D, Yan SS, Wu H (2004) ABAD directly links Abeta to mitochondrial toxicity in Alzheimer's disease. Science 304:448–452

Mancuso M, Conforti FL, Rocchi A, Tessitore A, Muglia M, Tedeschi G, Panza D, Monsurrò M, Sola P, Mandrioli J, Choub A, Delcorona A, Manca ML, Mazzei R, Sprovieri T, Filosto M, Salviati A, Valentino P, Bono F, Caracciolo M, Simone IL, Bella VL, Majorana G, Siciliano G, Murri L, Quattrone A (2004) Could mitochondrial haplogroups play a role in sporadic amyotrophic lateral sclerosis? Neurosci Lett 371:158–162

Manczak M, Anekonda TS, Henson E, Park BS, Quinn J, Reddy PH (2006) Mitochondria are a direct site of A beta accumulation in Alzheimer's disease neurons: implications for free radical generation and oxidative damage in disease progression. Hum Mol Genet 15:1437–1449

Martin LJ, Pan Y, Price AC, Sterling W, Copeland NG, Jenkins NA, Price DL, Lee MK (2006) Parkinson's disease alpha-synuclein transgenic mice develop neuronal mitochondrial degeneration and cell death. J Neurosci 26:41–50

Masui Y, Mozai T, Kakehi K (1985) Functional and morphometric study of the liver in motor neuron disease. J Neurol 232:15–19

Mecocci P, Macgarvey U, Beal MF (1994) Oxidative damage to mitochondrial DNA is increased in Alzheimer's disease. Ann Neurol 36(5):747–751

Menzies FM, Cookson MR, Taylor RW, Turnbull DM, Chrzanowska-Lightowlers ZMA, Dong L, Figlewicz DA, Shaw PJ (2002) Mitochondrial dysfunction in a cell culture model of familial amyotrophic lateral sclerosis. Brain 125:1522–1533

Mizuno Y, Suzuki K, Sone N, Saitoh T (1988) Inhibition of mitochondrial respiration by 1-methyl-4-phenyl-1,2,3,6-tetrahydropyridine (MPTP) in mouse brain in vivo. Neurosci Lett 91:349–353

Mosconi L (2005) Brain glucose metabolism in the early and specific diagnosis of Alzheimer's disease. FDG-PET studies in MCI and AD. Eur J Nucl Med Mol Imaging 32(4):486–510

Mosconi L, Brys M, Switalski R, Mistur R, Glodzik L, Pirraglia E, Tsui W, Santi SD, Leon MJD (2007) Maternal family history of Alzheimer's disease predisposes to reduced brain glucose metabolism. Proc Natl Acad Sci USA 104(48):19067–19072

Mosconi L, Mistur R, Switalski R, Brys M, Glodzik L, Rich K, Pirraglia E, Tsui W, Santi SD, Leon MJD (2009) Declining brain glucose metabolism in normal individuals with a maternal history of Alzheimer disease. Neurology 72:513–520

Murata T, Ohtsuka C, Terayama Y (2008) Increased mitochondrial oxidative damage and oxidative DNA damage contributes to the neurodegenerative process in sporadic amyotrophic lateral sclerosis. Free Radic Res 42:221–225

Mutisya EM, Bowling AC, Beal MF (1994) Cortical cytochrome oxidase activity is reduced in Alzheimer's disease. J Neurochem 63(6):2179–2184

Mytilineou C, Werner P, Molinari S, Di-Rocco A, Cohen G, Yahr MD (1994) Impaired oxidative decarboxylation of pyruvate in fibroblasts from patients with Parkinson's disease. J Neural Transm Parkinson's Dis Dement Sect 8(3):223–228

Nakano Y, Hirayama K, Terao K (1987) Hepatic ultrastructural changes and liver dysfunction in amyotrophic lateral sclerosis. Arch Neurol 44:103–106

Nemoto S, Fergusson MM, Finkel T (2005) SIRT1 functionally interacts with the metabolic regulator and transcriptional coactivator PGC-1{alpha}. J Biol Chem 280:16456–16460

Ng MC, Iacopino AM, Quintero EM, Marches F, Sonsalla PK, Liang CL, Speciale SG, German DC (1996) The neurotoxin MPTP increases calbindin-D28k levels in mouse midbrain dopaminergic neurons. Brain Res Mol Brain Res 36:329–336

Nicklas WJ, Vyas I, Heikkila RE (1985) Inhibition of NADH-linked oxidation in brain mitochondria by 1-methyl-4-phenyl-pyridine, a metabolite of the neurotoxin, 1-methyl-4-phenyl-1,2,5,6-tetrahydropyridine. Life Sci 36:2503–2508

Palacino JJ, Sagi D, Goldberg MS, Krauss S, Motz C, Wacker M, Klose J, Shen J (2004) Mitochondrial dysfunction and oxidative damage in parkin-deficient mice. J Biol Chem 279:18614–18622

Panov AV, Gutekunst CA, Leavitt BR, Hayden MR, Burke JR, Strittmatter WJ, Greenamyre JT (2002) Early mitochondrial calcium defects in Huntington's disease are a direct effect of polyglutamines. Nat Neurosci 5:731–736

Parker WD, Boyson SJ, Parks JK (1989) Abnormalities of the electron transport chain in idiopathic Parkinson's disease. Ann Neurol 26:719–723

Parker WD, Filley CM, Parks JK (1990a) Cytochrome oxidase deficiency in Alzheimer's disease. Neurology 40:1302–1303

Parker WD Jr, Boyson SJ, Luder AS, Parks JK (1990b) Evidence for a defect in NADH: ubiquinone oxidoreductase (complex I) in Huntington's disease. Neurology 40:1231–1234

Parker WD, Mahr NJ, Filley CM, Parks JK, Hughes D, Young DA, Cullum CM (1994) Reduced platelet cytochrome c oxidase activity in Alzheimer's disease. Neurology 44:1086–1090

Parker JA, Arango M, Abderrahmane S, Lambert E, Tourette C, Catoire H, Néri C (2005) Resveratrol rescues mutant polyglutamine cytotoxicity in nematode and mammalian neurons. Nat Genet 37:349–350

Parker WD, Parksa JK, Swerdlow RH (2008) Complex I deficiency in Parkinson's disease frontal cortex. Brain Res 1189:215–218

Payami H, Hoffbuhr K (1993) Lack of evidence for maternal effect in familial Alzheimer's disease. Genet Epidemiol 10:461–464

Pereira C, Santos MS, Oliveira C (1998) Mitochondrial function impairment induced by amyloid peptide on PC12 cells. Neuroreport 9:1749–1755

Pesah Y, Pham T, Burgess H, Middlebrooks B, Verstreken P, Zhou Y, Harding M, Bellen H, Mardon G (2004) Drosophila parkin mutants have decreased mass and cell size and increased sensitivity to oxygen radical stress. Development 131:2183–2194

Petit A, Kawarai T, Paitel E, Sanjo N, Maj M, Scheid M, Chen F, Gu Y, Hasegawa H, Salehi-Rad S, Wang L, Rogaeva E, Fraser P, Robinson B, George-Hyslop PS, Tandon A (2005) Wild-type PINK1 prevents basal and induced neuronal apoptosis, a protective effect abrogated by Parkinson disease-related mutations. J Biol Chem 280:34025–34032

Praticò D, Uryu K, Leight S, Trojanoswk JQ, Lee VM-Y (2001) Increased lipid peroxidation precedes amyloid plaque formation in an animal model of Alzheimer amyloidosis. J Neurosci 21:4183–4187

Raimondi A, Mangolini A, Rizzardini M, Tartari S, Massari S, Bendotti C, Francolini M, Borgese N, Cantoni L, Pietrini G (2006) Cell culture models to investigate the selective vulnerability of motoneuronal mitochondria to familial ALS-linked G93ASOD1. Eur J Neurosci 24:387–399

Ro L-S, Lai S-L, Chen C-M, Chen S-T (2003) Deleted 4977-bp mitochondrial DNA mutation is associated with sporadic amyotrophic lateral sclerosis: a hospital-based case-control study. Muscle Nerve 28:737–743

Rodgers JT, Lerin C, Haas W, Gygi SP, Spiegelman BM, Puigserver P (2005) Nutrient control of glucose homeostasis through a complex of PGC-1alpha and SIRT1. Nature 434:113–118

Rui Y, Tiwari P, Xie Z, Zheng JQ (2006) Acute Impairment of Mitochondrial Trafficking by beta–Amyloid Peptides in Hippocampal Neurons. J Neurosci 26:10480–10487

Sanberg PR, Fibiger HC, Mark RF (1981) Body weight and dietary factors in Huntington's disease patients compared with matched controls. Med J Aust 1:407–409

Sasaki S, Iwata M (1996) Impairment of fast axonal transport in the proximal axons of anterior horn neurons in amyotrophic lateral sclerosis. Neurology 47:535–540

Schapira AHV, Cooper JM, Dexter D, Jenner P, Clark JB, Marsden CD (1989) Mitochondrial complex I deficiency in Parkinson's disease. Lancet 1:1269

Schapira AHV, Holt IJ, Sweeney M, Harding AE, Jenner P, Marsden CD (1990) Mitochondrial DNA analysis in Parkinson's disease. Mov Disord 5(4):294–297

Scheuner D, Eckman C, Jensen M, Song X, Citron M, Suzuki N, Bird T, Hardy J, Hutton M, Kukull W, Larson E, Levy-Lahad E, Viitanen M, Peskind E, Poorkaj P, Schellenberg G, Tanzi R, Wasco W, Lannfelt L, Selkoe D, Younkin S (1996) Secreted amyloid beta-protein similar to that in the senile plaques of Alzheimer's disease is increased in vivo by the presenilin 1 and 2 and APP mutations linked to familial Alzheimer's disease. Nat Med 2:864–870

Sheehan JP, Swerdlow RH, Parker WD, Miller SW, Davis RE, Tuttle JB (1997) Altered calcium homeostasis in cells transformed by mitochondria from individuals with Parkinson's disease. J Neurochem 68:1221–1233

Shibata N, Nagai R, Uchida K, Horiuchi S, Yamada S, Hirano A, Kawaguchi M, Yamamoto T, Sasaki S, Kobayashi M (2001) Morphological evidence for lipid peroxidation and protein glycoxidation in spinal cords from sporadic amyotrophic lateral sclerosis patients. Brain Res 917:97–104

Siciliano G, D'avino C, Del Corona A, Barsacchi R, Kusmic C, Rocchi A, Pastorini E, Murri L (2002) Impaired oxidative metabolism and lipid peroxidation in exercising muscle from ALS patients. Amyotroph Lateral Scler Other Motor Neuron Disord 3:57–62

Silvestri L, Caputo V, Bellacchio E, Atorino L, Dallapiccola B, Valente EM, Casari G (2005) Mitochondrial import and enzymatic activity of PINK1 mutants associated to recessive parkinsonism. Hum Mol Genet 14:3477–3492

Simpson EP, Henry YK, Henkel JS, Smith RG, Appel SH (2004) Increased lipid peroxidation in sera of ALS patients: a potential biomarker of disease burden. Neurology 62:1758–1765

Smith TS, Swerdlow RH, Parker WD Jr, Bennett JP Jr (1994) Reduction of MPP(+)-induced hydroxyl radical formation and nigrostriatal MPTP toxicity by inhibiting nitric oxide synthase. Neuroreport 5:2598–2600

Song DD, Shults CW, Sisk A, Rockenstein E, Masliah E (2004) Enhanced substantia nigra mitochondrial pathology in human alpha-synuclein transgenic mice after treatment with MPTP. Exp Neurol 186:158–172

Spillantini MG, Schmidt ML, Lee VM-Y, Trojanowski JQ, Jakes R, Goedert M (1997) Alpha-synuclein in Lewy bodies. Nature 388:839–840

Sreedharan J, Blair IP, Tripathi VB, Hu X, Vance C, Rogelj B, Ackerley S, Durnall JC, Williams KL, Buratti E, Baralle F, De Belleroche J, Mitchell JD, Leigh PN, Al-Chalabi A, Miller CC, Nicholson G, Shaw CE (2008) TDP-43 mutations in familial and sporadic amyotrophic lateral sclerosis. Science 319:str. 1668–str. 1672

Sugars KL, Rubinsztein DC (2003) Transcriptional abnormalities in Huntington disease. Trends Genet 19:233–238

Swerdlow RH (2000) Role of mitochondria in Parkinson's disease. In: Molecular mechanisms of neurodegenerative diseases. Humana Press Inc, Totowa

Swerdlow RH (2007a) Is aging part of Alzheimer's disease, or is Alzheimer's disease part of aging? Neurobiol Aging 28:1465–1480

Swerdlow RH (2007b) Mitochondria in cybrids containing mtDNA from persons with mitochondriopathies. J Neurosci Res 85:3416–3428

Swerdlow RH (2007c) Pathogenesis of Alzheimer's disease. Clin Interv Aging 2:347–359

Swerdlow RH (2009) The neurodegenerative mitochondriopathies. J Alzheimers Dis 17:737–751

Swerdlow RH, Khan SM (2004) A "mitochondrial cascade hypothesis" for sporadic Alzheimer's disease. Med Hypotheses 63:8–20

Swerdlow RH, Khan SM (2009) The Alzheimer's disease mitochondrial cascade hypothesis: an update. Exp Neurol 218:308–315

Swerdlow RH, Kish SJ (2002) Mitochondria in Alzheimer's disease. Int Rev Neurobiol 53:341–385

Swerdlow RH, Parks JK, Miller SW, Davis RE, Tuttle JB, Trimmer PA, Sheehan JP, Bennett JP, Parker WD (1996a) Origin and functional consequences of the complex I defect in Parkinson's disease. Ann Neurol 40:663–671

Swerdlow RH, Parks JK, Miller SW, Pattee G, Davis RE, Parker WD (1996b) Evidence of genetic mitochondrial pathology in sporadic Amyotrophic Lateral Sclerosis. Soc Neurosci Abst 22:94.5

Swerdlow RH, Parks JK, Cassarino DS, Maguire DJ, Maguire RS, Bennett JP, Davis RE, Parker WD (1997) Cybrids in Alzheimer's disease: a cellular model of the disease? Neurology 49:918–925

Swerdlow RH, Parks JK, Cassarino DS, Trimmer PA, Miller SW, Maguire DJ, Sheehan JP, Maguire RS, Pattee G, Juel VC, Phillips LH, Tuttle JB, Bennett JP, Davis RE, Parker WD (1998) Mitochondria in sporadic amyotrophic lateral sclerosis. Exp Neurol 153:135–142

Swerdlow RH, Parks JK, Pattee G, Parker WD (2000) Role of mitochondria in amyotrophic lateral sclerosis. Amyotroph Lateral Scler Other Motor Neuron Disord 1:185–190

Swerdlow RH, Parker WD, Currie LJ, Bennett JP, Harrison MB, Trugman JM, Wooten GF (2001) Gender ratio differences between Parkinson's disease patients and their affected parents. Parkinsonism Relat Disord 7:129–133

Tanner CM, Goldman SM (1996) Epidemiology of Parkinson's disease. Neurol Clin 14:317–335

Trimmer PA, Bennett JP (2009) The cybrid model of sporadic Parkinson's disease. Exp Neurol 218:320–325

Trimmer PA, Borland MK, Keeney PM, Bennett JP, Parker WD (2004) Parkinson's disease transgenic mitochondrial cybrids generate Lewy inclusion bodies. J Neurochem 88:800–812

Valavanidis A, Vlachogianni T, Fiotakis C (2009) 8-hydroxy-2′ -deoxyguanosine (8-OHdG): a critical biomarker of oxidative stress and carcinogenesis. J Environ Sci Health C Environ Carcinog Ecotoxicol Rev 27:20–39

Valla J, Schneider L, Niedzielko T, Coon KD, Caselli R, Sabbagh MN, Ahern GL, Baxter L, Alexander G, Walker DG, Reiman EM (2006) Impaired platelet mitochondrial activity in Alzheimer's disease and mild cognitive impairment. Mitochondrion 6:323–330

Van Der Walt JM, Nicodemus KK, Martin ER, Scott WK, Nance MA, Watts RL, Hubble JP, Haines JL, Koller WC, Lyons K, Pahwa R, Stern MB, Colcher A, Hiner BC, Jankovic J, Ondo WG, Allen FH Jr, Goetz CG, Small GW, Mastaglia F, Stajich JM, Mclaurin AC, Middleton LT, Scott BL, Schmechel DE, Pericak-Vance MA, Vance JM (2003) Mitochondrial polymorphisms significantly reduce the risk of Parkinson disease. Am J Hum Genet 72:804–811

Vance C, Rogelj B, Hortobágyi T, De Vos KJ, Nishimura AL, Sreedharan J, Hu X, Smith B, Ruddy D, Wright P, Ganesalingam J, Williams KL, Tripathi V, Al-Saraj S, Al-Chalabi A, Leigh PN, Blair IP, Nicholson G, De Belleroche J, Gallo JM, Miller CC, Shaw CE (2009) Mutations in FUS, an RNA processing protein, cause familial amyotrophic lateral sclerosis type 6. Science 323:1208–1211

Velde CV, Miller TM, Cashman NR, Cleveland DW (2008) Selective association of misfolded ALS-linked mutant SOD1 with the cytoplasmic face of mitochondria. Proc Natl Acad Sci USA 105:4022–4027

Vielhaber S, Kunz D, Winkler K, Wiedemann FR, Kirches E, Feistner H, Heinze H-J, Elger CE, Schubert W, Kunz WS (2000) Mitochondrial DNA abnormalities in skeletal muscle of patients with sporadic amyotrophic lateral sclerosis. Brain 123:1339–1348

Vijayvergiya C, Beal MF, Buck J, Manfredi G (2005) Mutant superoxide dismutase 1 forms aggregates in the brain mitochondrial matrix of amyotrophic lateral sclerosis mice. J Neurosci 25:2463–2470

Vonsattel JP, Difiglia M (1998) Huntington disease. J Neuropathol Exp Neurol 57:369–384

Wang J, Xiong S, Xie C, Markesbery WR, Lovell MA (2005) Increased oxidative damage in nuclear and mitochondrial DNA in Alzheimer's disease. J Neurochem 93:953–962

Wang X, Su B, Fujioka H, Zhu X (2008a) Dymanin-like protein 1 reduction underlies mitochondrial morphology and distribution abnormalities in fibroblasts from sporadic Alzheimer's disease patients. Am J Pathol 173:470–482

Wang X, Su B, Siedlak SL, Moreira PI, Fujioka H, Wang Y, Casadesus G, Zhu X (2008b) Amyloid-beta overproduction causes abnormal mitochondrial dynamics via differential modulation of mitochondrial fission/fusion proteins. Proc Natl Acad Sci USA 105:19318–19323

Weydt P, Pineda VV, Torrence AE, Libby RT, Satterfield TF, Lazarowski ER, Gilbert ML, Morton GJ, Bammler TK, Strand AD, Cui L, Beyer RP, Easley CN, Smith AC, Krainc D, Luquet S, Sweet IR, Schwartz MW, La Spada AR (2006) Thermoregulatory and metabolic defects in Huntington's disease transgenic mice implicate PGC-1alpha in Huntington's disease neurodegeneration. Cell Metab 4:349–362

Wiedemann FR, Manfredi G, Mawrin C, Beal MF, Schon EA (2002) Mitochondrial DNA and respiratory chain function in spinal cords of ALS patients. J Neurochem 80:616–625

Wong-Riley M, Antuono P, Ho KC, Egan R, Hevner R, Liebl W, Huang Z, Rachel R, Jones J (1997) Cytochrome oxidase in Alzheimer's disease: biochemical, histochemical, and immunohistochemical analyses of the visual and other systems. Vision Res 37:3593–3608

Wooten GF, Currie LJ, Bennett JP, Harrison MB, Trugman JM, Parker WD (1997) Maternal inheritance in Parkinson's disease. Ann Neurol 41:265–268

Yang Y, Gehrke S, Imai Y, Huang Z, Ouyang Y, Wang J-W, Yang L, Beal MF, Vogel H, Lu B (2006) Mitochondrial pathology and muscle and dopaminergic neuron degeneration caused by inactivation of Drosophila Pink1 is rescued by Parkin. Proc Natl Acad Sci USA 103:10793–10798

Yao J, Irwin RW, Zhao L, Nilsen J, Hamilton RT, Brinton RD (2009) Mitochondrial bioenergetic deficit precedes Alzheimer's pathology in female mouse model of Alzheimer's disease. Proc Natl Acad Sci USA 106:14670–14675

Chapter 13
Mitochondria and Cancer: A Growing Role in Apoptosis, Cancer Cell Metabolism and Dedifferentiation

Roberto Scatena

Abstract At the beginning of the twentieth century, Otto Warburg demonstrated that cancer cells have a peculiar metabolism. These cells preferentially utilise glycolysis for energetic and anabolic purposes, producing large quantities of lactic acid. He defined this unusual metabolism "aerobic glycolysis". At the same time, Warburg hypothesised that a disruption of mitochondrial activities played a precise pathogenic role in cancer. Because of this so-called "Warburg effect", mitochondrial physiology and cellular respiration in particular have been overlooked in pathophysiological studies of cancer. Over time, however, many studies have shown that mitochondria play a fundamental role in cell death by apoptosis or necrosis. Moreover, metabolic enzymes of the Krebs cycle have also recently been recognised as oncosuppressors. Recently, a series of studies were undertaken to re-evaluate the role of oxidative mitochondrial metabolism in cancer cell growth and progression. Some of these data indicate that modulation of mitochondrial respiration may induce an arrest of cancer cell proliferation and differentiation (pseudodifferentiation) and/or or death, suggesting that iatrogenic manipulation of some mitochondrial activities may induce anticancer effects. Moreover, studying the role of mitochondria in cancer cell dedifferentiation/differentiation processes may allow further insight into the pathophysiology and therapy of so-called cancer stem cells.

Keywords Neoplasm metabolism • Warburg effect • Tumor markers • Cell Transformation • Neoplastic/genetics • Antineoplastic agents • Cancer stem cell

13.1 Introduction

The role of mitochondria in cancer has been disregarded for a long time because of laudable research by Otto Warburg (1883–1970), who was awarded the Nobel Prize in Physiology for his discovery of the nature and mode of action of the respiratory enzymes in 1931. Specifically, Warburg showed evidence for increased glycolysis both in solid tumour cells and leukaemia cells cultured in the presence of oxygen. Cancer cells process glucose through lactic acid fermentation, bypassing the entry of pyruvate into the citric acid cycle. These observations led Warburg to the hypothesis that such a metabolic alteration

R. Scatena (✉)
Institute of Biochemistry and Alinical Biochemistry, Department of Laboratory Medicine, Catholic University,
Largo A. Gemelli 8, 00168 Rome, Italy
e-mail: r.scatena@rm.unicatt.it

R. Scatena et al. (eds.), *Advances in Mitochondrial Medicine*, Advances in Experimental
Medicine and Biology 942, DOI 10.1007/978-94-007-2869-1_13,
© Springer Science+Business Media B.V. 2012

was due to bona fide respiratory disruption, and this critical metabolic event could be considered "the origin of the cancer cell" (Warburg 1925). Importantly, this increased glycolytic activity was similar to that observed in early embryonic cells. This latter observation led Warburg to conclude that cancer cells somehow resume a more primitive metabolic pattern (Warburg 1925). Intriguingly, this could be considered the original hypothesis of so-called cancer stem cells or stem-like cancer cells (CSCs).

13.2 Mitochondria and Cancer Cell Metabolism

It is now evident that cancer cells show various degrees of increased glycolysis, depending on the cell types and growth conditions. Generally, in the presence of oxygen, cancer cells produce about 60% of their ATP through glycolysis (Nakashima et al. 1984; Chen et al. 2007a, b), whereas normal cells seem to generate most of their ATP through mitochondrial oxidative phosphorylation using glucose, fatty acids, and other metabolic intermediates as energy sources. This increased dependency of cancer cells on the glycolytic pathway represents an important metabolic difference between normal and malignant cells and has been utilised for developing therapeutics and strategies to preferentially target cancer cells (Vander Heiden et al. 2010; Scatena et al. 2008). Interestingly, the Warburg effect represents the biological basis of positron emission tomography (PET), a nuclear medicine imaging technique widely used in the clinical diagnosis of cancer that is based on the fact that cancer cells have elevated glucose uptake (Koppenol et al. 2011).

Intriguingly, the real pathogenic role of this increased glycolysis, which is consistently observed in cancer cells, still remains controversial (Vander Heiden et al. 2009). A careful explanation of the real metabolism of cancer cells could represent a significant step in identifying more efficacious and specific targets for diagnostic and therapeutic purposes.

Various authors have suggested that switching to glycolysis could represent an advantageous adaptation for cancer cells; the following constitute the logic behind this hypothesis:

- glycolysis alone generates ATP more rapidly than glycolysis coupled to OXPHOS, although with a low efficiency (Jezek et al. 2010; Smolková et al. 2010);
- glycolysis generates carbon intermediates that are used for various anaplerotic pathways, such as fatty acid synthesis, maintenance of the non-essential amino acid pool during cell growth, and synthesis of nucleotide precursors for RNA and DNA (Bellance et al. 2009);
- more rapid glycolysis coupled to lowered OXPHOS efficiency triggers the accumulation of pyruvate and formation of lactate, which results in cellular acidification, and seems to favour cancer cell invasion (Wu et al. 2007);
- some of the accumulated pyruvate can be also redirected for lipid synthesis (Moreno-Sanchez et al. 2007);
- similarly, the decreased OXPHOS leads to citrate accumulation and export from the matrix, where it is converted to cytosolic acetyl-CoA and can be utilised for fatty acid and cholesterol synthesis (Moreno-Sanchez et al. 2007; Wellen et al. 2009);
- lower OXPHOS in cancer cells is accompanied by a decrease in mitochondrial biogenesis in general and of OXPHOS components in particular, achieving significant energetic savings for highly proliferating cells (Scatena et al. 2008, 2010).

The increased glucose uptake associated with the lowering of OXPHOS permits a greater utilisation of the pentose phosphate pathway. This produces ribose for *de novo* nucleic acid synthesis and NADPH, the main source of reducing equivalents for all anabolic pathways (Moreno-Sanchez et al. 2007; Marín-Hernández et al. 2011).

In summary, this altered metabolic state was considered to be the result of adaptation of cancer cells to the new, potentially anoxic environment of the neoplastic lesion via Hypoxia-inducible factor

(HIF) and/or Akt, implicating a reduction/damage of mitochondrial metabolism (Naumov et al. 2006; Deberardinis et al. 2008b). It is becoming clear that aerobic glycolysis in cancer cells is an epiphenomenon that results from a more complex metabolic rearrangement in which mitochondria play an active role. Thus, glycolysis and the Krebs cycle, beta oxidation, and anabolic metabolism in general adapt to respond to the new primary function of this cell (i.e., uncontrolled proliferation) by providing energy and building blocks for the synthesis of nucleotides and amino and fatty acids (Moreno-Sánchez et al. 2009).

Further data has demonstrated that glycolytic enzymes that are highly expressed in cancer cells (i.e., hexokinase II, lactate dehydrogenase A, glucose-6-phosphate isomerase) may possess different biological functions, acting as both facilitators and gatekeepers of malignancy (Kim and Dang 2005; Kondoh et al. 2005).

It has been postulated that cellular stress can induce expression of isoform II of hexokinase (HK II) in cancer cells, and this isoform plays a particular role in mitochondrial oxidative metabolism. In fact, HK II typically binds to voltage-dependent anion channels (VDAC), which are located on the outer mitochondrial membrane, allowing direct access of enzyme to ATP generated by ATP synthase that is transported across the inner-mitochondrial membrane by the adenine nucleotide translocator. In this way, rapid synthesis of glucose-6-phosphate can maintain a highly glycolytic metabolic flux in malignant cells (Scatena et al. 2003; Gatenby and Gillies 2004; Mathupala et al. 2006; Moreno-Sanchez et al. 2007). Accordingly, hexokinase has rapid access to mitochondria-generated ATP, is protected against feedback inhibition by glucose-6-phosphate and against proteolytic degradation, and above all, inhibits Bax-induced cytochrome-c release and apoptosis. Interestingly, binding of HK-II to VDAC in the outer mitochondrial membrane is enhanced by overexpression of the oncogenic kinase Akt due to negative regulation of the activity of glycogen synthase kinase-3-β (GSK-3-β) (Robey and Hay 2009).

These molecular data are consistent with clinical observations regarding a poorer prognosis in cancers with high glycolytic activity. In fact, much research has indicated that the aggressiveness of a cancer can be estimated by its bioenergetic signature, a protein ratio that correlates the expression of β-F1-ATPase of oxidative phosphorylation relative to the glycolytic GAPDH (Cuezva et al. 2002, 2004; Sánchez-Aragó and Cuezva 2011).

Therefore, we are proposing the re-evaluation of the Warburg effect because recent evidence relating glycolysis to the pentose phosphate pathway and to mitochondrial metabolism suggests the existence of abnormal metabolic status that is typical of proliferating cells. This altered metabolism in which glycolysis only represents the central metabolic signal transduction pathway would finely adapt overall cancer cell metabolism to the selection pressures of the cancer milieu, thus maintaining the homeostasis of the transformed cells and permitting to them to survive and proliferate (Costello and Franklin 2005; Shaw 2006; Kroemer and Pouyssegur 2008; Deberardinis et al. 2008a, b).

The oversimplified concept of enhanced glycolysis accompanied by negligible oxidative phosphorylation has too often been indiscriminately applied to all types of cancer. It is important to note that the fundamental genetic, biochemical and morphological heterogeneity of tumour cells may allow the application of the Warburg effect to all cancers, but not all areas of all tumours. Tumour cell types such as glioblastoma multiforme, astrocytoma, and certain forms of hepatomas utilise both glycolysis and oxidative phosphorylation to an equal extent for energy production (Lowry et al. 1983; Liu et al. 2001; Zu and Guppy 2004; Chen et al. 2009). More importantly, tumours such as bone sarcoma, lung carcinoma, breast cancer, skin melanoma, cervical, ovarian and uterine carcinomas all primarily use oxidative phosphorylation for the generation of ATP (Chen et al. 2009; Balaban and Bader 1984; Rodríguez-Enríquez et al. 2006; Kallinowski et al. 1989). However, some cancer cells can modify and adapt their energy metabolism in the passage from primary tumour to metastasis (Chen et al. 2007a, b).

The original hypothesis of a hypoxia-mediated disruption of oxidative phosphorylation is problematic because the concentration of oxygen in hypoxic regions of most human tumours seems to be above the Km O_2 of cytochrome c oxidase (Frezza and Gottlieb 2009). Therefore, it is likely that tumour oxidative metabolism should be unaffected by the level of hypoxia within the tumour microenvironment. Thus, it should be accepted that fast-growing tumours show a large increase in glycolytic flux even in the presence of high oxygen concentrations, and this increase in glycolytic capacity may not necessarily depend on a primary defect of the oxidative phosphorylation system (Bellance et al. 2009; Frezza and Gottlieb 2009; Marín-Hernández et al. 2011). In fact, enhanced tumour glycolysis may be operating in tandem with oxidative phosphorylation, with preferential utilisation of one pathway determined on the basis of the microenvironment energy requirements and biosynthetic capabilities (Frezza and Gottlieb 2009; Marín-Hernández et al. 2011). It is generally accepted that when rapidly growing tumours shift their ATP production to glycolysis in response to HIF-1 or other factors, mitochondrial activity slows down. Under these circumstances, mitochondria consume less oxygen, and their ATP production decreases. Interestingly, analysis of possible alterations in the oxidative phosphorylation machinery in some tumours revealed downregulation of the catalytic subunit of the mitochondrial ATP synthase (beta-F1-ATPase). This was observed in most human carcinomas. Remarkably, the expression level of the beta-F1-ATPase protein correlated inversely with the rate of aerobic glycolysis (Gogvadze et al. 2008). In fact, HIF-1 seems to suppress mitochondrial function in cancer cells, suggesting that it modulates the reciprocal relationship between glycolysis and oxidative phosphorylation. In our opinion, this dichotomy is an artefact: cancer cells have altered metabolism with a strong preference towards anaplerotic reactions, and mitochondrial metabolism finely adapts to the needs of proliferating transformed cells. In this situation, some metabolites are not progressively oxidised to CO_2 and water but utilised as substrates for various biosynthetic pathways; the levels of NADH and FADH2 go down, significantly reducing OXPHOS. In this case, proliferating cells do not always require high OXPHOS, and the level of oxygen consumption can be low.

A series of molecular studies have been performed to elucidate the mechanisms of this altered metabolism of cancer cells. For example, it has been demonstrated that HIF-1 stimulates expression of the lactate dehydrogenase A gene, which facilitates conversion of pyruvate into lactate. Moreover, mutation of p53 can suppress mitochondrial respiratory activity through downregulation of the Synthesis of Cytochrome c Oxidase 2 (SCO2) gene, the product of which is required for the assembly of cytochrome c oxidase (COX) of the mitochondrial respiratory chain (Gogvadze et al. 2008). Thus, mutations in p53 can suppress mitochondrial respiration and facilitate the shift of cellular energetic metabolism towards glycolysis. Moreover, p53 has recently been reported to block the pentose phosphate metabolic pathway that diverts glucose away from bioenergetic and into biosynthetic routes (Jiang et al. 2011).

Interestingly, Parra-Bonilla et al. (2010) showed that normal proliferating cells (pulmonary microvascular endothelial cells, PMVEC) display aerobic glycolysis during their growth, including glucose consumption and lactic acidosis, and this was dependent on the expression of LDH-A. This distinctive metabolic strategy seems necessary to sustain rapid growth, as limiting glucose or replacing glucose abolishes lactic acidosis and prevents rapid proliferation. Moreover, lactate plays a key role is sustaining PMVEC growth, as replenishing lactate even in the absence of extracellular glucose is sufficient to restore ATP levels and partially rescue cell growth.

Intriguingly, pharmacological inhibition of LDH-A has been shown to trigger oxidative stress in cancer cells similar to gene knockdown mediated by siRNA, resulting in necrotic cell death (Le et al. 2010). Reduction of LDHA activity is associated with elevation of the NADH/NAD + ratio, which is linked to increased reactive oxygen (Dang et al. 2011). Specifically, excess NADH could diminish upstream glycolytic flux, which requires recycled NAD+. Moreover, it may increase inappropriate respiratory complex I activity, ROS production, and consequently induce cell death.

Similar results have been published by Fantin et al. (2006). These authors showed that knockdown of lactate dehydrogenase A (LDH-A) expression by LDH-A short hairpin RNAs in tumour cell lines reactivates mitochondrial respiration, as measured by proton leakage and ATP turnover, and restores the normally depolarised state of mitochondrial membranes. In this situation, cancer cells can no longer oxidise NADH via LDH but must rely on the mitochondrial respiratory chain. Interestingly, this abrupt change in metabolism inhibits cell growth.

The complexity in the relationships between mitochondrial oxidative metabolism and glycolysis, in which HIF-1 is the key factor, was further emphasised by Semenza (2007). Semenza stressed that under hypoxic conditions, the subunit composition of COX is altered to optimise its activity; expression of the COX4–2 subunit is increased, whereas the COX4–1 subunit, which optimises COX activity under aerobic conditions, is degraded by activation of the mitochondrial protease LON.

Importantly, HIF-1alpha is also involved in the activation of numerous cellular processes including resistance to apoptosis, overexpression of drug efflux membrane pumps, vascular remodelling, angiogenesis and metastasis (Marín-Hernández et al. 2009). In cancer cells, HIF-1alpha induces overexpression and higher activity of several glycolytic protein isoforms that differ from those found in non-malignant cells, including transporters (GLUT1, GLUT3) and enzymes (HKI, HKII, PFK-L, ALD-A, ALD-C, PGK1, ENO-alpha, PYK-M2, LDH-A, PFKFB-3). The enhanced tumour glycolytic flux triggered by HIF-1alpha also involves changes in the kinetic patterns of isoforms of key glycolytic enzymes. The HIF-1alpha-induced isoforms provide cancer cells with reduced sensitivity to physiological inhibitors, lower affinity for products and higher catalytic capacity (Vmax) (Robey and Hay 2009; Marín-Hernández et al. 2011).

In conclusion, we have the following unanswered questions: is the Warburg effect really unique to cancer cells? And, above all, are mitochondria unnecessary organelles in cancer cells?

As mentioned, many studies have demonstrated a reduction in OXPHOS in different types of cancer cells. In contrast, other studies have revealed upregulation of OXPHOS components and a larger dependency of cancer cells on oxidative energy substrates for anabolism and energy production. This apparently conflicting data seems to find justification in differences in tumour size, hypoxia, and the sequence of oncogenes activated. In this respect, the roles of p53, C-MYC, Oct and RAS in the control of mitochondrial respiration and glutamine utilisation has been extensively validated (Bensaad and Vousden 2007; Yeung et al. 2008; Semenza 2009; Fan et al. 2010).

Thus, tumours of various bioenergetic types, from exclusively glycolytic to mainly OXPHOS, have been found with differing tumour stage, serial oncogene activation and microenvironment conditions. The importance of mitochondria in a dynamic view of tumour bioenergetics is clear.

In conclusion, if glycolysis really represents the key to cancer cell metabolism, mitochondria have a precise role in the metabolic flexibility of cancer cells that allows them to circumvent hostile microenvironments. The complexity of the interplay of this metabolism is, in some ways, demonstrated by the conflicting results obtained in experimental and clinical studies that have adopted glycolysis and/or mitochondrial inhibitors for therapeutic purposes (Scatena et al. 2008; Fulda et al. 2010; Martinez-Outschoorn et al. 2011; Alvero et al. 2011; Zhang et al. 2011; D'Souza et al. 2011).

Glutamine metabolism, mitochondria and cancer. Interestingly, the role of mitochondria in metabolic cancer flexibility was, in some way, already underscored by the well-known role of glutamine (Gln) in cancer cell proliferation. In fact, glutaminolysis and the Warburg effect are the two most noticeable metabolic features of tumour cells, but the biological significance of these processes in cell proliferation remains unknown. A widely-accepted hypothesis is that cancer cells use glutamine as a preferred carbon source for energy and reducing power. Specifically, since the 1950s, cancer biologists have recognised the importance of glutamine as a tumour nutrient. Glutamine contributes to essentially every core metabolic task of proliferating tumour cells, participating in bioenergetics, supporting cell defences against oxidative stress, and complementing glucose metabolism in the production of macromolecules. Interest in glutamine metabolism has been heightened further by the recent finding that c-*myc* controls glutamine uptake and degradation and that glutamine itself exerts influence over a number of signalling pathways that contribute to tumour growth (DeBerardinis and Cheng 2010).

It is well known that Gln, the most abundant free amino acid in humans, has a plasma concentration of about 1 mM, and this abundance allows it to serve as a major source of carbon and nitrogen. Gln can be appropriated by tumours and used as a substrate for proliferation of tumour cells to maintain pools of citric acid cycle (TCA) cycle intermediates, and its nitrogen can be used to produce nonessential amino acids, hexosamine, nucleotides, and other molecules. Thereby, many tumour cells may use glutamine to feed their anaplerotic reactions, as recently shown by Cheng et al. (2011); importantly, mitochondria have a central role in these anabolic pathways. In fact, the proximal reactions of glutaminolysis occur in the mitochondria. The first step is catalysed by phosphate-dependent glutaminases, which deamidate glutamine to form glutamate and ammonia. Physiologically, interconversion of glutamine and glutamate is typically bidirectional, with glutamine formation catalysed by glutamine synthetase. In tumours, however, the forward (toward glutamate) reaction is favoured by overexpression of glutaminases and/or suppression of glutamine synthetase (Shanware et al. 2011; Meng et al. 2010). Thereby, as alternative and/or better complement to glucose as the fuel for bioenergetic pathways, glutamine feeds the TCA cycle by providing α-ketoglutarate from glutamate. Recently, one isoform of the enzyme glutaminase (GLS1/KGA) was shown to act as an oncogene (Maddocks and Vousden 2011). Importantly, utilisation of glutamine as an anaplerotic precursor and source of NADPH results in the secretion of a large fraction of glutamine-derived carbon and nitrogen. Some of the secreted molecules (lactate, alanine) may subsequently be used as precursors for hepatic gluconeogenesis, ultimately providing more fuel for tumour metabolism (Deberardinis et al. 2008b).

Little is known about how tumour cells regulate glutaminase expression. Mammals have two major glutaminase activities, K-type (low Km for glutamine, inhibited by glutamate) and L-type (high Km, glutamate resistant) (Deberardinis et al. 2008b).

The human K-type enzyme is encoded by the GLS gene, which yields several mRNAs owing to alternative polyadenylation and splicing, and the L-type enzyme is encoded by GLS2. In general, tumour cells have K-type activity, although most cell lines express transcripts from both genes (Deberardinis et al. 2008a; Elgadi et al. 1999). This suggests that tumours can modulate glutaminase kinetics through relative levels of GLS and GLS2 gene products, resulting in the ability to optimise glutaminase activity despite local fluctuations in glutamine and glutamate concentrations (Deberardinis et al. 2008b).

Interestingly, the high rate of glutamine uptake in glutamine-dependent cells does not appear to solely result from its role as a nitrogen donor in nucleotide and amino acid biosynthesis. In addition, glutamine plays a required role in the uptake of essential amino acids and in maintaining activation of TOR (target of rapamycin) kinase. Moreover, in many cancer cells, glutamine is the primary mitochondrial substrate and is required for maintenance of mitochondrial membrane potential and integrity and for support of the NADPH production needed for redox control and macromolecular synthesis.

Recently, Gao et al. (2009) reported that the oncogenic transcription factor c-Myc, which is known to regulate microRNAs and stimulate cell proliferation, transcriptionally represses miR23a and miR23b, resulting in greater expression of their target protein, mitochondrial glutaminase (GLS) in human P-493 B lymphoma cells and PC3 prostate cancer cells. This effect leads to upregulation of glutamine catabolism. Glutaminase converts glutamine to glutamate, which is further catabolised through the TCA cycle for the production of ATP or serves as substrate for glutathione synthesis. Gao et al. (2009) concluded that the unique means by which Myc regulates glutaminase uncovers a previously unknown link between Myc regulation of microRNAs, glutamine metabolism, and energy and reactive oxygen species homeostasis. Intriguingly, these new data show that whereas cell cycle arrest, apoptosis, and senescence are traditionally thought to be the major functions of the tumour suppressor p53, this study revealed two further functions for this protein: regulation of cellular energy metabolism and antioxidant defence maintenance. Importantly, these latter activities seem to be related to glutaminase 2 (GLS2), a mitochondrial phosphate-activated glutaminase that is a previously uncharacterised p53 target gene. p53 seems to increase GLS2 expression under both non-stressed and stressed conditions. GLS2 regulates cellular energy metabolism by increasing production of glutamate and alpha-ketoglutarate, which in turn results in enhanced mitochondrial respiration and ATP generation. Furthermore, GLS2 regulates antioxidant defence function in cells by increasing reduced glutathione (GSH) levels and decreasing ROS levels, which in turn protects cells from oxidative stress-induced apoptosis. Consistent with these functions of GLS2, the activation of p53 increases the glutamate, alpha-ketoglutarate, and GSH levels and the mitochondrial respiration rate and decreases reactive oxygen species (ROS) levels in cells. Furthermore, GLS2 expression is lost or greatly decreased in hepatocellular carcinomas, and the overexpression of GLS2 greatly reduces tumour cell colony formation. These results demonstrated that GLS2 is a mediator of p53's role in energy metabolism and antioxidant defence, and this likely contributes to its role in tumour suppression (Puzio-Kuter 2011).

In conclusion, it is important to stress that Gln, which is regulated metabolically by mitochondria, is more than simply fuel for the cell growth engine, but rather a multi-functional regulator of several cellular activities linked to both physiological and pathological processes in mammals. In fact, Gln import supports mTORC1 activation by leucine and other amino acids, and Gln metabolism via glutaminolysis generates products that protect cells from the deleterious effects of ROS. Finally, Gln metabolism generates a diffusible product, ammonia, which may increase stress resistance in tumour tissues (Shanware et al. 2011).

Mitochondrial enzymes and cancer. The discoveries of oncogenic mutations in mitochondrial metabolic enzymes, such as fumarate hydratase (FH), succinate dehydrogenase (SDH) and isocitrate dehydrogenase 2 (IDH2), represents bona fide proof for a role of altered mitochondrial metabolism in cancer pathogenesis.

Fumarate hydratase is an enzymatic component of the TCA cycle. It catalyses the conversion of fumarate to malate.

Succinate dehydrogenase (SDH) (or succinate-coenzyme Q reductase or Complex II) is an enzyme complex that is bound to the inner mitochondrial membrane of mammalian mitochondria. SDH is the only enzyme that participates in both the citric acid cycle and the electron transport chain, and it catalyses the oxidation of succinate to fumarate with concomitant reduction of ubiquinone to ubiquinol.

Isocitrate dehydrogenase 2, also known as IDH2, is another enzyme of the TCA cycle. It catalyses the third step of the cycle, the oxidative decarboxylation of isocitrate, producing α-ketoglutarate and CO_2 while converting NAD+ to NADH. Other isoforms (IDH1 and 3) of the enzyme catalyse the same reaction; however, this reaction is unrelated to the TCA cycle and is carried out in the cytosol and uses NADP+.

Pollard et al. (2005) stated that the nuclear-encoded Krebs cycle enzymes FH and SDH act as tumour suppressors, and germline mutations in these genes predispose individuals to leiomyomas and renal cancer and to pheochromocytoma/paragangliomas. Pollard also showed that FH-deficient cells and tumours accumulated fumarate and, to a lesser extent, succinate. Fumarate competitively inhibits HIF prolyl hydroxylase, preventing prolyl hydroxylation of the HIF oxygen-dependent degradation domain and allowing HIF-α to escape recognition by the von Hippel-Lindau protein. Moreover, HIF-α stabilisation enables transcriptional activation of HIF target genes that promote tumour growth and vascularisation.

Somatic mutations of IDH1 (which is cytosolic) and IDH2 (which is mitochondrial) have been found in 80% of low-grade gliomas and 30% of karyotypically normal acute myelogenous leukaemias (Yan et al. 2009; Green and Beer 2010). Mutations affecting the catalytic sites of IDH1 and IDH2 are thought to be functionally equivalent. Interestingly, mutant IDH1 and IDH2 exhibit neo-enzymatic activity because they convert α-ketoglutarate to 2-hydroxyglutarate (2-HG), which in turn alters the homeostasis of α-ketoglutarate and reduces its availability as a substrate for the enzymes that methylate DNA and histones. Thus, tumourigenesis seems to be enhanced through the modification of the epigenome.

In conclusion, alterations in three enzymatic reactions have been reported to have genetically causal links to cancer formation: (1) Germline mutations in FH are associated with leiomyoma and renal cancer and potentially with other tumours. (2) Both germline and somatic mutations in any of the four subunits of SDH (SDHA, SDHB, SDHC, and SDHD) or the SDH assembly factor SDHAF2 are associated with paraganglioma, pheochromocytoma, and/or renal cancer. (3) Somatic mutations in either IDH1 or IDH2 are associated with gliomas or acute myelogenous leukaemia. While the FH and SDH mutations are typically loss-of-function mutations, and the genes involved behave genetically like tumour suppressors, the IDH mutations lead to a gain of NADPH-dependent α-ketoglutarate-reductase activity, which generates 2HG. Because one wild-type IDH allele is retained in tumours with IDH mutations, and no significant changes in α-ketoglutarate or isocitrate levels were observed in these tumours, it is safe to propose that IDH1/IDH2 mutations are oncogenic gain-of-function mutations (Yan et al. 2009).

Importantly, in all three types of these genetic-metabolic events, it appears that the underlying mechanism of tumourigenesis involves the accumulation of metabolites that convey oncogenic signals (oncometabolites). Some of this oncogenic activity might be attributed to hormone-like effects of these molecules. In fact, strong evidence indicates that the principal oncometabolic activities of succinate, fumarate and 2HG are related to the inhibition of the α-ketoglutarate-dependent dioxygenases, including:

(i)   JMJd3, which regulates chromatin structure;
(ii)   PHD3, which is involved in promoting neuronal apoptosis in response to NGF withdrawal;
(iii) PHD2, which primarily regulates HIFα stability;
(iv) aKG-dependent dioxygenase TET2, which is involved in hematopoietic cell differentiation (Frezza et al. 2011; Cairns et al. 2011).

Recently, Frezza et al. (2011) validated a new linear metabolic pathway beginning with glutamine uptake and ending with bilirubin excretion using a newly characterised genetically-modified kidney mouse cell line in which the FH gene (*Fh1*) is deleted. Specifically, this pathway for the biosynthesis and degradation of haem enables *Fh1*-deficient cells to use the accumulated TCA cycle metabolites, permitting partial mitochondrial NADH production. Interestingly, targeting this pathway renders *Fh1*-deficient cells non-viable while sparing wild-type *Fh1*-containing cells. This work, beyond identifying a new metabolic pathway that is induced in *Fh1*-deficient cells, stresses the role of fumarate as an oncometabolite and showed that inhibition of haem oxygenation is synthetically lethal when combined with *Fh1* deficiency, providing a new potential target for treating patients with renal cancer.

In conclusion, mitochondrial metabolism enzymes play a significant pathogenic role in cancer. This theory suggests interesting clinical applications in terms of prevention, early diagnosis and identification of more selective therapeutic targets. Moreover, these data underline the dynamic and bidirectional interactions between the metabolic status of the cell and its genetic profile and suggest that small metabolites may be novel and unexplored signalling units (Frezza et al. 2011). However, it should be stressed that such mitochondrial enzyme mutations are associated with different types of cancer with very different grades of aggressiveness. From a molecular point of view, studies must consider the relationships with other potential oncogenetic hits in cells that cooperate to determine the level of malignancy.

13.3 Mitochondrial Apoptosis and Cancer

Type I programmed cell death, also known as apoptosis, is a genetic pathway for rapid and efficient physiological killing of unnecessary or damaged cells; it was initially described by Kerr et al. (1972). It is well known that mitochondria have a well-defined role in the induction of the intrinsic pathway of apoptosis. Intrinsic apoptosis is characterised by the release of cytochrome c and SMAC (Second Mitochondrial Activator of Caspases) from the mitochondrial intermembrane space in response to a variety of noxious stimuli, including DNA damage, loss of adherence to the extracellular matrix (ECM), oncogene-induced proliferation, and growth factor deprivation, which causes the subsequent activation of caspases. Perturbations in the release of apoptosis-inducing proteins, which are regulated by pro- and anti-apoptotic members of the Bcl-2 family (e.g., Bcl-2, Bcl-XL, and Mcl-1), may have a role not only in the etiopathogenesis but also in the prognosis and therapy of different forms of cancer.

Indeed, it is well known that the permeability transition pore (PTP) and electrochemical gradient can play a role in the release of these apoptotis-inducing proteins.

There are about 20 known members of the BCL2 family, some of which are pro-apoptotic and others that are anti-apoptotic. They share common domains, termed BH1 to BH4. The first to be discovered, BCL2, was discovered as the oncogene at the common translocation site t(14;18) in follicular B-cell lymphoma. This translocation places the BCL2 gene under the control of the immunoglobulin heavy chain enhancer. Overexpression of BCL2 prevents apoptosis of follicular B-cells and is the initiating event in this relatively slow-growing cancer.

Interestingly, a fundamental mitochondrial step in the intrinsic pathway mediated by BAX and BAK consists of a change in the mitochondrial structure and function designated 'mitochondrial permeability transition' (MPT). At the contact sites between the outer and the inner mitochondrial membrane, pores are formed by a multiprotein complex, to which proteins from all mitochondrial compartments contribute. One crucial component is the adenine nucleotide translocator (ANT), which exchanges ADP/P for ATP across the inner mitochondrial membrane. The pores allow molecules smaller than 1,500 Da to pass through. This leads to a break-down of the mitochondrial transmembrane potential, since protons and other ions including Ca2+ can move freely across the membrane. In conjunction with the mitochondrial permeability transition, mitochondria release several proteins, mostly from the inter-membrane compartment, such as cytochrome c, SMAC/Diablo and the apoptosis-inducing factor (AIF, a caspase-independent death effector that also functions as an NADH and NADPH oxidase).

In the cytoplasm, molecules of cytochrome c associate with an equal number of APAF-1 proteins and form a large structure resembling the spokes of a wheel. It is therefore called the 'wheel of death' or 'apoptosome'. The apoptosome binds a stoichiometric number of the pro-protease pro-caspase 9 and supports its autocatalytic activation in an ATP-dependent process.

Importantly, induction of apoptosis by the intrinsic pathway requires inactivation of BCL2 and other anti-apoptotic proteins such as BCL-XL. These proteins are located at the mitochondrial membrane, probably forming heterodimers with BAX and BAK, pro-apoptotic members of the BCL2 family. Other members of the family are distinguished by containing only a BH3 domain and none of the other motifs.

As already mentioned, cellular stress of various kinds can induce apoptosis. In many cases, activation of TP53 is involved. Activated TP53 induces transcription of one or several pro-apoptotic BCL2 signalling proteins, such as NOXA or PUMA, and increases BAX while downregulating BCL2. The precise mechanisms by which the balance between proapoptotic and anti apoptotic factors is modified may differ according to cell type and type of cellular stress. The pro-apoptotic proteins induced by TP53 override anti-apoptotic signals to initiate the next step in the intrinsic apoptotic pathway, formation of pores in the mitochondria.

Cancers often have defects in the intrinsic apoptosis pathway. In fact, as already mentioned, Bcl-2 was discovered as an oncogene in human cancers. BCL-2 inhibits mitochondrial pathways of apoptosis through local effects at the mitochondrial and endoplasmic reticulum membranes. Increased expression of BCL-2 and the related anti-apoptotic proteins BCL-X(L), MCL-1, and BCL-W occurs in significant subsets of common cancer types and is generally correlated with poor responses to therapy. In human cancers, mechanisms to disable apoptosis include loss of function of the pro-apoptosis p53 tumour suppressor and gain of function of the anti-apoptotic and oncogenic Bcl-2.

In the last decade of the twentieth century, mitochondria from cancer cells were shown to be resistant to the induction of mitochondrial outer membrane permeabilisation (MOMP). Some authors hypothesised a mechanistic link between aerobic glycolysis and MOMP resistance.

The following hypothetical explanation may explain the simultaneous presence of the Warburg effect. Suppression of MOMP is provided by induced hexokinase II, which simultaneously increases glycolysis and inhibits MOMP when it associates with the voltage-dependent anion channel (VDAC) in the mitochondrial outer membrane. This interaction may be favoured by the cancer-specific over-expression of mitochondrion-binding hexokinase isoenzymes (Mathupala et al. 2006) or by activation of the Akt pathway, which stimulates the interaction between hexokinase and VDAC (Robey and Hay 2009).

Many drugs have been designed to induce apoptosis in cancer cells (Gogvadze et al. 2009). Indeed, it is conceivable to therapeutically induce MOMP (and hence apoptosis) in cancer cells by targeting mitochondrial membranes, members from the Bcl-2 family and components of the permeability transition pore complex (Debatin et al. 2002).

In addition, molecules can be designed that mimic the action of the pro-apoptotic mitochondrial protein Smac/DIABLO (Fulda and Debatin 2006) or that release the pro-apoptotic mitochondrial protein AIF from its inhibition by heat shock protein 70 (HSP70) (Galluzzi et al. 2006). Moll et al. (2006) proposed a particularly intriguing strategy to target anti-MOMP proteins such as Bcl-2, causing them to switch from an anti-apoptotic to a pro-apoptotic function. Another fascinating possibility is the development of drugs that target cytotoxic agents to a tumour specific surface receptor and then to mitochondria to induce MOMP (Fantin and Leder 2006). Several MOMP inducers or facilitators are currently undergoing clinical evaluation, but the fundamental problem of this class of powerful anticancer agents is selectivity. In fact, the therapeutic use of molecules capable of activating the apoptotic pathway must exclusively induce it in the target cells because the abnormal activation of apoptosis in healthy cells could cause dramatic and irreversible side effects. Because of this, it is necessary to understand the mechanisms of apoptosis resistance in cancer cells, specifically at the mitochondria level, to have a specific target for apoptosis-inducing anti-cancer therapy.

13.4 Mitochondria, Cancer, Reactive Oxygen Species (ROS) and Reactive Nitrogen Species (RNS)

Historically, it has been assumed that oxidative stress contributes to tumour initiation and progression mainly by inducing genomic instability. The main sources of free radicals in cells are by-products of oxidative metabolism. Free radical damage may affect nuclear and mitochondrial DNA, proteins, and lipids. Interestingly, recent data support a re-evaluation of free radical toxicity, suggesting that physiological levels of these chemical species can function as intracellular signal transducers and even oncosuppressors (Takahashi et al. 2006).

Most ROS are generated in cells by the mitochondrial respiratory chain. Mitochondrial ROS production is modulated largely by the rate of electron flow through respiratory chain complexes. Recently, it has become clear that under hypoxic conditions, the mitochondrial respiratory chain also produces nitric oxide (NO), which can generate other reactive nitrogen species (RNS). Although excess ROS and RNS can lead to oxidative and nitrosative stress, it is important to stress that moderate to low levels of both function in cellular signalling pathways. Especially important are the roles of these mitochondria-generated free radicals in hypoxic signalling pathways, which have important implications in cancer, inflammation and a variety of other diseases.

Thereby, the hypothetical pathogenic role of free radicals in degenerative diseases in general and cancer in particular may have been overestimated, and some conclusions may have been made based on laboratory artefacts (Herrnstadt et al. 2003; Salas et al. 2005).

Importantly, ROS and RNS acting as biological mediators can modulate mitogen activated protein kinases (MAPKs), fundamental components of phosphorylation signalling pathways involved in cell survival, proliferation and differentiation (Moncada and Erusalimsky 2002; Cadenas 2004).

In terms of cytotoxicity, the oxidation products formed during normal metabolic processes in cells include superoxide (O_2^-), hydrogen peroxide (H_2O_2), and hydroxyl radicals (OH). These are also produced in cells by radiation, and they are capable of damaging DNA and causing mutagenesis. Of these, the hydroxyl radical appears to be the primary DNA-damaging species, but it has a short half-life and high reactivity, so it must be generated in close proximity to DNA.

Singlet oxygen, which is produced by lipid peroxidation or by respiratory bursts from neutrophils, is also mutagenic and has a much longer half-life than the hydroxyl radical. Lipid peroxidation can also give rise to mutagenic products such as lipid epoxides, hydroperoxides, alkanyl and peroxyl radicals, and alpha and beta unsaturated aldehydes.

Cells have developed multiple mechanisms (enzymatic and non-enzymatic) to protect themselves from oxidative damage, including superoxide dismutase, catalase, glutathione peroxidase, glutathione-S-transferases, glutathione, ascorbic acid, tocopherols, and others. Hence, in cancer physiopathogenesis related to ROS, it is necessary to stress the pathophysiological role of the repair mechanisms as well. It is estimated that the human genome suffers about 10,000 "oxidative hits" to the DNA per cell per day. Moreover, parallel to cancer incidence, mutations accumulate with age, so that an "old" rat (2 years old) has twice as many DNA lesions per cell as a young rat. Furthermore, the frequency of somatic mutations found in human lymphocytes is about ninefold higher in the aged than in neonates.

Interestingly, caloric or protein restriction in the diet slows oxidative damage to proteins and DNA and decreases the rate of formation of neoplasms in rodents. Similar results are seen by dietary supplementation with antioxidants such as tocopherol (vitamin E), ascorbate (vitamin C), and carotenoids such as b-carotene, leading to the hypothesis that dietary intake of such substances could decrease the incidence of human cancer. This is supported by epidemiological data in humans. It should also be noted that one of the major sources of exogenous oxidant exposure is the oxides of nitrogen found in cigarette smoke.

Interestingly, oxidative and nitrosative stress may not only have a role in cancer pathogenesis but also in therapy. In fact, many anti-cancer agents utilise their molecular properties to generate high levels of reactive radical species that are capable of inducing lethal oxidative/nitrosative stress in cancer cells directly and/or indirectly by mitochondria disruption.

Recently a series of interesting studies have been published that have revisited the role of ROS/RNOS in the pathophysiology of cancer. For example, Martinez-Outschoorn et al. (2010) showed that an acute loss of stromal fibroblast Caveolin-1 expression causes a "lethal tumour micro-environment" by leading to mitochondrial dysfunction, oxidative stress and aerobic glycolysis in cancer-associated fibroblasts. This oxidative stress in these abnormal fibroblasts seems sufficient to induce genomic instability in adjacent cancer cells via a bystander effect. Interestingly, nitric oxide over-production, secondary to Cav-1 loss, seems to be the main cause for mitochondrial dysfunction in cancer-associated fibroblasts. In fact, treatment with anti-oxidants (such as N-acetyl-cysteine, metformin and quercetin) or NO inhibitors (L-NAME) was sufficient to reverse many of the cancer-associated fibroblast phenotypes. Importantly, these authors concluded that the effects of stromal oxidative stress can be laterally propagated and amplified and are effectively "contagious". They suggested that the effects spread from cell-to-cell like a virus and create an "oncogenic/mutagenic" field, thus promoting widespread DNA damage and facilitating the mutator phenotype of cancer cells.

As previously mentioned, the provocative research of Takahashi et al. (2006) showed that ROS have an unexpected role in inducing and maintaining senescence-induced tumour suppression. Specifically, the authors showed that the p16(INK4a)/Rb-pathway cooperates with mitogenic signals to induce elevated intracellular levels of ROS, thereby activating protein kinase C delta (PKCdelta) in senescent human cells. Once activated by ROS, PKCdelta promotes further generation of ROS, thus establishing a positive feedback loop to sustain ROS-PKCdelta signalling. This sustained activation of ROS-PKCdelta signalling irreversibly blocks cytokinesis, at least partly through reducing the level of WARTS (also known as LATS1).

Additionally, another study indicated that ROS are upregulated in tumours and can lead to aberrant induction of signalling networks that cause tumourigenesis and metastasis. In fact, Weinberg et al. (2010) showed that generation of ROS by mitochondrial metabolism allowed Kras-induced anchorage-independent growth in different experimental models of cancer growth through regulation of the ERK MAPK signalling pathway. Moreover, the major source of ROS generation required for this abnormal anchorage-independent growth was the Q(o) site of mitochondrial complex III. Furthermore, disruption of mitochondrial function by loss of the mitochondrial transcription factor A (TFAM) gene reduced tumourigenesis in an oncogenic Kras-driven mouse model of lung cancer, demonstrating that mitochondrial metabolism and mitochondrial ROS generation were essential for Kras-induced cell proliferation and tumourigenesis.

An interesting therapeutic approach exploiting relationships among cancer cells, ROS and abnormal antioxidant defences was suggested by Raj et al. (2011). Because malignant transformation frequently results in enhanced cellular oxidative stress, the authors tested a molecule capable of selectively inducing cancer cell death by increasing the level of ROS only in cells with a cancer genotype. Indeed, piperlongumine enhanced ROS accumulation only in cancer cells by targeting the stress response to ROS. Independent of the therapeutic implications, this study underlines an often neglected aspect of cancer cells, the induction of different antioxidant mechanisms. According to the authors, this induction does not appear to be related to the level of cell proliferation.

Finally, it is important to stress that the relationships among mitochondria, redox imbalance/ROS and cancer should be evaluated from the point of view of the so-called cancer stem cells or "stem-like cancer cells" hypothesis. These cells in fact possess properties similar to those of normal stem cells, in which redox balance plays an important role in the maintenance of self-renewal and, above all, differentiation.

13.5　Mitochondria, Mitochondrial DNA (mtDNA) Mutations and Cancer

Mitochondria contain circular molecules of DNA reminiscent of bacterial chromosomes, but the mitochondrial genome is much smaller. The mitochondrial DNA only codes for a few of the proteins and ribosomal RNA molecules needed in the mitochondrion, and most components are encoded by the nucleus. A dissertation about mitochondrial DNA is the subject of a different chapter in this monograph. Here, it should be stressed that the mitochondrial DNA of humans accumulates mutations much faster than the nuclear genes. In particular, mutations accumulate rapidly in the third codon position of structural genes and even faster in the intergenic regulatory regions. Specifically, most of the variability in human mitochondrial DNA occurs within the D-loop segment of the regulatory region. This means that mitochondrial DNA is frequently used for phylogenetic and forensic purposes.

The role of mtDNA mutations (intragenic deletions, missense and chain-terminating point mutations, alterations of homopolymeric sequences, etc.) in the pathophysiology of cancer is still controversial. In fact, some authors do not consider these mutations significant pathogenetic noxae in cancer but simply associated lesions or even effects of laboratory malpractice. Thus, the role of these mtDNA mutations and of their related mitochondrial respiratory dysfunctions in terms of ROS induction in carcinogenesis is not clear (Brandon et al. 2006).

The following examples demonstrate the contrasting data available on mtDNA. In gastrointestinal cancers, somatic mitochondrial D-loop mutations have been identified in 48% (15/31) of gastric tumour specimens (Wu et al. 2005) and in 39% (24/61) and 68% (13/19) of hepatocellular carcinomas by two different groups, respectively (Nomoto et al. 2002; Lee et al. 2004). In renal cancer, Horton et al. (1996) showed that 48.7% (19/39) of renal adenocarcinoma tissues contained a 294 bp in-frame deletion in the ND1 gene, resulting in truncated mRNA. In another study, depletion of mtDNA and loss of mRNA coding for ND3 was reported in 62% (8/13) of renal cell carcinoma samples. In another study, somatic mutations in the D-loop region were detected in 23% (7/31) of bladder cancer specimens and in 14% (3/21) of renal cancer specimens (Wada et al. 2006).

In breast cancer, somatic mtDNA mutations were found in fine needle aspirates from primary breast tumours in 61% (11/18) of patients (Parrella et al. 2001). Among these, 42% were deletions or insertions within the D-loop region, whereas the remaining were single-base substitutions throughout the genome. In an interesting comparative study on prostate, researchers sequenced the entire mitochondrial genome from 24 prostatectomy samples, including tumour, adjacent benign, and distant benign samples, and compared them with mtDNA from 12 histologically benign control samples and paired blood as the non-disease germline control (Parr et al. 2006). The authors found that 16 of 24 (66.7%) patients had mutations in all three tested prostate tissues: 22 of 24 (91.7%) had mutations in tumour samples, 19 of 24 (79.2%) had alterations in adjacent benign samples, and 22 of 24 (91.7%) displayed changes in distant benign samples. Analysis of the D-loop showed 34 substitution mutations in 21 of 29 (72%) prostate biopsy samples, although there were no differences in mutation load between malignant and symptomatic benign specimens.

Finally, an investigation of D-loop repetitive regions in melanoma by Deichmann et al. (2004) showed that 12% (4/34) of melanoma primary tumours and 20% (7/35) of cutaneous and subcutaneous metastases contained somatic mutations, seven of which were insertions, and two were deletions. These last data, in particular, do not suggest a direct role of mtDNA mutations in cancer pathogenesis. In fact, in melanoma, a particularly aggressive type of cancer, about 80% of metastasis and 82% of primary tumours did not contain significant mtDNA mutations. Further, in other cancers, mtDNA mutations are observed in less than 60% of cases.

However, some recent studies have taken the "bystander" point of view for mitochondrial DNA mutations. In the study of Ishikawa et al. (2008), the authors showed that by replacing the endogenous mtDNA in a mouse tumour cell line that was poorly metastatic with mtDNA from a cell line that was highly metastatic by cytoplasmic hybrid (cybrid) technology, the recipient tumour cells acquired the metastatic potential of the transferred mtDNA. Moreover, the mtDNA conferring high metastatic potential contained G13997A and 13885insC mutations in the gene encoding ND6. These mutations produced a deficiency in respiratory complex I activity and were associated with overproduction of reactive oxygen species (ROS). Pre-treatment of the highly metastatic tumour cells with ROS scavengers suppressed their metastatic potential in mice. These debated results seem to indicate that mtDNA mutations can contribute to tumour progression by enhancing the metastatic potential of tumour cells by promoting genetic instability directly and/or indirectly. Finally, for a diagnostic point of view, we should note the study of He et al. (2010). By digital sequencing of mtDNA genomes with a massively parallel sequencing-by-synthesis approach, the authors showed that the mtDNA of human cells, which was considered to be homogeneous, actually contains widespread heterogeneity (heteroplasmy). Moreover, the frequency of heteroplasmic variants varied considerably between different tissues in the same individual. In addition to the variants identified in normal tissues, cancer cells harboured further homoplasmic and heteroplasmic mutations that could also be detected in patient plasma, and this mutated mtDNA could be used as a cancer biomarker.

The study of Lueth et al. (2010) supported this data, identifying somatic mutations in 6 of 15 medulloblastoma samples by temporal temperature gel electrophoresis and direct sequencing. These changes were insertions, deletions, or substitutions restricted to the 303–315 bp poly-C tract of the D-loop region. Interestingly, three were changes from heteroplasmy to homoplasmy, two were changes from heteroplasmy to heteroplasmy and one mutation represented a change from homoplasmy to heteroplasmy. In addition, 25 distinct germline variations were identified. These results are in support on the high frequency of somatic mitochondrial mutations in medulloblastoma, but there are no data on the frequency of mitochondrial mutation in normal nervous tissue. Importantly, these somatic alterations were found only in the hypervariable D-loop region, supporting the idea that these control regions contain hot spots for both germline variations and somatic alterations of the mitochondrial genome.

13.6 Mitochondria, Heat Shock Proteins (HSPs) and Cancer

The complicated pathophysiology of HSPs in cancer seems particularly worthy of potential clinical targeting. In cancer, HSPs seem to have fundamental tumour promoting activities. HSP90 family members protect and maintain functionally aberrant conformations of point mutated or grossly altered proteins with oncogenic functions (i.e., the products of chromosomal translocation, such as Bcr-Abl, or point mutations, such as variants of the epidermal growth factor receptor). Another fundamental tumour-promoting activity of HSPs, which is mainly related to the HSP70 and −27 families, depends upon the strong inhibitory activities of these proteins in both mitochondrial and extra-mitochondrial programmed cell death (apoptosis) and cell senescence (Smith et al. 1998; Wang et al. 2000; Sur et al. 2008). This very efficient road block to programmed cell death not only synergises with the other tumour-promoting activities of HSPs (specifically chaperone properties) but has a significant role in the development of resistance to various cancer therapeutics (Ritossa 1962; Pockley 2001; Soti et al. 2005; Chen et al. 2007a, b).

Importantly, the ability of HSPs to interact with various signal transduction pathways, their chaperone properties and their anti-apoptotic effects render them facilitators of genetic variation in cancer. These attributes of HSPs favourably influence the promotion of other cancer properties, including local invasion, angiogenesis and, although somewhat contested, metastasis (Smith et al. 1998; Schmitt et al. 2007; Powers and Workman 2007; Zhou et al. 2004; Keezer et al. 2003; Hoang et al. 2000). In fact, HSPs are strongly induced in many different cancer cells and function to protect cells by blocking apoptosis during tumour progression. HSPs may also function to protect cells from other cancer characteristics such as genetic instability, ischemic stroma, the Warburg effect, and invasion and metastatic potential. This suggests a role in carcinogenesis also for mtHSPs, such as prohibitin, mortalin, HSP60/HSP10 complexes, and HSP-70 (Calderwood et al. 2006; Czarnecka et al. 2006). Specifically, mortalin, which is also known as mitochondrial HSP70, is known to be involved in cell cycle regulation, cellular senescence and immortalisation pathways. In fact, mortalin overexpression in colorectal adenocarcinoma was found to correlate with a poor prognosis (Dundas et al. 2005).

However, the relationships among HSPs, mitochondria and cancer are far from being clarified, as recently demonstrated by the study of Wadhwa et al. (2010), which found that the Drosophila melanogaster mitochondrial Hsp22 (DmHsp22) is preferentially up-regulated during aging. It is well known that its overexpression results in an extension of life span (>30%) (Morrow et al. 2004). Moreover, long lived flies expressing Hsp22 have increased resistance to oxidative stress and maintain locomotor activity longer. The authors evaluated the cross-species effects of Hsp22 expression in human cells. The results showed that DmHsp22 was functionally active in human cells. It extended the life span of normal fibroblasts, slowing the aging process as evidenced by lower levels of the senescence-associated betagalactosidase. Further, DmHsp22 expression in human cancer cells increased their malignant properties including anchorage-independent growth, tumour formation in nude mice, and resistance to a variety of anti-cancer drugs. Finally, DmHsp22 interacts with and inactivates the tumour suppressor protein p53.

13.7 Mitochondria, Calcium and Cancer

It is well known that mitochondria can accumulate calcium (Ca^{2+}). However, unlike the other organelles, such as the sarcoplasmic or endoplasmic reticula, mitochondria do not have large stores of Ca^{2+}. These concentrations, however, are sufficient for mitochondria to couple the cellular metabolic state with Ca^{2+} transport processes. They therefore control not only their own intra-organelle $[Ca^{2+}]$, but they also influence the entire cellular network of cellular Ca^{2+} signalling, including the endoplasmic reticulum, the plasma membrane, and the nucleus. That defines a central mitochondrial role in Ca^{2+} signalling and in inter-organelle communication as well. Moreover, by this fine tuning of the Ca^{2+} signal, mitochondria can modulate various enzymatic activities. In turn, these Ca^{2+} oscillations permit specific outcomes, such as regulation of gene transcription, cell cycle, apoptosis or proliferation and angiogenesis, all aspects relevant for tumourigenesis and tissue homeostasis.

The physiology and pathophysiology of calcium in mitochondria is the topic of a different chapter. Here, it is useful just to stress that some cancers are associated with the up- or downregulation of specific Ca^{2+} channels or pumps. For example, TRPM8 is upregulated in prostate cancer and SERCA3 is downregulated in colon cancer. These observations are stimulating significant research on various potential pharmacological agents that can modulate Ca^{2+} channels, pumps and exchangers with the aim of selectively targeting calcium-related cancer proliferation and/or cancer-induced inhibition of apoptosis. However, it is still unclear if these changes in the expression or activity of Ca^{2+} channels and pumps at the cellular and mitochondria levels have a causal role in cancer or not. For example, increased expression of plasma membrane Ca^{2+} channels may increase Ca^{2+} influx and promote Ca^{2+}-dependent proliferative pathways. Alternatively, altered activity or expression of specific Ca^{2+} channels and pumps might be an adaptive response or might offer a survival advantage, such as resistance to apoptosis. Indeed, caspase-resistant PMCA exogenously expressed in CHO cells results in a reduced rate of apoptosis and necrosis after treatment with staurosporine.

But is it really possible hypothesise a pathogenetic link among mitochondria, calcium and cancer?

It should be stressed that location, degree and temporal aspects of changes in free Ca^{2+} may influence different pathways related to carcinogenesis, such as:

- Motility: Ca^{2+} is implicated in cellular motility (an important aspect of tumour invasion and metastasis);
- Angiogenesis: Ca^{2+} is a key regulator in different signalling pathways that is important in angiogenesis (i.e., vascular endothelial growth factor (VEGF) can increase intracellular Ca^{2+} by inducing Ca^{2+} release from its stores);
- Genotoxicity: Ca^{2+} can modulate some aspects of DNA damage response pathways, which influence genomic stability and cell survival (i.e., it is a modulator of poly-(ADP-ribose) polymerase-1 (PARP1) activity);
- Transcription: Ca^{2+} levels directly and/or indirectly regulate transcription by influencing the downstream regulatory element antagonist modulator (DREAM) and the transcription factor NFAT (nuclear factor of activated T cells);
- Telomerase activity: The Ca^{2+} effector S100A8 can inhibit the activity of telomerase;
- Differentiation: Ca^{2+} signalling is implicated in differentiation/dedifferentiation processes either through the extracellular Ca^{2+}-sensing receptor and/or through alterations in intracellular Ca^{2+} ;
- Cell cycle: Ca^{2+} is a key regulator of the cell cycle, and hence proliferation, through various pathways including regulation of RAS activity, control of PTEN nuclear localisation, transcription of immediate early genes important in the G0–G1 transition, and last but not least facilitating the phosphorylation of the retinoblastoma protein in late G1;
- Apoptosis: programmed cell death is often linked to accumulation of excessive Ca^{2+} by the mitochondria with activation of mitochondrial membrane permeabilisation, while reduction in the Ca^{2+} content of the intracellular stores is associated with resistance to apoptosis.

However, the molecular mechanisms of the possible alterations in calcium level oscillations are not understood, particularly at the mitochondrial level. Interestingly, the recent identification of a 40 kDa protein that may be a mitochondrial calcium uniporter has opened new ideas on the role of mitochondria in cellular Ca^{2+} signalling. In fact, by characterisation of this protein, a better understanding of the physiology and pathophysiology at the molecular level would be possible. This would permit a better analysis, in addition to animal models, of all processes regulated by mitochondrial Ca^{2+} signals, such as aerobic metabolism and cell death, aspects that are typically altered in cancer cells.

13.8 Mitochondria and Cancer Cell Differentiation: An Illustrative Example

It is well-known that cancer cell can be induced to differentiate, which lowers proliferation, by different physical (temperature) and chemical agents (DMSO, retinoic acid, hybrid polar agents, HDCA inhibitors, and so on). The molecular mechanisms of this differentiation are debated. For some agents with potential therapeutic use, some molecular mechanisms have been elucidated. Although the connection between mitochondrial respiration and cancer cell dedifferentiation (i.e., pleomorphism, resistance to apoptosis, cell proliferation, metabolic shift, cell invasion, and genetic instability) is fundamental to cancer pathogenesis, the precise molecular relationships and regulatory processes are far from understood. Recent studies are re-examining mitochondrial function, especially cellular respiration, in cancer. However, a consensus among the findings has yet to be achieved (Modica-Napolitano and Singh 2004; Scatena et al. 1999, 2003, 2007; Felty and Roy 2005).

Herein we summarise important findings linking cellular respiration to cell differentiation in cancer. It is worth noting that this putative link may have crucial pharmacologic and clinical implications. For example, the work of Amuthan et al. (2002) showed mechanistic insight into how cancer progression and tumour invasion may be directly related to chemical damage of mtDNA that results in mitochondrial respiratory chain dysfunction, loss of mitochondrial membrane potential, and reduction of ATP synthesis. This mitochondrial derangement also causes calcium release into the cytoplasm, which activates a cell dedifferentiation program. This study showed in C2C12 myoblasts and human pulmonary carcinoma A549 cells that a mitochondrial stress-induced cell dedifferentiation program (by mtDNA depletion) can transform cells into a more aggressive phenotype with the following properties:

- induction of hexokinase, the enzyme that primes glucose by consuming ATP;
- induction of phosphoenolpyruvate carboxykinase (PEPCK), which regulates gluconeogenesis, glyceroneogenesis, and many other anaplerotic reactions;
- induction of tumour invasion markers (i.e., cathepsin L, TGF-β1, ERK1, ERK2, and calcineurin);
- induction of anti-apoptotic proteins (Bcl2 and Bcl-XL) and reduction of levels of the pro-apoptotic proteins Bid and Bax;
- reduction of cell growth and significant morphologic changes.

In summary, the findings of Amuthan et al. (2002) demonstrate that, at least in this set of experimental conditions, generic mitochondrial stress caused by mtDNA depletion alters cellular respiration and patterns of nuclear gene expression, thereby inducing tumourigenic properties.

Generally, mtDNA depletion renders cells more sensitive to apoptotic stimuli. Interestingly, Amuthan et al. (2002) explained that the outcome of the stress (cell dedifferentiation vs. apoptosis) could be related to the relative resistance to apoptosis and/or to the capacity of the adopted cellular models to efficiently buffer the secondary metabolic stresses. Furthermore, this combination of methodological approaches demonstrated mitochondria-to-nucleus stress signalling, through which alterations in cellular respiration have the ability to change nuclear gene expression and selectively promote the growth of more aggressive clones.

Other studies suggest that mitochondria can mediate the proliferative or inhibitory actions of physiologic or pharmacologic molecules that influence cellular respiration. It was recently reported that some "non-genomic" effects of oestrogens (i.e., effects mediated by mitochondria rather than oestrogen receptors) modulate the expression of nuclear cell cycle genes and human breast tumour growth. Specifically, oestrogens cause increased transcription of various complex subunits of the electron respiratory chain in mitochondria. Oestradiol treatment (0.5 nM for 6 days) caused a 16-fold increase in cytochrome oxidase II (COII) mRNA in rat pituitary tumour cells. Similarly, ethinyl oestradiol treatment (0.5–10 M for 40 h) caused a two- to three-fold increase in cytochrome oxidase I (COI), COII, and NADH dehydrogenase subunit I. Oestrogens seem to negatively affect mitochondria at the protein level as well. Several studies have shown that oestrogens can inhibit mitochondrial respiratory complexes I, II, III, IV, and V. This perturbation of the electron respiratory chain can induce mitochondrial ROS production, which promotes the generation and progression of some cancers via oxidative stress and/or ROS-related signalling pathways (Felty and Roy 2005). Given the suggested role of oestrogens in some cancers (i.e., breast cancer) and their carcinogenic activity, further evidence should be gathered to determine the relevance of these findings, particularly at the mitochondrial and nuclear levels.

The ability of lipophilic molecules to alter cellular respiration and cell differentiation/dedifferentiation processes is a neglected pathophysiologic facet of the mitochondrial respiratory chain. In fact, fibrates and their thiazolidinedione derivatives interact with many hydrophobic protein domains and especially with complex I subunits of the mitochondrial electron respiratory chain. This molecular interaction occurs both *in vitro* and *in vivo*, and it is rapid (<1 h from administration) and occurs in numerous cell types to varying degrees.

Specifically, *in vitro*, the following human cell lines have shown alteration of complex I and cell differentiation: K-562 human erythroleukaemia, HL-60 human myeloid leukaemia, U-937 human monocytic leukaemia, TE-671 human rhabdomyosarcoma, HepG2 human hepatocarcinoma, and SK-N-BE[2] human neuroblastoma (Scatena et al. 1999, 2003; Bottoni et al. 2005).

Importantly, the lipophilic properties of these molecules allow them to diffuse freely into lipid bilayers and especially mitochondria because of the interplay between their logD and mitochondrial electrochemical gradient, thereby altering the function of proteins embedded in membranes. One of the larger protein components of the mitochondria membranes is complex I (NADH-ubiquinone oxidoreductase, subunits >30, MW 850 kDa), which because of these features may act as the main lipophilic molecular sink in mitochondria (Scatena et al. 2007).

The rapid iatrogenic respiratory disruption caused by introduction of these lipophilic molecules has been shown to induce metabolic- and ROS-mediated stress that promotes differentiation in human tumour cell lines; mitochondrial HSPs have also been shown to be involved (Bottoni et al. 2009). In particular, the disruption of mitochondrial complex I may induce ROS production and impair NADH oxidation, resulting in an energetic shortage in cancer cells. Importantly, because complex I is only partially disrupted, the oxidative and energetic stress are generally non-lethal. Under these conditions, cell growth is hampered, and phenotypic features of differentiation may reappear. This suggests that these agent do not cause bona fide differentiation (i.e., by epigenetic modifications), but, by simply inducing significant metabolic and energetic stress, they impair the proliferative capacity of cancer cells. In this case, molecular activities typical of a their differentiated state return.

These observations necessitate a re-evaluation of the differentiation/dedifferentiation definition with significant pharmacological implications. In fact, the so-called drug-induced differentiation should be better defined as a drug induced "pseudodifferentiation". These results may justify the poor results obtained with some so-called differentiating agents (i.e., HDAC inhibitors) (Mai et al. 2005).

Moreover, these data confirm that fibrates and thiazolidinediones may inhibit complex I via excess PPAR activity, thus impairing NADH oxidation at the mitochondrial level, and may explain some of the pharmacologic activities of this class of drugs (i.e., anti-hyperlipidemia, insulin sensitisation). These findings also may account for some of the adverse side effects of fibrates and thiazolidinediones, including myocardiotoxicity, hepatotoxicity, and, most relevant to this discussion, peroxisome proliferation, carcinogenicity, and cancer differentiating properties, which are considered typical peroxisome proliferator activated receptor (PPAR)-alpha–mediated effects in rodents (Michalik et al. 2004).

In conclusion, stress-related differentiation in human tumour cell lines, including some human leukaemia cell lines, is a well-known occurrence (Richards et al. 1988). The differentiating activity of fibrates and thiazolidinediones on human tumour cell lines has been shown to be tightly correlated with the level of mitochondrial complex I disruption. This differentiating activity is independent of the expression level of PPARs, as well as the embryonic origin of the tissue.

Interestingly, fibrate/thiazolidinedione-induced differentiation is unusual; it is linked to the metabolic status of differentiated cells that shift toward a more glycolytic metabolism (paradoxical Warburg effect), thus demonstrating that the original neoplastic phenotype utilised mitochondria for energy. Moreover, metabolic parameters recorded during drug-induced cell differentiation (residual activity of the mitochondrial electron respiratory chain components glycerol 3-phosphate dehydrogenase and succinate dehydrogenase and levels of glycolytic and nonglycolytic acetate, pyruvate, and alanine) suggest that the so-called Warburg effect is really an epiphenomenon of a more complex metabolic rearrangement of the neoplastic cell. Notably, this cancer-associated metabolic rearrangement, induced by the cancer's rigid genetic selection program, is characterised by a high level of cell proliferation and diffusion. This high proliferation and diffusion is normally present only during embryonic and foetal development and seems to re-activate in cancer cells, underscoring the importance of the cancer stem cells hypothesis (i.e., stem-like cancer cells) and the original hypothesis of Warburg.

13.9 Conclusions

Discussing all that is known on the relationship between mitochondria and cancer is quite difficult. It is only possible to stress some aspects that underline the potential translational applications of intriguing pathophysiological links. Mitochondria are not innocent bystanders in cancer progression. They have various important pathogenetic roles with fundamental diagnostic, prognostic and therapeutic implications.

In particular, experimental and clinical data seem to confirm:

- A more active role of mitochondria in modulating the differentiated cellular phenotype and the pathogenetic significance of disruptions in oxidative metabolism in carcinogenesis
- The importance of the shift of cellular metabolism in cancer, resembling stem cell metabolism, to ensure that the new energetic and structural needs of neoplastic cells are met
- The role of NADH and the NADH/NAD+ ratio in the modulation of a signal transduction pathway that controls differentiation/dedifferentiation status
- The interplay of complex I and complex II of the mitochondrial respiratory chain to adapt cell metabolism to different physiopathologic conditions
- The value of an accurate morphofunctional definition of the so-called cancer stem cell, which may represent the real reservoir of a tumour

Elucidating the relationship between cancer cell oxidative metabolism and cellular differentiation state is fundamental not only for the field of oncology but also for stem cells.

References

Alvero AB, Montagna MK, Holmberg JC et al (2011) Targeting the mitochondria activates two independent cell death pathways in the ovarian cancer stem cells. Mol Cancer Ther 10:1385–1393

Amuthan G, Biswas G, Ananadatheerthavarada HK et al (2002) Mitochondrial stress-induced calcium signaling, phenotypic changes and invasive behavior in human lung carcinoma A549 cells. Oncogene 21:7839–7849

Balaban RS, Bader JP (1984) Studies on the relationship between glycolysis and (Na+ K+)-ATPase in cultured cells. Biochim Biophys Acta 804:419–426

Bellance N, Lestienne P, Rossignol R (2009) Mitochondria from bioenergetics to the metabolic regulation of carcinogenesis. Front Biosci 14:4015–4034

Bensaad K, Vousden KH (2007) P53: new roles in metabolism. Trends Cell Biol 17:286–291

Bottoni P, Giardina B, Martorana GE et al (2005) A two-dimensional electrophoresis preliminary approach to human hepatocarcinoma differentiation induced by PPAR-agonists. J Cell Mol Med 9:462–467

Bottoni P, Giardina B, Vitali A et al (2009) A proteomic approach to characterizing ciglitazone-induced cancer cell differentiation in Hep-G2 cell line. Biochim Biophys Acta 1794:615–626

Brandon M, Baldi P, Wallace DC (2006) Mitochondrial mutations in cancer. Oncogene 25:4647–4662

Cadenas E (2004) Mitochondrial free radical production and cell signaling. Mol Aspects Med 25:17–26

Cairns RA, Harris IS, Mak TW (2011) Regulation of cancer cell metabolism. Nat Rev Cancer 11:85–95

Calderwood SK, Khaleque MA, Sawyer DB et al (2006) Heat shock proteins in cancer: chaperones of tumorigenesis. Trends Biochem Sci 31:164–172

Chen EI, Hewel J, Krueger JS et al (2007a) Adaptation of energy metabolism in breast cancer brain metastases. Cancer Res 67:1472–1486

Chen Y, Voegeli TS, Liu PP et al (2007b) Heat shock paradox and a new role of heat shock proteins and their receptors as anti-inflammation targets. Inflamm Allergy Drug Targets 6:91–100

Chen ZX, Velaithan R, Pervaiz S (2009) MitoEnergetics and cancer cell fate. Biochim Biophys Acta 1787:462–467

Cheng T, Sudderth J, Yang C et al (2011) Pyruvate carboxylase is required for glutamine-independent growth of tumor cells. Proc Natl Acad Sci USA 108:8674–8679

Costello LC, Franklin RB (2005) Why do tumour cells glycolyse?': from glycolysis through citrate to lipogenesis. Mol Cell Biochem 280:1–8

Cuezva JM, Krajewska M, de Heredia ML et al (2002) The bioenergetic signature of cancer: a marker of tumor progression. Cancer Res 62:6674–6681

Cuezva JM, Chen G, Alonso AM et al (2004) The bioenergetic signature of lung adenocarcinomas is a molecular marker of cancer diagnosis and prognosis. Carcinogenesis 25:1157–1163

Czarnecka AM, Campanella C, Zummo G, Cappello F (2006) Mitochondrial chaperones in cancer: from molecular biology to clinical diagnostics. Cancer Biol Ther 5:714–720

D'Souza GG, Wagle MA, Saxena V, Shah A (2011) Approaches for targeting mitochondria in cancer therapy. Biochim Biophys Acta 1807:689–696

Dang CV, Hamaker M, Sun P et al (2011) Therapeutic targeting of cancer cell metabolism. J Mol Med (Berl) 89:205–212

Debatin KM, Poncet D, Kroemer G (2002) Chemotherapy: targeting the mitochondrial cell death pathway. Oncogene 21:8786–8803

DeBerardinis RJ, Cheng T (2010) Q's next: the diverse functions of glutamine in metabolism, cell biology and cancer. Oncogene 29:313–324

Deberardinis RJ, Lum JJ, Hatzivassiliou G, Thompson CB (2008a) The biology of cancer: metabolic reprogramming fuels cell growth and proliferation. Cell Metab 7:11–20

Deberardinis RJ, Sayed N, Ditsworth D, Thompson CB (2008b) Brick by brick: metabolism and tumor cell growth. Curr Opin Genet Dev 18:54–61

Deichmann M, Kahle B, Benner A et al (2004) Somatic mitochondrial mutations in melanoma resection specimens. Int J Oncol 24:137–141

Dundas SR, Lawrie LC, Rooney PH, Murray GI (2005) Mortalin is over-expressed by colorectal adenocarcinomas and correlates with poor survival. J Patholm 205:74–81

Elgadi KM, Meguid RA, Qian M et al (1999) Cloning and analysis of unique human glutaminase isoforms generated by tissue-specific alternative splicing. Physiol Genomics 1:51–62

Fan Y, Dickman KG, Zong WX (2010) Akt and c-Myc differentially activate cellular metabolic programs and prime cells to bioenergetic inhibition. J Biol Chem 285:7324–7333

Fantin VR, Leder P (2006) Mitochondriotoxic compounds for cancer therapy. Oncogene 25:4787–4797

Fantin VR, St-Pierre J, Leder P (2006) Attenuation of LDH-A expression uncovers a link between glycolysis, mitochondrial physiology, and tumor maintenance. Cancer Cell 9:425–434

Felty Q, Roy D (2005) Estrogen, mitochondria, and growth of cancer and non-cancer cells. J Carcinog 4:1–18

Frezza C, Gottlieb E (2009) Mitochondria in cancer: not just innocent bystanders. Semin Cancer Biol 19:4–11

Frezza C, Zheng L, Folger O et al (2011) Haem oxygenase is synthetically lethal with the tumour suppressor fumarate hydratase. Nature. doi:10.1038/nature10363

Fulda S, Debatin KM (2006) Extrinsic versus intrinsic apoptosis pathways in anticancer chemotherapy. Oncogene 25:4798–4811

Fulda S, Galluzzi L, Kroemer G (2010) Targeting mitochondria for cancer therapy. Nat Rev Drug Discov 9:447–464

Galluzzi L, Larochette N, Zamzami N, Kroemer G (2006) Mitochondria as therapeutic targets for cancer chemotherapy. Oncogene 25:4812–4830

Gao P, Tchernyshyov I, Chang TC et al (2009) c-Myc suppression of miR-23a/b enhances mitochondrial glutaminase expression and glutamine metabolism. Nature 458:762–765

Gatenby RA, Gillies RJ (2004) Why do cancers have high aerobic glycolysis? Nat Rev Cancer 4:891–899

Gogvadze V, Orrenius S, Zhivotovsky B (2008) Mitochondria in cancer cells: what is so special about them? Trends Cell Biol 18:165–173

Gogvadze V, Orrenius S, Zhivotovsky B (2009) Mitochondria as targets for cancer chemotherapy. Semin Cancer Biol 19:57–66

Green A, Beer P (2010) Somatic mutations of IDH1 and IDH2 in the leukemic transformation of myeloproliferative neoplasms. N Engl J Med 362:369–370

He Y, Wu J, Dressman DC et al (2010) Heteroplasmic mitochondrial DNA mutations in normal and tumour cells. Nature 464:610–614

Herrnstadt C, Preston G, Howell N (2003) Errors, phantoms and otherwise, in human mtDNA sequences. Am J Hum Genet 72:1585–1586

Hoang AT, Huang J, Rudra-Ganguly N et al (2000) A novel association between the human heat shock transcription factor 1 (HSF1) and prostate adenocarcinoma. Am J Pathol 156:857–864

Horton TM, Petros JA, Heddi A et al (1996) Novel mitochondrial DNA deletion found in a renal cell carcinoma. Genes Chromosomes Cancer 15:95–101

Ishikawa K, Takenaga K, Akimoto M (2008) ROS-generating mitochondrial DNA mutations can regulate tumor cell metastasis. Science 320:661–664

Jezek P, Plecitá-Hlavatá L, Smolková K, Rossignol R (2010) Distinctions and similarities of cell bioenergetics and the role of mitochondria in hypoxia, cancer, and embryonic development. Int J Biochem Cell Biol 42:604–622

Jiang P, Du W, Wang X et al (2011) p53 regulates biosynthesis through direct inactivation of glucose-6-phosphate dehydrogenase. Nat Cell Biol 13:310–316

Kallinowski F, Schlenger KH, Kloes M et al (1989) Tumor blood flow: the principal modulator of oxidative and glycolytic metabolism, and of the metabolic micromilieu of human tumor xenografts in vivo. Int J Cancer 44:266–272

Keezer SM, Ivie SE, Krutzsch HC et al (2003) Angiogenesis inhibitors target the endothelial cell cytoskeleton through altered regulation of heat shock protein 27 and cofilin. Cancer Res 63:6405–6412

Kerr JF, Wyllie AH, Currie AR (1972) Apoptosis: a basic biological phenomenon with wide-ranging implications in tissue kinetics. Br J Cancer 26:239–257

Kim JW, Dang CV (2005) Multifaceted roles of glycolytic enzymes. Trends Biochem Sci 30:142–150

Kondoh H, Lleonart ME, Gil J et al (2005) Glycolytic enzymes can modulate cellular life span. Cancer Res 65:177–185

Koppenol WH, Bounds PL, Dang CV (2011) Otto Warburg's contributions to current concepts of cancer metabolism. Nat Rev Cancer 11:325–337

Kroemer G, Pouyssegur J (2008) Tumor cell metabolism: cancer's Achilles' heel. Cancer Cell 13:472–482

Le A, Cooper CR, Gouw AM et al (2010) Inhibition of lactate dehydrogenase A induces oxidative stress and inhibits tumor progression. Proc Natl Acad Sci USA 107:2037–2042

Lee HC, Li SH, Lin JC et al (2004) Somatic mutations in the D-loop and decrease in the copy number of mitochondrial DNA in human hepatocellular carcinoma. Mutat Res 547:71–78

Liu H, Hu YP, Savaraj N et al (2001) Hypersensitization of tumor cells to glycolytic inhibitors. Biochemistry 40:5542–5547

Lowry OH, Berger SJ, Carter JG et al (1983) Diversity of metabolic patterns in human brain tumors: enzymes of energy metabolism and related metabolites and cofactors. J Neurochem 41:994–1010

Lueth M, von Deimling A, Pietsch T et al (2010) Medulloblastoma harbor somatic mitochondrial DNA mutations in the D-loop region. J Pediatr Hematol Oncol 32:156–159

Maddocks ODK, Vousden KH (2011) Metabolic regulation by p53. J Mol Med 89:237–245

Mai A, Massa S, Rotili D et al (2005) Exploring the connection unit in the HDAC inhibitor pharmacophore model: novel uracil-based hydroxamates. Bioorg Med Chem Lett 15:4656–4661

Marín-Hernández A, Gallardo-Pérez JC, Ralph SJ et al (2009) HIF-1alpha modulates energy metabolism in cancer cells by inducing over-expression of specific glycolytic isoforms. Mini Rev Med Chem 9:1084–1101

Marín-Hernández A, Gallardo-Pérez JC, Rodríguez-Enríquez S et al (2011) Modeling cancer glycolysis. Biochim Biophys Acta 1807:755–767

Martinez-Outschoorn UE, Balliet RM, Rivadeneira DB et al (2010) Oxidative stress in cancer associated fibroblasts drives tumor-stroma co-evolution: a new paradigm for understanding tumor metabolism, the field effect and genomic instability in cancer cells. Cell Cycle 9:3256–3276

Martinez-Outschoorn UE, Lin Z, Ko YH et al (2011) Understanding the metabolic basis of drug resistance: therapeutic induction of the Warburg effect kills cancer cells. Cell Cycle 10:2521–2528

Mathupala SP, Ko YH, Pedersen PL (2006) Hexokinase II: cancer's double-edged sword acting as both facilitator and gatekeeper of malignancy when bound to mitochondria. Oncogene 25:4777–4786

Meng M, Chen S, Lao T et al (2010) Nitrogen anabolism underlies the importance of glutaminolysis in proliferating cells. Cell Cycle 9:3921–3932

Michalik L, Desvergne B, Wahli W (2004) Peroxisome proliferator-activated receptor and cancers: complex stories. Nat Rev Cancer 4:61–70

Modica-Napolitano JS, Singh KK (2004) Mitochondrial dysfunction in cancer. Mitochondrion 4:755–762

Moll UM, Marchenko N, Zhang XK (2006) p53 and Nur77/TR3 - transcription factors that directly target mitochondria for cell death induction. Oncogene 25:4725–4743

Moncada S, Erusalimsky JD (2002) Does nitric oxide modulate mitochondrial energy generation and apoptosis? Nat Rev Mol Cell Biol 3:214–220

Moreno-Sanchez R, Rodriguez-Enriquez S, Marin-Hernandez A, Saavedra E (2007) Energy metabolism in tumor cells. FEBS J 274:1393–1418

Moreno-Sánchez R, Rodríguez-Enríquez S, Saavedra E et al (2009) The bioenergetics of cancer: is glycolysis the main ATP supplier in all tumor cells? Biofactors 35:209–225

Morrow G, Samson M, Michaud S, Tanguay RM (2004) Overexpression of the small mitochondrial Hsp22 extends Drosophila life span and increases resistance to oxidative stress. FASEB J 18:598–599

Nakashima RA, Paggi MG, Pedersen PL (1984) Contributions of glycolysis and oxidative phosphorylation to adenosine 5′-triphosphate production in AS-30D hepatoma cells. Cancer Res 44(12 Pt 1):5702–5706

Naumov GN, Bender E, Zurakowski D et al (2006) A model of human tumor dormancy: an angiogenic switch from the nonangiogenic phenotype. J Natl Cancer Inst 98:316–325

Nomoto S, Yamashita K, Koshikawa K et al (2002) Mitochondrial D-loop mutations as clonal markers in multicentric hepatocellular carcinoma and plasma. Clin Cancer Res 8:481–487

Parra-Bonilla G, Alvarez DF, Al-Mehdi AB et al (2010) Critical role for lactate dehydrogenase A in aerobic glycolysis that sustains pulmonary microvascular endothelial cell proliferation. Am J Physiol Lung Cell Mol Physiol 299:L513–L522

Parr RL, Dakubo GD, Crandall KA et al (2006) Somatic mitochondrial DNA mutations in prostate cancer and normal appearing adjacent glands in comparison to age-matched prostate samples without malignant histology. J Mol Diagn 8:312–319

Parrella P, Xiao Y, Fliss M et al (2001) Detection of mitochondrial DNA mutations in primary breast cancer and fine-needle aspirates. Cancer Res 61:7623–7626

Pockley AG (2001) Heat shock proteins in health and disease: therapeutic targets or therapeutics agents? Expert Rev Mol Med 3:1–21

Pollard PJ, Brière JJ, Alam NA et al (2005) Accumulation of Krebs cycle intermediates and over-expression of HIF1alpha in tumours which result from germline FH and SDH mutations. Hum Mol Genet 14:2231–2239

Powers MV, Workman P (2007) Inhibitors of the heat shock response: biology and pharmacology. FEBS Lett 581:3758–3769

Puzio-Kuter AM (2011) The role of p53 in metabolic regulation. Genes Cancer 2:385–391

Raj L, Ide T, Gurkar AU et al (2011) Selective killing of cancer cells by a small molecule targeting the stress response to ROS. Nature 475:231–234

Richards FM, Watson A, Hickman JA (1988) Investigation of the effects of heat shock and agents which induce a heat shock response on the induction of differentiation of HL-60 cells. Cancer Res 48:6715–6720

Ritossa F (1962) A new puffing pattern induced by temperature shock and DNP in drosophila. Cell Mol Life Sci 18:571–573

Robey RB, Hay N (2009) Is Akt the "Warburg kinase"?-Akt-energy metabolism interactions and oncogenesis. Semin Cancer Biol 19:25–31

Rodríguez-Enríquez S, Vital-González PA, Flores-Rodríguez FL et al (2006) Control of cellular proliferation by modulation of oxidative phosphorylation in human and rodent fast-growing tumor cells. Toxicol Appl Pharmacol 215:208–217

Salas A, Yao YG, Macaulay V et al (2005) A critical reassessment of the role of mitochondria in tumorigenesis. PLoS Med 2:296

Sánchez-Aragó M, Cuezva JM (2011) The bioenergetic signature of isogenic colon cancer cells predicts the cell death response to treatment with 3-bromopyruvate, iodoacetate or 5-fluorouracil. J Transl Med 9:19

Scatena R, Nocca G, Sole PD et al (1999) Bezafibrate as differentiating factor of human myeloid leukemia cells. Cell Death Differ 6:781–787

Scatena R, Bottoni P, Vincenzoni F et al (2003) Bezafibrate induces a mitochondrial derangement in human cell lines. Intriguing effects for a peroxisome proliferator. Chem Res Tox 16:1440–1447

Scatena R, Bottoni P, Martorana GE et al (2007) Mitochondria, ciglitazone and liver: a neglected interaction in biochemical pharmacology. Eur J Pharmacol 567:50–58

Scatena R, Bottoni P, Pontoglio A et al (2008) Glycolytic enzyme inhibitors in cancer treatment. Expert Opin Investig Drugs 17:1533–1545

Scatena R, Bottoni P, Pontoglio A, Giardina B (2010) Revisiting the Warburg effect in cancer cells with proteomics. The emergence of new approaches to diagnosis, prognosis and therapy. Proteomics Clin Appl 4:143–158

Schmitt E, Gehrmann M, Brunet M et al (2007) Intracellular and extracellular functions of heat shock proteins: repercussions in cancer therapy. J Leukoc Biol 81:15–27

Semenza GL (2007) Oxygen-dependent regulation of mitochondrial respiration by hypoxia-inducible factor 1. Biochem J 405:1–9

Semenza GL (2009) Regulation of cancer cell metabolism by hypoxia-inducible factor 1. Semin Cancer Biol 19:12–16

Shanware NP, Mullen AR, DeBerardinis RJ, Abraham RT (2011) Glutamine: pleiotropic roles in tumor growth and stress resistance. J Mol Med (Berl) 89:229–236

Shaw RJ (2006) Glucose metabolism and cancer. Curr Opin Cell Biol 18:598–608

Smith DF, Whitesell L, Katsanis E (1998) Molecular chaperones: biology and prospects for pharmacological intervention. Pharmacol Res 50:493–513

Smolková K, Bellance N, Scandurra F et al (2010) Mitochondrial bioenergetic adaptations of breast cancer cells to aglycemia and hypoxia. J Bioenerg Biomembr 42:55–67

Soti C, Nagy E, Giricz Z et al (2005) Heat shock proteins as emerging therapeutic targets. Br J Pharmacol 146:769–780

Sur R, Lyte PA, Southall MD (2008) Hsp27 regulates proinflammatory mediator release in keratinocytes by modulating NF-kappaB signaling. J Invest Dermatol 128:1116–1122

Takahashi A, Ohtani N, Yamakoshi K (2006) Mitogenic signalling and the p16INK4a-Rb pathway cooperate to enforce irreversible cellular senescence. Nat Cell Biol 8:1291–1297

Vander Heiden MG, Cantley LC, Thompson CB (2009) Understanding the Warburg effect: the metabolic requirements of cell proliferation. Science 324:1029–1033

Vander Heiden MG, Christofk HR, Schuman E et al (2010) Identification of small molecule inhibitors of pyruvate kinase M2. Biochem Pharmacol 79:1118–1124

Wada T, Tanji N, Ozawa A et al (2006) Mitochondrial DNA mutations and 8-hydroxy-2'-deoxyguanosine Content in Japanese patients with urinary bladder and renal cancers. Anticancer Res 26:3403–3408

Wadhwa R, Ryu J, Gao R et al (2010) Proproliferative functions of Drosophila small mitochondrial heat shock protein 22 in human cells. J Biol Chem 285:3833–3839

Wang XY, Chen X, Oh HJ et al (2000) Characterization of native interaction of hsp110 with hsp25 and hsc70. FEBS Lett 465:98–102

Warburg O (1925) Über den Stoffwechsel der Carcinomzelle. Klin Wochenschr 4:534–536

Weinberg F, Hamanaka R, Wheaton WW et al (2010) Mitochondrial metabolism and ROS generation are essential for Kras-mediated tumorigenicity. Proc Natl Acad Sci USA 107:8788–8793

Wellen KE, Hatzivassiliou G, Sachdeva UM et al (2009) ATP-citrate lyase links cellular metabolism to histone acetylation. Science 324:1076–1080

Wu CW, Yin PH, Hung WY et al (2005) Mitochondrial DNA mutations and mitochondrial DNA depletion in gastric cancer. Genes Chromosomes Cancer 44:19–28

Wu M, Neilson A, Swift AL et al (2007) Multiparameter metabolic analysis reveals a close link between attenuated mitochondrial bioenergetic function and enhanced glycolysis dependency in human tumor cells. Am J Physiol Cell Physiol 292:C125–C136

Yan H, Parsons DW, Jin G et al (2009) IDH1 and IDH2 mutations in gliomas. N Engl J Med 360:765–773

Yeung SJ, Pan J, Lee MH (2008) Roles of p53, MYC and HIF-1 in regulating glycolysis – the seventh hallmark of cancer. Cell Mol Life Sci 65:3981–3999

Zhang E, Zhang C, Su Y et al (2011) Newly developed strategies for multifunctional mitochondria-targeted agents in cancer therapy. Drug Discov Today 16:140–146

Zhou J, Schmid T, Frank R et al (2004) PI3K/Akt is required for heat shock proteins to protect hypoxia-inducible factor 1alpha from pVHL-independent degradation. J Biol Chem 279:13506–13513

Zu XL, Guppy M (2004) Cancer metabolism: facts, fantasy, and fiction. Biochem Biophys Res Commun 313:459–465

Part III
Mitochondria, Aging and Pharmacotoxicological Aspects

Chapter 14
Mitochondria and Aging

Hsin-Chen Lee and Yau-Huei Wei

Abstract Aging is a degenerative process that is associated with progressive accumulation of deleterious changes with time, reduction of physiological function and increase in the chance of disease and death. Studies in several species reveal a wide spectrum of alterations in mitochondria and mitochondrial DNA (mtDNA) with aging, including (1) increased disorganization of mitochondrial structure, (2) decline in mitochondrial oxidative phosphorylation (OXPHOS) function, (3) accumulation of mtDNA mutation, (4) increased mitochondrial production of reactive oxygen species (ROS) and (5) increased extent of oxidative damage to DNA, proteins, and lipids. In this chapter, we outline the common alterations in mitochondria of the aging tissues and recent advances in understanding the role of mitochondrial H_2O_2 production and mtDNA mutation in the aging process and lifespan determination. In addition, we discuss the effect of caloric restriction on age-associated mitochondrial changes and its role in longevity. Taking these findings together, we suggest that decline in mitochondrial energy metabolism, enhanced mitochondrial oxidative stress, and accumulation of mtDNA mutations are important contributors to human aging.

Keywords Aging • mtDNA • Mitochondria • ROS • Oxidative damage • Caloric restriction

14.1 Introduction

Aging is a degenerative process that is characterized by a time-dependent decline in physiological function and an increase in the chance of disease and death. The deleterious changes with time occur in all organisms that are believed to be associated with the metabolic activity and are influenced by

H.-C. Lee, Ph.D. (✉)
Institute of Pharmacology, School of Medicine, National Yang-Ming University,
No. 155, Sec. 2, Li-Nong St., Peitou, Taipei, Taiwan 112, Republic of China
e-mail: hclee2@ym.edu.tw

Y.-H. Wei
Department of Biochemistry and Molecular Biology, National Yang-Ming University,
Taipei, Taiwan, Republic of China

Department of Medicine, Mackay Medical College, Danshui, Taipei County, Taiwan, Republic of China

R. Scatena et al. (eds.), *Advances in Mitochondrial Medicine*, Advances in Experimental
Medicine and Biology 942, DOI 10.1007/978-94-007-2869-1_14,
© Springer Science+Business Media B.V. 2012

genetic and environmental factors. In the early 1950s, Harman considered factors which influenced aging and searched for factors capable of causing death that was present in every living organism, and proposed the "free radical theory of aging". He contended that free radicals, produced from normal metabolism, could be the cause of aging and aging-related degenerative diseases (Harman 1956). In 1972, he modified his theory and proposed that mitochondria are both the main source and a major target of free radicals, and the accumulation of damage with time leads to aging (Harman 1972). In 1980, Miquel and associates suggested that the progressive membrane damage in mitochondria of postmitotic cells by free radicals and lipid peroxides, as by-products of the reduction of oxygen during respiration, could cause an age-related decrease in the amount of functionally competent mitochondria with concomitant decline in cellular production of ATP and increased peroxide generation (Miquel et al. 1980). Linnane et al. (1989) further proposed that accumulation of somatic mutations in mitochondrial DNA (mtDNA) is a major contributor to human aging and degenerative diseases. The free radical theory of aging has thus been extended to the "Mitochondrial theory of aging".

Mitochondria are the main cellular energy sources that generate ATP through the process of respiration and oxidative phosphorylation (OXPHOS) in the inner membrane of mitochondria. The respiratory chain of the OXPHOS system is also the primary intracellular source of reactive oxygen species (ROS) and free radicals under normal physiological and pathological conditions. In addition, mitochondria play a central role in a variety of cellular processes, including β-oxidation of fatty acids, phospholipid biosynthesis, calcium signaling, and apoptosis.

Mitochondria contain their own DNA (mtDNA) and the mitochondrial genome is important in the maintenance of functionally competent organelle. Although the majority of the proteins involved in the OXPHOS are encoded by nuclear DNA, translated in the cytoplasm and are imported into the mitochondria, the mitochondrial genome codes for 2 rRNAs and 22 tRNAs which are required for intramitochondrial protein synthesis, and 13 polypeptides of the respiratory enzyme complexes required for normal function of the OXPHOS system. Distinct from nuclear DNA, mtDNA can be replicated independently of the cell cycle and is present in multiple copies within each cell. The actual number of mtDNA varies between cell types and is dependent on the energy demands within each cell. Any mutations in the mtDNA can co-exist with wild-type copies, a condition called heteroplasmy. The mutant mtDNAs do not exert a biochemical phenotype on a cell until the mutant load reach a certain level. The threshold of mutant/wild type can vary depending on the specific mutation and the cell type.

Mitochondrial theory of aging proposes that progressive accumulation of somatic mutations in mtDNA during an individual's lifetime causes a decline in mitochondrial bioenergetic function and is a contributory factor of aging. Under normal physiological conditions ROS are generated at very low levels during mitochondrial respiration. The complexes I and III of the respiratory chain are the main sites that electrons are leaked out to generate superoxide anions, which can be further converted to H_2O_2 and hydroxyl radicals. It has been estimated that 2–5% of oxygen consumed by mitochondria can be converted to ROS. Most of these ROS can be removed by antioxidants and free radical scavenging enzymes. However, some leakage in the antioxidant protection can damage DNA, proteins and lipids. Oxidative damage to mtDNA may lead to strand breaks of DNA and the occurrence of mutations in mtDNA. Accumulation of these mtDNA mutations could result in dysfunction of the respiratory chain, leading to increased ROS production in mitochondria and subsequent accumulation of more mtDNA mutations. This vicious cycle has been proposed to account for an increase in oxidative damage during aging, which leads to the progressive decline of cellular and tissue functions as a result of insufficient supply of energy and increased susceptibility to apoptosis (Linnane et al. 1989; Wei 1992; Lee and Wei 2007).

In the past decades, these aging theories have been extensively tested by many approaches and substantial supportive evidence has been gained from molecular and cellular biological studies. Studies from aging humans and animals have shown good correlations between aging, mitochondrial function decline, and accumulation of mtDNA mutations. However, although it is clear that oxidative damage increases during aging, the role of mitochondrial oxidative stress in the aging process remains controversial. This chapter reviews recent advances in the understanding of the roles that alterations of mitochondria and mtDNA may play in aging. In addition, the roles of ROS in aging-associated mitochondrial function decline and somatic mtDNA mutation, and the effect of caloric restriction on mitochondria in aging are discussed.

14.2 Changes of Mitochondrial Morphology with Age

Evidence based on electron microscopic studies has shown that mitochondrial disorganization accumulated with age in a variety of tissues, especially postmitotic cells such as neurons and muscle cells. Age-related changes in the muscle mitochondria of insects (e.g., flies) have been described, including a decrease in the number of mitochondria accompanied by an enlargement and more irregular structure of the remaining mitochondria, a loss of the stacked arrays of mitochondrial cristae, and a disruption of crystal packing with expansion of the intracristal space (Miquel et al. 1980). Similar age-related changes were also observed in the myocardium, the skeletal muscle, liver, kidney, and the cerebral cortex of mammals (e.g., mice, rats, and human subjects). The mitochondrial structural changes in these old organisms included a decrease in the total number of mitochondria, an increase in their size, and a decrease in the number of mitochondrial cristae (Miquel et al. 1980).

Recent work has shown that mitochondria are very dynamic organelles and maintain a constant remodeling of mitochondrial architecture, allowing morphological transitions from individual structures to complex tubular networks through fusion and fission (Chen and Chan 2009). It has been established that this dynamic structure is regulated by proteins controlling fission, such as hFis1 and Drp1, and fusion, such as mitofusin 1 and 2 (MFN1 and 2) and OPA1. These proteins appear to be critical for normal mitochondrial function and abnormalities in mitochondrial dynamics play an important role in the pathophysiology of neurodegenerative diseases (Chen and Chan 2009). Evidence reveals that the fission-related protein hFis1 has been associated with the process of senescence in mammalian cells (Lee et al. 2007). Using RNA interference to reduce hFis1 in mammalian cells, it was found that mitochondria become enlarged and flattened and these morphological changes are correlated with increased β-galactosidase activity, a marker of cell senescence, and decreased mitochondrial membrane potential, increased ROS generation and DNA damage. This suggests that hFis1 plays an important role in cell senescence and both the structure and dynamics of mitochondrial architecture are important factors involved in the cell senescence program. However, the role of proteins that regulate fission/fusion in aging warrants further investigation.

14.3 Mitochondrial OXPHOS Function Declines with Age

Bioenergetic studies of the human and animals have suggested that respiratory function of mitochondria declines in aging post-mitotic tissues. Immunohistochemical staining showed that cytochrome c oxidase (COX)-negative cardiomyocytes and muscle fibers are present in the heart, limb, diaphragm and extraocular muscle of normal elderly subjects, and that the number of COX-negative muscle fibers is increased with age in the human subjects (Müller-Höcker 1989, 1990; Müller-Höcker et al. 1993). Moreover, a decrease of COX proteins was observed in aged human brain (Ojaimi et al. 1999a). An age-related increase in the number of COX-negative muscle fibers was also found in fruit flies, *Drosophila melanogaster* (DiMauro et al. 2002).

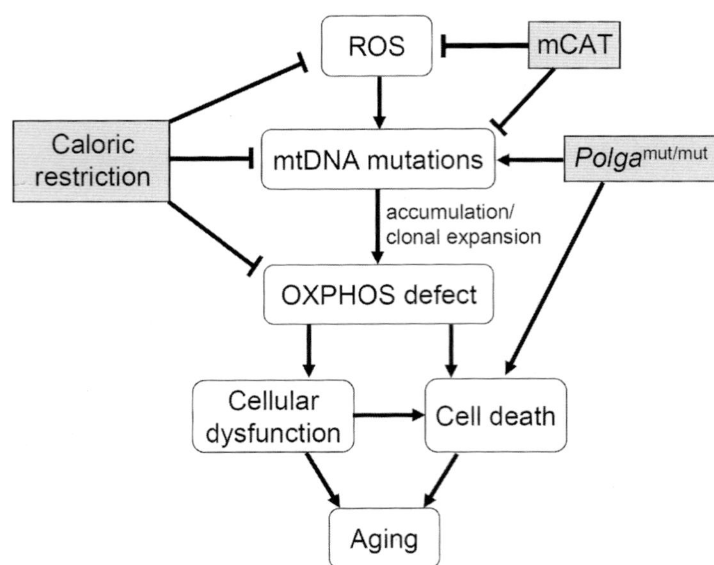

Fig. 14.1 Mitochondrial role in the aging process. There is increasing amount of evidence to suggest that accumulation of mitochondrial DNA (*mtDNA*) mutations with age plays a role in cellular dysfunction in many tissues. MtDNA mutations could be caused by increased oxidative stress. If a mutated mtDNA molecule is replicated and clonally expanded within a cell, this cell may become deficient in respiration and oxidative phosphorylation (*OXPHOS*). The compromised energy production could lead to cellular dysfunction and/or cell death, which may result in tissue dysfunction and onset of aging. Recent studies revealed that overexpressing human catalase localized to mitochondria (*mCAT*) can reduce mtDNA mutations in tissues during aging and increase the lifespan of transgenic mice. Mitochondrial DNA polymerase γ-mutated mice (*Polga^{mut/mut}*) can accumulate high level of mtDNA mutations and increased apoptosis in tissues and develop premature aging phenotype. In addition, caloric restriction has been demonstrated to be able to delay the onset of age-associated phenotypes and extend lifespan in diverse living organisms. It has also been found that caloric restriction is able to reduce the rate of mitochondrial ROS production, mtDNA mutations, and the abnormalities in the mitochondrial OXPHOS system. These lines of evidence have supported the concept that the decline in energy metabolism, ROS overproduction and accumulation of mtDNA mutations in tissue cells are important factors that contribute to the aging process

Numerous biochemical studies on isolated mitochondria revealed that the electron transport activities of respiratory enzyme complexes gradually decline with age in the brain, skeletal muscle, liver and skin fibroblasts of normal human subjects (Trounce et al. 1989; Yen et al. 1989; Cooper et al. 1992; Hsieh et al. 1994; Boffoli et al. 1994; Ojaimi et al. 1999b; Greco et al. 2003; Short et al. 2005). Similar age-related decline in the activities of respiratory enzymes was also demonstrated in the flight muscle of flies (Bulos et al. 1972, 1975), as well as in skeletal muscle, heart, liver of rats (Torii et al. 1992a, b; Takasawa et al. 1993; Sugiyama et al. 1993; Lesnefsky and Hoppel 2006) and dogs (Sugiyama et al. 1993), and in brain of rhesus monkeys (Bowling et al. 1993).

Age-related decrease in ADP-stimulated (State 3) respiration and respiratory control of isolated mitochondria were reported in flies (Martinez and McDaniel 1979) and in the myocardium of old rats (Murfitt and Sanadi 1978). The respiratory control ratio, OXPHOS efficiency, the rates of resting and ADP-stimulated respiration and ATP synthesis of isolated mitochondria were all found to decline, although with different degrees, with age in the skeletal muscle and liver (Trounce et al. 1989; Yen et al. 1989) and in human skin fibroblasts (Greco et al. 2003). The age-associated decrease in mitochondrial membrane potential, the driving force for OXPHOS and the increase in proton leakage of the respiratory chain were found to correlate with reduced ATP synthesis in tissues of old animals (Pieri et al. 1993; Hagen et al. 1997; Harper et al. 1998) and in skin fibroblasts from elderly subjects (Greco et al. 2003). A study further confirmed that the activities of mitochondrial respiratory enzymes and that mitochondrial ATP production rate are declined with age in muscle biopsies from 146 healthy subjects (Short et al. 2005).

One study assessed *in vivo* rates of mitochondrial oxidative metabolism by ^{13}C nuclear magnetic resonance (NMR) spectroscopy and phosphorylation activity by ^{31}P NMR and found approximately 40% reduction in oxidative phosphorylation activity of mitochondria in skeletal muscle of healthy elderly subjects as compared with that of the young controls (Petersen et al. 2003).

The age-associated decreases in mitochondrial respiratory proteins and OXPHOS function could be resulted from the decline in the rates of mtDNA transcription and mitochondrial protein synthesis. Many lines of evidence revealed that steady-state levels of mitochondrial RNA transcripts are decreased in old *D. melanogaster* (Calleja et al. 1993) and in various aging tissues of the human and animals (Gadaleta et al. 1990; Fernandez-Silva et al. 1991; Barrientos et al. 1997a, b). Moreover, an age-dependent decline in the rate of protein synthesis was observed in *D. melanogaster*, mouse liver and kidney (Marcus et al. 1982; Bailey and Webster 1984), and human skeletal muscle (Rooyackers et al. 1996) as well as skin fibroblasts (Greco et al. 2003). The age-related decrease in mitochondrial gene transcripts and proteins of human skeletal muscle was found to closely relate to the reduction of mtDNA content and the ATP production rate of mitochondria (Short et al. 2005).

Different lines of evidence from immunohistochemical staining, biochemical studies and *in vivo* investigations have supported the central idea that the decline in bioenergetic function of mitochondria plays an important role in aging (Fig. 14.1). The decline in mitochondrial respiratory function can lead to lower ATP production and more ROS formation in aged tissues.

14.4 MtDNA Mutations Accumulate with Age

Numerous molecular studies using polymerase chain reaction (PCR) or quantitative PCR techniques demonstrated that somatic mutations in mtDNA progressively accumulate with age in a variety of tissues of humans (Yen et al. 1991; Torii et al. 1992a, b; Lee et al. 1994a), rhesus monkeys (Schwarze et al. 1995) and rodents (Khaidakov et al. 2003). These age-related mtDNA mutations include large-scale deletions (Yen et al. 1991; Zhang et al. 1992; Lee et al. 1994a), tandem duplications (Lee et al. 1994b; Wei et al. 1996) and point mutations (Zhang et al. 1993; Münscher et al. 1993; Michikawa et al. 1999; Wang et al. 2001; Khaidakov et al. 2003). Many lines of studies have revealed that multiple deletions of mtDNA occur in the skeletal muscle, heart, and brain of aged human subjects and mice, and suggest that a broad spectrum of mtDNA deletions is accumulated with age. Many types of tandem duplications in the D-loop region of mtDNA were identified in a variety of tissues of elderly subjects (Lee et al. 1994b; Wei et al. 1996). Some pathogenic point mutations in the tRNA genes of mtDNA (Münscher et al. 1993; Zhang et al. 1993) and high levels of point mutations in the D-loop region of mtDNA (Michikawa et al. 1999; Wang et al. 2001) have also been found to accumulate with age in human tissues and cultured human skin fibroblasts.

It has been observed that terminally differentiated tissues with active oxidative metabolism, such as skeletal muscle, heart, and brain, accumulate relatively higher levels of mutant mtDNA during the aging process. Many of these mtDNA mutations start to occur after mid-1930s and accumulate with age in post-mitotic tissues of humans (Yen et al. 1991; Lee et al. 1994a). It is noteworthy that occurrence of mtDNA deletions was correlated with the reduction of mitochondrial respiratory chain enzyme activities in aging human skeletal muscles (Hsieh et al. 1994; Lezza et al. 1994).

Initially, most studies showed that the overall proportion of a specific mutant mtDNA is lower than a level of approximately 0.1% of total mtDNA molecules in any somatic tissue examined (Wei and Lee 2002). The levels are far lower than a threshold of mtDNA mutation (~80–100% of the mtDNA) required for the expression of a defective electron transport system in patients with mitochondrial myopathies (Shoubridge et al. 1990; Schon et al. 1994; He et al. 2002). However, it could be because most investigators screened for mtDNA mutations in the whole tissue rather than individual cells. The mutated mtDNA molecules may be unevenly distributed and can accumulate clonally in certain cells, causing a mosaic pattern of respiratory chain deficiency in somatic tissues during aging. Besides, the unevenly distributed mutant mtDNA molecules were largely diluted by wild-type mtDNA when the whole tissue was used to screen for mtDNA mutations. The idea was supported by some evidence that the proportion of mtDNA with a large-scale deletion was well correlated with that of COX-negative fibers in the same subjects (Kovalenko et al. 1997; Pesce et al. 2001). Using a single fiber PCR method or the laser-capture micro-dissection technique (Kopsidas et al. 1998; Cao et al. 2001; Wanagat et al. 2001), it was further demonstrated that COX-negative fibers in the skeletal muscle of normal elderly subjects and aged rats contain reduced levels of full-length mtDNA and high levels of mtDNA deletions.

Using both histological and polymerase chain reaction (PCR) analyses, it was shown that mtDNA deletions clonally accumulate to high levels within COX$^-$/SDH$^+$ regions (>90% of total mtDNA) in vastus lateralis muscle of human subjects aged 49–93 years (Bua et al. 2006). Moreover, the amplitude of decline in the levels of the deletion-containing mtDNA in the transition regions and in mitochondrial electron transport chain-normal regions immediately adjacent to the transition regions suggest that the accumulation of mtDNA deletions precedes the electron transport chain deficiency (Bua et al. 2006). The high levels of accumulated mtDNA deletion were also observed to link to enzymatic and morphological abnormalities of mitochondria such as fiber splitting, atrophy, and breakage in muscle fibers from aged rats (Herbst et al. 2007). These observations strongly support the notion that mtDNA deletions play a causal role in mitochondrial dysfunction of skeletal-muscle fibers with age, a process that ultimately leads to fiber loss.

Studies on the dissected substantia nigra of post-mortem human brains further revealed that very high levels of mtDNA deletions are present in dopaminergic neurons from very old individuals (Bender et al. 2006; Kraytsberg et al. 2006). Importantly, the proportion of mtDNA with deletions increased significantly with age and neurons containing over 60% of deleted mtDNA molecules were associated with a striking loss of COX activity. These findings suggest that mtDNA mosaic seems to parallel the occurrence of the bioenergy mosaic, and mtDNA mutations can reach rather high levels in the cells of elderly subjects. The accumulation of mtDNA mutations with age in tissues of human and rodents can cause adverse effects and may play a causal role in aging (Fig. 14.1).

Although actual mechanism for the formation of mtDNA deletions has remained unclear, oxidative damage-associated single- or double-strand DNA breaks might be involved in their formation. It has been shown that the proportion of mtDNA with deletions correlates with the level of oxidative modification (8-OHdG content) of mtDNA (Hayakawa et al. 1992). It has also been demonstrated that treatment of human skin fibroblasts with sublethal dose of oxidative stress results in the formation and accumulation of the common 4,977 bp deletion in mtDNA (Dumont et al. 2000). In addition to normal aging, environmental insults, such as UV irradiation (Pang et al. 1994; Yang et al. 1995; Berneburg et al. 1999), cigarette smoking (Fahn et al. 1998; Lee et al. 1999), and betel quid chewing (Lee et al. 2001), have been demonstrated to increase the levels of mtDNA with large-scale deletion. These studies suggest that oxidative damage to mtDNA is a major cause of instability and mutations (point mutation and deletion) of the mitochondrial genome in the tissues of elderly subjects (Linnane et al. 1989; Beckman and Ames 1998). These findings provided evidence to support the notion that ROS and free radicals play an important role in the mechanism underlying aging-associated somatic mutation of mtDNA.

14.5 Mitochondrial ROS Production Increases with Age

A majority of intracellular ROS are thought to be generated as byproducts of oxidation-reduction reactions in mitochondrial respiratory chain (Beckman and Ames 1998). Knowledge of how mitochondria produce ROS is based on the evidence from isolated mitochondria. During respiration, superoxide anions ($O_2^{\cdot-}$) and organic free radicals (e.g., ubisemiquinone and flavosemiquinone) are generated from mitochondria, mainly through Complex I and Complex III in the respiratory chain (Chance et al. 1979; Wei et al. 1981). Although it is still not clear about the actual rate of mitochondrial ROS production *in vivo*, it was estimated that about 2% of the oxygen consumed by isolated mitochondria from mammalian tissues is converted to ROS, including superoxide anions, hydrogen peroxide (H_2O_2), and hydroxyl radicals (Chance et al. 1979; Beckman and Ames 1998).

Evidence supporting the link of mitochondrial generation of superoxide anions and H_2O_2 to aging is provided by studies on isolated mitochondria of tissues from insects and mammals (Ku et al. 1993; Sohal et al. 1995). It was reported that the average lifespan of different species of flies is inversely correlated with the rate of mitochondrial superoxide anions and H_2O_2 generation (Sohal et al. 1995). Similar correlations were also observed in the comparison among different mammalian species, including mouse, hamster, rat, guinea pig, rabbits, pig, and cow (Ku et al. 1993). Moreover, the rates of ROS production from mitochondria are increased with age in the brain, heart, and kidney of mice (Sohal et al. 1994).

It has become clear that under resting conditions in which mitochondria are not actively making ATP, mitochondria exhibit a low rate of oxygen consumption, high membrane potential across the inner membrane, and high proportion of reduced electron carriers ($NADH/NAD^+$ ratio and $CoQH_2/CoQ$ ratio), the rates of ROS production from isolated mitochondria are high (Murphy 2009). This suggests that *in vivo* factors leading to these conditions will favor ROS production. However, the extent to which these situations arise *in vivo* with age is not clear.

14.6 Oxidative Damages Accumulate with Age

Several antioxidant enzymes and small-molecular-weight antioxidants within the cell and mitochondrion can cope with and dispose of most of ROS generated by aerobic metabolism under normal physiological conditions. The important antioxidant enzymes include manganese superoxide dismutase (MnSOD), copper/zinc superoxide dismutase (Cu/ZnSOD), glutathione peroxidase (GPx) and catalase. Superoxide anions can be dismutated to H_2O_2 by MnSOD and Cu/ZnSOD. MnSOD is located in the mitochondrial matrix and CuZnSOD is localized in the mitochondrial intermembrane space and cytosol (Okado-Matsumoto and Fridovich 2001; O'Brien et al. 2004; Inarrea et al. 2007). H_2O_2 can be scavenged by either GPx in the mitochondrial matrix or catalase in the cytosol. Although several studies on age-related changes in antioxidant enzymes have generated conflicting results (Sohal et al. 1994; Beckman and Ames 1998; Lu et al. 1999), it is generally accepted that a leakage of ROS from mitochondria and an excess production of ROS that overwhelms the antioxidant defense system can cause oxidative damage to cellular constituents, including nucleic acids, lipids, and proteins. As the major intracellular source of ROS, mitochondria are subjected to direct attack by ROS in animal and human cells. Moreover, superoxide anions in the intermembrane space might be released into the cytosol through the voltage-dependent anion channel (VDAC) (Han et al. 2003), and H_2O_2 can move across mitochondrial membranes into the cytosol to damage extra-mitochondrial constituents.

Many lines of evidence suggest that oxidative damage to nuclear DNA and mtDNA of tissue cells are increased with age of the mammals (Beckman and Ames 1998; Hamilton et al. 2001a, b). Some characteristics of mammalian mtDNA were thought to render it to be highly susceptible to oxidative damage, including its close proximity to the sites of ROS production from the respiratory chain, lack of protection by histones, and limited capacity for repair of DNA damage. It has been documented that the steady-state levels of oxidative modifications observed in mtDNA, especially 8-OH-dG, are several-fold higher than those in nuclear DNA (Richter et al. 1988; Ames et al. 1993; Barja and Herrero 2000; Hamilton et al. 2001a, b). The levels of oxidative modifications in mtDNA of the diaphragm and heart muscle were found to increase with the age of human subjects (Hayakawa et al. 1991, 1992). The age-associated oxidative damage to mtDNA was shown to correlate with mitochondrial glutathione oxidation in the liver, kidney and brain of rats and mice (de la Asuncion et al. 1996). In addition to modifications of the purine and pyrimidine bases, oxidative damage to DNA can lead to abasic sites, single- and double-strand breaks as well as cross-links to other DNA molecules. DNA damage accumulation can block the progression of DNA polymerase resulting in decreased amplification of the target sequence. Studies using a gene-specific DNA damage assay based on quantitative PCR revealed that mtDNA is more susceptible to oxidative damage than is nuclear DNA (Yakes and van Houten 1997), and that the mtDNA damage accumulates with age in post-mitotic tissues (Lin et al. 2003).

The hydroxyl radical is one of the most potent inducers of lipid peroxidation. It has been shown that the content of lipid peroxides in mitochondria is increased with age (Hruszkewycz 1992). The extent of lipid peroxidation was also correlated with alterations in mitochondrial respiration and OXPHOS activity, inner membrane barrier properties, maintenance of mitochondrial membrane potential, and mitochondrial Ca^{2+} buffering capacity (Britton et al. 1990; Albano et al. 1991; Bacon et al. 1993). Cardiolipin resides primarily in the inner membrane of mitochondria and the highly unsaturated nature of the fatty acyl chains in cardiolipin is required for optimal function of many of the proteins involved in mitochondrial respiratory chain. It has been shown that increased ROS production from mitochondria may result in oxidation and depletion of cardiolipin, as well as inhibition of COX activity (Paradies et al. 2000). Peroxidation of cardiolipin can impair the barrier function of the inner membrane and facilitate the detachment of cytochrome c from mitochondrial respiratory chain and contribute to apoptosis (Petrosillo et al. 2001).

On the other hand, it has been shown that the amounts of proteins with oxidative modifications, such as oxidation of the sulfhydryl groups of proteins or the formation of protein carbonyls, in mitochondria are increased with age (Sohal et al. 1994; Agarwal and Sohal 1995; Sohal 2002). The age-related increase in the level of oxidized proteins was also observed in human skin fibroblasts and the mitochondrial fraction accumulated higher levels of protein carbonyl than the whole-cell lysate of these skin fibroblasts (Miyoshi et al. 2006). This increase in the level of proteins with oxidative modification correlated with a decline in the intracellular ATP level (Miyoshi et al. 2006). Aconitase and adenine nucleotide translocase (ANT) have been found to be the preferred targets of oxidative damage to mitochondrial proteins during aging of the animals (Gardner et al. 1994; Yan et al. 1997; Yan and Sohal 1998). In addition, DNA polymerase γ was shown as one of the major targets of oxidative damage in mitochondrial matrix, which may contribute to a reduction in mtDNA replication and DNA repair activities in mitochondria (Graziewicz et al. 2002). Oxidative modification of proteins can alter protein structure and/or result in a loss of their normal function, which might lead to further ROS production from mitochondria.

14.7 Role of Mitochondrial ROS in Aging

The evidence that mitochondrial ROS production and accumulation of oxidative damage increase with age corroborates the possibility that mitochondrial ROS cause adverse effects in aging. To investigate the importance of mitochondrial ROS in aging, several genetics approaches have been used.

Studies of animals deficient in MnSOD have provided evidence to substantiate the role of mitochondrial superoxide anions in aging. Mice deficient in the MnSOD exhibited neonatal lethality in association with dilated cardiomyopathy and lipid accumulation in the liver (Li et al. 1995; Melov et al. 1999). These mice also displayed severe mitochondrial dysfunction and enhanced oxidative damage to mitochondria (Li et al. 1995; Melov et al. 1999). The $Sod2^{+/-}$ mice showed partially reduced (30–80%) scavenging activity for superoxide anions in all tissues throughout life and had an increased oxidative damage to mitochondria as compared with the $Sod2^{+/+}$ mice (Williams et al. 1998; Kokoszka et al. 2001; Van Remmen et al. 2003; Mansouri et al. 2006). However, the activities of respiratory enzyme Complex I and ATP synthase were not significantly reduced in old Sod2$^{+/-}$ mice compared with age-matched wild-type mice (Mansouri et al. 2006). In addition, several aging biomarkers, such as cataract formation, defective immune response, and formation of glycoxidation products such as carboxymethyl lysine and pentosidine in skin collagen, change with age in the similar extent in both wild-type mice and the Sod2$^{+/-}$ mice (van Remmen et al. 2003). Importantly, the life spans of the Sod2$^{+/-}$ mice were not shorter than those of wild-type mice, which suggest that increased mitochondrial superoxide anions production is not sufficient for acceleration of the aging process (van Remmen et al. 2003).

On the other hand, it was shown that transgenic mice that over-expressed a mitochondrially localized version of the human catalase (mCAT) exhibit prolonged median and maximum lifespan (Schriner et al. 2005). The extension of lifespan was associated with a specifically increased H_2O_2-scavenging activity in mitochondria and attenuated oxidative damage to mtDNA, as well as reduced accumulations of deletion and point mutation of mtDNA in heart and muscle tissues (Schriner et al. 2005; Vermulst et al. 2007, 2008). The results suggest that mitochondrial H_2O_2 plays an important role in aging and determination of lifespan of the animals (Fig. 14.1).

14.8 Consequences of Somatic mtDNA Mutations in Aging

Human mitochondrial genome codes for 13 polypeptides, which are crucial components of the OXPHOS system, and two rRNAs (12S and 16S) and 22 tRNAs essential for protein synthesis in mitochondria. Because of the crucial role of mitochondrial genome in the OXPHOS function, accumulation of mtDNA mutations can result in energy crisis, oxidative stress or cell death, which may contribute to aging phenotype.

The causal role of mtDNA mutations in mammalian aging is supported by the studies using mtDNA mutator mice harboring homozygous genetic defects in the proofreading exonuclease activity of mitochondrial DNA polymerase γ (Polg A) (Trifunovic et al. 2004; Kujoth et al. 2005). These mtDNA mutator mice were found to accumulate elevated levels of mtDNA mutations, including point mutations and deletions. There was a mosaic pattern with COX deficiency, an accumulation of abnormal mitochondria, and a progressive reduction of respiratory chain enzyme activities and mitochondrial ATP production rate in the hearts of the mtDNA mutator mice (Trifunovic et al. 2004). Importantly, the mtDNA mutator mice had a reduced lifespan and exhibited accelerated onset of aging-related phenotypes such as weight loss, reduced subcutaneous fat, alopecia (hair loss), kyphosis (curvature of the spine), loss of muscle mass (sarcopenia), osteoporosis, anemia, thymic involution, testicular atrophy associated with the depletion spermatogonia, reduced fertility, loss of intestinal crypts, heart enlargement and hearing loss (Trifunovic et al. 2004; Kujoth et al. 2005). These findings have provided strong evidence to support the notion that accelerating the mtDNA mutation rate can result in premature aging.

According to the mitochondrial theory of aging, these accumulated mtDNA mutations may compromise the integrity of the electron transport chain and increase the formation of ROS, creating a vicious cycle of mutagenesis that continuously amplifies the production of cytotoxic oxygen free radicals. However, it was found that despite increased mutational load in mtDNA, mitochondria from these mtDNA mutator mice did not show increased oxidative stress (Kujoth et al. 2005). Levels of H_2O_2, markers of oxidative damage to DNA (8-OH-dG), proteins (protein carbonyls) and lipids (F2-isoprostanes) were not significantly different in the somatic tissues between mutant and wild-type mice. In addition, mouse embryonic fibroblasts from mtDNA mutator mice exhibited normal rate of ROS production and did not show increased sensitivity to oxidative stress (Trifunovic et al. 2005). There were no significant changes in the levels of antioxidant enzymes, protein carbonyls, and aconitase enzyme activity in tissues from the mtDNA mutator mice. These findings indicate that there was no or only minor oxidative stress in tissues from these mice (Trifunovic et al. 2005).

Therefore, although the mtDNA mutator mice accumulated mtDNA mutations and exhibited severe respiratory chain dysfunction, accelerated development of aging phenotype through mtDNA mutations can occur in the absence of increased ROS production or oxidative stress. However, this does not rule out the possibility that mtDNA mutation is downstream of mitochondrial ROS generation.

Evidence from mouse embryonic fibroblasts derived from the mtDNA mutator mice revealed that accelerated aging in the mice is not associated with an intrinsic defect in cellular proliferation or accelerated cellular senescence (Kujoth et al. 2005). Instead, the tissue dysfunction and pathological changes in the mtDNA mutator mice were found to associate with the extent of apoptosis (Kujoth et al. 2005). The levels of apoptotic markers (e.g., caspase 3 activation) were found to increase more rapidly during aging in the mutator mice as compared with wild-type mice. These results suggest that age-related accumulation of mtDNA mutations in normal or Plog A mutant mice promote apoptosis and contribute to the decline of physiological function, which may be an important mechanism of aging in mammals (Fig. 14.1).

The mtDNA mutator mice have high levels of point mutations and deletions of mtDNA. Recent studies debated whether point mutations or deletions of mtDNA are the driving force behind premature aging in the mtDNA mutator mice (Vermulst et al. 2007, 2008; Edgar et al. 2009). Distinct from the mtDNA mutator mice with homozygous defects in the proofreading-deficient *Polga* allele (*Polga*$^{mut/mut}$), heterozygous mice (*Polga*$^{+/mut}$) did not show the features of accelerated aging and a significant reduction in the mean lifespan (Trifunovic et al. 2004; Kujoth et al. 2005). Using a more sensitive assay, Vermulst et al. (2007) found that heterozygous mice (*Polga*$^{+/mut}$) displayed more than 100-fold increase in the point mutation frequency without manifesting features of premature aging and thus suggested mtDNA point mutations do not limit the lifespan of normal mice. The same group further reported that mtDNA deletions are associated with a number of age-related pathologies of the mtDNA mutator mice, which suggest that mtDNA deletions drive premature aging in the mtDNA mutator mice (Vermulst et al. 2008). On the other hand, Edgar et al. (2009) reported that mitochondrial protein synthesis is unimpaired but the stability of several respiratory chain complexes is severely impaired in the mtDNA mutator mice. They suggested that random point mutations in mtDNA are the driving force behind premature aging in mtDNA mutator mice through causing amino acid substitutions in mtDNA-encoded respiratory chain subunits, which leads to decreased stability of the respiratory enzyme complexes and progressive decline of respiratory chain function (Edgar et al. 2009). In addition, it was found that the mtDNA mutator mice harbor linear mtDNAs (Trifunovic et al. 2004). Bailey et al. (2009) provided evidence that the linear mtDNAs were derived from replication intermediates and suggested that the mtDNA mutator mice display elevated replication pausing and chromosomal breakage at fragile sites of mtDNA and the perturbed mtDNA replication is likely to contribute to the pathophysiologic features of the mtDNA mutator mice.

The mtDNA mutator mice provided genetic evidence linking mtDNA mutations to aging phenotypes and shortened lifespan. However, the mechanism by which accelerated mtDNA mutation rate results in premature aging has remained unclear. It is an open question whether certain types of mtDNA mutations are particularly important for human aging and whether the functional impact of mtDNA mutations in mice is the same as those observed in the mammals and humans (Khrapko and Vijg 2009).

14.9 Effect of Caloric Restriction on Mitochondria in Aging

Caloric restriction, a reduction in caloric intake of 20–40% without malnutrition, is the only experimental manipulation that could delay the onset of age-associated phenotypes and extend the average and maximum lifespan in several living organisms ranging from yeast and nematodes to rodents and monkeys (Bordone and Guarente 2005). Caloric restriction could also reduce the incidence of age-related diseases including diabetes, cancer, cardiovascular disease, brain atrophy, immune deficiencies and mortality in rhesus monkeys (Roth et al. 2004; Colman et al. 2009).

Studies using oligonucleotide-based microarrays to analyze age-associated transcriptional changes in different species revealed that genes involved in mitochondrial energy metabolism showed similar age-related changes (Park and Prolla 2005; Zahn et al. 2007). A meta-analysis of age-related gene expression profiles using 27 datasets from mice, rats, and the human has identified several common signatures of aging, including increased expression of genes involved in inflammation and immune responses, and reduced expression of genes associated with mitochondrial energy metabolism (de Magalhães et al. 2009). Importantly, most of the age-associated alterations in gene expression can be completely or partially prevented by caloric restriction (Park and Prolla 2005). These studies in diverse species suggest that dysregulation of mitochondrial energy metabolism is a hallmark of aging, and that caloric restriction-induced metabolic reprogramming plays a critical role in its retardation of the aging process.

It has been proposed that caloric restriction increased longevity by metabolic changes linking to reducing ROS production and decreasing cellular damage (Sohal and Weindruch 1996; Gredilla and Barja 2005). It was reported that mitochondria isolated from caloric-restricted rodents exhibited a reduction in ROS production and a lower steady-state levels of oxidative stress as compared with animals fed on the ad libitum diet (Sohal et al. 1994; Gredilla et al. 2001; López-Torres et al. 2002; Sanz et al. 2005; Hagopian et al. 2005). Aging-related increases in the levels of oxidative damage to mtDNA, proteins and lipids in mitochondria were attenuated or prevented in caloric-restricted animals (Lass et al. 1998; Gredilla et al. 2001; López-Torres et al. 2002; Sanz et al. 2005).

In addition, caloric restriction significantly reduced the age-dependent decline of mitochondrial respiratory capacity (Sohal et al. 1994; Hagopian et al. 2005). It was demonstrated that caloric restriction attenuated the abnormalities of mitochondrial electron transport chain, but did not affect the length or associated fiber atrophy of the muscle with mitochondrial abnormalities (Bua et al. 2004). This suggests that calorie restriction affects the onset but not the progression of electron transport chain abnormalities, which thus limits a process that ultimately results in fiber breakage and fiber loss. Moreover, it was reported that caloric restriction reduces age-related accumulation of mtDNA deletions in skeletal muscle and liver of caloric-restricted rats (Lee et al. 1998; Cassano et al. 2004).

Based on the above-mentioned studies in several species, we suggest that caloric restriction changes energy metabolism, and this altered metabolic state can reduce mitochondrial ROS production and oxidative damage, prevent the formation of mtDNA mutation, and reduce abnormalities in mitochondrial electron transport chain as well as ATP synthesis, which retard the aging process and extend life span (Fig. 14.1). It awaits further study to elucidate the underlying mechanism by which caloric restriction leads to the reprogramming of energy metabolism.

14.10 Concluding Remarks

In this chapter, we have outlined several common mitochondrial changes in the aging process, which include increased disorganization of mitochondrial structure, progressive decline in mitochondrial OXPHOS function, accumulation of mtDNA mutations, as well as increased mitochondrial ROS production and oxidative damage. These age-associated changes in mitochondria are well correlated with the deteriorative processes of tissues in aging. Convincing evidence from several genetic approaches supports the causal role of mitochondrial H_2O_2 production and mtDNA mutation in the aging process and determination of lifespan of animals. In addition, it has been shown that caloric restriction without malnutrition can modulate energy metabolism of mitochondria and prevents or attenuates most of these age-associated mitochondrial changes, and thereby slow down the aging process and extends lifespan in diverse organisms.

Although abundant experimental data have been gathered in the past decade to support the concept that decline in mitochondrial energy metabolism, ROS overproduction and accumulation of mtDNA mutations in tissue cells are important contributors to human aging, the detailed mechanisms by which these biochemical events cause human aging have remained to be established. Gaining insights into the execution and regulation of these key events in aging will help us to better understand the age-related alterations in the structure and function of mitochondria as well as dysregulation of mtDNA metabolism in the aging process. It is also crucial to unravel the changes in the signaling pathways between the nucleus and mitochondria in aging tissue cells in order to elucidate the molecular mechanism of aging and to better manage aging and age-related diseases in the human.

References

Agarwal S, Sohal RS (1995) Differential oxidative damage to mitochondrial proteins during aging. Mech Ageing Dev 85:55–63

Albano E, Bellomo G, Parola M, Carini R, Dianzani MU (1991) Stimulation of lipid peroxidation increases the intracellular calcium content of isolated hepatocytes. Biochim Biophys Acta 1091:310–316

Ames BN, Shigenaga MK, Hagen TM (1993) Oxidants, antioxidants, and the degenerative diseases of aging. Proc Natl Acad Sci USA 90:7915–7922

Bacon BR, O'Neill R, Britton RS (1993) Hepatic mitochondrial energy production in rats with chronic iron overload. Gastroenterology 105:1134–1140

Bailey PJ, Webster GC (1984) Lowered rates of protein synthesis by mitochondria isolated from organisms of increasing age. Mech Ageing Dev 24:233–241

Bailey LJ, Cluett TJ, Reyes A, Prolla TA, Poulton J, Leeuwenburgh C, Holt IJ (2009) Mice expressing an error-prone DNA polymerase in mitochondria display elevated replication pausing and chromosomal breakage at fragile sites of mitochondrial DNA. Nucleic Acids Res 37:2327–2335

Barja G, Herrero A (2000) Oxidative damage to mitochondrial DNA is inversely related to maximum life span in the heart and brain of mammals. FASEB J 14:312–318

Barrientos A, Casademont J, Cardellach F, Ardite E, Estivill X, Urbano-Marquez A, Fernandez-Checa JC, Nunes V (1997a) Qualitative and quantitative changes in skeletal muscle mtDNA and expression of mitochondrial-encoded genes in the human aging process. Biochem Mol Med 62:165–171

Barrientos A, Casademont J, Cardellach F, Estivill X, Urbano-Marquez A, Nunes V (1997b) Reduced steady-state levels of mitochondrial RNA and increased mitochondrial DNA amount in human brain with aging. Mol Brain Res 52:284–289

Beckman KB, Ames BN (1998) The free radical theory of aging matures. Physiol Rev 78:547–581

Bender A, Krishnan KJ, Morris CM, Taylor GA, Reeve AK, Perry RH, Jaros E, Hersheson JS, Betts J, Klopstock T, Taylor RW, Turnbull DM (2006) High levels of mitochondrial DNA deletions in substantia nigra neurons in aging and Parkinson disease. Nat Genet 38:515–517

Berneburg M, Grether-Beck S, Kurten V, Ruzicka T, Briviba K, Sies H, Krutmann J (1999) Singlet oxygen mediates the UVA-induced generation of the photoaging-associated mitochondrial common deletion. J Biol Chem 274:15345–15349

Boffoli D, Scacco SC, Vergari R, Solarino G, Santacroce G, Papa S (1994) Decline with age of the respiratory chain activity in human skeletal muscle. Biochim Biophys Acta 1226:73–82

Bordone L, Guarente L (2005) Calorie restriction, SIRT1 and metabolism: understanding longevity. Nat Rev Mol Cell Biol 6:298–305

Bowling AC, Mutisya EM, Walker LC, Price DL, Cork LC, Beal MF (1993) Age-dependent impairment of mitochondrial function in primate brain. J Neurochem 60:1964–1967

Britton RS, O'Neill R, Bacon BR (1990) Hepatic mitochondrial malondialdehyde metabolism in rats with chronic iron overload. Hepatology 11:93–97

Bua E, McKiernan SH, Aiken JM (2004) Calorie restriction limits the generation but not the progression of mitochondrial abnormalities in aging skeletal muscle. FASEB J 18:582–584

Bua E, Johnson J, Herbst A, Delong B, McKenzie D, Salamat S, Aiken JM (2006) Mitochondrial DNA-deletion mutations accumulate intracellularly to detrimental levels in aged human skeletal muscle fibers. Am J Hum Genet 79:469–480

Bulos B, Shukla S, Sacktor B (1972) Bioenergetic properties of mitochondria from flight muscle of aging blowflies. Arch Biochem Biophys 149:461–469

Bulos B, Shukla S, Sacktor B (1975) Bioenergetics of mitochondria from flight muscles of aging blowflies: partial reactions of oxidation and phosphorylation. Arch Biochem Biophys 166:639–644

Calleja M, Pena P, Ugalde C, Ferreiro C, Marco R, Garesse R (1993) Mitochondrial DNA remains intact during Drosophila aging, but the levels of mitochondrial transcripts are significantly reduced. J Biol Chem 268:18891–18897

Cao Z, Wanagat J, McKiernan SH, Aiken JM (2001) Mitochondrial DNA deletion mutations are concomitant with ragged red regions of individual, aged muscle fibers: analysis by laser-capture microdissection. Nucleic Acids Res 29:4502–4508

Cassano P, Lezza AM, Leeuwenburgh C, Cantatore P, Gadaleta MN (2004) Measurement of the 4,834-bp mitochondrial DNA deletion level in aging rat liver and brain subjected or not to caloric restriction diet. Ann N Y Acad Sci 1019:269–273

Chance B, Sies H, Boveris A (1979) Hydroperoxide metabolism in mammalian organs. Physiol Rev 59:527–605

Chen H, Chan DC (2009) Mitochondrial dynamics fusion, fission, movement, and mitophagy in neurodegenerative diseases. Hum Mol Genet 18:R169–R176

Colman RJ, Anderson RM, Johnson SC, Kastman EK, Kosmatka KJ, Beasley TM, Allison DB, Cruzen C, Simmons HA, Kemnitz JW, Weindruch R (2009) Caloric restriction delays disease onset and mortality in rhesus monkeys. Science 325:201–204

Cooper JM, Mann VM, Schapira AH (1992) Analyses of mitochondrial respiratory chain function and mitochondrial DNA deletion in human skeletal muscle: effect of ageing. J Neurol Sci 113:91–98

de la Asuncion JG, Millán A, Pla R, Bruseghini L, Esteras A, Pallardó FV, Sastre J, Viña J (1996) Mitochondrial glutathione oxidation correlates with age-associated oxidative damage to mitochondrial DNA. FASEB J 10:333–338

de Magalhães JP, Curado J, Church GM (2009) Meta-analysis of age-related gene expression profiles identifies common signatures of aging. Bioinformatics 25:875–881

DiMauro S, Tanji K, Bonilla E, Pallotti F, Schon EA (2002) Mitochondrial abnormalities in muscle and other aging cells: classification, causes, and effects. Muscle Nerve 26:597–607

Dumont P, Burton M, Chen QM, Gonos ES, Frippiat C, Mazarati JB, Eliaers F, Remacle J, Toussaint O (2000) Induction of replicative senescence biomarkers by sublethal oxidative stresses in normal human fibroblast. Free Radic Biol Med 28:361–373

Edgar D, Larsson NG, Trifunovic A (2009) Point mutations are causing progeroid phenotypes in the mtDNA mutator mouse. Cell Metab 10:131–138

Fahn HJ, Wang LS, Kao SH, Chang SC, Huang MH, Wei YH (1998) Smoking-associated mitochondrial DNA mutations and lipid peroxidation in human lung tissues. Am J Respir Cell Mol Biol 19:901–909

Fernandez-Silva SP, Petruzzela V, Fracasso F, Gadaleta MN, Cantatore P (1991) Reduced synthesis of mtRNA in isolated mitochondria of senescent rat brain. Biochem Biophys Res Commun 176:645–653

Gadaleta MN, Petruzzella V, Renis M, Fracasso F, Cantatore P (1990) Reduced transcription of mitochondrial DNA in the senescent rat. Tissue dependence and effect of L-carnitine. Eur J Biochem 187:501–506

Gardner PR, Nguyen DD, White CW (1994) Aconitase is a sensitive and critical target of oxygen poisoning in cultured mammalian cells and in rat lungs. Proc Natl Acad Sci USA 91:12248–12252

Graziewicz MA, Day BJ, Copeland WC (2002) The mitochondrial DNA polymerase as a target of oxidative damage. Nucleic Acids Res 30:2817–2824

Greco M, Villani G, Mazzucchelli F, Bresolin N, Papa S, Attardi G (2003) Marked aging-related decline in efficiency of oxidative phosphorylation in human skin fibroblasts. FASEB J 17:1706–1708

Gredilla R, Barja G (2005) Minireview: the role of oxidative stress in relation to caloric restriction and longevity. Endocrinology 146:3713–3717

Gredilla R, Sanz A, Lopez-Torres M, Barja G (2001) Caloric restriction decreases mitochondrial free radical generation at complex I and lowers oxidative damage to mitochondrial DNA in the rat heart. FASEB J 15:1589–1591

Hagen TM, Yowe DL, Bartholomew JC, Wehr CM, Do KL, Park JY, Ames BN (1997) Mitochondrial decay in hepatocytes from old rats: membrane potential declines, heterogeneity and oxidants increase. Proc Natl Acad Sci USA 94:3064–3069

Hagopian K, Harper ME, Ram JJ, Humble SJ, Weindruch R, Ramsey JJ (2005) Long-term calorie restriction reduces proton leak and hydrogen peroxide production in liver mitochondria. Am J Physiol Endocrinol Metab 288:E674–E684

Hamilton ML, Guo Z, Fuller CD, Van Remmen H, Ward WF, Austad SN, Troyer DA, Thompson I, Richardson A (2001a) A reliable assessment of 8-oxo-2-deoxyguanosine levels in nuclear and mitochondrial DNA using the sodium iodide method to isolate DNA. Nucleic Acids Res 29:2117–2126

Hamilton ML, Van Remmen H, Drake JA, Yang H, Guo ZM, Kewitt K, Walter CA, Richardson A (2001b) Does oxidative damage to DNA increase with age? Proc Natl Acad Sci USA 98:10469–10474

Han D, Antunes F, Canali R, Rettori D, Cadenas E (2003) Voltage-dependent anion channels control the release of the superoxide anion from mitochondria to cytosol. J Biol Chem 278:5557–5563

Harman D (1956) Ageing: theory based on free radical and radiation chemistry. J Gerontol 11:298–300

Harman D (1972) The biological clock: the mitochondria. J Am Geriatr Soc 20:145–147

Harper ME, Monemdjou S, Ramsey JJ, Weindruch R (1998) Age-related increase in mitochondrial proton leak and decrease in ATP turnover reactions in mouse hepatocytes. Am J Physiol 275:E197–E206

Hayakawa M, Torii K, Sugiyama S, Tanaka M, Ozawa T (1991) Age-associated accumulation of 8-hydroxydeoxyguanosine in mitochondrial DNA of human diaphragm. Biochem Biophys Res Commun 179:1023–1029

Hayakawa M, Hattori K, Sugiyama S, Ozawa T (1992) Age-associated oxygen damage and mutations in mitochondrial DNA in human heart. Biochem Biophys Res Commun 189:979–985

He L, Chinnery PF, Durham SE, Blakely EL, Wardell TM, Borthwick GM, Taylor RW, Turnbull DM (2002) Detection and quantification of mitochondrial DNA deletions in individual cells by real-time PCR. Nucleic Acids Res 30:e68

Herbst A, Pak JW, McKenzie D, Bua E, Bassiouni M, Aiken JM (2007) Accumulation of mitochondrial DNA deletion mutations in aged muscle fibers: evidence for a causal role in muscle fiber loss. J Gerontol A Biol Sci Med Sci 62:235–245

Hruszkewycz AM (1992) Lipid peroxidation and mtDNA degeneration. A hypothesis. Mutat Res 275:243–248

Hsieh RH, Hou JH, Hsu HS, Wei YH (1994) Age-dependent respiratory function decline and DNA deletions in human muscle mitochondria. Biochem Mol Biol Int 32:1009–1022

Inarrea P, Moini H, Han D, Rettori D, Aguiló I, Alava MA, Iturralde M, Cadenas E (2007) Mitochondrial respiratory chain and thioredoxin reductase regulate intermembrane Cu. Zn-superoxide dismutase activity: implications for mitochondrial energy metabolism and apoptosis. Biochem J 405:173–179

Khaidakov M, Heflich RH, Manjanatha MG, Myers MB, Aidoo A (2003) Accumulation of point mutations in mitochondrial DNA of aging mice. Mutat Res 526:1–7

Khrapko K, Vijg J (2009) Mitochondrial DNA mutations and aging: devils in the details? Trends Genet 25:91–98

Kokoszka JE, Coskun P, Esposito LA, Wallace DC (2001) Increased mitochondrial oxidative stress in the Sod2 (+/−) mouse results in the age-related decline of mitochondrial function culminating in increased apoptosis. Proc Natl Acad Sci USA 98:2278–2283

Kopsidas G, Kovalenko SA, Kelso JM, Linnane AW (1998) An age-associated correlation between cellular bioenergy decline and mtDNA rearrangements in human skeletal muscle. Mutat Res 421:27–36

Kovalenko SA, Kopsidas G, Kelso JM, Linnane AW (1997) Deltoid human muscle mtDNA is extensively rearranged in old age subjects. Biochem Biophys Res Commun 232:147–152

Kraytsberg Y, Kudryavtseva E, McKee AC, Geula C, Kowall NW, Khrapko K (2006) Mitochondrial DNA deletions are abundant and cause functional impairment in aged human substantia nigra neurons. Nat Genet 38:518–520

Ku HH, Brunk UT, Sohal RS (1993) Relationship between mitochondrial superoxide and hydrogen peroxide production and longevity of mammalian species. Free Radic Biol Med 15:621–627

Kujoth GC, Hiona A, Pugh TD, Someya S, Panzer K, Wohlgemuth SE, Hofer T, Seo AY, Sullivan R, Jobling WA, Morrow JD, van Remmen H, Sedivy JM, Yamasoba T, Tanokura M, Weindruch R, Leeuwenburgh C, Prolla TA (2005) Mitochondrial DNA mutations, oxidative stress, and apoptosis in mammalian aging. Science 309:481–484

Lass A, Sohal BH, Weindruch R, Forster MJ, Sohal RS (1998) Caloric restriction prevents age-associated accrual of oxidative damage to mouse skeletal muscle mitochondria. Free Radic Biol Med 25:1089–1097

Lee HC, Wei YH (2007) Oxidative stress, mitochondrial DNA mutation, and apoptosis in aging. Exp Biol Med 232:592–606

Lee HC, Pang CY, Hsu HS, Wei YH (1994a) Differential accumulations of 4,977 bp deletion in mitochondrial DNA of various tissues in human ageing. Biochim Biophys Acta 1226:37–43

Lee HC, Pang CY, Hsu HS, Wei YH (1994b) Ageing-associated tandem duplications in the D-loop of mitochondrial DNA of human muscle. FEBS Lett 354:79–83

Lee CM, Aspnes LE, Chung SS, Weindruch R, Aiken JM (1998) Influences of caloric restriction on age-associated skeletal muscle fiber characteristics and mitochondrial changes in rats and mice. Ann N Y Acad Sci 854:182–191

Lee HC, Lim ML, Lu CY, Liu VW, Fahn HJ, Zhang C, Nagley P, Wei YH (1999) Concurrent increase of oxidative DNA damage and lipid peroxidation together with mitochondrial DNA mutation in human lung tissues during aging-smoking enhances oxidative stress on the aged tissues. Arch Biochem Biophys 362:309–316

Lee HC, Yin PH, Yu TN, Chang YD, Hsu WC, Kao SY, Chi CW, Liu TY, Wei YH (2001) Accumulation of mitochondrial DNA deletions in human oral tissues-Effects of betel quid chewing and oral cancer. Mutat Res 493:67–74

Lee S, Jeong SY, Lim WC, Kim S, Park YY, Sun X, Youle RJ, Cho H (2007) Mitochondrial fission and fusion mediators, hFis1 and OPA1, modulate cellular senescence. J Biol Chem 282:22977–22983

Lesnefsky EJ, Hoppel CL (2006) Oxidative phosphorylation and aging. Ageing Res Rev 5:402–433

Lezza AM, Boffoli D, Scacco S, Cantatore P, Gadaleta MN (1994) Correlation between mitochondrial DNA 4977-bp deletion and respiratory chain enzyme activities in aging human skeletal muscles. Biochem Biophys Res Commun 205:772–779

Li Y, Huang TT, Carlson EJ, Melvo S, Ursell PC, Olson JL, Noble LJ, Yoshimura MP, Berge C, Chan PH, Wallace DC, Epstein CJ (1995) Dilated cardiomyopathy and neonatal lethality in mutant mice lacking manganese superoxide dismutase. Nat Genet 11:376–381

Lin PH, Lee SH, Su CP, Wei YH (2003) Oxidative damage to mitochondrial DNA in atrial muscle of patients with atrial fibrillation. Free Radic Biol Med 35:1310–1318

Linnane AW, Marzuki S, Ozawa T, Tanaka M (1989) Mitochondrial DNA mutations as an important contributor to aging and degenerative disease. Lancet 334:642–645

López-Torres M, Gredilla R, Sanz A, Barja G (2002) Influence of aging and long-term caloric restriction on oxygen radical generation and oxidative DNA damage in rat liver mitochondria. Free Radic Biol Med 32:882–889

Lu CY, Lee HC, Fahn HJ, Wei YH (1999) Oxidative damage elicited by imbalance of free radical scavenging enzymes is associated with large-scale mtDNA deletions in aging human skin. Mutat Res 423:11–21

Mansouri A, Muller FL, Liu Y, Ng R, Faulkner J, Hamilton M, Richardson A, Huang TT, Epstein CJ, Van Remmen H (2006) Alterations in mitochondrial function, hydrogen peroxide release and oxidative damage in mouse hind-limb skeletal muscle during aging. Mech Ageing Dev 127:298–306

Marcus DL, Ibrahim NG, Freedman ML (1982) Age-related decline in the biosynthesis of mitochondrial inner membrane proteins. Exp Gerontol 17:333–341

Martinez AO, McDaniel RG (1979) Mitochondrial heterosis in aging *Drosophila* hybrids. Exp Gerontol 14:231–238

Melov S, Coskun P, Patel M, Tuinstra R, Cottrell B, Jun AS, Zastawny TH, Dizdaroglu M, Goodman SI, Huang TT, Miziorko H, Epstein CJ, Wallace DC (1999) Mitochondrial disease in superoxide dismutase 2 mutant mice. Proc Natl Acad Sci USA 96:846–851

Michikawa Y, Mazzucchelli F, Bresolin N, Scarlato G, Attardi G (1999) Aging-dependent large accumulation of point mutations in the human mtDNA control region for replication. Science 286:774–779

Miquel J, Economos AC, Fleming J, Johnson JE Jr (1980) Mitochondrial role in cell aging. Exp Gerontol 15:575–591

Miyoshi N, Oubrahim H, Chock PB, Stadtman ER (2006) Age-dependent cell death and the role of ATP in hydrogen peroxide-induced apoptosis and necrosis. Proc Natl Acad Sci USA 103:1727–1731

Müller-Höcker J (1989) Cytochrome *c* oxidase deficient cardiomyocytes in the human heart-an age-related phenomenon: a histochemical ultracytochemical study. Am J Pathol 134:1167–1173

Müller-Höcker J (1990) Cytochrome *c* oxidase deficient fibers in the limb muscle and diaphragm of man without muscular disease: an age-related alteration. J Neurol Sci 100:14–21

Müller-Höcker J, Seibel P, Schneiderbanger K, Kadenbach B (1993) Different *in situ* hybridization patterns of mitochondrial DNA in cytochrome *c* oxidase-deficient extraocular muscle fibers in the elderly. Virchows Arch 422:7–15

Münscher C, Rieger T, Müller-Höcker J, Kadenbach B (1993) The point mutation of mitochondrial DNA characteristic for MERRF disease is found also in healthy people of different ages. FEBS Lett 317:27–30

Murfitt RR, Sanadi DR (1978) Evidence for increased degeneration of mitochondria in old rats. A brief note. Mech Ageing Dev 8:197–201

Murphy MP (2009) How mitochondria produce reactive oxygen species. Biochem J 417:1–13

O'Brien KM, Dirmeier R, Engle M, Poyton RO (2004) Mitochondrial protein oxidation in yeast mutants lacking manganese-(MnSOD) or copper- and zinc-containing superoxide dismutase (CuZnSOD): evidence that MnSOD and CuZnSOD have both unique and overlapping functions in protecting mitochondrial proteins from oxidative damage. J Biol Chem 279:51817–51827

Ojaimi J, Masters CL, McLean C, Opeskin K, McKelvie P, Byrne E (1999a) Irregular distribution of cytochrome *c* oxidase protein subunits in aging and Alzheimer's disease. Ann Neurol 46:656–660

Ojaimi J, Masters CL, Opeskin K, McKelvie P, Byrne E (1999b) Mitochondrial respiratory chain activity in the human brain as a function of age. Mech Ageing Dev 111:39–47

Okado-Matsumoto A, Fridovich I (2001) Subcellular distribution of superoxide dismutases (SOD) in rat liver: Cu. Zn-SOD in mitochondria. J Biol Chem 276:38388–38393

Pang CY, Lee HC, Yang JH, Wei YH (1994) Human skin mitochondrial DNA deletions associated with light exposure. Arch Biochem Biophys 312:534–538

Paradies G, Petrosillo G, Pistolese M, Ruggiero FM (2000) The effect of reactive oxygen species generated from the mitochondrial electron transport chain on the cytochrome *c* oxidase activity and on the cardiolipin content in bovine heart submitochondrial particles. FEBS Lett 466:323–326

Park SK, Prolla TA (2005) Lessons learned from gene expression profile studies of aging and caloric restriction. Ageing Res Rev 4:55–65

Pesce V, Cormio A, Fracasso F, Vecchiet J, Felzani G, Lezza AM, Cantatore P, Gadaleta MN (2001) Age-related mitochondrial genotypic and phenotypic alterations in human skeletal muscle. Free Radic Biol Med 30:1223–1233

Petersen KF, Befroy D, Dufour S, Dziura J, Ariyan C, Rothman DL, DiPietro L, Cline GW, Shulman GI (2003) Mitochondrial dysfunction in the elderly: possible role in insulin resistance. Science 300:1140–1142

Petrosillo G, Ruggiero FM, Pistolese M, Paradies G (2001) Reactive oxygen species generated from the mitochondrial electron transport chain induce cytochrome *c* dissociation from beef-heart submitochondrial particles via cardiolipin peroxidation. Possible role in the apoptosis. FEBS Lett 509:435–438

Pieri C, Recchioni R, Moroni F (1993) Age-dependent modifications of mitochondrial trans-membrane potential and mass in rat splenic lymphocytes during proliferation. Mech Ageing Dev 70:201–212

Richter C, Park JW, Ames BN (1988) Normal oxidative damage to mitochondrial and nuclear DNA is extensive. Proc Natl Acad Sci USA 85:6465–6467

Rooyackers OE, Adey DB, Ades PA, Nair KS (1996) Effect of age on in vivo rates of mitochondrial protein synthesis in human skeletal muscle. Proc Natl Acad Sci USA 93:15364–15369

Roth GS, Mattison JA, Ottinger MA, Chachich ME, Lane MA, Ingram DK (2004) Aging in rhesus monkeys: relevance to human health interventions. Science 305:1423–1426

Sanz A, Caro P, Ibañez J, Gómez J, Gredilla R, Barja G (2005) Dietary restriction at old age lowers mitochondrial oxygen radical production and leak at complex I and oxidative DNA damage in rat brain. J Bioenerg Biomembr 37:83–90

Schon EA, Hirano M, DiMauro S (1994) Mitochondrial encephalomyopathies: clinical and molecular analysis. J Bioenerg Biomembr 26:291–299

Schriner SE, Linford NJ, Martin GM, Treuting P, Ogburn CE, Emond M, Coskun PE, Ladiges W, Wolf N, Van Remmen H, Wallace DC, Rabinovitch PS (2005) Extension of murine life span by overexpression of catalase targeted to mitochondria. Science 308:1909–1911

Schwarze SR, Lee CM, Chung SS, Roecker EB, Weindruch R, Aiken JM (1995) High levels of mitochondrial DNA deletions in skeletal muscle of old rhesus monkeys. Mech Ageing Dev 83:91–101

Short KR, Bigelow ML, Kahl J, Singh R, Coenen-Schimke J, Raghavakaimal S, Nair KS (2005) Decline in skeletal muscle mitochondrial function with aging in humans. Proc Natl Acad Sci USA 102:5618–5623

Shoubridge EA, Karpati G, Hastings KE (1990) Deletion mutants are functionally dominant over wild-type mitochondrial genomes in skeletal muscle fiber segments in mitochondrial disease. Cell 62:43–49

Sohal RS (2002) Role of oxidative stress and protein oxidation in the aging process. Free Radic Biol Med 33:37–44

Sohal RS, Weindruch R (1996) Oxidative stress, caloric restriction, and aging. Science 273:59–63

Sohal RS, Ku HH, Agarwal S, Forster MJ, Lal H (1994) Oxidative damage, mitochondrial oxidant generation, and antioxidant defenses during aging and in response to food restriction in the mouse. Mech Ageing Dev 74:121–133

Sohal RS, Sohal BH, Orr WC (1995) Mitochondrial superoxide and hydrogen peroxide generation, protein oxidative damage, and longevity in different species of flies. Free Radic Biol Med 19:499–504

Sugiyama S, Takasawa M, Hayakawa M, Ozawa T (1993) Changes in skeletal muscle, heart and liver mitochondrial electron transport activities in rats and dogs of various ages. Biochem Mol Biol Int 30:937–944

Takasawa M, Hayakawa M, Sugiyama S, Hattori K, Ito T, Ozawa T (1993) Age-associated damage in mitochondrial function in rat heart. Exp Gerontol 28:269–280

Torii K, Sugiyama S, Takagi K, Satake T, Ozawa T (1992a) Age-related decrease in respiratory muscle mitochondrial function in rats. Am J Respir Cell Mol Biol 6:88–92

Torii K, Sugiyama S, Tanaka M, Takagi K, Hanaki Y, Iida K, Matsuyama M, Hirabayashi N, Uno H, Ozawa T (1992b) Ageing-associated deletions of human diaphragmatic mitochondrial DNA. Am J Respir Cell Mol Biol 6:543–549

Trifunovic A, Wredenberg A, Falkenberg M, Spelbrink JN, Rovio AT, Bruder CE, Bohlooly-Y M, Gidlof S, Oldfors A, Wibom R, Tornell J, Jacobs HT, Larsson NG (2004) Premature ageing in mice expressing defective mitochondrial DNA polymerase. Nature 429:417–423

Trifunovic A, Hansson A, Wredenberg A, Rovio AT, Dufour E, Khvorostov I, Spelbrink JN, Wibom R, Jacobs HT, Larsson NG (2005) Somatic mtDNA mutations cause aging phenotypes without affecting reactive oxygen species production. Proc Natl Acad Sci USA 102:17993–17998

Trounce I, Byrne E, Marzuki S (1989) Decline in skeletal muscle mitochondrial respiratory chain function: possible factor in ageing. Lancet 334:637–639

Van Remmen H, Ikeno Y, Hamilton M, Pahlavani M, Wolf N, Thorpe SR, Alderson NL, Baynes JW, Epstein CJ, Huang TT, Nelson J, Strong R, Richardson A (2003) Life-long reduction in MnSOD activity results in increased DNA damage and higher incidence of cancer but does not accelerate aging. Physiol Genomics 16:29–37

Vermulst M, Bielas JH, Kujoth GC, Ladiges WC, Rabinovitch PS, Prolla TA, Loeb LA (2007) Mitochondrial point mutations do not limit the natural lifespan of mice. Nat Genet 39:540–543

Vermulst M, Wanagat J, Kujoth GC, Bielas JH, Rabinovitch PS, Prolla TA, Loeb LA (2008) DNA deletions and clonal mutations drive premature aging in mitochondrial mutator mice. Nat Genet 40:392–394

Wanagat J, Cao Z, Pathare P, Aiken JM (2001) Mitochondrial DNA deletion mutations colocalize with segmental electron transport system abnormalities, muscle fiber atrophy, fiber splitting, and oxidative damage in sarcopenia. FASEB J 15:322–332

Wang Y, Michikawa Y, Mallidis C, Bai Y, Woodhouse L, Yarasheski KE, Miller CA, Askanas V, Engel WK, Bhasin S, Attardi G (2001) Muscle-specific mutations accumulate with aging in critical human mtDNA control sites for replication. Proc Natl Acad Sci USA 98:4022–4027

Wei YH (1992) Mitochondrial DNA alterations as ageing-associated molecular events. Mutat Res 275:145–155

Wei YH, Lee HC (2002) Oxidative stress, mitochondrial DNA mutation, and impairment of antioxidant enzymes in aging. Exp Biol Med 227:671–682

Wei YH, Scholes CP, King TE (1981) Ubisemiquinone radicals from the cytochrome b-c_1 complex of mitochondrial electron transport chain-Demonstration of QP-S radical formation. Biochem Biophys Res Commun 99:1411–1419

Wei YH, Pang CY, You BJ, Lee HC (1996) Tandem duplications and large-scale deletions of mitochondrial DNA are early molecular events of human aging process. Ann N Y Acad Sci 786:82–101

Williams MD, Van Remmen H, Conrad CC, Huang TT, Epstein CJ, Richardson A (1998) Increased oxidative damage is correlated to altered mitochondrial function in heterozygous manganese superoxide dismutase knockout mice. J Biol Chem 273:28510–28515

Yakes FM, van Houten B (1997) Mitochondrial DNA damage is more extensive and persists longer than nuclear DNA damage in human cells following oxidative stress. Proc Natl Acad Sci USA 94:514–519

Yan LJ, Sohal RS (1998) Mitochondrial adenine nucleotide translocase is modified oxidatively during aging. Proc Natl Acad Sci USA 95:12896–12901

Yan LJ, Levine RL, Sohol RS (1997) Oxidative damage during aging targets mitochondrial aconitase. Proc Natl Acad Sci USA 94:11168–11172

Yang JH, Lee HC, Wei YH (1995) Photoageing-associated mitochondrial DNA length mutations in human skin. Arch Dermatol Res 287:641–648

Yen TC, Chen YS, King KL, Yeh SH, Wei YH (1989) Liver mitochondrial respiratory functions decline with age. Biochem Biophys Res Commun 165:994–1003

Yen TC, Su JH, King KL, Wei YH (1991) Ageing-associated 5 kb deletion in human liver mitochondrial DNA. Biochem Biophys Res Commun 178:124–131

Zahn JM, Poosala S, Owen AB, Ingram DK, Lustig A, Carter A, Weeraratna AT, Taub DD, Gorospe M, Mazan-Mamczarz K, Lakatta EG, Boheler KR, Xu X, Mattson MP, Falco G, Ko MS, Schlessinger D, Firman J, Kummerfeld SK, Wood WH 3rd, Zonderman AB, Kim SK, Becker KG (2007) AGEMAP: a gene expression database for aging in mice. PLoS Genet 3:e201

Zhang C, Baumer A, Maxwell RJ, Linnane AW, Nagley P (1992) Multiple mitochondrial DNA deletions in an elderly human individual. FEBS Lett 297:34–38

Zhang C, Linnane AW, Nagley P (1993) Occurrence of a particular base substitution (3243 A to G) in mitochondrial DNA of tissues of ageing humans. Biochem Biophys Res Commun 195:1104–1110

Chapter 15
Mitochondria and Drugs

Roberto Scatena

Abstract Mitochondria play a central role in the life and death of cells. They are not merely the centre for energy metabolism, but are also the headquarters for different catabolic and anabolic processes, calcium fluxes, and various signalling pathways. Mitochondria maintain homeostasis in the cell by interacting with reactive oxygen-nitrogen species and responding adequately to different stimuli. In this context, the interaction of pharmacological agents with mitochondria is an aspect of molecular biology that is too often disregarded, not only in terms of toxicology but also from a therapeutic point of view, especially considering the potential therapeutic applications related to the modulation of mitochondrial activity.

At the mitochondrial level, there are several potential drug targets that can lead to toxicity, but only for few of them, a real clinical counterpart has been demonstrated. Recently, antiviral nucleoside analogues have shown mitochondrial toxicity through the inhibition of DNA polymerase-gamma. Other drugs targeted to different components of the mitochondrial channels can disrupt ion homeostasis or affect the mitochondrial permeability transition pore. Many molecules are known inhibitors of the mitochondrial electron transport chain, interfering with one or more of the complexes in the respiratory chain. Some drugs, including non-steroidal anti-inflammatory drugs (NSAIDs), may lead to uncoupling of oxidative phosphorylation, while the mitochondrial toxicity of other drugs seems to depend on the production of free radicals, although this mechanism has yet to be defined. Besides toxicity, other drugs have been targeted to mitochondria to treat mitochondrial dysfunctions. Many drugs have been recently developed to target the mitochondria of cancer cells in order to trigger apoptosis or necrosis. The aim of this chapter is to underline the role of mitochondria in pharmacology and toxicology, stressing all the potential therapeutic approaches being due to iatrogenic modulation of the multitude of mitochondrial activities

Keywords Apoptosis • Cancer metabolism • Degenerative diseases • Drug effects • Free radicals • Mitochondrial diseases • Nitric oxide • Toxic effects

R. Scatena, MD (✉)
Institute of Biochemistry and Clinical Biochemistry, Department of Laboratory Medicine,
Catholic University School of Medicine, Largo A. Gemelli 8, 00168 Rome, Italy
e-mail: r.scatena@rm.unicatt.it

R. Scatena et al. (eds.), *Advances in Mitochondrial Medicine*, Advances in Experimental Medicine and Biology 942, DOI 10.1007/978-94-007-2869-1_15,
© Springer Science+Business Media B.V. 2012

15.1 Introduction

In recent years, there has been extraordinary progress in mitochondrial science that has further outlined the critical role of mitochondria in cell biology, cell and tissue pathophysiology, and the diagnosis and therapeutic treatment of different human diseases, such as ischaemic diseases, diabetes, some forms of neurodegeneration, and cancer (Duchen 2004; Scatena et al. 2007a, b; Giorgi et al. 2011).

Mitochondrial physiology and pathophysiology is notably complex, and the role of these organelles in bioenergetics is also linked to other essential functions, such as anabolic metabolism, the balance of redox potential, cell death and differentiation, and mitosis. In addition to these basic functions, mitochondria are associated with more specialized cell activities, including calcium homeostasis and thermogenesis, reactive oxygen species (ROS) and reactive nitrogen species (RNS), signalling, maintenance of ion channels, and the transport of metabolites. The basis of different congenital mitochondrial diseases on a molecular level is equally complex and heterogeneous, making mitochondrial pathophysiology difficult to investigate (Hamm-Alvarez and Cadenas 2009; Cardoso et al. 2010).

This field is made even more challenging by recent evidence that suggests mitochondrial structure and function is dynamic. Specifically, mitochondria possess many interesting properties, such as the ability to fuse or divide, move along microtubules and microfilaments, or undergo turnover, and these unique properties are often overlooked in research. Undoubtedly, much is still unknown about the mutual interactions between mitochondrial energetics, biogenesis, dynamics and degradation (Lenaz et al. 2006; Detmer and Chan 2007).

In the clinic, research has shown a significant relationship between mitochondrial metabolic abnormalities and tumours found in renal carcinomas, glioblastomas, paragangliomas or skin leiomyoma, which has led to the discovery of new genes, oncogenes and oncometabolites involved in the regulation of cellular and mitochondrial energy production with a particular focus on reevaluating the Warburg effect (Fulda et al. 2010; Ralph et al. 2010; Solaini et al. 2011). Furthermore, the examination of rare neurological diseases, such as Charcot-Marie Tooth type 2a, autosomal dominant optic atrophy, lethal mitochondrial and peroxisomal fission, and spastic paraplegia have suggested the involvement of MFN2, OPA1/3, DRP1 or paraplegin in the auxiliary control of mitochondrial energy production (Benard et al. 2010; Du and Yan 2010; Zhu 2010). Advances in the understanding of mitochondrial apoptosis have suggested a supplementary role for Bcl2 or Bax in the regulation of mitochondrial respiration and dynamics, which has led to the investigation of alternative mechanisms of energy regulation (Benard et al. 2010). Finally, different metabolic diseases, such as diabetes, obesity, non-alcoholic fatty liver disease (NAFLD) and the more general metabolic syndrome underline the role of a dysfunctional uncoupling protein (UCP)-mitochondria relationship in pathogenesis (Dalgaard 2011; Richard and Picard 2011; Pessayre 2007; De Souza et al. 2007).

Because mitochondria can be either primary or secondary targets of therapeutic compounds, (Szewczyk and Wojtczak 2002; Wallace 2003) it is often difficult to foresee and understand all of the drugs' potential effects on mitochondrial pathophysiology, and some aspects of drug-mitochondria interactions are often underestimated.

A poor understanding of mitochondrial pharmacology can lead to increased or aggravated toxicity, but it can also camouflage positive effects induced by therapeutic drugs that target mitochondria.

More attention should be devoted to the toxic and therapeutic effects of drugs on mitochondria, due to these peculiar aspects of mitochondrial pharmacology.

Although there is a growing consensus of the vital role mitochondria play in medicine, a relatively small number of translational studies on the diversified pathophysiology of these organelles has been carried out.

In the future, the design of unique mitochondrial drug targets will allow for the manipulation of mitochondrial function and the selective protection or destruction of affected cells in a variety of diseases.

15.2 Mitochondria: The Structural and Functional Characteristics of Mitochondria as Potential Targets in Pharmacotoxicology

Many structural and functional properties of mitochondria should be considered as drug targets of particular pharmacotoxicological value, such as:

- Peculiar metabolic pathways (e.g., the Krebs cycle, fatty acid metabolism, the urea cycle, haem biosynthesis, cardiolipin and lipid biosynthesis and metabolism, ubiquinol biosynthesis, and the biosynthesis of Fe–S centres).
- Peculiar transport mechanisms inside and outside of the organelle (e.g., voltage-dependent anion channels (VDAC), the ADP/ATP translocator, various mitochondrial carrier proteins, cation transport, calcium transport, and the mitochondrial permeability transition pore).
- The system of uncoupling proteins (UCPs).
- The mitochondrial genome, which consists of a small circular chromosome and a total of 37 genes.
- The characteristic two-lipid bilayer membrane in which the outer membrane delineates the organelle and is structurally similar to other cell membranes (i.e., rich in cholesterol and permeable to ions), while the inner membrane, which isolates the matrix, is virtually devoid of cholesterol, is rich in cardiolipin (which binds electron transport chain proteins) and is impermeable to ions.

Maintaining the impermeability of the inner mitochondrial membrane is critical for mitochondrial function. This impermeability enables the generation of the electrochemical gradient that supplies the proton motive force for ATP generation. The peculiar structure of the mitochondrial matrix (i.e., an alkaline and negatively charged interior with a series of specific channels and carrier proteins) is organized to perform and finely coordinate distinct mitochondrial activities. Interestingly, the unique physicochemical characteristics of the mitochondrial matrix (mainly $\Delta\psi$ and a pH ≈ 8) may facilitate the selective accumulation of different xenobiotics in the matrix and/or in the inner mitochondrial membrane by an efficient trapping effect (Murphy and Smith 2000; Szewczyk and Wojtczak 2002; Suski et al. 2011). As a consequence, lipophilic compounds of cationic character and even weak acids in anionic forms can accumulate in mitochondria. In particular, weak acids in undissociated forms can penetrate the inner mitochondrial membrane freely, while, once inside the alkaline matrix, their protons dissociate, rendering them less membrane-permeable and trapping them inside the organelle (Scatena et al. 2004a, b). This effect of mitochondrial drug storage may impact the determination of pharmacokinetic parameters (e.g., the distribution volume, plasma concentration and half-life). Moreover, as these acidic and lipophilic xenobiotics progressively accumulate inside mitochondria, they can inhibit mitochondrial function and affect membrane permeability. Depending on the extent of damage and the number of mitochondria affected, the cell could then undergo a loss in energy, leading to localized damage of the $\Delta\psi$ of some mitochondria or even necrosis. The build-up of weak acids in the mitochondrial matrix and subsequent decrease in pH could result in the protonation of xenobiotics, rendering them freely permeable in the cell and capable of entering other mitochondria, causing a chain reaction that leads to increased mitochondrial damage (Scatena et al. 2003, 2004a, b).

Another fundamental aspect of mitochondria is their unique DNA, which contains a total of 37 genes. Thirteen of these genes encode proteins that are unique components of the electron transport chain, while the remaining genes encode for 22 tRNAs and two ribosomal RNAs that are used in the two subunits of the mitochondrial ribosome. The presence of its own DNA renders the mitochondrion fully capable of synthesizing at least some of the proteins needed for energy generation (the remaining are the products of translocation of nuclear proteins synthesized in the cytosol), but this condition also makes mitochondria susceptible to DNA damage (Lewis et al. 2006).

Unlike nuclear DNA, mitochondrial DNA is not protected by histone proteins, and it is located in close proximity to sites at which reactive oxygen species (ROS) are routinely generated. In general, DNA repair processes are less efficient in mitochondria compared with nuclear DNA repair. The result is that mitochondrial DNA is more likely to undergo mutation than nuclear DNA; in fact, the mutation rate is estimated to be at least 10–20 times higher for mitochondrial DNA than for nuclear DNA (Brandon et al. 2006).

Mitochondrial DNA does undergo replication, and, to a certain extent, DNA repair is performed by base excision. A single DNA polymerase (pol-γ) is responsible for both DNA replication and base excision in mitochondria (as compared to nuclear DNA, which is maintained by at least nine different polymerases). Although pol-γ is a nuclear protein, it does not function outside of mitochondria; thus, any mutation or inhibition of this enzyme is manifested only in mitochondrial DNA (Brandon et al. 2006).

All of these findings underscore the fact that mitochondria are potential primary or secondary targets of xenobiotics. However, the interaction between mitochondria and their components (i.e., mitochondrial DNA, respiratory chain complexes, biomembranes with different transporters, or matrix metabolic enzymes) with xenobiotics should not always be considered negative. In fact, recent data show an unexpected therapeutic potential for the pharmacological modulation of mitochondrial activity (Murphy and Smith 2000; Don and Hogg 2004; Drose et al. 2006; Duchen 2004; Scatena et al. 2003, 2004a, b).

Many chemicals have been shown to interact with different mitochondrial molecules (Wallace and Starkov 2000; Szewczyk and Wojtczak 2002; Don and Hogg 2004; Oliveira 2011), but a thorough description of all the known interactions is beyond the scope of this chapter. Here, our aim is to underline the role of mitochondria and their subcompartments in pharmacotoxicology, describing, when possible, the molecular basis of the adverse and/or therapeutic effects. Knowledge of the role mitochondria play in pharmacotoxicology could be used to understand better the incidence of iatrogenic mitochondriopathies, and eventually provide therapeutic indications for many diseases, such as ischaemia/reperfusion injury, neurodegenerative diseases, cancer, metabolic syndromes, and hyperlipidaemia.

15.3   The Toxicological Aspect of Mitochondria and Drugs

Mitochondrial dysfunction has been shown to be a significant adverse effect for a variety of currently-marketed drugs

One example, idiosyncratic drug-induced liver injury (DILI) is a major clinical problem and poses a considerable challenge for drug development, as an increasing number of successfully launched drugs or new potential drugs have been implicated in DILI in subsets of susceptible patients. Although the incidence of DILI for a particular drug treatment is low, the outcome of the disorder can be serious (as shown dramatically in the case of troglitazone and cerivastatin) (Scatena et al. 2003; Schaefer et al. 2004; Jaeschke 2007; Ong et al. 2007). Unfortunately, the prediction of DILI has remained poor, both in terms of patients at risk and the effect of new chemical entities, and this topic has interesting ramifications for pharmacogenetics. The underlying mechanisms and determinants of susceptibility have remained largely ill-defined. The mitochondrial hypothesis suggests that mitochondrial damage in heteroplasmic cells, although initially silent, gradually reaches a critical threshold and abruptly triggers liver injury. This hypothesis is consistent with findings indicating that the onset of idiosyncratic DILI is typically delayed (by weeks or months), that older patients, especially women, are at risk, and that these drugs are targeted to the liver and clearly exhibit a hazard to mitochondria both in vitro and in vivo (Russmann et al. 2010).

In general, mitochondria play a critical role in supplying the cell with the bulk of its ATP via oxidative phosphorylation; thus, any cell type or tissue with a high aerobic energy requirement (such as the liver) is more likely to be affected by mitochondrial damage.

Additionally, there are several specialized metabolic processes (fatty acid β oxidation, urea synthesis, haem synthesis) that are conducted by enzymes in the mitochondrial matrix, and tissues that rely heavily on these processes are also frequently targeted by mitochondrial toxins. For these reasons, common syndromes associated with mitochondrial toxicity include lactic acidosis, cardiac and skeletal myopathy, peripheral, central and optic neuropathy, retinopathy, ototoxicity, enteropathy, pancreatitis, diabetes, hepatic steatosis, and haematotoxicity. Combinations of these disorders (or different manifestations of toxicity in different individuals treated with the same compound) are not uncommon and are strong indicators that the underlying mechanism of toxicity involves the mitochondria. In addition, when cells are divided, the apportionment of mitochondria between them is random, a condition referred to as heteroplasmy. As such, one daughter cell may contain primarily normal mitochondria, while the other cell receives a disproportionate share of damaged mitochondria, resulting in an uneven distribution of damaged cells within a tissue.

As discussed previously, different functional and/or structural targets that could be affected by drug toxicity can be identified at the mitochondrial level:

15.3.1 Mitochondrial DNA (mtDNA)

Research on the mitochondrial genome has provided tremendous insight into mitochondrial replication, mitochondrial disorders, and, subsequently, mitochondrial drug toxicity. However, some aspects of the latter topic remain unclear. For example, it is still unclear how impairment of the mitochondrial polymerase by nucleoside analogues results in drastically different phenotypes (Lewis et al. 2003).

Moreover, there are many drugs capable of targeting the mitochondrial genome, but the molecular mechanism for damage is less understood.

Because of its similarity to translation in bacteria, mtDNA translation is similarly vulnerable to inhibition by some antibiotics. In addition, ethanol is a well-known exogenous agent capable of oxidative damage of mtDNA (Deschamps et al. 1994). In the last few years, it has become evident that the mechanism of mtDNA replication, which is required for normal mitochondrial maintenance and duplication, is inhibited by a relatively new class of drugs used to treat AIDS, the so-called nucleotide reverse transcriptase inhibitors (NRTI). These drugs damaged mtDNA by inhibiting its synthesis. The biomedical value of this topic alone deserves a specific chapter in this book; here, we briefly stress the effect of the uptake of these nucleoside analogue compounds into cells and their phosphorylation to the triphosphate active form (Lewis et al. 2006). Thus, these active nucleotide triphosphates can be used as substrates by retroviral reverse transcriptase, but it is their incorporation into nascent DNA chains that results in chain termination and DNA damage. The triphosphate forms of these analogues have also been shown to be potential substrates for γ polymerase, the unique mitochondrial DNA polymerase, and incorporation of these analogues can similarly result in chain termination during mitochondrial DNA replication (Lewis et al. 2006). The additional effects on mitochondrial DNA synthesis result from the fact that conversion of the monophosphorylated forms to the triphosphates is extremely inefficient within mitochondria, leading to a strong (millimolar) build-up of these monophosphorylated forms in the mitochondrial matrix and adverse effects on mitochondrial DNA synthesis. These effects include inhibition of the exonuclease function of γ polymerase (resulting in decreased replication fidelity) and also, as was recently shown for the drug azidothymidine (AZT), a significant inhibition of thymidine phosphorylation, depleting reserves of thymidine triphosphate (Lewis et al. 2006). This dysfunction in DNA pol-γ, inducing a progressive depletion of mtDNA, disrupts the synthesis of essential proteins in the mitochondrial respiratory chain (Lewis et al. 2003). Consequently, this disruption results in a drop in ATP synthesis and leaking of electrons with an increased production of free radical species. Studies of NRTIs in enzyme assays and cell culture demonstrate that these drugs affect mitochondrial DNA polymerase in the following order: zalcitabine > didanosine > stavudine > lamivudine > zidovudine > abacavir (Lewis et al. 2006). In vitro investigations have also documented the impairment of mitochondrial adenylate kinase and the adenosine diphosphate/adenosine triphosphate translocator by NRTIs

(Lund and Wallace 2004). Inhibition of DNA polymerase gamma and other mitochondrial enzymes can gradually lead to serious mitochondrial dysfunction and cytotoxicity. The clinical manifestations of NRTI-induced mitochondrial toxicity resemble those of inherited mitochondrial diseases, such as hepatic steatosis, lactic acidosis, myopathy, peripheral neuropathy, and, intriguingly, nephrotoxicity. Fat redistribution syndrome, also known as HIV-associated lipodystrophy, is another side effect that is, in part, attributed to NRTI therapy (Lewis et al. 2003, 2006). The morphological and metabolic complications of HIV-associated lipodystrophy are similar to those of the mitochondrial disorder known as multiple symmetric lipomatosis, suggesting that mitochondrial toxicity may be the underlying mechanism for this disorder (Lewis et al. 2003; White et al. 2005).

Recent evidence has shown that the telomerase enzyme and its catalytic subunit, the telomerase reverse transcriptase (TERT), are further possible genomic targets in mitochondria. The telomerase is important for the maintenance of telomere length in the nucleus. Haendeler et al. (2009) provided evidence for a mitochondrial localization of TERT, and these authors showed that mitochondrial TERT exerted a novel protective function by binding to mtDNA and protecting it against oxidative stress-induced damage. These protective effects positively influenced complex I activity.

15.3.2 *Mitochondrial Respiratory Chain (MRC)*

In spite of the peculiar physicochemical and biological properties of the electron respiratory chain, direct drug-induced disruption of the MRC is often overlooked in the pathogenesis of drug-related disorders. In reality, drugs can target all four of the protein complexes in the respiratory chain. Often, disruption of the MRC is associated with a significant generation of free radical species, as the electron transport chain becomes unstable, which, in turn, may cause serious cellular damage. In fact, reactive oxygen species (ROS) and reactive nitrogen species (RNS) are closely linked to degenerative diseases, such as Alzheimer's disease, Parkinson's disease, neuronal death, including ischaemic and haemorrhagic stroke, acute and chronic degenerative cardiac myocyte death, and cancer. As a byproduct of oxidative phosphorylation, a steady stream of ROS and RNS is produced in mitochondria, and these species can potentially cause damage to all cellular components. ROS- and RNS-mediated alteration and fragmentation of biomolecule structure and oxidation of amino acid side chains are tangible risks of oxidative phosphorylation. Escape of ROS and RNS from the MRC results in the activation of cytosolic stress pathways, DNA damage, and upregulation of JNK, p38, and p53. Moreover, incomplete scavenging of ROS and RNS particularly affects the mitochondrial lipid cardiolipin (CL), triggering the release of mitochondrial cytochrome c and activating the intrinsic death pathway (Hatefi 1985; Harold 1986; Ho et al. 2005).

Many molecules that are well-known inhibitors of different mitochondrial complexes may be involved in iatrogenic mitochondriopathies. Some of these toxic compounds (rotenone, antimycin, cyanide, oligomycin, and mixothiazol) have been widely used in research to analyse the function of bio-energetic machinery in mitochondria and the electron transport chain and have already been the subject of numerous and exhaustive reviews and books (Fleischer 1979; Ernster 1984; Hatefi 1985,). Interactions of clinical interest include drugs that interact with the MRC, and these drugs have been less studied, but several drugs are well-known to act by partially inhibiting, either directly and/or indirectly, metabolites and different components of the MRC, particularly the drugs amiodarone, perhexiline, flutamide, and anthralin (Deschamps et al. 1994; Fromenty et al. 1990; Fau et al. 1994; Foody et al. 2006). However, the molecular mechanisms by which these drugs impair the MRC are not fully clear. Two hypotheses have been postulated: (1) a direct inhibition of a protein subunit of one (or more than one) of the enzyme complexes, and (2) scavenging of electrons from the MRC by drugs that act as electron acceptors (Krahenbuhl 2001; Scatena et al. 2003, 2007).

To further clarify the importance of this phenomenon, it is useful to discuss the evidence for chemically induced Parkinson's disease by accidental poisoning from MPTP (1-methyl-4-phenyl-

1,2,5,6-tetrahydropiridine), which is produced as an impurity in batches of the illegally made "synthetic heroin" MPPP (1-methyl-4-phenyl-4-propion-oxypiperidine). In particular, the metabolite of MPTP, MPP+, seems to affect preferentially complex I of the mitochondrial oxidative phosphorylation pathway in dopaminergic neurons (Krueger et al. 1990). Experimental and clinical data showed that iatrogenic Parkinson's disease is characterized by the same neuropathological features of the idiopathic form (i.e., loss of substantia nigra dopaminergic neurons, formation of Lewy bodies, accumulation of neuromelanin in microglia and the extracellular matrix) (Fahn and Sulzer 2005). Many other miscellaneous molecules are considered complex I inhibitors, some of which are well-established drugs, such as papaverine, meperidine, cinnarizine, amytal, haloperidol, ketoconazole and its analogues (Singer and Gutman 1971; Filser and Werner 1988; Subramanyan et al. 1990; Veitch and Hue 1994; Morikawa et al. 1996.). These molecules have been described as having the common structural motif of a cyclic head plus a hydrophobic tail (Degli Esposti 1998; Miyoshi 1998; Drose et al. 2006; Duchen 2004). Interestingly, this typical structure is also present in another class of therapeutic agents, the so-called fibrates (clofibric acid, bezafibrate, and gemfibrozil) and in some of their derivatives, the thiazolidinediones (ciglitazone, troglitazone, and pioglitazone). Our studies (Scatena et al. 2003, 2004a, b, 2005, 2007), recently confirmed by Brunmair et al. (2004a, b), showed that these compounds can also induce inhibition of mitochondrial complex I that leads to the metabolic consequences typical of their pharmacological activities (hypolipidaemic and hypoglycaemic effects), and this could, in turn, explain some of their toxic effects (rhabdomyolisis, acute liver failure), which resemble inherited mitochondriopathies.

In conclusion, more than 60 different types of compounds are well-known inhibitors of complex I, and this number continues to grow. Interestingly, this tendency of xenobiotics to disrupt complex I (mitochondrial NADH ubiquinone oxidoreductase; EC 1.6.5.3) could depend on the intricate structure of this enzymatic complex, which consists of at least 40 different polypeptides that are strongly embedded in the inner mitochondrial membrane. This characteristic predisposes complex I to vulnerability to lipophilic molecules (Degli Esposti 1998; Miyoshi 1998; Don and Hogg 2004).

In addition to being susceptible to inhibition by drugs, complex I is also a secondary target of nitric oxide in general and nitrogen radical species in particular, and this property should be kept in mind when patients are treated with NO-donor drugs, particularly those that are new (Moncada and Erusalimsky 2002; Brown and Borutaite 2004; Carreras et al. 2004; Scatena et al. 2005).

Complex II of the electron respiratory chain (succinate dehydrogenase, or SDH) is less commonly studied in mitochondrial pharmacotoxicology, which is surprising, considering that it plays an additional role in the Krebs cycle. Apart from the common inhibitors usually employed in experimental studies (e.g., malonate, carboxin, 3-nitropropionic acid, etc), it is important to point out that some cis-crotonalide fungicides, diazoxide, chloramphenicol succinate, anthracycline drugs, and, more recently, some fluoroquinolones are complex II inhibitors, which are also inhibitory to other mitochondrial components, as previously reported (Wallace and Starkov 2000; Szewczyk and Wojtczak 2002). Recent reports about the role of SDH (or one of its subunits B, C or D) in susceptibility to tumours sheds opens up the possibility of oncosuppression and/or oncopromotion by mitochondria (Bayley et al. 2005; Gottlieb and Tomlinson 2005; Perumal et al. 2005; Stenthilnathan et al. 2006). The mechanism behind tumour promotion by SDH (and also by fumarate hydratase, or FH) has been ascribed to an intriguing metabolic signalling pathway, which starts with the physiological substrates of these enzymes (e.g., succinate and fumarate). In fact, these metabolites accumulate in mitochondria, owing to the inactivation and/or low activity of SDH and FH; therefore, they leak out to the cytosol and inhibit a family of prolyl hydroxylase enzymes (PHDs). This inhibition, in turn, may render neoplastic cells more resistant to apoptotic signals and activate a pseudohypoxic response (mediated by hypoxia inducible factor, HIF) that enhances glycolysis (Pollard et al. 2005). Other authors point to a different pathogenic mechanism which mainly involves oxidative stress. In particular, dysfunction of SDH seems to cause a mitochondrial overproduction of superoxide anion (O_2^-), and this mitochondrially generated oxidative stress can contribute to nuclear DNA damage, mutagenesis and, ultimately, tumourigenesis (Ishii et al. 2005).

Considering the potential value of these findings for pathophysiology and pharmacotoxicology, together with the recent publication describing a role of ROS as tumour suppressors and senescent inducers (Takahashi et al. 2006), a more defined understanding of the molecular mechanisms at the basis of SDH- and FH-mediated tumour suppression will lead to better insight into the link between cancer and mitochondria and carcinogenesis in general.

For complex III (ubiquinol and cytochrome c oxidoreductase; EC 1.10.2.2), there is a large number of inhibitors acting at different levels (myxothiazol, antimycin A), which until now, have not shown any outstanding clinical value (Wallace and Starkov 2000; Szewczyk and Wojtczak 2002), although complex III is reputed to be the major site for superoxide production in normal conditions and in disease states.

On the contrary, there are a number of well-known entities that fatally inhibit complex IV (cytochrome c oxidase), such as cyanide or hydrosulfide poisoning or carbon monoxide intoxication. More important, although not yet fully understood, are the effects arising from the interaction of nitric oxide (NO) and peroxynitrite (ONOO-) with cytochrome c oxidase, as well as with all of the other mitochondrial components in general (Scatena et al. 2010). NO mainly interacts at physiological levels with cytochrome c oxidase by competitively and reversibly inhibiting its activity (Brown and Borutaite 2004), thus altering the electrochemical gradient, which could affect calcium uptake, regulating such processes as mitochondrial transition pore (MTP) opening and the release of pro-apoptotic proteins (Ho et al. 2005). However, it is generally accepted that NO has a direct effect on the permeability transition pore complex (Figueroa et al. 2006). Moreover, high or persistent levels of NO in mitochondria could also promote the formation of mitochondrial oxidants, such as peroxynitrite, either extra- or intra-mitochondrially, leading to oxidative damage, most notably in complexes I and II of the electron transport chain, but also in ATPase, aconitase and Mn-superoxide dismutase (Moncada and Erusalimsky 2002; Radi et al. 2002). These findings should be taken into account during pharmacological treatment with new and old NO donors because the kinetics of NO-release in these drugs is rather difficult to regulate, which can result in abrupt changes in NO concentration to levels higher than normal (Brown and Borutaite 2004; Scatena et al. 2010).

The inhibition of complex IV by local anaesthetic drugs, such as dibucaine and lidocaine, appears less important from a clinical point of view; however, drug inhibition does show an interesting positive correlation with the degree of lipophilicity (Don and Hogg 2004; Krahenbuhl 2001).

Some polycationic molecules can interact with mobile electron carriers, leading to potential mitochondrial dysfunction induced by the interplay between biomembranes and/or cytochrome oxidase with cytochrome c (Indig et al. 2000; Callahan and Kopecek 2006; Yip et al. 2006). As an example of this, a dramatic toxic effect related to cerivastatin was characterized by severe episodes of rhabdomyolysis and secondary acute renal failure and was caused by the high dosage formulation of this statin (administered alone or in association with fibrates). Cerivastatin is an HMG-CoA reductase inhibitor but also reduces the endogenous synthesis of coenzyme Q, an effect that is often disregarded and may promote mitochondrial dysfunction of both complex I and II in predisposed patients with bioenergetic mitochondrial dysfunction from concomitant diseases, concurrent mitoxicant pharmacological treatment (e.g., treatment with fibrates), slow drug inactivation, or other pharmacogenomic conditions (Schaefer et al. 2004; Foody et al. 2006; Davidson et al. 2006).

Another class of chemical agents capable of MRC disruption are claimed to act as alternate electron acceptors (AeA) by extracting electrons from intermediates in the respiratory chain in competition with their natural substrates. These substances may also alter the redox cycle, passing electrons back to the respiratory chain at a later point, thus bypassing sites in the chain essential for energy generation. Compounds that are known to do this are the quinones, such as doxorubicin, menadione and paraquat. In particular, menadione, or vitamin K3, is a well-known electron respiratory chain uncoupling agent which functions by shunting electrons from complex I directly to complex IV, and its toxicity comes from the production of free radicals and a dramatic decrease in ATP (Shneyvays et al. 2005). Doxorubicin, a potent and broad-spectrum antineoplastic agent, is characterized by an intriguing myocardiotoxicity that seems to depend, at least in part, on its capability to trigger a redox cycle by interacting with components of the mitochondrial respiratory chain. Doxorubicin, or one of its metabolites, can accept one electron from complex I, generating a highly unstable semiquinone free radical intermediate that, in turn, can undergo three possible fates: (1) reduction to the corresponding hydroquinone, (2) formation of a covalent adduct with DNA and proteins, and (3) transfer of the unpaired electron to another acceptors (i.e., glutathione, thiol groups, haem proteins, tocopherols, ascorbic acid, and/or oxygen directly) (Wallace et al. 2000, 2003).

Importantly, many of the drugs capable of disrupting the MRC also induce the formation of reactive intermediates by mitochondrial-specific processes, many of which are often considered to be the molecular basis for cellular and/or molecular damage. There are also xenobiotics capable of inducing ROS generation without directly disrupting the MRC, examples of which are haloalkenyl cysteine conjugates, such as hexachlorobutadiene (which forms reactive thiols after activation by the mitochondrial enzyme β lyase), 4-thiaalkanoates (activated by fatty acid β oxidase) and valproic acid (activated by acyl-CoA synthase) (Nadanaciva and Will 2011; Price et al. 2011).

15.3.3 Mitochondrial Oxidative Phosphorylation

Compounds that dissipate the proton gradient between the intramembrane space and the mitochondrial matrix interact at the oxphos level. They can, in fact, act as direct protonophores, shuttling hydrogen ions into the matrix (2,4-dinitrophenol is the classic example), or they may act as ionophores and exchange hydrogen ions for other mono- or divalent cations, or they may even increase the permeability of the inner membrane in general. The dissipation of the proton gradient without ATP generation can result in the generation of heat and, in extreme conditions, the onset of malignant hyperthermia syndrome (Duchen 2004). In this set of compounds that dissipate the proton gradient, we can include most of the NSAIDs, such as aspirin, diclofenac, and nimesulide (the pathogenesis of NSAID-related enteropathy involves intestinal damage from alteration of the intercellular junctions by uncoupling of mitochondrial oxidative phosphorylation) (Leite et al. 2001), but also some anti-tumour drugs and anti-psychotic, hypolipidaemic, and anti-mycotic compounds, as well. Interestingly, for all these drugs the main structure-activity relationship is based on the presence of a lipophilic weak acid moiety (Fleischer 1979; Moreno-Sanchez et al. 1999; Raza et al. 2011).

Other xenobiotics may disrupt oxphos by direct inhibition of the ATP synthase. The majority of these molecules are mycotoxins, such as oligomycin, but there are other well-known drugs that have this effect, such as propanolol, local anaesthetics and diethylstilbestrol. In particular, the pharmacological activities of propanolol should be carefully reevaluated, especially considering its typical side effect of reduction in cardiac output (Wagner et al. 2008; Minamiyama et al. 2010; Nadanaciva and Will 2011).

15.3.4 Mitochondrial Metabolic Processes

Catabolic and anabolic pathways in mitochondria can certainly be affected by different xenobiotics. In this chapter, we previously described some drugs that are able to induce tricarboxylic acid cycle dysfunction by interacting with SDH and FH. The potential toxicological value of these adverse interactions should not be underestimated, considering the etiopathogenic role of congenital abnormalities of these enzymes in serious forms of neurodegenerative diseases and cancer.

Evidence reported by Nulton-Persson et al. (2004) showed that treatment with salicylic acid and, to a lesser extent, acetylsalicylate increased the rate of uncoupled respiration in isolated cardiac mitochondria in agreement with previous findings (Moreno-Sanchez et al. 1999). However, under the experimental conditions employed, a loss in state 3 respiration resulted from inhibition of the Krebs cycle enzyme α-ketoglutarate dehydrogenase (KGDH). In particular, kinetic analysis revealed that salicylic acid acts as a competitive inhibitor at the α-ketoglutarate binding site. On the contrary, acetylsalicylate inhibited the enzyme in a non-competitive manner, consistent with interaction with the α-ketoglutarate binding site followed by enzyme catalysed acetylation.

Furthermore, it was also observed that cyclosporine reduced the concentrations of Krebs cycle intermediates in a time-dependent manner and inhibited mitochondrial oxidative phosphorylation at the level of ATP synthase. The real mechanism of such metabolic dysfunctions is still debated, and hypotheses include energetic failure, reduced protein synthesis and real enzymatic inhibition (Christians et al. 2004).

Isoniazid overdosage is an example of a drug interaction that may be related to metabolic dysfunction in mitochondria. At first glance, the effects of isoniazid overdosage are easily mistaken for a case of diabetic ketoacidosis, but further analysis suggests that the inhibition of pyruvate conversion to lactate and the interference with NADH synthesis in the Krebs cycle could contribute to the lactic acidosis observed in isoniazid intoxication, although the exact mechanism is still controversial. Surprisingly, serum isoniazid levels are not found to correlate with isoniazid toxicity and treatment (Alvarez and Guntupalli 1995; Tafazoli et al. 2008).

Another fundamental metabolic pathway that is often affected by xenobiotics is beta-oxidation. Numerous drugs (tetracycline derivatives, some NSAIDs such as ibuprofen and irprofen, glucocorticoids, antidepressants such as amineptine and tianeptinesome, some statins, fibrates, estrogens, and some antiarrhythmics and antianginal drugs, such as amiodarone and perhexiline) can either directly and/or indirectly disrupt mitochondrial fatty acid oxidation with considerable safety concerns, especially those affecting the liver (Szewczyk and Wojtczak 2002; Wallace 2003; Scatena et al. 2003, 2007; Vickers 2009). The precise molecular mechanisms serving as the basis of this dysfunction are not, however, clearly established. The pathogenesis associated with adverse effects of these drugs often appears secondary to MRC disruption that heavily hampers NADH and/or $FADH_2$ oxidation. Regarding the aforementioned fibrates and thiazolidinediones, it is interesting to note that our data, confirmed by Brunmair et al. (2004a, b), showed that the disruption of glucose metabolism and/or beta-oxidation correlates significantly with the level of complex I inhibition. In addition, Vickers et al. (2006) showed a direct inhibition by etomoxir of the mitochondrial beta-oxidation rate-limiting enzyme carnitine palmitoyltransferase I, and this inhibition was associated with oxidative stress, inflammation and apoptosis in the liver.

15.3.5 Mitochondrial Protein Synthesis

The close similarity between bacterial and mitochondrial ribosomes makes the latter a potential target for bacteriostatic antibiotics, such as chloramphenicol, aminoglycosides, tetracycline, and the newest family, the oxazolidizones (McKee et al. 2006). For the latter class, a direct correlation has been demonstrated between the bacterial MIC90, the IC50 for mitochondrial protein synthesis, and the potential for mammalian toxicity seen both in the clinical and toxicological studies, suggesting that this toxicity is manifested as a consequence of effects on mitochondria (Wallace and Starkov 2000; McKee et al. 2006). Interestingly, since the FDA approval of the oxazolidinone antibiotic linezolid, a number of papers surfaced reporting of lactic acidosis, peripheral and optic neuropathy, thrombocytopenia and pure red cell aplasia resulting from prolonged use, all of which are syndromes commonly associated with mitochondrial injury (McKee et al. 2006). It is worth noting that antibiotic inhibition of mammalian mitochondrial protein synthesis is often disregarded by not considering synergistic pharmacological interactions with other mitochondria toxicants.

A conclusion could be that the development of future antibiotics will have to evaluate potential mitochondrial toxicity.

15.3.6 Mitochondrial Channels and the Mitochondrial Permeability Transition Pore

A number of well-known drugs (e.g., potassium channel openers such as nicorandil and diazoxide, antidiabetic and antitumor sulphonylureas) modify the activity of different mitochondrial channels with fundamental roles of maintaining electrolyte homeostasis in mitochondria. These drugs interact with different components of the various ion channels, but the potential toxic effects and/or therapeutic applications of these mitochondrial channel alterations are not yet clearly defined. Similar considerations could be made for drugs interacting with or modulating components of the mitochondrial permeability transition pore, such as binding of cyclophilin D by cyclosporine A, binding of lonidamine to adenine nucleotide transferase (ANT), or drugs that bind to the mitochondrial benzodiazepine receptor, the toxic effects of which are still controversial in the clinic. The permeability transition pore is a high conductivity, nonspecific pore in the inner mitochondrial membrane that is composed of proteins that link the inner and outer mitochondrial membranes. When opened as a result of exposure to high calcium or inorganic phosphate, NAD(P)H, alkaline compounds, reactive oxygen species, and low molecular weight substrates can freely penetrate the mitochondrial matrix, carrying along water and resulting in mitochondrial swelling and the release of cytochrome c to the cytosol. Cytochrome c release triggers a cascade of events that lead either to apoptosis (in ATP-replete cells) or necrosis (in ATP-depleted cells). The toxicity of t-butyl-hydroperoxide and valproic acid and the chronic hepatotoxicity of diclofenac and other NSAIDs are mediated by this mechanism (Renner et al. 2003; Bouchier-Hayes et al. 2005), but, in general, the opening of this peculiar mitochondrial pore is a common end event brought on by different cell and mitochondrial toxicants.

Specifically, a recent study showed that NSAIDs, including low-dose aspirin, can induce small bowel injury by uncoupling of oxidative phosphorylation, and this uncoupling depends on the opening of the mitochondrial permeability transition pore. Interestingly, bile acids and tumour necrosis factor-α also seem to cooperate to open the permeability transition pore. The opening of the permeability transition pore induces the release of cytochrome c from the mitochondrial matrix into the cytosol, which triggers a cascade of events that leads to cell death. In conclusion, these mitochondrial disorders may play particularly important roles in early stages of bowel injury caused by NSAIDs (Scarpignato and Hunt 2010).

The controversy in the literature surrounding is an example of the debate on drugs and mitochondrial channels. According to Sklaska et al. (2005), sulphonylureas induce mitochondrial swelling, lower the mitochondrial membrane potential, and allow for the efflux of calcium from the matrix, mostly by activating the mitochondrial permeability transition pore. In contrast, Fernandes et al. (2004) suggest that sulphonylureas interfere with mitochondrial bioenergetics mainly by permeabilizing the inner mitochondrial membrane to chloride and promoting the transport of chloride and potassium into mitochondria.

15.4 Mitochondria and Drugs: The Therapeutic Potential

Indeed, recent advances in mitochondrial biology have allowed for the selective targeting of drugs to mitochondria to modulate and manipulate their function and genomics for therapeutic purposes. A wide range of seemingly unrelated disorders (schizophrenia, bipolar disease, dementia, Alzheimer's disease, epilepsy, migraine headaches, strokes, neuropathic pain, Parkinson's disease, ataxia, transient ischaemic attack, cardiomyopathy, coronary artery disease, chronic fatigue syndrome, fibromyalgia, retinitis pigmentosa, diabetes, hepatitis C, and primary biliary cirrhosis) have similar underlying pathophysiological mechanisms, namely, the aberrant production of reactive oxygen species that results in mitochondrial DNA damage and ultimately, mitochondrial dysfunction. Therefore, antioxidant therapies hold promise for improving mitochondrial performance.

Due to the active redox environment and the excess of NADH and ATP at the inner mitochondrial membrane, a broad range of agents, including electron acceptors, electron donors, and hydrid acceptors can be used to influence the biochemical pathways related to the release of ROS and RNS. For example, a key therapeutic value could be used to enrich for selective redox modulators at their target sites. Hoye et al. (2008) used conjugating nitroxides with relatively high affinity for mitochondrial membranes to prevent superoxide production. Specifically, a modified gramicidin S segment was used for this purpose and was proven to be effective in cells and with cardiolipin oxidation in mitochondria and protected cells against a range of pro-apoptotic triggers, such as actinomycin D, radiation, and staurosporine. More importantly, these mitochondria-targeted nitroxide/gramicidin conjugates were able to protect against apoptosis in vivo by preventing cardiolipin oxidation induced by intestinal haemorrhagic shock. The authors also proposed an alternative chemistry-based approach to targeting mitochondria with proteins and peptides, as well as by attaching therapeutic payloads to lipophilic cationic compounds, such as sulfonylureas, anthracyclines, and other agents with proven or hypothetical affinities for mitochondria.

A more classical therapeutic approach is based on the use of antioxidants. In particular, coenzyme Q10 (CoQ10, 2,3-dimethoxy-5-methyl-6-decaprenyl-1,4-benzoquinone), a fat-soluble quinone with a side chain of 10 isoprenoid units, was the first drug adopted for targeting mitochondria. In fact, besides its physiological function as an electron carrier, CoQ10 also seems to stabilize mitochondrial respiratory chain complexes and to act as a potent scavenger of oxygen free radicals. Based on these molecular activities, CoQ10 has been applied with beneficial effects to the therapy of different congenital oxidative phosphorylation diseases. Interestingly, some positive effects have also been reported with neurodegenerative disorders in general and with Alzheimer disease in particular, although these results have not been confirmed (Kooncumchoo et al. 2006; Schaars and Stalenhoef 2008). Also, menadione and phylloquinone (vitamin K compounds that are well-known uncouplers of the electron respiratory chain), either alone or in combination with ascorbate, have been adopted for use in different congenital oxidative phosphorylation diseases, particularly in complex III dysfunctions, presumably because their mechanism of action consists of shunting electrons from complex I directly to complex IV (Scatena et al. 2007a, b).

15.4.1 Mitochondrial Channel Modulators

Many mammalian cells have two distinct types of ATP-sensitive potassium/K_{ATP} channels: the classic ones involve the surface membrane (sK_{ATP}), while the others involve the mitochondrial inner membrane (mitoK-ATP). Cardiac mitoK-ATP channels play a pivotal role in ischaemic preconditioning and, thus, are interesting drug targets. Unfortunately, the molecular structure of mitoK-ATP channels is not well-known, in contrast to sK_{ATP} channels, which consist of pore-forming subunits (Kir6.1 or Kir6.2) and a sulfonylurea receptor (SUR1, SUR2A, or SUR2B). Recently, it has been observed that some drugs behave as potassium channel openers (KCOs) that are capable of acting at the level of cellular membranes, including mitochondrial membranes, meaning that their pharmacological activity can be ascribed to mitochondrial ion modulation, as well (O'Rourke 2000; Szewczyk et al. 2010). These compounds, which include cromakalim, nicorandil and pinacidil, were found to modulate K1 channels, both in smooth muscle cell membranes and in mitochondria that displayed anti-anginal (nicorandil) or antihypertensive (cromakalim and pinacidil) profiles. Therapeutic activity at the mitochondrial level has also been reported for a variety of older antihypertensive agents, notably diazoxide and minoxidil sulphate, which may influence the activity of mitoK-ATP channels. Moreover, it has been recently observed that diazoxide decreases succinate oxidation in a dose-dependent manner, albeit at higher concentrations than those necessary to activate mitoK-ATP. Thus, it has been proposed that the cardioprotective effects of diazoxide may result from inhibition of SDH and a decrease in respiration, rather than from the opening of mitoK-ATP channels (Wang et al. 2001). Consistent with the findings that SDH is part of a protein complex capable of transporting K+, it has also been proposed that SDH regulates mitoK-ATP by physical interaction with the ionophore and not by its role in oxidative phosphorylation. Such data, once confirmed, could allow for the development of therapeutic strategies for different degenerative diseases and would underline the potential therapeutic role of mitoK-ATP modulation (Eguchi et al. 2009; Frantz and Wipf 2010).

15.4.2 Drug Targeting of Mitochondria as Anticancer Therapy

At present, there is an ongoing reevaluation of cell metabolism in general and cancer cell oxidative metabolism. The Warburg effect has been used to explain the metabolism of cancer since 1920. Some assumptions of Otto Warburg have been misinterpreted. In particular, aerobic glycolysis is erroneously thought to be upregulated in cancer cells because mitochondrial respiration in these cells is seriously impaired. It is becoming clear that the amount of lactic acid produced by cancer cells is two orders of magnitude higher than that produced by normal tissue, and this enhanced production of lactic acid is not at the expense of respiration. The interaction between drugs and mitochondria is worth mentioning in this section, as it could have striking possibilities for cancer therapy.

In fact, if the physicochemical and biological properties of mitochondria predispose them to damage by toxic agents, then these same properties could be used to target mitochondria as a selective anticancer therapy.

There are many potential anticancer targets in mitochondria, and their dysfunction could trigger cell apoptosis or necrosis pathways. Mitochondria are the main regulators of apoptotic cell death, mediating both extrinsic (cell-surface receptor mediated) and intrinsic apoptotic pathways.

Several molecular mechanisms are the basis for mitochondrial toxicity by different xenobiotics, and some of these can be and/or already are being utilized in cancer therapy, such as:

1. The inhibition of mtDNA synthesis by targeting of topoisomerase II with etoposide and its analogues, cisplatin, and 5-fluorouracil and analogues, or by targeting polymerase γ with the aforementioned NRTIs.
2. Disruption of the electron respiratory chain either by: (a) directly altering a single complex with drugs such as rotenone and analogues, arsenic trioxide (for Complex I), tamoxifen (for complexes III and IV), or genistein, 17α, and β-estradiol (for ATP synthase); (b) indirect generation of free radical species by the same agents that disrupt the electron respiratory chain, by impairing complex I and III; and (c) using photosensitizers or inhibitors of intrinsic antioxidant defences of mitochondria (i.e. as the SOD inhibitor 2 metoxyestradiol) (Dias and Bailly 2005).
3. Alteration of the mitochondrial permeability transition pore (MPTP) by interfering in different ways with the physiological function of this fundamental mitochondrial structure (i.e., using lonidamine and arsenic trioxide for adenine nucleotide translocase, cyclosporine A for cyclophilin D, or PK 11195 for the peripheral benzodiazepine receptor)
4. Inhibition of metabolic pathways other than glycolysis, such as the Krebs cycle and/or beta oxidation;
5. Opening of potassium channels by analogues of dequalinium, diazoxide, and amiodarone, which increase the permeability of the mitochondrial membrane to protons or potassium and induce a decrease of the mitochondrial membrane potential, resulting in the swelling of mitochondria, a decrease in ATP synthesis and the release of cytochrome c .
6. Bcl-2/Bcl-X$_L$ inhibition or Bax/Bak activation by antisense Bcl-2/ Bcl-X$_L$ drugs or by a single chain antibody which can sensitize apoptosis resistant cancer cells to chemotherapy (Don and Hogg 2004; Fulda et al. 2010; Ralph et al. 2010; Rohlena et al. 2011; Solaini et al. 2011).

The last two classes of anticancer targets represent interesting and innovative therapeutic approaches in which mitochondria are the primary targets. However, these therapies are not yet in the preclinical phase, and the real therapeutic index must be accurately evaluated before speculations can be made about their applications to cancer.

Before anticancer drugs target the induction of apoptosis and/or necrosis in cancer cells, experiments should be carried out first with neoplastic cells and to confirm the effect on mitochondria. As discussed previously in this chapter, some authors suggest that positively charged amphipathic molecules can be attracted by and penetrate into mitochondria in response to their highly negative membrane potential, and this response should be even more apparent in neoplastic cells, which have a more elevated cytoplasma/mitochondrial membrane potential than differentiated cells. This strategy represents the best compromise to target specifically pro-apoptotic drugs to cancer cells, but it should be kept in mind that the in vivo situation in cancer presents an extreme variability in the biological environment, thus risking exposure of patients to possible dangerous and dramatic side effects (Renner et al. 2003; Fulda et al. 2010; Giorgi et al. 2011; Lemarie and Grimm 2011).

Last, but not least, we envisage that the discovery of the so called "cancer stem cell" will revolutionize research on cancer cell metabolism because these cells, which may exhibit peculiar functional characteristics, could show a metabolism completely different from that of differentiated high cells (Scatena et al. 2011).

15.5 Conclusions

The structural and functional complexity of mitochondria justifies the growing pharmacological interest in this organelle. However, although many interesting and exhaustive reviews have been published, experimental studies with real clinical applications are scarce.

The future of mitochondrial pharmacology appears committed to the treatment of glucidic and lipidic metabolism and energy expenditure disorders. In fact, recent experimental and clinical research has been focused on molecular disruption of mitochondria and the pathogenesis of some of these inherited or acquired metabolic diseases (some mitochondrial forms of non-insulin-dependent diabetes mellitus, metabolic syndrome, and hyperlipoproteinaemias). The data from these studies seem to be confirmed by experimental evidence showing that it is possible to modulate glucose and /or fatty acid oxidation at the cellular level by pharmaceuticals. A similar approach to modulation of the expression and/or activity of the so-called UCPs (uncoupling proteins) of different tissues in general, or of adipose tissue in particular, could represent a new and revolutionary approach to pharmacological treatment of obesity (Harper et al. 2001; Woo et al. 2009). On this note, it is interesting that pharmacological research is developing new and more potent PPAR-ligands (type δ, in particular) for this specific clinical indication that exploit the capability to induce the expression of genes required for fatty acid catabolism and adaptive thermogenesis (Wang et al. 2003; Ooi et al. 2011). Considering the adverse side effects of some PPAR-ligands, an accurate analysis of the potential interactions of these compounds with mitochondria seems obligatory (Lopez-Soriano et al. 2006).

Recent data seem to indicate that mitochondria in cancer do not merely represent effectors of apoptosis, but have a more complex role in oncogenesis and oncosuppression (Scatena et al. 2008; de Moura et al. 2010; Czarnecka et al. 2010). Specifically, analysis of cancer cell metabolism is leading to a modification of the original concept of the Warburg effect that regarded mitochondria as simply damaged cell structures that cause a toxic release of ROS. At present, researches are rethinking the role of mitochondria in cancer metabolism, as an oxidative metabolism capable of adapting itself to the demands of uncontrolled cell proliferation. Experimental data (Scatena et al. 2003, 2004) clearly indicate that an iatrogenic disruption of the electron respiratory chain can induce differentiation or, more interestingly, a pseudo-differentiation in various human neoplastic cell lines, suggesting there are even more potential roles of mitochondria in the regulation of cancer cell homeostasis.

The possibility of modulating the activity of the mitochondrial electron respiratory chain by the so-called NO-releasing drugs can be further expanded to include potential therapeutic applications in mitochondrial medicine, although we should always be wary of causing undesired toxic effects, as drug-mitochondria interactions often are not carefully considered (Moncada and Erusalimsky 2002; Scatena et al. 2005).

In conclusion, aside from its functional role as an organelle, mitochondria represent, from a pharmacological point of view, a potential drug target with unexplored therapeutic and toxicological potential. The progress of mitochondrial medicine in the near future will shed light on this particular topic and provide a rich scientific background from which valid translational research can be realized.

References

Alvarez FG, Guntupalli KK (1995) Isoniazid overdose: four case reports and review of the literature. Intensive Care Med 21:641–644

Bayley JP, Devilee P, Taschner PE (2005) The SDH mutation database: an online resource for succinate dehydrogenase sequence variants involved in pheochromocytoma, paraganglioma and mitochondrial complex II deficiency. BMC Med Genet 6:39

Benard G, Bellance N, Jose C et al (2010) Multi-site control and regulation of mitochondrial energy production. Biochim Biophys Acta 1797:698–709

Bouchier-Hayes L, Lartigue L, Newmeyer DD (2005) Mitochondria: pharmacological manipulation of cell death. J Clin Invest 10:2640–2647

Brandon M, Baldi P, Wallace DC (2006) Mitochondrial mutations in cancer. Oncogene 25:4647–4662

Brown GC, Borutaite V (2004) Inhibition of mitochondrial respiratory complex I by nitric oxide, peroxynitrite and S-nitrosothiols. Biochim Biophys Acta 1658:44–49

Brunmair B, Lest A, Staniek K (2004a) Fenofibrate impairs rat mitochondrial function by inhibition of respiratory complex I. J Pharmacol Exp Ther 311:109–114

Brunmair B, Staniek K, Gras F (2004b) Thiazolidinediones, like metformin, inhibit respiratory complex I: a common mechanism contributing to their antidiabetic actions? Diabetes 53:1052–1059

Callahan J, Kopecek J (2006) Semitelechelic HPMA copolymers functionalized with triphenylphosphonium as drug carriers for membrane transduction and mitochondrial localization. Biomacromolecules 7:2347–2356

Cardoso AR, Queliconi BB, Kowaltowski AJ (2010) Mitochondrial ion transport pathways: role in metabolic diseases. Biochim Biophys Acta 1797:832–838

Carreras MC, Franco MC, Peralta JG, Poderoso JJ (2004) Nitric oxide, complex I, and the modulation of mitochondrial reactive species in biology and disease. Mol Aspects Med 25:125–139

Christians U, Gottschalk S, Miljus J (2004) Alterations in glucose metabolism by cyclosporine in rat brain slices link to oxidative stress: interactions with mTOR inhibitors. Br J Pharmacol 143:388–396

Czarnecka AM, Czarnecki JS, Kukwa W (2010) Molecular oncology focus - is carcinogenesis a 'mitochondriopathy'? J Biomed Sci 25:17–31

Dalgaard LT (2011) Genetic variance in uncoupling protein 2 in relation to obesity, type 2 diabetes, and related metabolic traits: focus on the functional -866G>A promoter variant (rs659366). J Obes 2011:340241

Davidson MH, Clark JA, Glass LM, Kanumalla A (2006) Statin safety: an appraisal from the adverse event reporting system. Am J Cardiol 97:32C–43C

de Moura MB, dos Santos LS, Van Houten B (2010) Mitochondrial dysfunction in neurodegenerative diseases and cancer. Environ Mol Mutagen 51:391–405

De Souza CT, Araújo EP, Stoppiglia LF (2007) Inhibition of UCP2 expression reverses diet-induced diabetes mellitus by effects on both insulin secretion and action. FASEB J 21:1153–1163

Degli Esposti M (1998) Inhibitors of NADH-ubiquinone reductase: an overview. Biochim Biophys Acta 1364: 222–235

Deschamps D, DeBeco V, Fisch C et al (1994) Inhibition by perhexiline of oxidative phosphorylation and the beta-oxidation of fatty acids: possible role in pseudoalcoholic liver lesions. Hepatology 19:948–961

Detmer SA, Chan DC (2007) Functions and dysfunctions of mitochondrial dynamics. Nat Rev Mol Cell Biol 8:870–879

Dias N, Bailly C (2005) Drugs targeting mitochondrial functions to control tumor cell growth. Biochem Pharmacol 70:1–12

Don AS, Hogg PJ (2004) Mitochondria as cancer drug targets. Trends Mol Med 10:372–378

Drose S, Brandt U, Hanley PJ (2006) K+-independent actions of diazoxide question the role of inner membrane KATP channels in mitochondrial cytoprotective signaling. J Biol Chem 281:23733–23739

Du H, Yan SS (2010) Mitochondrial medicine for neurodegenerative diseases. Int J Biochem Cell Biol 42:560–572

Duchen MR (2004) Mitochondria in health and disease: perspectives on a new mitochondrial biology. Mol Aspects Med 25:365–451

Eguchi Y, Takahari Y, Higashijima N (2009) Nicorandil attenuates FeCl(3)-induced thrombus formation through the inhibition of reactive oxygen species production. Circ J 73:554–561

Ernster L (1984) Bioenergetics. Elsevier Science Publishers, Amsterdam, The Netherlands

Fahn S, Sulzer D (2005) Neurodegeneration and neuroprotection in Parkinson disease. NeuroRx 1:139–154

Fau D, Eugene D, Berson A (1994) Toxicity of the antiandrogen flutamide in isolated rat hepatocytes. J Pharmacol Exp Ther 269:954–962

Fernandes MA, Santos MS, Moreno AJ (2004) Glibenclamide interferes with mitochondrial bioenergetics by inducing changes on membrane ion permeability. J Biochem Mol Toxicol 18:162–169

Figueroa S, Oset-Gasque MJ, Arce C (2006) Mitochondrial involvement in nitric oxide-induced cellular death in cortical neurons in culture. J Neurosci Res 83:441–449

Filser M, Werner S (1988) Pethidine analogues, a novel class of potent inhibitors of mitochondrial NADH: ubiquinone reductase. Biochem Pharmacol 37:2551–2558

Fleischer S and Parcker L (1979) Biomembranes, Part F: bioenergetics: oxidative phosphorylation, Methods in enzymol. Academic Press, New York

Foody JM, Rathore SS, Galusha D (2006) Hydroxymethylglutaryl-CoA reductase inhibitors in older persons with acute myocardial infarction: evidence for an age-statin interaction. J Am Geriatr Soc 3:421–430

Frantz MC, Wipf P (2010) Mitochondria as a target in treatment. Environ Mol Mutagen 51:462–475

Fromenty B, Fisch C, Berson A (1990) Dual effect of amiodarone on mitochondrial respiration. Initial protonophoric uncoupling effect followed by inhibition of the respiratory chain at the levels of complex I and complex II. J Pharmacol Exp Ther 255:1377–1384

Fulda S, Galluzzi L, Kroemer G (2010) Targeting mitochondria for cancer therapy. Nat Rev Drug Discov 9:447–464

Giorgi C, Agnoletto C, Bononi A et al (2011) Mitochondrial calcium homeostasis as potential target for mitochondrial medicine. Mitochondrion (in press)

Gottlieb E, Tomlinson IP (2005) Mitochondrial tumour suppressors: a genetic and biochemical update. Nat Rev Cancer 5:857–866

Haendeler J, Dröse S, Büchner N et al (2009) Mitochondrial telomerase reverse transcriptase binds to and protects mitochondrial DNA and function from damage. Arterioscler Thromb Vasc Biol 29:929–935

Hamm-Alvarez S, Cadenas E (2009) Mitochondrial medicine and therapeutics, Part II. Preface. Adv Drug Deliv Rev 61:1233

Harold F (1986) The Vital Force: A Study of Bioenergetics, W.H. Freeman & Co., New York

Harper JA, Dickinson K, Brand MD (2001) Mitochondrial uncoupling as a target for drug development for the treatment of obesity. Obes Rev 2:255–265

Hatefi Y (1985) The mitochondrial electron transport and oxidative phosphorylation system. Annu Rev Biochem 54:1015–1069

Ho WP, Chen TL, Chiu WT et al (2005) Nitric oxide induces osteoblast apoptosis through a mitochondria-dependent pathway. Ann NY Acad Sci 1042:460–470

Hoye AT, Davoren JE, Wipf P et al (2008) Targeting mitochondria. Acc Chem Res 41:87–97

Indig GL, Anderson GS, Nichols MG et al (2000) Effect of molecular structure on the performance of triarylmethane dyes as therapeutic agents for photochemical purging of autologous bone marrow grafts from residual tumor cells. J Pharm Sci 89:88–99

Ishii T, Yasuda K, Akatsuka A et al (2005) A mutation in the SDHC gene of complex II increases oxidative stress, resulting in apoptosis and tumorigenesis. Cancer Res 65:203–209

Jaeschke H (2007) Troglitazone hepatotoxicity: are we getting closer to understanding idiosyncratic liver injury? Toxicol Sci 97:1–3

Kooncumchoo P, Sharma S, Porter J et al (2006) Coenzyme Q(10)provides neuroprotection in iron-induced apoptosis in dopaminergic neurons. J Mol Neurosci 28:125–141

Krahenbuhl S (2001) Mitochondria: important target for drug toxicity? J Hepatol 34:334–336

Krueger MJ, Singer TP, Casida JE, Ramsay RR (1990) Evidence that the blockade of mitochondrial respiration by the neurotoxin 1-methyl-4-phenylpyridinium (MPP+) involves binding at the same site as the respiratory inhibitor, rotenone. Biochem Biophys Res Commun 169:123–128

Leite AZ, Sipahi AM, Damiao AO et al (2001) Protective effect of metronidazole on uncoupling mitochondrial oxidative phosphorylation induced by NSAID: a new mechanism. Gut 2:163–167

Lemarie A, Grimm S (2011) Mitochondrial respiratory chain complexes: apoptosis sensors mutated in cancer? Oncogene 30:3985–4003

Lenaz G, Baracca A, Fato R et al (2006) New insights into structure and function of mitochondria and their role in aging and disease. Antioxid Redox Signal 8:417–437

Lewis W, Day BJ, Copeland WC (2003) Mitochondrial toxicity of NRTI antiviral drugs: an integrated cellular perspective. Nat Rev Drug Discov 10:812–822

Lewis W, Kohler JJ, Hosseini SH et al (2006) Antiretroviral nucleosides, deoxynucleotide carrier and mitochondrial DNA: evidence supporting the DNA pol gamma hypothesis. AIDS 5:675–684

Lopez-Soriano J, Chiellini C, Maffei M et al (2006) Roles of skeletal muscle and peroxisome proliferator-activated receptors in the development and treatment of obesity. Endocr Rev 27:318–329

Lund KC, Wallace KB (2004) Direct, DNA pol-gamma-independent effects of nucleoside reverse transcriptase inhibitors on mitochondrial bioenergetics. Cardiovasc Toxicol 4:217–228

McKee EE, Ferguson M, Bentley AT, Marks TA (2006) Inhibition of mammalian mitochondrial protein synthesis by oxazolidinones. Antimicrob Agents Chemother 50:2042–2049

Minamiyama Y, Ichikawa H, Takemura S et al (2010) Generation of reactive oxygen species in sperms of rats as an earlier marker for evaluating the toxicity of endocrine-disrupting chemicals. Free Radic Res 44:1398–1406

Miyoshi H (1998) Structure-activity relationships of some complex I inhibitors. Biochim Biophys Acta 1364:236–244

Moncada S, Erusalimsky JD (2002) Does nitric oxide modulate mitochondrial energy generation and apoptosis? Nat Rev Mol Cell Biol 3:214–219

Moreno-Sanchez R, Bravo C, Vasquez C et al (1999) Inhibition and uncoupling of oxidative phosphorylation by non-steroidal anti-inflammatory drugs: study in mitochondria, submitochondrial particles, cells, and whole heart. Biochem Pharmacol 57:743–752

Morikawa N, Nakagawa-Hattori Y, Mizuno Y (1996) Effect of dopamine, dimethoxyphenylethylamine, papaverine, and related compounds on mitochondrial respiration and complex I activity. J Neurochem 66:1174–1181

Murphy MP, Smith RAJ (2000) Drug delivery to mitochondria: the key to mitochondrial medicine. Adv Drug Deliv Rev 41:235–250

Nadanaciva S, Will Y (2011) New insights in drug-induced mitochondrial toxicity. Curr Pharm Des 17:2100–2112

Nulton-Persson AC, Szweda LI, Sadek HA (2004) Inhibition of cardiac mitochondrial respiration by salicylic acid and acetylsalicylate. J Cardiovasc Pharmacol 44:591–595

O'Rourke B (2000) Myocardial K_{ATP} channels in preconditioning. Circ Res 87:845–855

Oliveira PJ (2011) Mitochondria as a drug target in health and disease. Curr Drug Targets 12:761

Ong MM, Latchoumycandane C, Boelsterli UA (2007) Troglitazone-induced hepatic necrosis in an animal model of silent genetic mitochondrial abnormalities. Toxicol Sci 97:205–213

Ooi EM, Watts GF, Sprecher DL et al (2011) Mechanism of action of a Peroxisome Proliferator-Activated Receptor (PPAR)-delta agonist on lipoprotein metabolism in dyslipidemic subjects with central obesity. J Clin Endocrinol Metab 96:E1568–E1576

Perumal SS, Shanthi P, Sachdanandam P (2005) Therapeutic effect of tamoxifen and energy-modulating vitamins on carbohydrate-metabolizing enzymes in breast cancer. Cancer Chemother Pharmacol 56:105–114

Pessayre D (2007) Role of mitochondria in non-alcoholic fatty liver disease. J Gastroenterol Hepatol 22:S20–S27

Pollard PJ, Brière JJ, Alam NA et al (2005) Accumulation of Krebs cycle intermediates and over-expression of HIF1α in tumours which result from germline FH and SDH mutations. Hum Mol Genet 14:2231–2239

Price KE, Pearce RE, Garg UC et al (2011) Effects of valproic acid on organic acid metabolism in children: a metabolic profiling study. Clin Pharmacol Ther 89:867–874

Radi R, Cassina A, Hodara R (2002) Nitric oxide and peroxynitrite interactions with mitochondria. Biol Chem 383:401–409

Ralph SJ, Rodríguez-Enríquez S, Neuzil J, Moreno-Sánchez R (2010) Bioenergetic pathways in tumor mitochondria as targets for cancer therapy and the importance of the ROS-induced apoptotic trigger. Mol Aspects Med 31:29–59

Raza H, John A, Benedict S (2011) Acetylsalicylic acid-induced oxidative stress, cell cycle arrest, apoptosis and mitochondrial dysfunction in human hepatoma HepG2 cells. Eur J Pharmacol 668:15–24

Renner K, Amberger A, Konwalinka G et al (2003) Changes of mitochondrial respiration, mitochondrial content and cell size after induction of apoptosis in leukemia cells. Biochim Biophys Acta 1642:115–123

Richard D, Picard F (2011) Brown fat biology and thermogenesis. Front Biosci 16:1233–1260

Rohlena J, Dong LF, Ralph SJ, Neuzil J (2011) Anticancer drugs targeting the mitochondrial electron transport chain. Antioxid Redox Signal 15:2951–74

Russmann S, Jetter A, Kullak-Ublick GA (2010) Pharmacogenetics of drug-induced liver injury. Hepatology 52: 748–761

Scarpignato C, Hunt RH (2010) Nonsteroidal antiinflammatory drug-related injury to the gastrointestinal tract: clinical picture, pathogenesis, and prevention. Gastroenterol Clin North Am 39:433–464

Scatena R, Bottoni P, Vincenzoni F et al (2003) Bezafibrate induces a mitochondrial derangement in human cell lines. Intriguing effects for a peroxisome proliferator. Chem Res Toxicol 16:1440–1447

Scatena R, Bottoni P, Martorana GE et al (2004a) Mitochondrial respiratory chain dysfunction, a non receptor-mediated effect of synthetic PPAR-ligands. Biochemical and pharmacological implications. Biochem Biophys Res Commun 319:967–973

Scatena R, Martorana GE, Bottoni P, Giardina B (2004b) Mitochondrial dysfunction by synthetic ligands of peroxisome proliferator activated receptors (PPARs). IUBMB Life 56:477–482

Scatena R, Bottoni P, Martorana GE, Giardina B (2005) Nitric oxide donor drugs: an update on pathophysiology and therapeutic potential. Expert Opin Investig Drugs 14:835–846

Scatena R, Bottoni P, Botta G et al (2007a) The role of mitochondria in pharmacotoxicology: a reevaluation of an old, newly emerging topic. Am J Physiol Cell Physiol 293:C12–C21

Scatena R, Bottoni P, Martorana GE et al (2007b) Mitochondria, ciglitazone and liver: a neglected interaction in biochemical pharmacology. Eur J Pharmacol 567:50–58

Scatena R, Bottoni P, Giardina B (2008) Mitochondria, PPARs, and cancer: is receptor-independent action of PPAR agonists a key? PPAR Res 2008:256251

Scatena R, Bottoni P, Pontoglio A, Giardina B (2010) Pharmacological modulation of nitric oxide release: new pharmacological perspectives, potential benefits and risks. Curr Med Chem 17:61–73

Scatena R, Bottoni P, Pontoglio A, Giardina B (2011) Cancer stem cells: the development of new cancer therapeutics. Expert Opin Biol Ther 11:875–892

Schaars CF, Stalenhoef AF (2008) Effects of ubiquinone (coenzyme Q10) on myopathy in statin users. Curr Opin Lipidol 19:553–557

Schaefer WH, Lawrence JW, Loughlin AF et al (2004) Evaluation of ubiquinone concentration and mitochondrial function relative to cerivastatin-induced skeletal myopathy in rats. Toxicol Appl Pharmacol 194:10–23

Shneyvays V, Leshem D, Shmist Y et al (2005) Effects of menadione and its derivative on cultured cardiomyocytes with mitochondrial disorders. J Mol Cell Cardiol 1:149–158

Singer TP, Gutman M (1971) The DPNH dehydrogenase of the mitochondrial respiratory chain. Adv Enzymol Relat Areas Mol Biol 34:79–153

Skalska J, Debska G, Kunz WS, Szewczyk A (2005) Antidiabetic sulphonylureas activate mitochondrial permeability transition in rat skeletal muscle. Br J Pharmacol 145:785–791

Solaini G, Sgarbi G, Baracca A (2011) Oxidative phosphorylation in cancer cells. Biochim Biophys Acta 1807:534–542

Senthilnathan P, Padmavathi R, Magesh V, Sakthisekaran D (2006) Modulation of TCA cycle enzymes and electron transport chain systems in experimental lung cancer Life Sci 78:1010–1014

Subramanyam B, Rollema H, Woolf T, Castagnoli N Jr (1990) Identification of a potentially neurotoxic pyridinium metabolite of haloperidol in rats. Biochem Biophys Res Commun 166:238–244

Suski J, Lebiedzinska M, Machado NG et al (2011) Mitochondrial tolerance to drugs and toxic agents in ageing and disease. Curr Drug Targets 12:827–849

Szewczyk A, Wojtczak L (2002) Mitochondria as a pharmacological target. Pharmacol Rev 54:101–127

Szewczyk A, Kajma A, Malinska D et al (2010) Pharmacology of mitochondrial potassium channels: dark side of the field. FEBS Lett 584:2063–2069

Tafazoli S, Mashregi M, O'Brien PJ (2008) Role of hydrazine in isoniazid-induced hepatotoxicity in a hepatocyte inflammation model. Toxicol Appl Pharmacol 229:94–101

Takahashi A, Ohtani N, Yamakoshi K et al (2006) Mitogenic signalling and the p16INK4a-Rb pathway cooperate to enforce irreversible cellular senescence. Nat Cell Biol 8:1291–1297

Veitch K, Hue L (1994) Flunarizine and cinnarizine inhibit mitochondrial complexes I and II: possible implication for parkinsonism. Mol Pharmacol 45:158–163

Vickers AE (2009) Characterization of hepatic mitochondrial injury induced by fatty acid oxidation inhibitors. Toxicol Pathol 37:78–88

Vickers AEM, Bentley P, Fisher RL (2006) Consequences of mitochondrial injury induced by pharmaceutical fatty acid oxidation inhibitors is characterized in human and rat liver slices. Toxicol In Vitro 20:1173–1182

Wagner BK, Kitami T, Gilbert TJ et al (2008) Large-scale chemical dissection of mitochondrial function. Nat Biotechnol 26:343–351

Wallace KB (2003) Doxorubicin-induced cardiac mitochondrionopathy. Pharmacol Toxicol 93:105–115

Wallace KB, Starkov AA (2000) Mitochondrial targets of drugs toxicity. Annu Rev Pharmacol Toxicol 40:353–388

Wang S, Cone J, Liu Y (2001) Dual roles of mitochondrial K_{ATP} channels in diazoxide-mediated protection in isolated rabbit hearts. Am J Physiol 280:H246–H256

Wang YX, Lee CH, Tiep S et al (2003) Peroxisome-proliferator-activated receptor delta activates fat metabolism to prevent obesity. Cell 113:159–170

White KL, Margot NA, Ly JK et al (2005) A combination of decreased NRTI incorporation and decreased excision determines he resistance profile of HIV-1 K65R RT. AIDS 19:1751–1760

Woo MN, Jeon SM, Shin YC et al (2009) Anti-obese property of fucoxanthin is partly mediated by altering lipid-regulating enzymes and uncoupling proteins of visceral adipose tissue in mice. Mol Nutr Food Res 53:1603–1611

Yip KW, Ito E, Mao X et al (2006) Potential use of alexidine dihydrochloride as an apoptosis-promoting anticancer agent. Mol Cancer Ther 5:2234–2240

Zhu X (2010) Mitochondrial dysfunction: mitochondrial diseases and pathways with a focus on neurodegeneration. Preface. Biochim Biophys Acta 1802:1

Chapter 16
Iatrogenic Mitochondriopathies: A Recent Lesson from Nucleoside/Nucleotide Reverse Transcriptase Inhibitors

George P.H. Leung

Abstract The use of nucleoside/nucleotide reverse transcriptase inhibitors (NRTIs) has revolutionized the treatment of infection by human immunodeficiency virus (HIV) and hepatitis-B virus. NRTIs can suppress viral replication in the long-term, but possess significant toxicity that can seriously compromise treatment effectiveness. The major toxicity of NRTIs is mitochondrial toxicity. This manifests as serious side effects such as myopathy, peripheral neuropathy and lactic acidosis. In general, it is believed that the mitochondrial pathogenesis is closely related to the effect of NRTIs on mitochondrial DNA polymerase-γ. Depletion and mutation of mitochondrial DNA during chronic NRTI therapy may lead to cellular respiratory dysfunction and release of reactive oxidative species, resulting in cellular damage. It is now apparent that the etiology is far more complex than originally thought. It appears to involve multiple mechanisms as well as host factors such as HIV *per se*, inborn mitochondrial mutation, and sex. Management of mitochondrial toxicity during NRTI therapy remains a challenge. Interruption of NRTI therapy and substitution of the causative agents with alternative better-tolerated NRTIs represents the mainstay of management for mitochondrial toxicity and its clinical manifestations. A range of pharmacological approaches has been proposed as treatments and prophylaxes.

Keywords NRTIs • Mitochondrial toxicity • Polymerase-γ • DNA depletion • Reactive oxygen species

16.1 Introduction

All cells except erythrocytes contain mitochondria. Mitochondria are small organelles located in the cellular cytoplasm. A single cell may contain hundreds-to-thousands of mitochondria (particularly cells with high-energy demands). Each mitochondrion contains 2–10 copies of mitochondrial DNA (mtDNA), which is almost exclusively maternally inherited (Wiesner et al. 1992). mtDNA is particularly susceptible to mutation due to the lack of several enzymes for DNA repair (Graziewicz et al. 2006). The mutation rate of mtDNA can be more than tenfold higher than that of nuclear DNA (Wallace 1992). Each mitochondrion has a double-lipid membrane, with an inner membrane folded into numerous cristae surrounding the matrix space. The inner membrane of the mitochondrion contains

G.P.H. Leung (✉)
Department of Pharmacology and Pharmacy, The University of Hong Kong, Hong Kong, China
e-mail: gphleung@hkucc.hku.hk

R. Scatena et al. (eds.), *Advances in Mitochondrial Medicine*, Advances in Experimental Medicine and Biology 942, DOI 10.1007/978-94-007-2869-1_16,
© Springer Science+Business Media B.V. 2012

Table 16.1 Clinical syndromes reported to be associated with NRTIs-induced mitochondrial toxicity

NRTIs	Clinical syndromes reported associated with mitochondrial toxicity	References
Abacavir	Negligible	Hervey and Perry (2000)
Adefovir	Nephotoxicity	Izzedine et al. (2004), Tanji et al. (2001)
Didanosine	Skeletal myopathy	Allaouchiche et al. (1999), Bissuel et al. (1994)
	Lactic acidosis and hepatic steatosis	Dalakas et al. (1990)
	Peripheral neuropathy	Cepeda and Wilks (2000), Dolin et al. (1995), Famularo et al. (1997)
	Pancreatitis	Allaouchiche et al. (1999), Dolin et al. (1995)
Emtricitabine	Negligible	Modrzejewski and Herman (2004)
Entecavir	Negligible	Amarapurkar (2007)
Lamivudine	Rare myopathy and pancreatitis	Adani et al. (2005), Tuon et al. (2008)
Stavudine	Skeletal myopathy	Miller et al. (2000), Mokrzycki et al. (2000)
	Lactic acidosis and hepatic steatosis	Miller et al. (2000), Mokrzycki et al. (2000)
	Peripheral neuropathy	Cepeda and Wilks (2000), Ronan et al. (2000)
Telbivudine	Rare myopathy and neuropathy	Fleischer and Lok (2009), Zhang et al. (2008)
Tenovir	Nephrotoxicity	Izzedine et al. (2009)
Zalcitabine	Skeletal myopathy	Benbrik et al. (1997)
	Lactic acidosis and hepatic steatosis	Vrouenraets et al. (2002)
	Peripheral neuropathy	Famularo et al. (1997), Fichtenbaum et al. (1995)
Zidovudine	Skeletal myopathy	Chariot et al. (1999), Dalakas et al. (1990), Dolin et al. (1995)
	Lactic acidosis and hepatic steatosis	Bissuel et al. (1994), Blanche et al. (1999), Chariot et al. (1999)
	Peripheral neuropathy	Dolin et al. (1995), Famularo et al. (1997)
	Cardiomyopathy	Domanski et al. (1995), Lipshultz et al. (2000)
	Pancreatitis	Chariot et al. (1999), Dolin et al. (1995)
	CNS degenerative disease	Blanche et al. (1999)

an oxidative phosphorylation (OXPHOS) system that provides most of the energy to cells (~95% of the ATP requirements of the cell). Mitochondria also play an important part in the progression and regulation of apoptosis as well as calcium homeostasis.

Mitochondrial dysfunction has been implicated in numerous disorders (e.g., neurological and cardiovascular) as well as drug-induced toxicities (Amacher 2005). A typical example of the latter occurs during treatment of infection by the human immunodeficiency virus (HIV) (Moyle 2005). Current guidelines in the United States recommend highly active antiretroviral therapy (HAART) in HIV patients. The regimen involves two nucleoside/nucleotide reverse transcriptase inhibitors (NRTIs) with a protease inhibitor. An alternative regimen involves three NRTIs. HAART has reduced morbidity and mortality due to HIV as well as the incidence of opportunistic infections, but the adverse effects associated with HAART (particularly with the use of NRTIs) are likely to pose a significant obstacle to long-term pharmacotherapy.

As early as 1988, it was found that HIV patients treated with high doses of the NRTI zidovudine developed skeletal muscle myopathies (Gertner et al. 1989). These adverse drug reactions were shown to be mitochondria-related after histological and electron microscopic examination of biopsy tissues. Tagged red fibers were evident, as was accumulation of mitochondria with paracrystalline inclusion in the subsarcolemmal space (Dalakas et al. 1990). Reduced levels of mitochondrial DNA, RNA and proteins were also observed in these patients, but these problems were reversible in 50% of patients withdrawn from the drug (Dagan et al. 2002). These findings led to the hypothesis that inhibition of mtDNA replication due to NRTIs may be the principal cause. In addition to myopathy, lactic acidosis, cadiomyopathy, hepatic steatosis, nephrotoxicity and neuropathy have been associated with NRTI therapy (Table 16.1). The clinical and morphological manifestations of these diseases very closely resemble those observed in various genetic mitochondrial disorders (Zeviani and Di Donato 2004).

This chapter aims to review the pharmacological mechanisms and pathways involved in the mitochondrial toxicity associated with NRTI use. Strategies to manage these sequelae and the future direction of pharmacological research are also outlined.

16.2 Pharmacology of NRTIs

The drug target of NRTIs is the RNA-dependent DNA polymerase viral reverse transcriptase. This enzyme is essential for viral replication because the virus can use it to copy the RNA retrovirus genome into double-stranded DNA. Once the viral DNA is integrated, cellular RNA polymerase copies it back into RNA to make full-length genomic RNA and mRNAs that encode the various viral proteins. The commonest NRTIs used clinically are abacavir, adefovir, didanosine, emtricitabine, entecavir, lamivudine, stavudine, telbivudine, tenofovir, zalcitabine and zidovudine (Fig. 16.1). Abacavir, didanosine, emtricitabine, stavudine, zalcitabine and zidovudine demonstrate efficacy for HIV infection, whereas adefovir, entecavir and telbivudine are used in the therapy of hepatitis-B infection. Lamivudine and tenofovir are used in the treatment of infection by HIV and hepatitis-B.

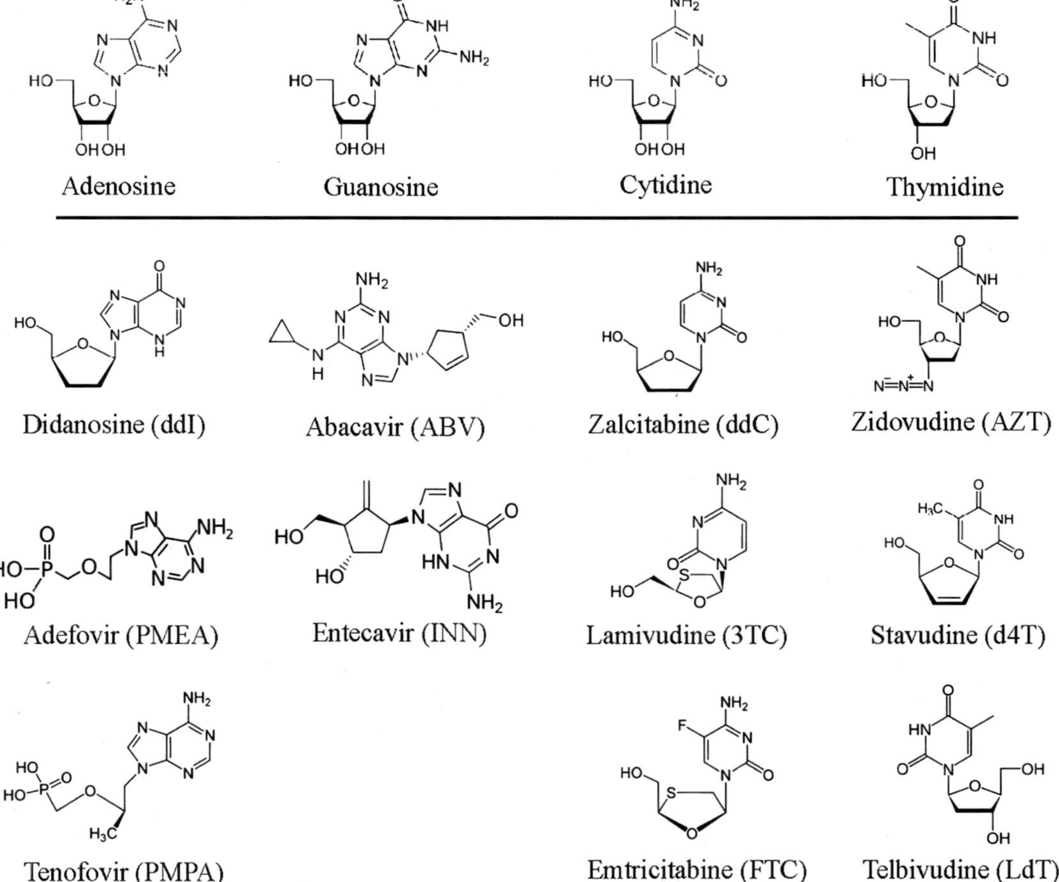

Fig. 16.1 Chemical structures of the nucleic acids and nucleoside/nucleotide reverse transcriptase inhibitors

NRTIs are derivatives of adenosine, cytidine, guanosine, and thymidine. As such, they provide an alternative substrate for viral reverse transcriptase. The important chemical modification of these compounds is the 3′-OH group of the deoxyribose sugar, which normally forms the 5- to 3-phosphoester bond with the next nucleic acid. The lack of an available 3′-OH group (or in the case of zidovudine, modification to an azido group (N_3)), prevents the attachment of subsequent nucleic acids by viral reverse transcriptase. Therefore, NRTIs can impair reverse transcription in two ways by: (i) competing with endogenous nucleic acids for incorporation; and (ii) prematurely terminating chain elongation once incorporated.

To serve as the substrates for viral reverse transcriptase, NRTIs must be in triphosphorylated forms. Metabolic activation (phosphorylation) occurs only if NRTIs are transported across plasma membranes and accumulate intracellularly. In general, NRTIs are too hydrophilic to diffuse into cells in large quantities. Most NRTIs (except tenofovir and adefovir) are nucleoside analogs, so are probably transported into cells by unique nucleoside transport systems rather than by diffusion (Leung and Tse 2007). Characterization of nucleoside uptake into human cells has led to the assumption that nucleoside transport can be mediated by at least nine systems. There are four equilibrative nucleoside transporters (ENTs); these are sodium-independent-facilitated systems and transport nucleosides down the concentration gradient. There are five human concentrative nucleoside transporters (CNTs); these are sodium-dependent systems and can transport nucleosides against a concentration gradient. Besides their thermodynamic properties (equilibrative or concentrative), these systems differ in their relative substrate specificity, pharmacological properties, and expression patterns in tissues and cells (Leung and Tse 2007). It has been reported that ENT1 can transport low concentrations of the antiviral drugs zalcitabine and didanosine but does not transport zidovudine. ENT2 transports zidovudine, zalcitabine and didanosine at a greater level than ENT1. ENT3 is a transporter of intracellular organelles, so its role in transporting nucleoside across plasma membrane is negligible. ENT4 mainly transports adenosine and organic cations across the plasma membrane, but the selectivity of nucleoside drugs to ENT4 has not been investigated. CNT1 can transport zidovudine and didanosine, but not lamivudine and zalcitabine. Didanosine is a substrate of CNT2, but zidovudine and zalcitabine are not substrates. CNT3 can transport zidovudine, zalcitabine and didanosine. In addition to CNT1-3, there are two other concentrative nucleoside transport systems: N4 and N5. The selectivity of the N4 and N5 systems to nucleoside drugs is not known.

Besides ENTs and CNTs, organic anion transporters (OATs), organic cation transporters (OCTs), peptide transporters (PEPTs) and multidrug-resistant proteins (MRPs) can transport NRTIs such as zidovudine, didanosine and zalcitabine (Chen and Nelson 2000; Han et al. 1998; Leung and Bendayan 1999; Wada et al. 2000). Tenofovir and adefovir are nucleotides so they are poor substrates of ENTs or CNTs. Evidence has demonstrated that adefovir and tenofovir can be transported by OAT1 and OAT3 (Uwai et al. 2007) as well as MRP4 (Imaoka et al. 2007). The relative contributions of ENTs, CNTs, OATs, OCTs, PEPTs and MRPs to the cellular transport of NRTIs has yet to be investigated, but is probably dependent upon the abundances and affinities of the transporters involved.

A schematic diagram of the intracellular phosporylation and activation of NRTIs is shown in Fig. 16.2. This stepwise activation process is mediated by a coordinated series of enzymes. Zidovudine, stavudine and telbivudine are initially phosphorylated by thymidine kinase to their monophosphorylated (MP) derivatives zidovudine-MP, stavudine-MP and telbivudine-MP, respectively; the corresponding diphosphate (DP) of zidovudine, stavudine and telbivudine is formed by deoxythymidine-MP kinase (Hsu et al. 2007). The first step in the phosphorylation of emitricitabine, lamivudine, and zalcitabine is catalyzed by deoxycytidine kinase. The second step is catalyzed by deoxycytidine-MP kinase to form the corresponding DP (Balzarini 1994). Cytidylyl transferase can add choline or ethanolamine to zalcitabine-DP, forming the liponucleotide adducts zalcitabine-DP choline and zalcitabine-DP ethanolamine, respectively (Rossi et al. 1999). These metabolites appear to be unique to zalcitabine. Didanosine is initially phosphorylated by 5′-nucleotidase to form didanosine-MP. It is then deaminated to form dideoxyadenosine-MP. Phosphorylation of dideoxyadenosine-MP to

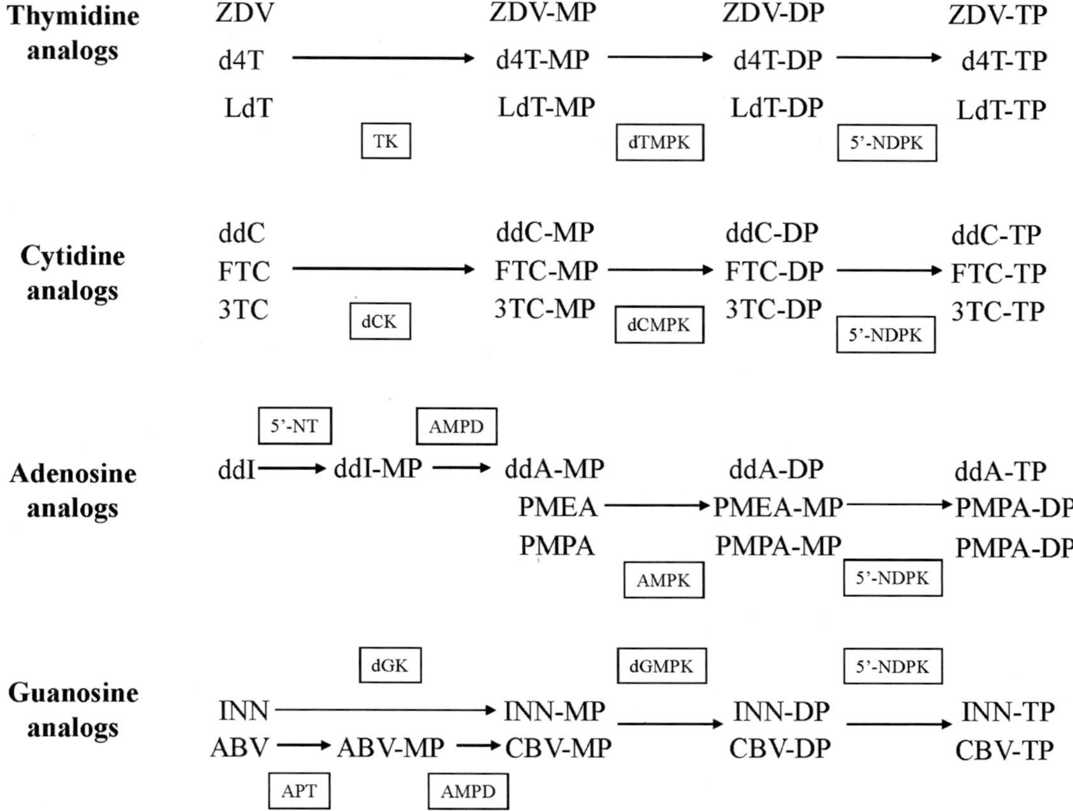

Fig. 16.2 *Host-cell-mediated sequential enzymatic phosphorylation steps required for activating the nucleoside/nucleotide reverse transcriptase inhibitors to the triphosphate moieties.* *ABV* abacavir, *AMPD* adenosine monophosphate deaminase, *AMPK* adenosine monophosphate kinase, *APT* adenosine phosphotransferase, *CBV* carbovir, *dCK* deoxycytidine kinase, *dCMPK* deoxycytidine monophosphate kinase, *ddA* 2,3-dideoxyadenosine, *ddC* zalcitabine, *ddI* didanosine, *DP* diphosphate, *dGK* deoxyguanosine kinase, *dGMPK* deoxyguanosin monophosphate kinase, *d4T* stavudine, *FTC* emtricitabine, *INN* entecavir, *MP* monophosphate, *LdT* telbivudine, *PMEA* adefovir (PMEA-MP and PMEA-DP are a diphosphate and triphosphate analogues, respectively), *PMPA* tenofovir (PMPA-MP and PMPA-DP are a diphosphate and triphosphate analogues, respectively), *TK* thymidine kinase, *dTMPK* deoxythymidine monophospahte kinase, *TP* triphosphate, *ZDV* zidovudine, *3TC* lamivudine, *5′-NDPK* 5′-nucleoside diphosphate kinase, *5′-NT* 5′-nucleotidase

dideoxyadenosine-DP is catalyzed by adenosine-MP kinase (Johnson and Fridland 1989). Unlike nucleoside analogs which are converted into nucleotide analogs by the body, tenofovir and adefovir are monophosphates already so they are directly phosphorylated by adenosine-MP kinase to form tenofovir-MP and adefovir-MP, respectively (Merta et al. 1992). Entecavir is phosphorylated by deoxyguanosine kinase (dGK) to form entecavir-MP, which is subsequently converted to entecavir-DP by deoxyguanosine-MP kinase (Yamanaka et al. 1999). Abacavir has a unique intracellular phosphorylation pathway that first involves addition of a phosphate group by adenosine phosphotransferase to form abacavir-MP; deamination of abacavir-MP forms carbovir-MP, which is subsequently phosphorylated to form carbovir-DP (Faletto et al. 1997). The final step in phosphorylation (which is probably common to all NRTIs) is catalyzed by nucleoside diphosphate kinase (Balzarini 1994). The triphosphate forms of NRTIs are the active moieties that carry out the antiviral action.

The intracellular phosphorylation of NRTIs is subject to enzymatic and cellular regulation. For example, deoxythymidine-MP kinase is the rate-limiting enzyme for zidovudine activation (Balzarini et al. 1989). Nucleoside diphosphate kinase may represent a second rate-limiting enzyme in the final production of zidovudine-TP (Bourdais et al. 1996). *In-vitro* studies have demonstrated that the intracellular concentration is zidovudine-MP >> zidovudine-DP > zidovudine-TP (Balzarini et al. 1989), reflecting the "enzymatic bottlenecks" that occur with this drug. Unlike zidovudine, the rate-limiting enzyme for stavudine phosphorylation is thymidine kinase. Intracellular concentrations of stavudine-MP, stavudine-DP, and stavudine-TP *in vitro* are similar and relatively low because the rate-limiting enzyme occurs at the initial phosphorylation step (Balzarini et al. 1989). The difference in rate-limiting enzymes has important clinical implications. For instance, increases in the plasma concentrations of stavudine are unlikely to cause further elevation of intracellular stavudine-MP concentrations, whereas increases in the plasma concentrations of zidovudine can probably cause an increase in intracellular formation of zidovudine-MP. The formation of zidovudine-MP plays a crucial role in inhibiting the proofreading function of DNA polymerase-γ, resulting in mtDNA mutation (please see Sect. 16.4.2).

Cellular regulation of NRTI activation is also dependent upon whether the cell is post-mitotic (resting) or active. Resting cells preferentially phosphorylate lamivudine, zalcitabine, and didanosine, whereas activated cells preferentially phosphorylate thymidine analogs such as stavudine and zidovudine (Gao et al. 1993, 1994). Cytosolic thymidine kinase-1 (TK1) is highly expressed during the S-phase of the cell cycle and probably accounts for the latter effect (Munch-Petersen and Tyrsted 1977; Sakamoto et al. 1984). There have been no reports of cell cycle-regulated expression of thymidine kinase-2 (TK2), and its activity appears to be constitutively expressed (Munch-Petersen and Tyrsted 1977). In dividing cells, only 1–5% of the activity of thymidine kinase is TK2 but, in quiescent cells (e.g., non-proliferating lymphocytes), all thymidine kinase activity is reliant upon TK2 (Arnér et al. 1992; Munch-Petersen 1984).

16.3   Entry of NRTIs into Mitochondria

The existence of phosphorylated NRTIs in mitochondria may explain the toxicity profile of this drug class. Phosphorylated NRTIs in the mitochondria can be derived from two sources. First, it is known that the NRTIs can be phosphorylated in the cytosol by the mechanisms described above, and these phosphorylated derivatives can be transported into the mitochondria by the deoxynucleoside carriers (DNCs) (Dolce et al. 2001) or by as-yet-unidentified transport systems (Bridges et al. 1999). Several studies have suggested that DNCs link the mitochondrial toxicity of NRTIs to their mitochondrial import. An *in-vitro* study showed that zidovudine could not generate mitochondrial toxicity during exposure of isolated mitochondria to zidovudine. Instead, zidovudine was extremely toxic to mitochondria in activated whole cells compared with resting whole cells, which may indicate significant NRTI phosphate shuttling into mitochondria to elicit toxicity (Sales et al. 2001). Studies in transgenic mice have shown that overexpression of DNCs in the heart enhances zidovudine-, didanosine- and lamivudine-induced mitochondrial dysfunction in cardiomyocytes (Lewis et al. 2005, 2006). However, conflicting results have also been reported. Lam and co-workers demonstrated that overexpression of DNCs did not sensitize cells to the depletion of mtDNA caused by zalcitabine and didanosine (Lam et al. 2005). Downregulation of DNC expression by small interfering RNA was also ineffective in changing the effects of NRTIs on mtDNA depletion (Lam et al. 2005). These results argued the contribution of DNCs to the mitochondrial toxicity of NRTIs, so further investigation is required.

Some phosphorylating enzymes are specific to the mitochondria (e.g., TK2 and dGK) (Al-madhoun et al. 2004; Jullig and Eriksson 2000; Wang and Eriksson 2003). Therefore, an alternative source of NRTI phosphate in mitochondria is the non-phosphorylated NRTIs that may be directly transported into the mitochondria and then phosphorylated there (Barile et al. 1997). ENT1 is present on mitochondrial membranes (Lai et al. 2004). One study demonstrated that overexpression of ENT1 facilitates the entry of fialuridine (a NRTI that was originally designed as a therapy for hepatitis-B virus infection but was withdrawn because of high toxicity) into mitochondria and enhances mitochondrial toxicity (Lai et al. 2004). The presence of ENT1 on mitochondrial membranes can explain the mitochondrial toxicity of NRTIs that are substrates of ENT1, but it cannot fully account for the mitochondrial toxicity of other NRTIs (such as zidovudine) that are poor substrates of ENT1. Therefore, other nucleoside transporters are probably located on the mitochondrial membrane. It has been reported that part of the uridine uptake into human liver mitochondria is resistant to 10 nM nitrobenzylthioinosine, but is inhibited by 10 µM nitrobenzylthioinosine (Lai, et al. 2004), which is a typical characteristic of ENT2 and ENT3 (Ward et al. 2000; Baldwin et al. 2005). ENT3 was recently found to be localized to mitochondria and certain NRTIs such as lamivudine, zalcitabine zidovudine, stavudine and didanosine were good substrates for this transporter (Govindarajan et al. 2009; Baldwin et al. 2005). In addition to ENT1 and ENT3, mitochondria may contain other novel transporters, but further study is required to confirm this possibility.

16.4 Mechanisms of Mitochondrial Toxicity Induced by NRTIs

16.4.1 Inhibition of DNA Polymerase-γ and mtDNA Depletion

In addition to viral reverse transcriptase, it is well established that NRTIs can incorporate and inhibit human cellular DNA polymerase. There are five major human cellular DNA polymerases: α, β, σ, ε and γ. DNA polymerase-γ is located in the mitochondrion, but the remaining polymerases are located in the nucleus. DNA polymerase-α and DNA polymerase-ε are responsible for nuclear DNA transcription, whereas the primary function of DNA polymerase-β and DNA polymerase-σ is DNA repair. Each of these polymerases can inadvertently incorporate NRTIs instead of endogenous nucleotides. The general affinity of NRTIs to these polymerases is DNA polymerase-γ > DNA polymerase-β > DNA polymerase-α = DNA polymerase-ε (Kakuda 2000).

The major and most widely accepted hypothesis accounting for NRTI-induced mitochondrial toxicity is the inhibition of DNA polymerase-γ (Lewis et al. 2003). Phosphorylated forms of NRTIs hamper mtDNA synthesis by acting as competitive substrates to endogenous nucleotides and chain terminators at the nucleotide-binding site of DNA polymerase-γ because NRTIs lack the 3′-OH group necessary for further elongation of the mtDNA strand (Lim and Copeland 2001). The mtDNA polymerase-γ is crucial for mtDNA replication (Graziewicz et al. 2006), so inhibition of DNA polymerase-γ leads to mtDNA depletion. Depletion of mtDNA has been detected in cell models and animal models exposed to NRTIs (Lewis et al. 1992; Gerschenson and Poirier 2000; Walker et al. 2002). Reductions in mtDNA levels in tissues such as subcutaneous adipose tissue (Shikuma et al. 2001), skeletal muscle (Casademont et al. 1996), peripheral blood monocytes (Cherry et al. 2003), liver (Chariot et al. 1999; Walker et al. 2003) and placenta (Shiramizu et al. 2003) were also found in HIV-infected patients undergoing NRTI treatment. This mtDNA depletion coincides with aberrant mitochondrial morphology (Dagan et al. 2002).

A reduction of mtDNA content decreases the synthesis of mtDNA-encoded protein subunits of the OXPHOS system (Duong Van Huyen et al. 2006). A disruption of the OXPHOS system causes a reduction in ATP production and an increase in electron leakage from the electron-transport chain, which enhances the generation of reactive oxygen species (ROS) (Lewis and Dalakas 1995; Velsor et al. 2004). The increase in the concentration of ROS damages proteins, lipids and mtDNA, setting off a cascade of further oxidative damage to cells (Fig. 16.3).

Among the seven NRTIs approved for treatment of HIV infection, the relative potency in inhibiting mitochondrial DNA polymerase-γ is zalcitabine >> didanosine > stavudine > zidovudine >>>> tenofovir, lamivudine, emtricitabine and abacavir (Birkus et al. 2002; Martin et al. 1994). *In-vitro* studies have demonstrated that, with respect to the five NRTIs approved for treatment of hepatitis-B (lamivudine, adefovir, entecavir, telbivudine and tenofovir), their strengths of inhibition of DNA polymerase-γ

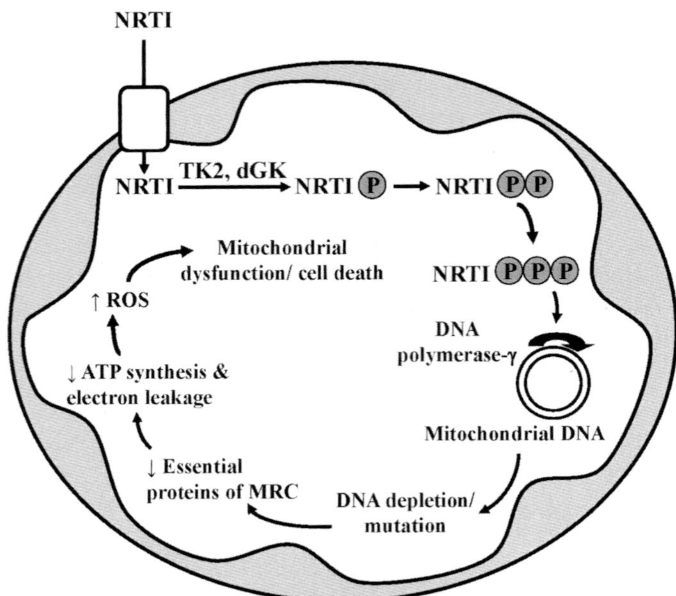

Fig. 16.3 *Mechanism leading to the mitochondrial toxicity of nucleoside and nucleotide reverse transcriptase inhibitors.* Nucleoside/nucleotide reverse transcriptase inhibitors (*NRTIs*) are transported into the mitochondria. They are phosphorylated by the mitochondrial-specific thymidine kinase-2 (*TK2*) or deoxyguanosine kinase (*dGK*), and then by other nucleotide kinases. *DNA polymerase-γ*, the mitochondrial DNA polymerase, is inhibited by the 5′-triphosphate derivatives of NRTIs. The resultant depletion and/or mutation of mitochondrial DNA then interferes the synthesis of essential proteins of the mitochondrial respiratory chain (*MRC*). The consequent disruption of the electron respiratory chain leads to the decreased *ATP synthesis* and causes electron leakage, resulting in the increase generation of reactive oxygen species (*ROS*). ROS damage the mitochondria and cause cell death

are substantially lower than those seen with zalcitabine, didanosine, stavudine and zidovudine (Birkus et al. 2003; Mazzucco et al. 2008; Venhoff et al. 2007). In particular, entecavir has demonstrated little evidence of mitochondrial toxicity compared with other NRTIs even at concentrations as high as 100-fold of the maximum concentration observed in humans (Mazzucco et al. 2008). Except for one case report (Fodale et al. 2005), lamivudine is, in general, believed to exhibit no significant mitochondrial toxic effect, and only causes mild myopathy and neuropathy. One factor that may be important for the lower toxicity profile of lamivudine is related to the exonuclease activity of DNA polymerase-γ. DNA polymerase-γ consists of a catalytic subunit of polymerase and 30–50 exonuclease activity (Falkenberg et al. 2007). NRTIs can usually persist in the mtDNA strands because of the inefficient activity of DNA polymerase-γ exonuclease (Hanes and Johnson 2008; Lewis et al. 2003; Kakuda 2000). An exception is lamivudine, which is more efficiently removed by DNA polymerase-γ exonuclease activity than other NRTIs (Gray et al. 1995).

It has been argued that the relatively less effective incorporation of zidovudine-TP into mtDNA cannot fully explain the mitochondrial toxicities of zidovudine (Elimadi et al. 1997), so zidovudine may have other cellular targets. Zidovudine has been shown to inhibit TK2 (McKee et al. 2004; Rylova et al. 2005) and nucleoside diphosphate kinase (Valenti et al. 1999), thus preventing the complete conversion of thymidine to deoxythymidine triphosphate (dTTP). It is known that dTTP concentrations are critical and rate-limiting to mtDNA replication (Song et al. 2005). Therefore, reduction in dTTP pools by inhibition of TK2 may explain the reduced mtDNA content in zidovudine-treated cells and tissues (Morris et al. 2009). Nevertheless, conflicting results also showed the lack of an effect of zidovudine on the dTTP pool in preadipocyte 3T3-F442a cells (Lynx et al. 2009).

16.4.2 Mutation of mtDNA

The hypothesis of mtDNA mutation is supported by studies showing that certain NRTIs can efficiently inhibit the exonuclease function of DNA polymerase-γ (Lim and Copeland 2001; Wu et al. 2009). For instance, zidovudine-MP is known to accumulate at high concentrations intracellularly, whereas the concentrations of the triphosphate form are found to be only 2 μM (Frick et al. 1988; Furman et al. 1986). This zidovudine-MP inhibits the exonuclease function as efficiently as its normal counterpart deoxythymidine-MP at concentrations predicted to occur in the cell (Lim and Copeland. 2001). Inhibition of DNA polymerase-γ proofreading by inactivation of exonuclease activity may result in lower replication fidelity, and an increase in mutations within mtDNA (Kunkel and Mosbaugh 1989). Zidovudine has been reported to be mutagenic in animal and cellular models (Meng et al. 2000; Sussman et al. 1999). Mutations of mtDNA were also demonstrated in 5 out of 26 patients undergoing NRTI therapy in which novel variations in the mtDNA sequence were found to arise within individuals (Martin et al. 2003). Similar to mtDNA depletion, mutations of mtDNA cause a wide range of mitochondrial diseases owing to the resulting defects in the OXPHOS system (Wallace 1992). When the OXPHOS system is disrupted, electrons can leak into the mitochondrial matrix, react with oxygen, and form ROS (Esposito et al. 1999).

16.4.3 Oxidative Stress

ROS are produced physiologically by the OXPHOS system of mitochondria in which ~2–4% of electron flux results in the reduction of oxygen to superoxide. In addition to superoxide, another ROS generated from mitochondria is hydrogen peroxide, which is rapidly formed from superoxide by dismutation. ROS are very reactive towards biomolecules. Upon oxidative attack of biomolecules, various types of damage can be generated: (1) lipid peroxidation (which leads to the generation of highly reactive aldehyde byproducts); (2) oxidation of SH groups (which causes protein aggregation); (3) oxidation of amino-acid side-chains form carbonyl groups (which target proteins for degradation); (4) oxidation of the sugar in nucleic acids (which leads to breakage of the phosphodiester backbone); and (5) oxidation of the bases in nucleic acids, with the concomitant formation of a plethora of base modifications that can be mutagenic or cytotoxic.

It has been reported that ROS, peroxynitrite formation, lipid peroxidation, and oxidation of cellular proteins are increased in the hearts of zidovudine-treated rats (Szabados et al. 1999). Via measurement of 8-hydroxyguanosine levels, oxidative stress has been demonstrated in cells isolated from the urine of zidovudine-treated patients or mice (de la Asuncion et al. 1998). Zidovudine also induces ROS formation in choriocarcinoma cells and primary explant cultures from human placentas (Collier et al. 2003). The increase in ROS production is probably due to the depletion and/or mutation of mtDNA as described above. Nonetheless, zidovudine can also directly cause a decrease in the expression of complex IV of the OXPHOS system, even in the absence of mtDNA depletion (Pan-Zhou et al. 2000). Besides, zidovudine may stimulate production of superoxide anion via inhibition of phosphate transport in rat heart mitochondria (Valenti et al. 2002). In addition, zidovudine may compete with nicotinamide adenine dinucleotide (NADH) directly at complex I (Lund and Wallace 2004). Zidovudine consistently exerted a dose-dependent inhibitory effect on NADH-linked respiration and cytochrome c reductase activity (Modica-Napolitano 1993). One study has shown that the short-term cardiotoxicity of zalcitabline may be partially induced by ROS-mediated signaling through activation of the poly- and mono-ADP-ribosylation reaction and depression of levels of heat-shock protein 70 (Skuta et al. 1999). This represents a new mtDNA-independent mechanism for NRTI-induced cellular damage.

16.4.4 Inhibition of Energy-Supplying Reactions

Depletion and mutation of mtDNA, and oxidative stress are incorporated into a pathophysiological continuum related to energy depletion. Mitochondrial bioenergetics can also be impaired by NRTIs via other mechanisms. For instance, complex I activity and superoxide production are modulated through cAMP-dependent phosphorylation, suggesting a mechanism through which NRTIs may affect mitochondrial respiration via kinase-dependent protein phosphorylation (Lund and Wallace 2008). It has been reported that zidovudine can bind to adenylate kinase, an enzyme involved in ATP formation (Barile et al. 1994). In addition, zidovudine may competitively inhibit ADP/ATP antiports in mitochondria (Barile et al. 1997).

16.4.5 Apoptosis

NRTIs may trigger mitochondrial-induced apoptosis (Hashimoto et al. 1997). A significant reduction in the levels of the anti-apoptotic protein Bcl-2, release of cytochrome *c*, and an increase in levels of caspase-3 protein have been demonstrated if mitochondria are treated with zalcitabine (Opii et al. 2007). These results suggest that oxidative stress-induced apoptosis may be a possible mechanistic pathway to explain the role of NRTIs in cellular toxicity. A possible pathway of apoptosis may involve the stimulation of apoptotic protease activating factor-1 (Apaf-1) by cytochrome *c*. Activation of Apaf-1 is known to stimulate caspase-9, which can cleaves procaspase-3 to form caspase-3, an apoptosis-related cysteine peptidase (Thornberry and Lazebnik 1998).

16.5 Risk Factors for the Development of Mitochondrial Toxicity Induced by NRTIs

16.5.1 Advanced HIV Disease

Increased intracellular concentrations of NRTIs have been found in patients with low CD4+ T-cell counts, and the concentrations were seen to decrease if the CD4+ T-cell count and immune activation improved (Anderson et al. 2004; Barry et al. 1994). Consistently, NRTI-associated peripheral neuropathy is twofold more common in persons with CD4+ T-cell counts of <100 cells/mm^3 than it is in persons with higher CD4+ T-cell counts (Moyle 2000). An elevated state of cellular activation in patients with advanced disease may be a biological mechanism for increased NRTI phosphorylation. In line with this notion, increased total TK activity has recently been associated with cellular activation of NRTIs in HIV infection (Turriziani et al. 2005).

HIV infection and advanced HIV disease are also associated with highly elevated concentrations of pro-inflammatory and cell-activation markers such as pro-inflammatory serum cytokines and molecules, interferon, tissue necrosis factor (TNF), and soluble TNF receptor type-2 (Godfried et al. 1993; Hestdal et al. 1997; Kestens et al. 1994). Treatment of advanced disease significantly reduces the concentration of these cell-activation markers, which corresponds well to the reduction in the intracellular level of NRTI phosphate (Anderson et al. 2003; Behbahani et al. 2000). It points to a possible relationship between pro-inflammatory cellular activation and the intracellular pharmacology and toxicity of NRTIs. To add weight to this notion, one study assessed the total levels of zidovudine phosphate in the PBMCs of patients who were initially treated with zidovudine alone followed by the cytokine granulocyte-macrophage colony-stimulating factor (GM-CSF)+zidovudine. A trend of increase in zidovudine phosphate levels was observed during GM-CSF + zidovudine combination therapy (Scadden et al. 1996). In line with this, *in-vitro* studies have shown that cells treated with phytohemagglutinin or GM-CSF can generate 2- to 1,150-fold higher triphosphate concentrations of zalcitabine, lamivudine, stavudine, zidovudine, and didanosine than resting cells (Gao et al. 1993, 1994; Perno et al. 1992). In a clinical trial on fialuridine (investigational nucleoside analog for hepatitis-B treatment), 7 out of 15 patients suffered serious fialuridine toxicity: patients required liver transplantation or died. Analyses of liver biopsy specimens obtained before initiation of fialuridine treatment showed that the inflammation scores for these seven patients were significantly higher (McKenzie et al. 1995).

16.5.2   Inborn Mitochondrial Variant

Pre-existing mutations in mtDNA and nuclear DNA may predispose mitochondria to toxicity. A R964C mutation in the gene encoding DNA polymerase-γ has been found in a woman with stavudine-associated lactic acidosis, suggesting a higher risk of mitochondrial toxicity due to the pre-existing mutation in this gene (Yamanaka et al. 2007). This R964C mutation may affect the ability of DNA polymerase-γ to discriminate between natural nucleotide substrates and nucleotide analogs such as stavudine-TP (Bailey et al. 2009). In addition, studies have shown that mitochondrial haplogroup T is associated with a higher risk for peripheral neuropathy in patients treated with stavudine and didanosine (Hulgan et al. 2005), whereas mitochondrial haplogroup J possibly protects patients from lipoatrophy (Hendrickson et al. 2009; Hulgan et al. 2008). A recent study in the Indonesian population demonstrated that TNF-α 1,031*2 variant may be a risk factor for NRTI-associated peripheral neuropathy (Affandi et al. 2008).

16.5.3   Sex

One study found that intracellular zidovudine-TP and lamivudine-TP concentrations were 2.3- and 1.6-fold higher in women than in men, respectively (Anderson et al. 2003). These data provide insight that is consistent with epidemiological studies showing a higher incidence of NRTI-induced lipodystrophy, lactic acidosis and pancreatitis in women than in men (Bolhaar and Karstaedt 2007; Currier 2007; Moyle et al. 2002).

16.5.4   Comorbidities and Concomitant Medications

It has been reported that patients co-infected with HIV and hepatitis-C treated with ribavirin in combination with didanosine have a substantial risk for lactic acidosis (Bani-Sadr et al. 2005; Butt 2003; Moreno et al. 2004). In addition, interferon-α may aggravate myalgia due to telbivudine treatment (Zhang et al. 2008). Protease inhibitors may also act synergistically with NRTIs to enhance the neurotoxic effects of the latter (Lichtenstein et al. 2005; Smyth et al. 2007).

A higher incidence of NRTI-induced pancreatitis and peripheral neuropathy was observed in patients receiving hydroxyurea (a ribonucleotide reductase inhibitor sometimes used as an adjunct to didanosine in combination antiretroviral therapies) (Frank et al. 2004). An *in-vitro* study showed that hydroxyurea increases pancreatic cell toxicity in the presence of a high concentration of didanosine (Foli et al. 2001). The mechanism underlying this interaction may involve the production of endogenous deoxynucleotides. Endogenous deoxynucleotides are produced from two sources: (i) reduction of nucleotides to form deoxynucleotides (the *de-novo* pathway) and (ii) sequential phosphorylation of deoxynucleosides to deoxynucleotides (the salvage pathway). Hydroxyurea inhibits ribonucleotide reductase (the enzyme responsible for the reduction of nucleotides to deoxynucleotides), thereby halting the *de-novo* pathway. Corresponding decrease in endogenous deoxynucleotide pools in the cytoplasm may create a condition favoring NRTI triphosphates to incorporate to DNA polymerase-γ (Moore et al. 2000; Kewn et al. 2000). This hypotheisis was critizized by Hoggard and co-workers (Hoggard et al. 2002), who claimed that hydroxyurea does not affect measurable pools of endogenous nucleosides *in vivo*.

16.5.5 *Other Risk Factors for NRTI Toxicity*

Older age is a risk factor of NRTI-associated peripheral neuropathy, and is probably associated with accumulated mtDNA mutations (Hill et al. 2007; Hulgan et al. 2005). Other proposed risk factors for NRTI-associated toxicity include white race, diabetes mellitus, and decreased creatinine clearance (Anderson et al. 2004; Peltier and Russell 2006; Smyth et al. 2007).

16.6 Treatment and Prevention of NRTI-Associated Mitochondriopathy

Maintaining a high index of suspicion for NRTI-induced mitochondrial toxicities is critical. Early detection of symptoms such as myopathy and lactic acidosis may be ensured by close monitoring of muscle enzymes, liver enzymes and lactate levels in blood. Hepatic steatosis can be detected by computed tomography. Supportive care is necessary if patients are severely ill. For instance, in the case of lactic acidosis, hemodialysis and intravenous administration of bicarbonate are needed to improve acidosis. Patients often develop respiratory failure due to the severe acidosis, so ventilation may also be required.

Development of inexpensive, simple and non-invasive diagnostic tests for routine screening and monitoring of mitochondrial toxicity is essential for patients on NRTI therapy. Quantity and quality (i.e., level of mutations) of mtDNA can be assessed by sequencing, analyses of deletions, or real-time polymerase chain reaction. These techniques have shown that mtDNA levels were significantly lower in patients with "symptomatic hyperlactatemia" taking NRTIs, and that discontinuing therapy led to an increase in mtDNA (Côté et al. 2002). Other data indicated that a significant decrease in mtDNA copies per cell was detected in placenta and cord blood from HIV-positive women on NRTI therapy (Shiramizu et al. 2003). Although mtDNA content can be precisely measured in almost all human cells, quantification of mtDNA content must only address if the therapy influences DNA polymerase-γ. As mentioned above, NRTIs may affect mitochondrial functions by altering mitochondrial enzymes other than DNA polymerase-γ, so the impact of these alterations on mitochondria will be missed if only mtDNA content is assessed. Most importantly, reduced mtDNA content along with normal mtRNA levels encoded by mitochondrial genes has been observed, suggesting possible upregulatory mechanisms for mitochondrial transcription (Miró et al. 2004). Therefore, even though quantitative assays are, in general, technically simple, functional assays for mitochondria are equally important and necessary. Additionally, NRTI-induced mitochondrial injury is tissue- and drug-specific (Cherry et al. 2006), probably due to variable activation of NRTIs in different tissues (Rylova et al. 2007). Therefore, measurement of the changes in mtDNA in one tissue may not accurately reflect conditions in other tissues. In theory, determination of mtDNA levels in easily accessible PBMCs may permit prediction of the risk of symptoms such as polyneuropathy, liver steatosis, and hyperlactatemia.

Unfortunately, studies have not shown an association between mtDNA levels in PBMCs and the development of NRTI-induced toxic symptoms such as lipoatrophy or lactic acidosis (Cherry et al. 2002; McComsey et al. 2002, 2005). Tissue sampling (e.g., muscle and liver) is invasive and impractical for routine clinical use. There is a lack of convenient and reliable non-invasive diagnostic tests for predicting mitochondrial toxicities.

Management of mitochondrial toxicity during antiviral therapy with NRTIs remains a challenge but fortunately mitochondrial toxicity is usually reversible. The major treatment option for patients suffering from NRTI-induced toxicity is a change of antiretroviral agents. Change of NRTIs has been effective in reducing toxicity for zidovudine-associated anemia, neuropathy and even lipodystrophy (Carr et al. 2002; McComsey et al. 2004). Abacavir, lamivudine, emtricitabine and tenofovir have not been associated with significant mitochondrial toxicity based on *in-vitro* and clinical experience and may therefore represent the best replacement drugs. An alternative is to use a NRTI-sparing regimen such as dual protease inhibitors + non-NRTIs (Negredo et al. 2009). For lactic acidosis or other progressive and severe symptoms that carry considerable morbidity and mortality, NRTIs as well as the entire regimen should be stopped immediately for a certain period before restarting the antiviral treatment with other, less toxic NRTIs (Lonergan et al. 2004). Nevertheless, recurrence of lactic acidosis was reported in one patient immediately after the introduction of an alternative antiviral regimen (Brinkman and ter Hofstede 1999). Such cases should (if possible) be cared for with a longer therapy interruption to enable more complete resolution.

A range of nutritional supplements such as riboflavin, thiamine, ubiquinones (i.e., co-enzyme Q10), and L-carnitine has been proposed to reduce the incidence of NRTI-induced mitochondrial toxicity. Riboflavin is a precursor to important cofactors in the electron transport chain. Theoretically, riboflavin deficiency could impair oxidative phosphorylation, whereas its administration could improve respiratory-chain activity (Fouty et al. 1998). Thiamine is a coenzyme to pyruvate dehydrogenase that catalyzes formation of acetyl CoA from pyruvate for entry into the citric acid cycle. Thus, deficiency of this cofactor could also impair oxidative phosphorylation. It has been reported that serum lactate levels were normalized after the administration of thiamine in a patient with hepatic steatosis and severe lactic acidosis receiving NRTIs (Schramm et al. 1999). Similar to thiamine, dichloroacetate (activator of pyruvate dehydrogenase) has been reported to be a potential therapeutic agent for reducing NRTI-associated hyperlactatemia (Shaer and Rastegar 2000). Coenzyme Q is an important carrier of electrons in the respiratory chain. Coenzyme Q was shown to resolve symptoms in a patient treated with NRTIs and who developed moderate lactic acidosis and hepatic steatosis (Lenzo et al. 1997). Patients with NRTI-associated peripheral neuropathy had reduced levels of serum L-carnitine, which was not seen in asymptomatic HIV-positive controls (Famularo et al. 1997). The protective effect of L-carnitine against NRTI toxicity has been demonstrated in *in-vitro* models (Rossi et al. 1999; Semino-Mora et al. 1994). A randomized clinical study also demonstrated that L-carnitine could reduce oxidative stress and maintain mitochondrial membrane potential, thereby providing a protective effect against apoptosis in lymphocytes of individuals receiving zidovudine and didanosine (Moretti et al. 2002). Treatment with L-carnitine also results in a significant reduction in neuropathic pain experienced by patients after long-term NRTI treatment (Hart et al. 2004). Treatment with L-Carnitine may counteract NRTI toxicity by two major mechanisms: (i) it may reduce mtDNA damage by a direct antioxidant effect (Tesco et al. 1992), and (ii) it facilitates mitochondrial homeostasis of acetyl CoA and promotes long-chain free fatty-acid transport across mitochondrial membranes (Bremer 1990).

An association was found between ROS and mitochondrial toxicity, so antioxidants are thought to be beneficial in reducing mitochondrial toxicity. A pilot trial of antioxidants such as vitamin C, vitamin E and N-acetyl cysteine was carried out in HIV-infected subjects with lipoatrophy. The results showed that the waist-to-hip ratio was significantly decreased (although other anthropometric measurements were unchanged) (McComsey et al. 2003). Vitamins C and E were shown to reduce zidovudine-induced myopathy (McComsey and Morrow 2003). In addition to the nutritional supplements and antioxidants mentioned above, the cardioprotective drug mildronate can effectively prevent zidovudine-induced degenerative and inflammatory events in cardiac muscle in experimental animals (Klusa et al. 2006). Mildronate has been shown to inhibit carnitine palmitoyl transferase-1 in rat mitochondria (Dambrova et al. 2002), and it therefore lowers the amount of activated free fatty acids which have detergent-like activity. It is proposed that mildronate may protect mitochondrial membranes from damage by free fatty acids.

Theoretically, therapeutic agents that have an effect on purine pools and pyrimidine pools should be avoided in HIV-infected patients treated with NRTIs. Examples of such substances are leflunomide, and inhibitors of tetrahydrofolate reductase (e.g., methotrexate, aminopterin, pyrimethamine, and trimethoprim). The anti-herpes drug brivudin-A should not be used with NRTIs because one study showed that one of its metabolites inhibits dihydropyrimidine dehydrogenase, and thus may adversely affect the intracellular balance of natural pyrimidines and stavudine (De Clercq 2004). It has been reported that uridine may attenuate the mtDNA depletion and prevent apoptosis caused by pyrimidine-type NRTIs such as stavudine and zidovudine (Lebrecht et al. 2008; Setzer et al. 2008). The mechanism of the protective effects of uridine is incompletely understood (Walker and Venhoff 2005). Severe depletion of mtDNA and secondary respiratory chain dysfunction is thought to diminish the availability of intracellular pyrimidines because a normal electron flux through the respiratory chain is required for the activity of dihydroorotate dehydrogenase (DHODH), an enzyme that is essential for *de-novo* synthesis of pyrimidine (Gattermann et al. 2004). Intramitochondrial deficiency of pyrimidine could then induce or contribute to even more profound mtDNA depletion by allowing triphosphorylated pyrimidine NRTIs to compete more efficiently with their natural pyrimidine counterparts at DNA polymerase-γ. It is hypothesized that exogenous uridine supplementation may replenish the intracellular pyrimidine pools distal from DHODH through the salvage pathway (Walker and Venhoff 2005). Alternatively, uridine and/or its metabolites may compete with pyrimidine NRTIs at carriers permitting their intramitochondrial import, or at enzymes responsible for their intracellular activation (Kakuda 2000). Uridine is well tolerated by humans, and data have not indicated any negative effect of uridine on the antiretroviral efficacy of NRTIs. Therefore, supplementation with uridine may be a promising strategy to prevent or treat problems caused by NRTI-induced toxicity.

Prevention of mitochondrial dysfunction could be possible using knowledge of the pharmacology of NRTIs. The discovery and use of abacavir, emtricitabine and entecavir (which are specific to viral reverse transcriptase but not to host mitochondrial DNA polymerase-γ) has been a great step forward. Several amino-acid residues in the active site of DNA polymerase-γ are known to be responsible for the selection of incoming endogenous nucleotides and NRTIs. The Tyr951 residue has the largest role in selection of dideoxynucleosides, stavudine-TP, and possibly lamivudine-TP and carbovir-TP. Tyr955 and Glu895 appear to interact to form a steric block against endogenous nucleotides, as well as to interact with the rigid sugar rings of stavudine-TP and carbovir-TP (Lim et al. 2003). In addition, slight modification of the chemical structure of NRTIs can have a significant impact on their affinity for DNA polymerase-γ. For instance, NRTIs with a fluoro substitution at the ribose showed a markedly reduced effect on mtDNA compared with that of unsubstituted NRTIs (Cihlar et al. 2008; Tsai et al. 1994). This information could be very useful for the rational design of more effective antiviral inhibitors that do not cause deleterious effects on mtDNA replication. Another possible measure to prevent mitochondrial toxicity is to prevent the entry of NRTIs into mitochondria. To achieve this, we must first identify the difference between nucleoside transporters in the plasma membrane and in the mitochondrial membrane. A good example is ENT3, which is a nucleoside transporter predominantly localized on the mitochondria but not on the plasma membrane (Govindarajan et al. 2009). Consequently, we could design nucleoside analogs that are specific to nucleoside transporters in the plasma membrane and do not interact with those in the mitochondria. Alternatively, specific inhibitors could be used to block mitochondrial nucleoside transporters (Leung and Tse 2007).

16.7   Conclusion

Most of the clinical manifestations of NRTI toxicities resemble mitochondrial diseases, and histologic evidence demonstrates abnormal mitochondria and/or mtDNA depletion in affected tissues. Several studies have shown that NRTI triphosphates can competitively inhibit mtDNA polymerase-γ. This effect may in turn decrease the number and functions of mitochondrial respiratory chain proteins, cause energy depletion, induce oxidative stress, increase mutation in mtDNA, and result in mitochondrial and/or tissue failure. Clinical syndromes that may be mediated by NRTI-induced mitochondrial toxicity include myopathies, hyperlactatemia, hepatic steatosis, peripheral neuropathy, and cardiomyopathy.

The mechanisms involved and the clinical relevance of NRTI-induced mitochondrial toxicity is more complicated than we may expect. To fully understand the pathogenesis of mitochondrial dysfunction, correlation between clinical observations, tissue biopsies, and assessment of mitochondrial function in humans is necessary. Risk factors for NRTI-associated toxicity also warrant further study because their clinical implications are important. For instance, current guidelines in the United States recommend a strategy of early administration of NRTIs to NRTI-naive patients (Panel on Antiretroviral Guidelines for Adults and Adolescents 2008). However, according to these guidelines, patients may also choose to postpone therapy, and providers may elect to defer therapy, based on clinical and/or psychosocial factors on a case-by-case basis. Postponing therapy may predispose patients with advanced HIV disease to increased NRTI toxicity. More studies are required to address the possible association between inflammatory cytokines and cellular NRTI pharmacology in patients. Drug–drug interactions involved in the treatment regimen of infection by HIV and hepatitis is another important topic. Further studies are also required to confirm if NRTI triphosphate levels are higher in women than in men. These issues may become more significant because women constitute most of the HIV-infected population in certain regions (e.g., sub-Saharan Africa) (Dabis and Ekpini 2002).

Patients established on therapy must be monitored closely for emerging signs and symptoms of mitochondrial toxicity. Various nutritional supplements and drugs such as riboflavin, co-enzyme Q10, L-carnitine, thiamine, dichloroacetate, antioxidants, uridine and mildronate have been proposed to reduce NRTI-associated toxicity. In general, the manifestations of NRTI-associated mitochondrial toxicity are (at least in part) reversible upon discontinuation of the causative agents. However, choosing agents that appear to have a low risk of these toxicities and avoiding use of combinations with overlapping mitochondrial toxicities remains the best means of limiting the incidence of these problems.

References

Adani GL, Baccarani U, Risaliti A, Bresadola F, Della Rocca G, Viale P (2005) Rhabdomyolysis due to Lamivudine administration in a liver transplant recipient. Am J Transplant 5(3):634

Affandi JS, Price P, Imran D, Yunihastuti E, Djauzi S, Cherry CL (2008) Can we predict neuropathy risk before stavudine prescription in a resource-limited setting? AIDS Res Hum Retroviruses 24(10):1281–1284

Allaouchiche B, Duflo F, Cotte L, Mathon L, Chassard D (1999) Acute pancreatitis with severe lactic acidosis in an HIV infected patient on didanosine therapy. J Antimicrob Chemother 44(1):137–138

Al-Madhoun AS, Tjarks W, Eriksson S (2004) The role of thymidine kinases in the activation of pyrimidine nucleoside analogues. Mini Rev Med Chem 4(4):341–350

Amacher DE (2005) Drug-associated mitochondrial toxicity and its detection. Curr Med Chem 12(16):1829–1839

Amarapurkar DN (2007) Telbivudine: a new treatment for chronic hepatitis B. World J Gastroenterol 13(46): 6150–6155

Anderson PL, Kakuda TN, Kawle S, Fletcher CV (2003) Antiviral dynamics and sex differences of zidovudine and lamivudine triphosphate concentrations in HIV-infected individuals. AIDS 17(15):2159–2168

Anderson PL, Kakuda TN, Lichtenstein KA (2004) The cellular pharmacology of nucleoside- and nucleotide-analogue reverse-transcriptase inhibitors and its relationship to clinical toxicities. Clin Infect Dis 38(5):743–753

Arnér ES, Spasokoukotskaja T, Eriksson S (1992) Selective assays for thymidine kinase 1 and 2 and deoxycytidine kinase and their activities in extracts from human cells and tissues. Biochem Biophys Res Commun 188(2):712–718

Bailey CM, Kasiviswanathan R, Copeland WC, Anderson KS (2009) R964C mutation of DNA polymerase gamma imparts increased stavudine toxicity by decreasing nucleoside analog discrimination and impairing polymerase activity. Antimicrob Agents Chemother 53(6):2610–2612

Baldwin SA, Yao SY, Hyde RJ, Ng AM, Foppolo S, Barnes K, Ritzel MW, Cass CE, Young JD (2005) Functional characterization of novel human and mouse equilibrative nucleoside transporters (hENT3 and mENT3) located in intracellular membranes. J Biol Chem 280(16):15880–15887

Balzarini J (1994) Metabolism and mechanism of antiretroviral action of purine and pyrimidine derivatives. Pharm World Sci 16(2):113–126

Balzarini J, Herdewijn P, De Clercq E (1989) Differential patterns of intracellular metabolism of 2′,3′-didehydro-2′,3′-dideoxythymidine (d4T) and 3′-azido-2′,3′-dideoxythymidine (AZT), two potent anti-HIV compounds. J Biol Chem 264(11):6127–6133

Bani-Sadr F, Carrat F, Pol S, Hor R, Rosenthal E, Goujard C, Morand P, Lunel-Fabiani F, Salmon-Ceron D, Piroth L, Pialoux G, Bentata M, Cacoub P, Perronne C, ANRS Hc02-Ribavic Study Team (2005) Risk factors for symptomatic mitochondrial toxicity in HIV/hepatitis C virus-coinfected patients during interferon plus ribavirin-based therapy. J Acquir Immune Defic Syndr 40(1):47–52

Barile M, Valenti D, Hobbs GA, Abruzzese MF, Keilbaugh SA, Passarella S, Quagliariello E, Simpson MV (1994) Mechanisms of toxicity of 3′-azido-3′-deoxythymidine. Its interaction with adenylate kinase. Biochem Pharmacol 48(7):1405–1412

Barile M, Valenti D, Passarella S, Quagliariello E (1997) 3′-Azido-3′-deoxythmidine uptake into isolated rat liver mitochondria and impairment of ADP/ATP translocator. Biochem Pharmacol 53(7):913–920

Barry M, Wild M, Veal G, Back D, Breckenridge A, Fox R, Beeching N, Nye F, Carey P, Timmins D (1994) Zidovudine phosphorylation in HIV infected patients and seronegative volunteers. AIDS 8(8):F1–F5

Behbahani H, Landay A, Patterson BK, Jones P, Pottage J, Agnoli M, Andersson J, Spetz AL (2000) Normalization of immune activation in lymphoid tissue following highly active antiretroviral therapy. J Acquir Immune Defic Syndr 25(2):150–156

Benbrik E, Chariot P, Bonavaud S, Ammi-Saïd M, Frisdal E, Rey C, Gherardi R, Barlovatz-Meimon G (1997) Cellular and mitochondrial toxicity of ziduvodine (AZT), didanosine(ddl) and zalcitabine(ddC) on cultured human cells. J Neurol Sci 149(1):19–25

Birkus G, Hajek M, Kramata P, Votruba I, Holy A, Otova B (2002) Tenofovir diphosphate is a poor substrate and a weak inhibitor of rat DNA polymerases alpha, delta, and epsilon. Antimicrob Agents Chemother 46(3):1610–1613

Birkus G, Gibbs CS, Cihlar T (2003) Comparative effects of adefovir and selected nucleoside inhibitors of hepatitis B virus DNA polymerase on mitochondrial DNA in liver and skeletal muscle cells. J Viral Hepat 10(1):50–54

Bissuel F, Bruneel F, Habersetzer F, Chassard D, Cotte L, Chevallier M, Bernuau J, Lucet JC, Trepo C (1994) Fulminant hepatitis with severe lactate acidosis in HIV-infected patients on didanosine therapy. J Intern Med 235(4):367–372

Blanche S, Tardieu M, Rustin P, Slama A, Barret B, Firtion G, Ciraru-Vigneron N, Lacroix C, Rouzioux C, Mandelbrot L, Desguerre I, Rötig A, Mayaux MJ, Delfraissy JF (1999) Persistant mitochondrial dysfunction and perinatal exposure to antiretroviral nucleoside analogues. Lancet 354(9184):1084–1089

Bolhaar MG, Karstaedt AS (2007) A high incidence of lactic acidosis and symptomatic hyperlactatemia in women receiving highly active antiretroviral therapy in Soweto, South Africa. Clin Infect Dis 45(2):254–260

Bourdais J, Biondi R, Sarfati S, Guerreiro C, Lascu I, Janin J, Véron M (1996) Cellular phosphorylation of anti-HIV nucleosides. J Biol Chem 271(14):7887–7890

Bremer J (1990) The role of carnitine in intracellular metabolism. J Clin Chem Clin Biochem 28(5):297–301

Bridges EG, Jiang Z, Cheng YC (1999) Characterization of a dCTP transport activity reconstituted from human mitochondria. J Biol Chem 274(8):4620–4625

Brinkman K, ter Hofstede HJ (1999) Mitochondrial toxicity of nucleoside analogue reverse transcriptase inhibitors: lactic acidosis, risk factors and therapeutic options. AIDS Rev 1:141–148

Butt AA (2003) Fatal lactic acidosis and pancreatitis associated with ribavirin and didanosine therapy. AIDS Read 13(7):344–348

Carr A, Workman C, Smith DE, Hoy J, Hudson J, Doong N, Martin A, Amin J, Freund J, Law M, Cooper DA, Mitochondrial Toxicity (MITOX) Study Group (2002) Abacavir substitution for nucleoside analogs in patients with HIV lipoatrophy: a randomized trial. JAMA 288(2):207–215

Casademont J, Barrientos A, Grau JM, Pedrol E, Estivill X, Urbano-Marquez A, Nunes V (1996) The effect of zidovudine on skeletal muscle mtDNA in HIV-1 infected patients with mild or no muscle dysfunction. Brain 119(Pt 4):1357–1364

Cepeda A, Wilks D (2000) Excess peripheral neuropathy in patients treated with hydroxyurea plus didanosine and stavudine for HIV infection. AIDS 14(3):332–333

Chariot P, Drogou I, de Lacroix-Szmania I, Eliezer-Vanerot MC, Chazaud B, Lombes A, Schaeffer A, Zafrani ES (1999) Zidovudine-induced mitochondrial disorder with massive liver steatosis, myopathy, lactic acidosis, and mitochondrial DNA depletion. J Hepatol 30(1):156–160

Chen R, Nelson JA (2000) Role of organic cation transporters in the renal secretion of nucleosides. Biochem Pharmacol 60(2):215–219

Cherry CL, Gahan ME, McArthur JC, Lewin SR, Hoy JF, Wesselingh SL (2002) Exposure to dideoxynucleosides is reflected in lowered mitochondrial DNA in subcutaneous fat. J Acquir Immune Defic Syndr 30(3):271–277

Cherry CL, McArthur JC, Hoy JF, Wesselingh SL (2003) Nucleoside analogues and neuropathy in the era of HAART. J Clin Virol 26(2):195–207

Cherry CL, Nolan D, James IR, McKinnon EJ, Mallal SA, Gahan ME, Lal L, McArthur JC, Wesselingh SL (2006) Tissue-specific associations between mitochondrial DNA levels and current treatment status in HIV-infected individuals. JAcquir Immune Defic Syndr 42(4):435–440

Cihlar T, Ray AS, Boojamra CG, Zhang L, Hui H, Laflamme G, Vela JE, Grant D, Chen J, Myrick F, White KL, Gao Y, Lin KY, Douglas JL, Parkin NT, Carey A, Pakdaman R, Mackman RL (2008) Design and profiling of GS-9148, a novel nucleotide analog active against nucleoside-resistant variants of human immunodeficiency virus type 1, and its orally bioavailable phosphonoamidate prodrug, GS-9131. Antimicrob Agents Chemother 52(2):655–665

Collier AC, Helliwell RJ, Keelan JA, Paxton JW, Mitchell MD, Tingle MD (2003) 30-Azido-30-deoxythymidine (AZT) induces apoptosis and alters metabolic enzyme activity in human placenta. Toxicol Appl Pharmacol 192(2):164–173

Côté HC, Brumme ZL, Craib KJ, Alexander CS, Wynhoven B, Ting L, Wong H, Harris M, Harrigan PR, O'Shaughnessy MV, Montaner JS (2002) Changes in mitochondrial DNA as a marker of nucleoside toxicity in HIV-infected patients. N Engl J Med 346(11):811–820

Currier JS (2007) Sex differences in antiretroviral therapy toxicity: lactic acidosis, stavudine, and women. Clin Infect Dis 45(11):261–262

Dabis F, Ekpini ER (2002) HIV-1/AIDS and maternal and child health in Africa. Lancet 359(9323):2097–2104

Dagan T, Sable C, Bray J, Gerschenson M (2002) Mitochondrial dysfunction and antiretroviral nucleoside analog toxicities: what is the evidence. Mitochondrion 1(5):397–412

Dalakas MC, Illa I, Pezeshkpour GH, Laukaitis JP, Cohen B, Griffin JL (1990) Mitochondrial myopathy caused by long-term zidovudine therapy. N Engl J Med 322(16):1098–1105

Dambrova M, Liepinsh E, Kalvinsh I (2002) Mildronate: cardioprotective action through carnitine-lowering effect. Trends Cardiovasc Med 12(6):275–279

De Clercq E (2004) Discovery and development of BVDU (brivudin) as a therapeutic for the treatment of herpes zoster. Biochem Pharmacol 68(12):2301–2315

de la Asuncion JG, del Olmo ML, Sastre J, Millan A, Pellin A, Pallardo FV, Vina J (1998) AZT treatment induces molecular and ultrastructural oxidative damage to muscle mitochondria. Prevention by antioxidant vitamins. J Clin Invest 102(1):4–9

Dolce V, Fiermonte G, Runswick MJ, Palmieri F, Walker JE (2001) The human mitochondrial deoxynucleotide carrier and its role in the toxicity of nucleoside antivirals. Proc Natl Acad Sci USA 98(5):2284–2288

Dolin R, Amato DA, Fischl MA, Pettinelli C, Beltangady M, Liou SH, Brown MJ, Cross AP, Hirsch MS, Hardy WD, Mildvan D, Blair DC, Powderly WG, Para MF, Fife KH, Steigbigel RT, Smaldone L, AIDS Clinical Trials Group (1995) Zidovudine compared with didanosine in patients with advanced HIV-1 infection and little or no previous experience with zidovudine. Arch Intern Med 155(9):961–974

Domanski MJ, Sloas MM, Follmann DA, Scalise PP 3rd, Tucker EE, Egan D, Pizzo PA (1995) Effect of zidovudine and didanosine treatment on heart function in children infected with human immunodeficiency virus. J Pediatr 127(1):137–146

Duong Van Huyen JP, Batisse D, Heudes D, Belair MF, Piketty C, Gonzalez-Canali G, Weiss L, Kazatchkine MD, Bruneval P (2006) Alteration of cytochrome oxidase subunit I labeling is associated with severe mitochondriopathy in NRTI-related hepatotoxicity in HIV patients. Mod Pathol 19(10):1277–1288

Elimadi A, Morin D, Albengres E, Chauvet-Monges AM, Allain V, Crevat A, Tillement JP (1997) Differential effects of zidovudine and zidovudine triphosphate on mitochondrial permeability transition and oxidative phosphorylation. Br J Pharmacol 121(7):1295–1300

Esposito LA, Melov S, Panov A, Cottrell BA, Wallace DC (1999) Mitochondrial disease in mouse results in increased oxidative stress. Proc Natl Acad Sci USA 96(9):4820–4825

Faletto MB, Miller WH, Garvey EP, St Clair MH, Daluge SM, Good SS (1997) Unique intracellular activation of the potent anti-human immunodeficiency virus agent 1592U89. Antimicrob Agents Chemother 41(5):1099–1107

Falkenberg M, Larsson NG, Gustafsson CM (2007) DNA replication and transcription in mammalian mitochondria. Annu Rev Biochem 76:679–699

Famularo G, Moretti S, Marcellini S, Trinchieri V, Tzantzoglou S, Santini G, Longo A, De Simone C (1997) Acetyl-carnitine deficiency in AIDS patients with neurotoxicity on treatment with antiretroviral nucleoside analogues. AIDS 11(2):185–190

Fichtenbaum CJ, Clifford DB, Powderly WG (1995) Risk factors for dideoxynucleoside-induced toxic neuropathy in patients with the human immunodeficiency virus infection. J Acquir Immune Defic Syndr Hum Retrovirol 10(2): 169–174

Fleischer RD, Lok AS (2009) Myopathy and neuropathy associated with nucleos(t)ide analog therapy for hepatitis B. J Hepatol 51(4):787–791

Fodale V, Mazzeo A, Praticò C, Aguennouz M, Toscano A, Santamaria LB, Vita G (2005) Fatal exacerbation of peripheral neuropathy during lamivudine therapy: evidence for iatrogenic mitochondrial damage. Anaesthesia 60(8):806–810

Foli A, Benvenuto F, Piccinini G, Bareggi A, Cossarizza A, Lisziewicz J, Lori F (2001) Direct analysis of mitochondrial toxicity of antiretroviral drugs. AIDS 15(13):1687–1694

Fouty B, Frerman F, Reves R (1998) Riboflavin to treat nucleoside analogue-induced lactic acidosis. Lancet 352(9124):291–292

Frank I, Bosch RJ, Fiscus S, Valentine F, Flexner C, Segal Y, Ruan P, Gulick R, Wood K, Estep S, Fox L, Nevin T, Stevens M, Eron JJ Jr, ACTG 307 Protocol Team, (2004) Activity, safety, and immunological effects of hydroxyurea added to didanosine in antiretroviral-naive and experienced HIV type 1-infected subjects: a randomized, placebo-controlled trial, ACTG 307. AIDS Res Hum Retroviruses 20(9):916–926

Frick LW, Nelson DJ, St Clair MH, Furman PA, Krenitsky TA (1988) Effects of 3'-azido-3'-deoxythymidine on the deoxynucleotide triphosphate pools of cultured human cells. Biochem Biophys Res Commun 154(1):124–129

Furman PA, Fyfe JA, St Clair MH, Weinhold K, Rideout JL, Freeman GA, Lehrman SN, Bolognesi DP, Broder S, Mitsuya H, Barry DW (1986) Phosphorylation of 3'-azido-3'-deoxythymidine and selective interaction of the 5'-triphosphate with human immunodeficiency virus reverse transcriptase. Proc Natl Acad Sci USA 83(21):8333–8337

Gao WY, Shirasaka T, Johns DG, Broder S, Mitsuya H (1993) Differential phosphorylation of azidothymidine, dideoxy-cytidine, and dideoxyinosine in resting and activated peripheral blood mononuclear cells. J Clin Invest 91(5):2326–2333

Gao WY, Agbaria R, Driscoll JS (1994) Mitsuya H. Divergent anti-human immunodeficiency virus activity and ana-bolic phosphorylation of 2,3-dideoxynucleoside analogs in resting and activated human cells. J Biol Chem 269(17):12633–12638

Gattermann N, Dadak M, Hofhaus G, Wulfert M, Berneburg M, Loeffler ML, Simmonds HA (2004) Severe impairment of nucleotide synthesisthrough inhibition of mitochondrial respiration. Nucleosides Nucleotides Nucleic Acids 23(8–9):1275–1279

Gerschenson M, Poirier MC (2000) Fetal patas monkeys sustain mitochondrial toxicity as a result of in utero zidovudine exposure. Ann N Y Acad Sci 918:269–281

Gertner E, Thurn JR, Williams DN, Simpson M, Balfour HH Jr, Rhame F, Henry K (1989) Zidovudine-associated myopathy. Am J Med 86(6 Pt 2):814–818

Godfried MH, van der Poll T, Jansen J, Romijn JA, Schattenkerk JK, Endert E, van Deventer SJ, Sauerwein HP (1993) Soluble receptors for tumour necrosis factor: a putative marker of disease progression in HIV infection. AIDS 7(1):33–36

Govindarajan R, Leung GP, Zhou M, Tse CM, Wang J, Unadkat JD (2009) Facilitated mitochondrial import of antiviral and anticancer nucleoside drugs by human equilibrative nucleoside transporter-3. Am J Physiol Gastrointest Liver Physiol 296(4):G910–G922

Gray NM, Marr CL, Penn CR, Cameron JM, Bethell RC (1995) The intracellular phosphorylation of (-)-2'-deoxy-3'-thiacytidine (3TC) and the incorporation of 3TC 5'-monophosphate into DNA by HIV-1 reverse transcriptase and human DNA polymerase gamma. Biochem Pharmacol 50(7):1043–1051

Graziewicz MA, Longley MJ, Copeland WC (2006) DNA polymerase gamma in mitochondrial DNA replication and repair. Chem Rev 106(2):383–405

Han H, de Vrueh RL, Rhie JK, Covitz KM, Smith PL, Lee CP, Oh DM, Sadée W, Amidon GL (1998) Amino acid esters of antiviral nucleosides, acyclovir, and AZT are absorbed by the intestinal PEPT1 peptide transporter. Pharm Res 15(8):1154–1159

Hanes JW, Johnson KA (2008) Exonuclease removal of dideoxycytidine (zalcitabine) by the human mitochondrial DNA polymerase. Antimicrob Agents Chemother 52(1):253–258

Hart AM, Wilson AD, Montovani C, Smith C, Johnson M, Terenghi G, Youle M (2004) Acetyl-l-carnitine: a pathogen-esis based treatment for HIV-associated antiretroviral toxic neuropathy. AIDS 18(11):1549–1560

Hashimoto KI, Tsunoda R, Okamoto M, Shigeta S, Baba M (1997) Stavudine selectively induces apoptosis in HIV type 1-infected cells. AIDS Res Hum Retroviruses 13(2):193–199

Hendrickson SL, Kingsley LA, Ruiz-Pesini E, Poole JC, Jacobson LP, Palella FJ, Bream JH, Wallace DC, O'Brien SJ (2009) Mitochondrial DNA haplogroups influence lipoatrophy after highly active antiretroviral therapy. J Acquir Immune Defic Syndr 51(2):111–116

Hervey PS, Perry CM (2000) Abacavir: a review of its clinical potential in patients with HIV infection. Drugs 60(2):447–479

Hestdal K, Aukrust P, Müller F, Lien E, Bjerkeli V, Espevik T, Frøland SS (1997) Dysregulation of membrane-bound tumor necrosis factor-α and tumor necrosis factor receptors on mononuclear cells in human immunodeficiency virus type 1 infection: low percentage of p75-tumor necrosis factor receptor positive cells in patients with advanced dis-ease and high viral load. Blood 90(7):2670–2679

Hill A, Ruxrungtham K, Hanvanich M, Katlama C, Wolf E, Soriano V, Milinkovic A, Gatell J, Ribera E (2007) Systematic review of clinical trials evaluating low doses of stavudine as part of antiretroviral treatment. Expert Opin Pharmacother 8(5):679–688

Hoggard PG, Kewn S, Maherbe A, Wood R, Almond LM, Sales SD, Gould J, Lou Y, De Vries C, Back DJ, Khoo SH, CHARM Study Group (2002) Time-dependent changes in HIV nucleoside analogue phosphorylation and the effect of hydroxyurea. AIDS 16(18):2439–2446

Hsu CH, Hu R, Dutschman GE, Yang G, Krishnan P, Tanaka H, Baba M, Cheng YC (2007) Comparison of the phosphorylation of 4′-ethynyl 2′,3′-dihydro-3′-deoxythymidine with that of other anti-human immunodeficiency virus thymidine analogs. Antimicrob Agents Chemother 51(5):1687–1693

Hulgan T, Haas DW, Haines JL, Ritchie MD, Robbins GK, Shafer RW, Clifford DB, Kallianpur AR, Summar M, Canter JA (2005) Mitochondrial haplogroups and peripheral neuropathy during antiretroviral therapy: an adult AIDS clinical trials group study. AIDS 19(13):1341–1349

Hulgan T, Tebas P, Canter JA, Mulligan K, Haas DW, Dubé M, Grinspoon S, Robbins GK, Motsinger AA, Kallianpur AR, AIDS Clinical Trials Group 384 and A5005s Study Teams (2008) Hemochromatosis gene polymorphisms, mitochondrial haplogroups, and peripheral lipoatrophy during antiretroviral therapy. J Infect Dis 197(6):858–866

Imaoka T, Kusuhara H, Adachi M, Schuetz JD, Takeuchi K, Sugiyama Y (2007) Functional involvement of multidrug resistance-associated protein 4 (MRP4/ABCC4) in the renal elimination of the antiviral drugs adefovir and tenofovir. Mol Pharmacol 71(2):619–627

Izzedine H, Hulot JS, Launay-Vacher V, Marcellini P, Hadziyannis SJ, Currie G, Brosgart CL, Westland C, Arterbrun S, Deray G, Adefovir Dipivoxil International 437 Study Group, Adefovir Dipivoxil International 438 Study Group (2004) Renal safety of adefovir dipivoxil in patients with chronic hepatitis B: Two double-blind, randomized, placebo-controlled studies. Kidney Int 66(6):1153–1158

Izzedine H, Harris M, Perazella MA (2009) The nephrotoxic effects of hAArT. Nat Rev Nephrol 5(10):563–573

Johnson MA, Fridland A (1989) Phosphorylation of 2′,3′-dideoxyinosine by cytosolic 5′-nucleotidase of human lymphoid cells. Mol Pharmacol 36(2):291–295

Jullig M, Eriksson S (2000) Mitochondrial and submitochondrial localization of human deoxyguanosine kinase. Eur J Biochem 267(17):5466–5472

Kakuda TN (2000) Pharmacology of nucleoside and nucleotide reverse transcriptase inhibitor-induced mitochondrial toxicity. Clin Ther 22(6):685–708

Kestens L, Vanham G, Vereecken C, Vandenbruaene M, Vercauteren G, Colebunders RL, Gigase PL (1994) Selective increase of activation antigens HLA-DR and CD38 on CD4+ CD45RO+T lymphocytes during HIV-1 infection. Clin Exp Immunol 95(4):436–441

Kewn S, Hoggard PG, Sales SD, Johnson MA, Back DJ (2000) The intracellular activation of lamivudine (3TC) and determination of 2′-deoxycytidine-5′-triphosphate (dCTP) pools in the presence and absence of various drugs in HepG2 cells. Br J Clin Pharmacol 50(6):597–604

Klusa V, Pupure J, Isajevs S, Rumaks J, Gordjushina V, Kratovska A, Taivans I, Svirskis S, Viksna L, Kalvinsh I (2006) Protection of azidothymidine-induced cardiopathology in mice by mildronate, a mitochondria-targeted drug. Basic Clin Pharmacol Toxicol 99(4):323–328

Kunkel TA, Mosbaugh DW (1989) Exonucleolytic proofreading by a mammalian DNA polymerase. Biochemistry 28(3):988–995

Lai Y, Tse CM, Unadkat JD (2004) Mitochondrial expression of the human equilibrative nucleoside transporter 1 (hENT1) results in enhanced mitochondrial toxicity of antiviral drugs. J Biol Chem 279(6):4490–4497

Lam W, Chen C, Ruan S, Leung CH, Cheng YC (2005) Expression of deoxynucleotide carrier is not associated with the mitochondrial DNA depletion caused by anti-HIV dideoxynucleoside analogs and mitochondrial dNTP uptake. Mol Pharmacol 67(2):408–416

Lebrecht D, Deveaud C, Beauvoit B, Bonnet J, Kirschner J, Walker UA (2008) Uridine supplementation antagonizes zidovudine-induced mitochondrial myopathy and hyperlactatemia in mice. Arthritis Rheum 58(1):318–326

Lenzo NP, Garas BA, French MA (1997) Hepatic steatosis and lactic acidosis associated with stavudine treatment in an HIV patient: a case report. AIDS 11(10):1294–1295

Leung S, Bendayan R (1999) Role of P-glycoprotein in the renal transport of dideoxynucleoside analog drugs. Can J Physiol Pharmacol 77(8):625–630

Leung GP, Tse CM (2007) The role of mitochondrial and plasma membrane nucleoside transporters in drug toxicity. Expert Opin Drug Metab Toxicol 3(5):705–718

Lewis W, Dalakas MC (1995) Mitochondrial toxicity of antiviral drugs. Nat Med 1(5):417–422

Lewis W, Gonzalez B, Chomyn A, Papoian T (1992) Zidovudine induces molecular, biochemical, and ultrastructural changes in rat skeletal muscle mitochondria. J Clin Invest 89(4):1354–1360

Lewis W, Day BJ, Copeland WC (2003) Mitochondrial toxicity of NRTI antiviral drugs: an integrated cellular perspective. Nat Rev Drug Discov 2(10):812–822

Lewis W, Haase CP, Miller YK, Ferguson B, Stuart T, Ludaway T, McNaught J, Russ R, Steltzer J, Santoianni R, Long R, Fiermonte G, Palmieri F (2005) Transgenic expression of the deoxynucleotide carrier causes mitochondrial damage that is enhanced by NRTIs for AIDS. Lab Invest 85(8):972–981

Lewis W, Kohler JJ, Hosseini SH, Haase CP, Copeland WC, Bienstock RJ, Ludaway T, McNaught J, Russ R, Stuart T, Santoianni R (2006) Antiretroviral nucleosides, deoxynucleotide carrier and mitochondrial DNA: evidence supporting the DNA pol gamma hypothesis. AIDS 20(5):675–684

Lichtenstein KA, Armon C, Baron A, Moorman AC, Wood KC, Holmberg SD, HIV Outpatient Study Investigators (2005) Modification of the incidence of drug-associated symmetrical peripheral neuropathy by host and disease factors in the HIV outpatient study cohort. Clin Infect Dis 40(1):148–157

Lim SE, Copeland WC (2001) Differential incorporation and removal of antiviral deoxynucleotides by human DNA polymerase gamma. J Biol Chem 276(26):23616–23623

Lim SE, Ponamarev MV, Longley MJ, Copeland WC (2003) Structural determinants in human DNA polymerase gamma account for mitochondrial toxicity from nucleoside analogs. J Mol Biol 329(1):45–57

Lipshultz SE, Easley KA, Orav EJ, Kaplan S, Starc TJ, Bricker JT, Lai WW, Moodie DS, Sopko G, McIntosh K, Colan SD (2000) Absence of cardiac toxicity of zidovudine in infants. Pediatric pulmonary and cardiac complications of vertically transmitted HIV infection study group. N Engl J Med 343(11):759–766

Lonergan JT, McComsey GA, Fisher RL, Shalit P, File TM Jr, Ward DJ, Williams VC, Hessenthaler SM, Lindsey L, Hernandez JE, for the ESS40010 (TARHEEL) Study Team (2004) Lack of recurrence of hyperlactatemia in HIV-infected patients switched from stavudine to abacavir to zidovudine. J Acquir Immune Defic Syndr 36(4):935–942

Lund KC, Wallace KB (2004) Direct, DNA pol-gamma-independent effects of nucleoside reverse transcriptase inhibitors on mitochondrial bioenergetics. Cardiovasc Toxicol 4(3):217–228

Lund KC, Wallace KB (2008) Adenosine 3′,5′-cyclic monophosphate (cAMP)-dependent phosphoregulation of mitochondrial complex I is inhibited by nucleoside reverse transcriptase inhibitors. Toxicol Appl Pharmacol 226(1): 94–106

Lynx MD, LaClair DD, McKee EE (2009) Effects of zidovudine and stavudine on mitochondrial DNA of differentiating 3 T3-F442a cells are not associated with imbalanced deoxynucleotide pools. Antimicrob Agents Chemother 53(3):1252–1255

Martin JL, Brown CE, Matthews-Davis N, Reardon JE (1994) Effects of antiviral nucleoside analogs on human DNA polymerases and mitochondrial DNA synthesis. Antimicrob Agents Chemother 38(12):2743–2749

Martin AM, Hammond E, Nolan D, Pace C, Den Boer M, Taylor L, Moore H, Martinez OP, Christiansen FT, Mallal S (2003) Accumulation of mitochondrial DNA mutations in human immunodeficiency virus-infected patients treated with nucleoside-analogue reversetranscriptase inhibitors. Am J Hum Genet 72(3):549–560

Mazzucco CE, Hamatake RK, Colonno RJ, Tenney DJ (2008) Entecavir for treatment of hepatitis B virus displays no in vitro mitochondrial toxicity or DNA polymerase gamma inhibition. Antimicrob Agents Chemother 52(2):598–605

McComsey GA, Morrow JD (2003) Lipid oxidative markers are significantly increased in lipoatrophy, but not in sustained asymptomatic hyperlactatemia. J Acquir Immune Defic Syndr 34(1):45–49

McComsey G, Tan DJ, Lederman M, Wilson E, Wong LJ (2002) Analysis of mitochondrial DNA genome in the peripheral blood leukocytes of HIV-infected patients with of without lipoatrophy. AIDS 16(4):513–518

McComsey G, Southwell H, Gripshover B, Salata R, Valdez H (2003) Effect of antioxidants on glucose metabolism and plasma lipids in HIV-infected subjects with lipoatrophy. J Acquir Immune Defic Syndr 33(5):605–607

McComsey GA, Ward DJ, Hessenthaler SM, Sension MG, Shalit P, Lonergan JT, Fisher RL, Williams VC, Hernandez JE, Trial to Assess the Regression of Hyperlactatemia and to Evaluate the Regression of Established Lipodystrophy in HIV-1-Positive Subjects (TARHEEL; ESS40010) Study Team (2004) Improvement in lipoatrophy associated with highly active antiretroviral therapy in human immunodeficiency virus-infected patients switched from stavudine to abacavir or zidovudine: the results of the TARHEEL study. Clin Infect Dis 38(2):263–270

McComsey G, Bai RK, Maa JF, Seekins D, Wong LJ (2005) Extensive investigations of mitochondrial DNA genome in treated HIV-infected subjects: beyond mitochondrial DNA depletion. J Acquir Immune Defic Syndr 39(2):181–188

McKee EE, Bentley AT, Hatch M, Gingerich J, Susan-Resiga D (2004) Phosphorylation of thymidine and AZT in heart mitochondria: elucidation of a novel mechanism of AZT cardiotoxicity. Cardiovasc Toxicol 4(2):155–167

McKenzie R, Fried MW, Sallie R, Conjeevaram H, Di Bisceglie AM, Park Y, Savarese B, Kleiner D, Tsokos M, Luciano C, Pruett T, Stotka JL, Straus SE, Hoofnagle JH (1995) Hepatic failure and lactic acidosis due to fialuridine (FIAU), an investigational nucleoside analogue for chronic hepatitis B. N Engl J Med 333(17):1099–1105

Meng Q, Grosovsky AJ, Shi X, Walker VE (2000) Mutagenicity and loss of heterozygosity at the APRT locus in human lymphoblastoid cells exposed to 3′-azido-3′-deoxythymidine. Mutagenesis 15(5):405–410

Merta A, Votruba I, Jindrich J, Holý A, Cihlár T, Rosenberg I, Otmar M, Herve TY (1992) Phosphorylation of 9-(2-phosphonomethoxyethyl)adenine and 9-(S)-(3-hydroxy-2-phosphonomethoxypropyl)adenine by AMP(dAMP) kinase from L1210 cells. Biochem Pharmacol 44(10):2067–2077

Miller KD, Cameron M, Wood LV, Dalakas MC, Kovacs JA (2000) Lactic acidosis and hepatic steatosis associated with use of stavudine: report of four cases. Ann Intern Med 133(3):192–196

Miró O, López S, Rodríguez de la Concepción M, Martínez E, Pedrol E, Garrabou G, Giralt M, Cardellach F, Gatell JM, Vilarroya F, Casademont J (2004) Upregulatory mechanisms compensate for mitochondrial DNA depletion in asymptomatic individuals receiving stavudine plus didanosine. J Acquir Immune Defic Syndr 37(5):1550–1555

Modica-Napolitano JS (1993) AZT causes tissue-specific inhibition of mitochondrial bioenergetic function. Biochem Biophys Res Commun 194(1):170–177

Modrzejewski KA, Herman RA (2004) Emtricitabine: a once-daily nucleoside reverse transcriptase inhibitor. Ann Pharmacother 38(6):1006–1014

Mokrzycki H, Harris C, May H, Laut J, Palmisano J (2000) Lactic acidosis associated with stavudine administration: a report of five cases. Clin Infect Dis 30(1):198–200

Moore RD, Wong WM, Keruly JC, McArthur JC (2000) Incidence of neuropathy in HIV-infected patients on monotherapy versus those on combination therapy with didanosine, stavudine and hydroxyurea. AIDS 14(3):273–278

Moreno A, Quereda C, Moreno L, Perez-Elías MJ, Muriel A, Casado JL, Antela A, Dronda F, Navas E, Bárcena R, Moreno S (2004) High rate of didanosine-related mitochondrial toxicity in HIV/HCV-coinfected patients receiving ribavirin. Antivir Ther 9(1):133–138

Moretti S, Famularo G, Marcellini S, Boschini A, Santini G, Trinchieri V, Lucci L, Alesse E, De Simone C (2002) L-carnitine reduces lymphocyte apoptosis and oxidative stress in HIV-1-infected subjects treated with zidovudine and didanosine. Antioxid Redox Signal 4(3):391–403

Morris GW, Iams TA, Slepchenko KG, McKee EE (2009) Origin of pyrimidine deoxyribonucleotide pools in perfused rat heart: implications for 3'-azido-3'-deoxythymidine-dependent cardiotoxicity. Biochem J 422(3):513–520

Moyle G (2000) Clinical manifestations and management of antiretroviral nucleoside analog-related mitochondrial toxicity. Clin Ther 22(8):911–936

Moyle G (2005) Mechanisms of HIV and nucleoside reverse transcriptase inhibitor injury to mitochondria. Antivir Ther 10(Suppl 2):M47–M52

Moyle GJ, Datta D, Mandalia S, Morlese J, Asboe D, Gazzard BG (2002) Hyperlactatemia and lactic acidosis during antiretroviral therapy: relevance, reproducibility and possible risk factors. AIDS 16(10):1341–1349

Munch-Petersen B (1984) Differences in the kinetic properties of thymidine kinase isoenzymes in unstimulated and phytohemagglutinin-stimulated human lymphocytes. Mol Cell Biochem 64(2):173–185

Munch-Petersen B, Tyrsted G (1977) Induction of thymidine kinases in phytohaemagglutinin-stimulated human lymphocytes. Biochim Biophys Acta 478(3):364–375

Negredo E, Miró O, Rodríguez-Santiago B, Garrabou G, Estany C, Masabeu A, Force L, Barrufet P, Cucurull J, Domingo P, Alonso-Villaverde C, Bonjoch A, Morén C, Pérez-Alvarez N, Clotet B, MULTINEKA Study Group (2009) Improvement of mitochondrial toxicity in patients receiving a nucleoside reverse-transcriptase inhibitor-sparing strategy: results from the Multicenter Study with Nevirapine and Kaletra (MULTINEKA). Clin Infect Dis 49(6):892–900

Opii WO, Sultana R, Abdul HM, Ansari MA, Nath A, Butterfield DA (2007) Oxidative stress and toxicity induced by the nucleoside reverse transcriptase inhibitor (NRTI)–2',3'-dideoxycytidine (ddC): relevance to HIV-dementia. Exp Neurol 204(1):29–38

Panel on Antiretroviral Guidelines for Adults and Adolescents (2008) Guidelines for the use of antiretroviral agents in HIV-1-infected adults and adolescents. Department of Health and Human Services (DHHS), Bethesda, p 139

Pan-Zhou XR, Cui L, Zhou XJ, Sommadossi JP, Darley-Usmar VM (2000) Differential effects of antiretroviral nucleoside analogs on mitochondrial function in HepG2 cells. Antimicrob Agents Chemother 44(3):496–503

Peltier AC, Russell JW (2006) Advances in understanding drug-induced neuropathies. Drug Saf 29(1):23–30

Perno CF, Cooney DA, Gao WY, Hao Z, Johns DG, Foli A, Hartman NR, Caliò R, Broder S, Yarchoan R (1992) Effects of bone marrow stimulatory cytokines on human immunodeficiency virus replication and the antiviral activity of dideoxynucleosides in cultures of monocyte/macrophages. Blood 80(4):995–1003

Ronan A, Lipman C, Johnson A, Breen RA (2000) Increased incidence of peripheral neuropathy with co-administration of stavudine and isoniazid in HIV-infected individuals. AIDS 14(5):615–616

Rossi L, Serafini S, Schiavano GF, Casabianca A, Vallanti G, Chiarantini L, Magnani M (1999) Metabolism, mitochondrial uptake and toxicity of 2',3'-dideoxycytidine. Biochem J 344(Pt 3):915–920

Rylova SN, Albertioni F, Flygh G, Eriksson S (2005) Activity profiles of deoxynucleoside kinases and 5'-nucleotidases in cultured adipocytes and myoblastic cells: insights into mitochondrial toxicity of nucleoside analogs. Biochem Pharmacol 69(6):951–960

Rylova SN, Mirzaee S, Albertioni F, Eriksson S (2007) Expression of deoxynucleoside kinases and 5'-nucleotidases in mouse tissues: implications for mitochondrial toxicity. Biochem Pharmacol 74(1):169–175

Sakamoto S, Iwama T, Tsukada K, Utsunomiya J, Kawasaki T, Okamoto R (1984) Increased activity of thymidine kinase isozyme in human colon tumor. Carcinogenesis 5(2):183–185

Sales SD, Hoggard PG, Sunderland D, Khoo S, Hart CA, Back DJ (2001) Zidovudine phosphorylation and mitochondrial toxicity in vitro. Toxicol Appl Pharmacol 177(1):54–58

Scadden DT, Pickus O, Hammer SM, Stretcher B, Bresnahan J, Gere J, McGrath J, Agosti JM (1996) Lack of in vivo effect of granulocyte-macrophage colony-stimulating factor on human immunodeficiency virus type 1. AIDS Res Hum Retroviruses 12(12):1151–1159

Schramm C, Wanitschke R, Galle PR (1999) Thiamine for the treatment of nucleoside analogue-induced severe lactic acidosis. Eur J Anaesthesiol 16(10):733–735

Semino-Mora MC, Leon-Monzon ME, Dalakas MC (1994) Effect of L-carnitine on the zidovudine-induced destruction of human myotubes. Part II: Treatment with L-carnitine improves AZTinduced changes and prevents further destruction. Lab Invest 71(5):773–781

Setzer B, Lebrecht D, Walker UA (2008) Pyrimidine nucleoside depletion sensitizes to the mitochondrial hepatotoxicity of the reverse transcriptase inhibitor stavudine. Am J Pathol 172(3):681–690

Shaer AJ, Rastegar A (2000) Lactic acidosis in the setting of antiretroviral therapy for the acquired immunodeficiency syndrome. A case report and review of the literature. Am J Nephrol 20(4):332–338

Shikuma CM, Hu N, Milne C, Yost F, Waslien C, Shimizu S, Shiramizu B (2001) Mitochondrial DNA decrease in subcutaneous adipose tissue of HIV-infected individuals with peripheral lipoatrophy. AIDS 15(14):1801–1809

Shiramizu B, Shikuma KM, Kamemoto L, Gerschenson M, Erdem G, Pinti M, Cossarizza A, Shikuma C (2003) Placenta and cord blood mitochondrial DNA toxicity in HIV-infected women receiving HAART during pregnancy. J Acquir Immune Defic Syndr 32(4):370–374

Skuta G, Fischer GM, Janaky T, Kele Z, Szabo P, Tozser J, Sumegi B (1999) Molecular mechanism of the short-term cardiotoxicity caused by 2′,3′-dideoxycytidine (ddC): modulation of reactive oxygen species levels and ADP-ribosylation reactions. Biochem Pharmacol 58(12):1915–1925

Smyth K, Affandi JS, McArthur JC, Bowtell-Harris C, Mijch AM, Watson K, Costello K, Woolley IJ, Price P, Wesselingh SL, Cherry CL (2007) Prevalence of and risk factors for HIV-associated neuropathy in Melbourne, Australia 1993–2006. HIV Med 8(6):367–373

Song S, Pursell ZF, Copeland WC, Longley MJ, Kunkel TA, Mathews CK (2005) DNA precursor asymmetries in mammalian tissue mitochondria and possible contribution to mutagenesis through reduced replication fidelity. Proc Natl Acad Sci USA 102(14):4990–4995

Sussman HE, Olivero OA, Meng Q, Pietras SM, Poirier MC, O'Neill JP, Finette BA, Bauer MJ, Walker VE (1999) Genotoxicity of 3′-azido-3′-deoxythymidine in the human lymphoblastoid cell line, TK6: relationships between DNA incorporation, mutant frequency, and spectrum of deletion mutations in HPRT. Mutat Res 429(2):249–259

Szabados E, Fischer GM, Toth K, Csete B, Nemeti B, Trombitas K, Habon T, Endrei D, Sumegi B (1999) Role of reactive oxygen species and poly-ADP-ribose polymerase in the development of AZT-induced cardiomyopathy in rat. Free Radic Biol Med 26(3–4):309–317

Tanji N, Tanji K, Kambham N, Markowitz GS, Bell A, D'agati VD (2001) Adefovir nephrotoxicity: possible role of mitochondrial DNA depletion. Hum Pathol 32(7):734–740

Tesco G, Latorraca S, Piersanti P, Piacentini S, Amaducci L, Sorbi S (1992) Protection from oxygen radical damage in human diploid fibroblasts by acetyl-L-carnitine. Dementia 3:58–60

Thornberry NA, Lazebnik Y (1998) Caspases: enemies within. Science 281(5381):1312–1316

Tsai CH, Doong SL, Johns DG, Driscoll JS, Cheng YC (1994) Effect of anti-HIV 2′-beta-fluoro-2′,3′-dideoxynucleoside analogs on the cellular content of mitochondrial DNA and on lactate production. Biochem Pharmacol 48(7):1477–1481

Tuon FF, Guastini CM, Boulos MI (2008) Acute pancreatitis associated with lamivudine therapy for chronic B hepatitis. Braz J Infect Dis 12(4):263

Turriziani O, Butera O, Gianotti N, Parisi SG, Mazzi R, Girardi E, Iaiani G, Antonelli L, Lazzarin A, Antonelli G (2005) Thymidine kinase and deoxycytidine kinase activity in mononuclear cells from antiretroviral-naive HIV-infected patients. AIDS 19(5):473–479

Uwai Y, Ida H, Tsuji Y, Katsura T, Inui K (2007) Renal transport of adefovir, cidofovir, and tenofovir by SLC22A family members (hOAT1, hOAT3, and hOCT2). Pharm Res 24(4):811–815

Valenti D, Barile M, Quagliariello E, Passarella S (1999) Inhibition of nucleoside diphosphate kinase in rat liver mitochondria by added 3′-azido-3′-deoxythymidine. FEBS Lett 444(2–3):291–295

Valenti D, Atlante A, Barile M, Passarella S (2002) Inhibition of phosphate transport in rat heart mitochondria by 3′-azido-3′-deoxythymidine due to stimulation of superoxide anion mitochondrial production. Biochem Pharmacol 64(2):201–206

Velsor LW, Kovacevic M, Goldstein M, Leitner HM, Lewis W, Day BJ (2004) Mitochondrial oxidative stress in human hepatoma cells exposed to stavudine. Toxicol Appl Pharmacol 199(1):10–19

Venhoff N, Setzer B, Melkaoui K, Walker UA (2007) Mitochondrial toxicity of tenofovir, emtricitabine, and abacavir alone and in combination with additional nucleoside reverse transcriptase inhibitors. Antivir Ther 12(7):1075–1085

Vrouenraets SM, Treskes M, Regez RM, Troost N, Smulders YM, Weigel HM, Frissen PH, Brinkman K (2002) Hyperlactataemia in HIV-infected patients: the role of NRTI-treatment. Antivir Ther 7(4):239–244

Wada S, Tsuda M, Sekine T, Cha SH, Kimura M, Kanai Y, Endou H (2000) Rat multispecifi c organic anion transporter 1 (rOAT1) transports zidovudine, acyclovir, and other antiviral nucleoside analogs. J Pharmacol Exp Ther 294(3):844–849

Walker UA, Venhoff N (2005) Uridine in the prevention and treatment of NRTI related mitochondrial toxicity. Antivir Ther 10(supp 2):M117–M123

Walker UA, Setzer B, Venhoff N (2002) Increased long-term mitochondrial toxicity in combinations of nucleoside analogue reverse-transcriptase inhibitors. AIDS 16(16):2165–2173

Walker UA, Bäuerle J, Laguno M, Murillas J, Mauss S, Schmutz G, Setzer B, Miquel R, Gatell JM, Mallolas J (2003) Depletion of mitochondrial DNA in liver under antiretroviral therapy with didanosine, stavudine, or zalcitabine. Hepatology 39(2):311–317

Wallace DC (1992) Mitochondrial genetics: a paradigm for aging and degenerative diseases? Science 256(5057):628–632

Wang L, Eriksson S (2003) Mitochondrial deoxyguanosine kinase mutations and mitochondrial DNA depletion syndrome. FEBS Lett 554(3):319–322

Ward JL, Sherali A, Mo ZP, Tse CM (2000) Kinetic and pharmacological properties of cloned human equilibrative nucleoside transporters, ENT1 and ENT2, stably expressed in nucleoside transporter-defi cient PK15 cells. Ent2 exhibits a low affi nity for guanosine and cytidine but a high affi nity for inosine. J Biol Chem 275(12):8375–8381

Wiesner RJ, Ruegg JC, Morano I (1992) Counting target molecules by exponential polymerase chain reaction: copy number of mitochondrial DNA in rat tissues. Biochem Biophys Res Commun 183(2):553–559

Wu Y, Li N, Zhang T, Wu H, Huang C, Chen D (2009) Mitochondrial DNA base excision repair and mitochondrial DNA mutation in human hepatic HuH-7 cells exposed to stavudine. Mutat Res 664(1–2):28–38

Yamanaka G, Wilson T, Innaimo S, Bisacchi GS, Egli P, Rinehart JK, Zahler R, Colonno RJ (1999) Metabolic studies on BMS-200475, a new antiviral compound active against hepatitis B virus. Antimicrob Agents Chemother 43(1): 190–193

Yamanaka H, Gatanaga H, Kosalaraksa P, Matsuoka-Aizawa S, Takahashi T, Kimura S, Oka S (2007) Novel mutation of human DNA polymerase gamma associated with mitochondrial toxicity induced by anti-HIV treatment. J Infect Dis 195(10):1419–1425

Zeviani M, Di Donato S (2004) Mitochondrial disorders. Brain 127(Pt10):2153–2172

Zhang XS, Jin R, Zhang SB, Tao ML (2008) Clinical features of adverse reactions associated with telbivudine. World J Gastroenterol 14(22):3549–3553

Chapter 17
Dysfunction of Mitochondrial Respiratory Chain Complex I in Neurological Disorders: Genetics and Pathogenetic Mechanisms

Vittoria Petruzzella, Anna Maria Sardanelli, Salvatore Scacco, Damiano Panelli, Francesco Papa, Raffaella Trentadue, and Sergio Papa

Abstract This chapter covers genetic and biochemical aspects of mitochondrial bioenergetics dysfunction in neurological disorders associated with complex I defects. Complex I formation and functionality in mammalian cells depends on coordinated expression of nuclear and mitochondrial genes, post-translational subunit modifications, mitochondrial import/maturation of nuclear encoded subunits, subunits interaction and stepwise assembly, and on proteolytic processing. Examples of complex I dysfunction are herein presented: homozygous mutations in the nuclear *NDUFS1* and *NDUFS4* genes for structural components of complex I; an autosomic recessive form of encephalopathy associated with enhanced proteolytic degradation of complex I; familial cases of Parkinson associated to mutations in the *PINK1* and *Parkin* genes, in particular, homoplasmic mutations in the *ND5* and *ND6* mitochondrial genes of the complex I, coexistent with mutation in the *PINK1* gene. This knowledge, besides clarifying molecular aspects of the pathogenesis of hereditary diseases, can also provide hints for understanding the involvement of complex I in neurological disorders, as well as for developing therapeutical strategies

Keywords Complex I • mtDNA mutation • NDUFS4 • NDUFS1 • Parkin • PINK1

17.1 Introduction

With more than 1,000 contributions to its proteome, it is conceivable that a remarkable number of defects may be disclosed within mitochondria, though the term "mitochondrial disease" is scholastically restricted to defects of oxidative phosphorylation (OXPHOS OxPhos) and energy metabolism. The concept of

V. Petruzzella • S. Papa (✉)
Department of Basic Medical Sciences, Section of Medical Biochemistry, University of Bari,
Policlinico, P.zza G. Cesare, 70124 Bari, Italy

Institute of Biomembranes and Bioenergetics (IBBE), Italian Research Council,
(CNR), Bari, Italy
e-mail: s.papa@biochem.uniba.it

A.M. Sardanelli • S. Scacco • D. Panelli • R. Trentadue
Department of Basic Medical Sciences, Section of Medical Biochemistry,
University of Bari, Policlinico, P.zza G. Cesare, 70124 Bari, Italy

F. Papa
Department of Dental Sciences and Surgery, University of Bari, Bari, Italy

R. Scatena et al. (eds.), *Advances in Mitochondrial Medicine*, Advances in Experimental
Medicine and Biology 942, DOI 10.1007/978-94-007-2869-1_17,
© Springer Science+Business Media B.V. 2012

"mitochondrial disease" was initially introduced in 1962 by Luft et al. but only in the late 1980s, the first group of disorders related to mutations in the mitochondrial DNA (mtDNA) was identified. After 20 years, we define a novel field that goes by the name of "Mitochondrial Medicine". Combining the epidemiological data on paediatric and adult population it can be estimated that the minimum prevalence of a primary mitochondrial diseases is at least 1 in 5,000 (Scheffler et al. 2004). It is believed that best estimates predict that at least one individual in 200 may harbour a pathogenic mtDNA point mutation (Elliott et al. 2008). Since mitochondria are ubiquitous, any organ of the body can be affected; neuropathies, myopathies, or their combination are typical, and injures to the hepatic, gastrointestinal, renal, hematopoietic and endocrine systems may also occur.

Importantly, it emerged in the past decade that an increasing number of degenerative diseases of the central nervous system, are associated with defects of mitochondrial function. Although the underlying genetic bases of well-known disorders such as Huntington disease (HD), hereditary spastic paraplegia (HSP), Friedreich ataxia (FRDA), familial forms of Parkinson disease (PD), Alzheimer disease (AD), and amyotrophic lateral sclerosis (ALS), have been in part identified, the associated pathogenetic mechanisms giving rise to the various clinical features of these diseases remain largely unclear. Since neurons are highly dependent on oxidative energy metabolism, a unified mechanism of neurodegeneration based on dysfunction in mitochondrial energy metabolism has been proposed (Lin and Beal 2006). The correct functioning of the OXPHOS OxPhos system is fundamental for the generation of most of the cellular ATP and its impairment may have consequences on other functions such as the maintenance of calcium homeostasis and production of reactive oxygen species (ROS). Relevant to these aspects are the documented defects of Complex I in sporadic (Orth and Schapira 2001; Pagliarini et al. 2008) and familial Parkinson disease (PD) (Piccoli et al. 2008a, b; Papa et al. 2009a), HSP (Atorino et al. 2003), FRDA (Orth and Schapira 2001), as well as in ageing (Papa 1996; Ventura et al. 2002) and type 2 non insulin-dependent diabetes mellitus (NIDDM) (Civitarese and Ravussin 2008).

Isolated complex I (NADH-ubiquinone oxidoreductase; EC 1.6.5.3) deficiency is the most frequently encountered among the so called "primary" defects of mitochondrial energy metabolism (Smeitink et al. 2001) and the spectrum of clinical and neuroimaging manifestations grows rapidly. The involvement of complex I in many diseases can be due to the following: (i) it is the largest among the respiratory chain complexes; (ii) the NADH-ubiquinone oxidoreductase activity of the complex contributes for 40% to the generation of the mitochondrial proton-motive force, utilized for ATP synthesis and transport processes; (iii) it is a major contributor to reactive oxygen species production in the cell.

Complex I is the largest enzyme of the mammalian OXPHOS OxPhos system. With a molecular weight of $\sim 1 \times 10^6$ Da, it contains a series of redox centers (one FMN, seven FeS-centers and two protein bound semiquinone/quinol couples) which catalyze the stepwise transfer of electrons from NADH to ubiquinone, coupled to the translocation of $4H^+/2e^-$ from the mitochondrial matrix to the cytosol (Walker 1992; Ohnishi 1998; Papa et al. 1999, 2007; Yagi and Matsuno-Yagi 2003; Friedrich and Böttcher 2004; Ohnishi and Salerno 2005; Brandt 2006; Sazanov and Hinchliffe 2006). During this process, direct electron leakage to oxygen may occur, which makes complex I a main site of cellular superoxide production (Duchen 2004). The catalytic core of the complex comprises 14 evolutionary conserved subunits which can be divided in two distinct groups: seven predominantly hydrophilic subunits of the membrane-extrinsic arm, which in humans are encoded by the nuclear *NDUFV1*, *NDUFV2*, *NDUFS1-3*, *NDUFS7* and *NDUFS8* genes, and seven highly hydrophobic subunits of the membrane intrinsic arm dominated by transmembrane helices, encoded by the mitochondrial ND1–ND6 and ND4L genes (Hirst et al. 2003; Yagi and Matsuno-Yagi 2003; Brandt 2006; Papa et al. 2007). The other subunits are termed "accessory", though a few appear to be essential for the assembly of the complex and may vary between species (Scacco et al. 2003; Antonicka et al. 2003; Hirst et al. 2003; Scheffler et al. 2004). Several assembly chaperones have also been identified in the eukaryotic enzyme, which facilitate the proper build-up and stability of the complex (Vogel et al. 2007). Complex I activity in mammalian cells depends on: (i) coordinated expression of nuclear and mitochondrial genes; (ii) post-translational subunit modifications; (iii) mitochondrial import/maturation of nuclear encoded subunits; (iv) subunits interaction and stepwise assembly; (v) proteolytic processing. Understanding the mechanisms of the biogenesis of complex I, energy transduction, and reactive oxygen species production in complex I is crucial for understanding its role in disease, and for the development of effective therapies.

17.2 Complex I Dysfunction in Primary Mitochondrial Neurological Diseases

Complex I deficiency starts mostly at birth or early childhood, and in general this failure results in multisystem disorders with a fatal outcome (Robinson 1998; Kirby et al. 1999; Loeffen et al. 2000). The most affected tissues are usually those with a high-energy demand, such as brain, heart, kidney, and skeletal muscle. Leigh syndrome (LS) (Leigh 1951) and Leigh-like disease are the most common phenotypes associated with an isolated complex I deficiency, totalling up to 50% of the cases (Rahman et al. 1996; Robinson 1998; Loeffen et al. 2000; Janssen et al. 2004). Leigh disease is an early-onset, generally fatal neurodegenerative disorder that is typically characterized by the observation of symmetrical necrosis lesions and capillary proliferation in the brainstem, medulla oblongata, and variable regions of the central nervous system. Neuroradiological evidence at brain Magnetic Resonance Imaging (MRI) of bilateral, symmetric hyperintensities in basal ganglia along with white matter hyperluciencies offers the possibility of a premortem diagnosis. Clinical signs and symptoms include muscular hypotonia, dystonia, developmental delay, abnormal eye movements, seizures, respiratory distress, failure-to-thrive and lactic acidemia (Loeffen et al. 2000). In addition to LS, isolated complex I deficiency is associated with progressive leukoencephalopathy, fatal infantile lactic acidosis, neonatal hypertrophic cardiomyopathy with lactic acidosis, leucodystrophy with macrocephaly and hepatopathy with renal tubulopathy (Pitkanen et al. 1996; Loeffen et al. 2000; Bugiani et al. 2004). Although for clinical purpose the identification and classification of complex I deficient children is extremely desirable, it is very difficult or even arbitrary to establish clinical phenotypes or syndromes for nuclear-encoded complex I deficiency other than Leigh or Leigh-like disease and it is not accepted that certain clinical features can exclusively be linked to specific defects in complex I subunits.

Structural integrity of complex I is essential to maintain its functionality. Therefore, alterations in one of its 'building bricks' may lead to catalytic problems or instability of the complete assembly. To date, disease causing mutations have been described in all of the seven mtDNA-encoded subunits and 12 of the nuclear DNA (nDNA)-encoded subunits (van den Heuvel et al. 1998; Loeffen et al. 1998, 2001; Schuelke et al. 1999; Triepels et al. 1999; Petruzzella et al. 2001, 2003; Bénit et al. 2001, 2003, 2004; Kirby et al. 2004; Berger et al. 2008; Hoefs et al. 2008; Papa et al. 2009b). Whilst variants occurring in mtDNA-encoded subunits are maternally inherited or seem to arise *de novo*, most of the defects in nDNA-subunits are inherited in an autosomal recessive mode of transmission. However, X-linked inheritance has also been described (Fernandez-Moreira et al. 2007). Mutations in assembly factors NDUFAF2, NDUFAF1, C6orf66, C8orf38, and C20orf7 have also been reported (Ogilvie et al. 2005; Dunning et al. 2007; Pagliarini et al. 2008; Saada et al. 2008; Sugiana et al. 2008). An even wider genetic heterogeneity and an ever expanding number of mutations are expected in both mtDNA *ND* genes and in nDNA *NDUF* genes as well as in supporting chaperone genes.

Genetic and biochemical observations on the pathogenic mechanism of mutations of *NDUFS4* and *NDUFS1* genes (Papa et al. 2001; Petruzzella et al. 2001; Scacco et al. 2003; Iuso et al. 2006) have highlighted different mechanisms by which the mitochondrial bioenergetic function may be altered in hereditary neurological diseases. Mutations in the *NDUFS4* and *NDUFS1* genes are each associated with encephalopathies with different clinical features (Bugiani et al. 2004). Missense mutations in *NDUFS1* (75 kDa FeS subunit) seem to be associated with a less severe encephalopathy, as result of significant but incomplete depression of the content and enzymatic activity of complex I and enhanced

ROS production, effects which are partially counteracted by cAMP addition. Mature complex is found to be partially converted to a small form, apparently by proteolytic degradation promoted by the same ROS produced as a consequence of the mutated 75 kDa subunit (Papa et al. 2009b). Under this *scenario*, treatment with β-adrenergic agonists and antioxidants could exert a beneficial effect on the clinical course of the disease.

The consequences of mutations in the nuclear gene *NDUFS4* of complex I have been studied at transcriptional and protein levels in cultured fibroblasts from children affected by severe encephalo-myopathies (Petruzzella et al. 2001; Papa et al. 2001; Scacco et al. 2003; Iuso et al. 2006). The mutations were: a base duplication at position 466–470 in exon 5 (van den Heuvel et al. 1998), which destroyed the RVSTK phosphorylation site in the carboxy terminus; a single base deletion at position 289/290 in exon 3, introducing a premature termination codon (PTC) (Budde et al. 2000); and a non-sense mutation in the first exon causing premature termination of the protein (Petruzzella et al. 2001). At protein level, not only in the case of the premature termination but also in the other two cases, the entire NDUFS4 subunit was not detectable in the patient's fibroblasts thus resulting in a non-functional lower molecular weight subcomplex, not responsive to cAMP activation (Papa et al. 2001). At transcriptional level, a different behaviour was observed for the three mutations in *NDUFS4* gene: the deletion at position 289/290 in exon 3 elicited the mRNA degradation by nonsense mediated decay (NMD), a mechanism of quality control of transcription (Isken and Maquat 2007). The 5 bp duplication at position 466/470 in the fifth-exon, did not have any effect on transcript abundance although the overall protein was not detected (Papa et al. 2001); lastly, the 44G → A non sense muta-tion in the first exon, leaded to the disappearance of the mature protein, as expected, but the introduc-tion of a PTC very close to the AUG start codon, rather than eliciting NMD degradation, upregulated three PTC containing alternative transcripts (Petruzzella et al. 2005; Panelli et al. 2008). These three alternative transcripts are normally produced in normal cells but their level is kept low by RNA sur-veillance mechanisms. Two of them are degraded in the cytosol by NMD, whereas the level of a third transcript is down-regulated directly in the nucleus (Panelli et al. 2008). In another patient, harbouring a homozygous splice acceptor site mutation in intron 1 (IV Snt-1, G → A) in the *NDUFS4* gene, only an exon 2 skipped-transcript was detected (Panelli et al. 2008). Overall, these data suggest that the accumulation of the aberrant alternative transcripts can represent another deleterious event contribut-ing to the pathogenetic mechanism of the mutations in neurological patients. In summary, the *NDUFS4* mutations, which were associated with earlier onset and severe disease course resulted in: (i) disap-pearance of the 18 kDa (AQDQ) protein; (ii) block of the last step in the assembly of the complex; (iii) full suppression of the NADH-ubiquinone oxidoreductase activity; (iv) loss of cAMP promotion of the activity; (v) loss of Pasteur effect with enhanced glycolitic activity and chronic lactic acidosis; (vi) accumulation of unproductive alternative transcripts of the gene.

Two male sibs affected by inherited progressive cerebral atrophy with lactic acidosis and drug resis-tant epilepsy, have highlighted a new phenotype of isolated complex I deficiency (Papa et al. 2009b). In primary fibroblast cultures from both children, along with decline of the NADH-ubiquinone oxidoreductase activity, a low content of a complete complex I, but no free subcomplexes, were detected. Mutational analysis of all the 45 structural genes of complex I did not show any causative mutation. The addition to the patient's fibroblast culture of a cocktail of protease inhibitors did rescue the steady state level of complex I subunits as well as the NADH-ubiquinone oxidoreductase activity. Experiments of *in vitro* import of the NDUFS4 precursor in mitochondria isolated from fibroblasts of the two chil-dren showed that although the binding of the precursor at the organelle surface was only partially affected, the mature form of the imported protein within mitochondria was detectable only when the import assay was carried out in the presence of protease inhibitors (Papa et al. 2009b). These results indicate that in the patients' fibroblasts complex I is exposed to protease digestion within mitochondria. The genetic determinants and the biochemical mechanisms leading to this enhanced proteolytic activity remain to be elucidated.

17.3 Complex I Dysfunction in Parkinson's Disease

Parkinson disease (PD), one of the most common neurodegenerative disease, is characterized by loss of dopaminergic neurons in *substantia nigra* and complex movement disorders (Lang and Lozano 1998). For most cases of PD, which are sporadic and age-related, the causes of the disease remain unclear although involvement of genetic and environmental factors is evident (Farrer 2006). Mutations in more than ten genes have, so far, been identified as responsible for familial forms of Parkinsonism (Thomas and Beal 2007; Fitzgerald and Plun-Favreau 2008). These mutations are associated with rare autosomal dominant (ADP) or autosomal recessive Parkinsonism (ARP). There is substantial evidence pointing to a critical role of mitochondrial dysfunction in the pathogenesis of Parkinson. Some of the genes associated with familial Parkinsonism do in fact impinge, directly or indirectly, on mitochondrial dynamics and function (Papa et al. 2009a). It has, on the other hand, been known for long time that exposure of animal laboratories to inhibitors of the mitochondrial NADH-ubiquinone oxidoreductase reproduces characteristic PD features, like nigrostriatal dopaminergic degeneration and α-synuclein citoplasmatic aggregates (Büeler 2009). Decreased activity of complex I and oxidative damage of subunits of the complex (Keeney et al. 2006) have been found in *substantia nigra*, as well as other brain regions (Parker et al. 2008), in autoptic samples from PD patients (Schapira 2008; Büeler 2009). Oxidative damage of complex I might be promoted in *substantia nigra* by the increased level of free radicals generated in dopamine metabolism (Chinta and Andersen 2008). Oxidative damage of mitochondria and defects in their autophagic degradation can be particularly detrimental in dopaminergic neurons of *substantia nigra*, if, like in mice, also in humans, these cells have *per se* a low mitochondrial content (Büeler 2009).

17.3.1 PINK1 Familial Parkinson

Recent work provides evidence showing contribution of mitochondrial dysfunction, in particular of complex I, in the onset and clinical course of familial cases of Parkinson associated to mutations in the *PINK1* (Fig. 17.1) and *Parkin* genes. The PINK1 kinase appears to be involved in the degradation of unfolded or oxidized mitochondrial proteins (Gandhi et al. 2006; Pridgeon et al. 2007; Plun-Favreau et al. 2007), autophagy of damaged mitochondria (Clark et al. 2006; Schapira 2008; Narendra et al. 2008; McBride 2008) and mitochondrial fission/fusion (Yang et al. 2008). PINK1 with an N-terminal mitochondrial targeting sequence (Fig. 17.1) is essentially localized in mitochondria. It has been reported from time to time that PINK1 is associated with the inner membrane (Silvestri et al. 2005; Gandhi et al. 2006; Pridgeon et al. 2007), the intermembrane space (Silvestri et al. 2005; Pridgeon et al. 2007; Plun-Favreau et al. 2007) and the outer membrane (Zhou et al. 2008). The catalytic domain of the outer membrane PINK1 faces the cytosolic space (Zhou et al. 2008) where it phosphorylates the E3 ubiquitin ligase Parkin (Kim et al. 2008; Matsuda et al. 2010), product of the *PARK2* gene, whose mutations represent the first most common cause of autosomal recessive Parkinsonism (Kitada et al. 1998). Parkin phosphorylation promotes its translocation from cytosol to mitochondria (Kim et al. 2008; Matsuda et al. 2010), where it appears to participate to autophagy of damaged mitochondria (Clark et al. 2006; Schapira 2008; Narendra et al. 2008; McBride 2008). PINK1 has also been reported to phosphorylate TRAP1 (HSP75) (Pridgeon et al. 2007) and to regulate, through an indirect phosphorylation mechanism, the protease HtrA2 (Plun-Favreau et al. 2007), both these proteins being involved in quality control of oxidized mitochondrial proteins. Since TRAP1 and HtrA2 reside in the intramitochondrial space, it is possible that PINK1 can partition between the outer and the inner mitochondrial location in response to the prevailing cellular conditions (see also Plun-Favreau et al. 2007).

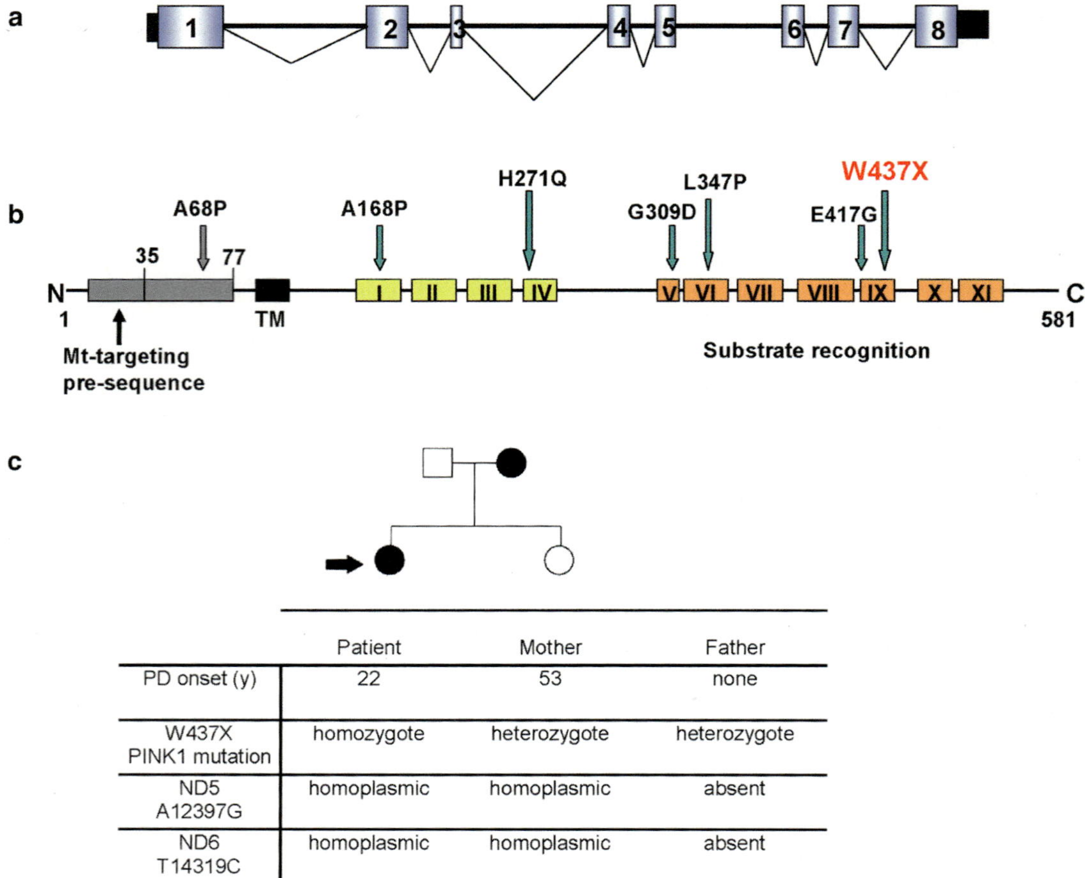

	Patient	Mother	Father
PD onset (y)	22	53	none
W437X PINK1 mutation	homozygote	heterozygote	heterozygote
ND5 A12397G	homoplasmic	homoplasmic	absent
ND6 T14319C	homoplasmic	homoplasmic	absent

Fig. 17.1 Structure of the gene (*PARK6*) (**a**) coding for the PTEN induced kinase 1 (PINK1) protein (**b**) localized in the inner mitochondrial membrane. In (**b**), the domains of the PINK1 protein (from ExPASy Proteomics Server; http://www.expasy.org/) and the mutations found in patients with familial Parkinson are shown. (**c**) PINK1 G1311A (W437X) mutation in the alleles and *ND5* and *ND6* mutations in the patient studied and her parents. Onset age of clinical manifestations of the disease is also shown (See also Papa et al. 2009b)

Different mutations in the *PINK1* gene have been detected in ARP and PD cases with an early onset (Valente et al. 2004; Bonifati et al. 2005; Criscuolo et al. 2006; Zadikoff et al. 2006) (Fig. 17.1). Even if the heterozygous state of subjects carrying *PINK1* mutations does not generally evolve towards the disease, in some cases it does, albeit with a later onset (Zadikoff et al. 2006; Abou-Sleiman et al. 2006a). This would suggest that dysfunction of PINK1 may promote the disease in combination with other acquired or inherited defect(s). Papa et al. have characterized the mitochondrial genotype and function in a female patient carrying a homozygous W437X *PINK1* mutation (Piccoli et al. 2008a, b), which results in a C-terminus truncated kinase with depressed activity (Fig. 17.1) (Sim et al. 2006). The same mutation was present in the heterozygous state in both the patient's parents (Piccoli et al. 2008b; Papa et al. 2009b) (see Fig. 17.1c). The fibroblasts of the homozygous W437X patient showed a significant depression of the endogenous respiratory activity. The patient's fibroblasts exhibited normal specific activities of complex I and III of the respiratory chain. The specific activity of complex IV was also normal when assayed with added cytochrome c, but depressed when assayed with ascorbate plus TMPD, a condition that depends on the endogenous mitochondrial content of cytochrome *c*. The content of cytochrome *c* was, in fact, markedly reduced in the patient's fibroblasts (Piccoli et al. 2008a).

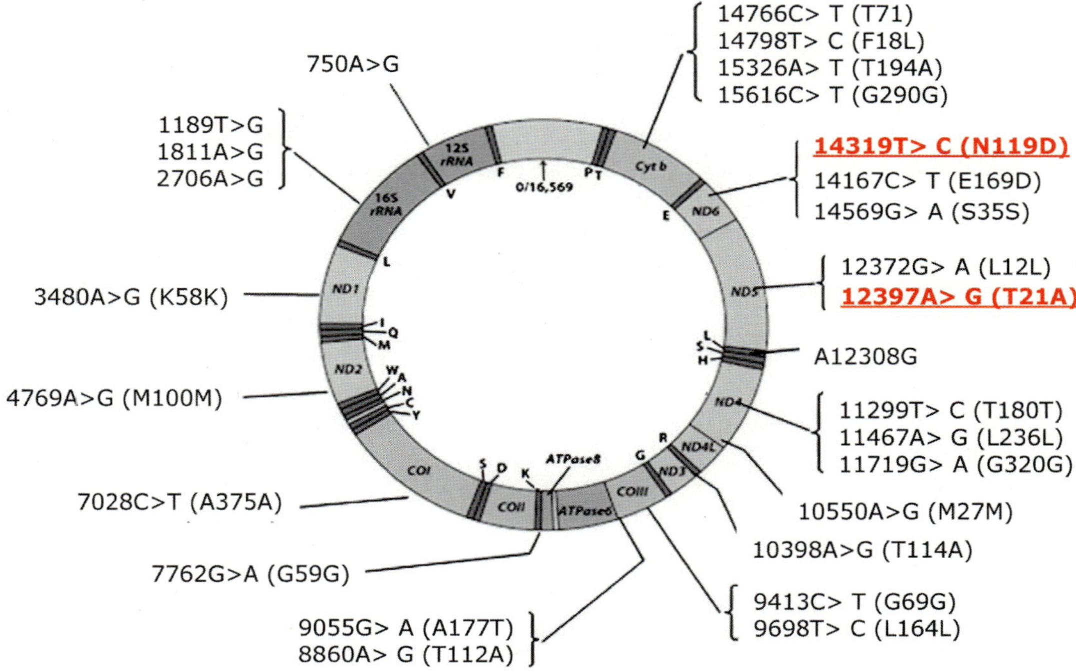

Fig. 17.2 Results of the mutational analysis of the entire mtDNA of the Parkinson patient with homozygous G1311A mutation in the *PINK1* gene. The SNCs m.A12397G and m.T14319.C, identified in the *ND5* and *ND6* genes respectively, are *underlined* (See also Piccoli et al. 2008b)

Patient's fibroblasts presented significant accumulation of H_2O_2 and of oxygen superoxide in the mitochondrial matrix (Piccoli et al. 2008a). DPI, which binds irreversibly to the prosthetic flavin moiety of redox enzymes, including complex I (Majander et al. 1994), prevented the accumulation of H_2O_2 in the patient's fibroblasts (Piccoli et al. 2008a). Depressed production of ATP by mitochondrial oxidative phosphorylation and the concomitant ROS accumulation, detected in the patient's fibroblasts, could both result from the combined impact of complex I dysfunction (Piccoli et al. 2008b), and the decreased mitochondrial content of cytochrome c (Piccoli et al. 2008a). The *PINK1* mutation can be responsible for the decrease of mitochondrial cytochrome *c* content. Defective phosphorylation by the mutated PINK1 kinase activity of TRAP1 has been reported to abrogate a protective effect exerted by this chaperone protein in preventing cytochrome c release from mitochondria (Pridgeon et al. 2007).

Sequence analysis of mtDNA of the homozygous patient's fibroblasts showed a number of single nucleotide changes (SNCs) disseminated throughout the entire mtDNA (Fig. 17.2). All but two were already reported as known polymorphisms (http://www.mitomap.org). These two SNCs were m. A12397G and m.T14319C in the *ND5* and *ND6* genes, respectively. Notably, both were homoplasmic (Piccoli et al. 2008b). The *ND5* and *ND6* mutations were also found in the homoplasmic state in the mtDNA of the patient's mother blood. Conversely, the same analysis carried out on the patient's father blood resulted in a normal ND5 and ND6 genotype (Piccoli et al. 2008b). Collectively these results demonstrate that the homoplasmic mtDNA mutations found in the patient coexisted with the *PINK1* mutation at birth and were inherited from the mother, who carried the same homoplasmic mtDNA mutations. The mother, heterozygous for the *PINK1* mutation, presented a Parkinson syndrome in her 50s. Thus the mtDNA mutation predisposed the *PINK1* heterozygous subject to a relatively late development of the disease. In the patient, the homozygous *PINK1* mutation, anticipated the decay of mitochondrial functions associated with the coexistent homoplasmic mutations in the *ND5* and *ND6* genes, with an early PD onset (age 22 years). The *PINK1* heterozygous mutation, in the absence of *ND5* and *ND6* mutations, would not result in Parkinsonism, as the case of the father still exempt from the disease in his 70s.

Various *ND6* mutations leading to aminoacid changes have been found, associated with mitochondrial diseases (Carelli et al. 1999; Chinnery et al. 2001). Some of these mutations result in changes in the kinetics parameters of complex I (Carelli et al. 1999; Chinnery et al. 2001) and/or production of oxygen free radicals (Gonzalo et al. 2005; Ishikawa et al. 2008). Site directed mutagenesis in the NuoJ subunit (counterpart of the mammalian ND6) of E. *coli* complex I, indicated that the NuoJ subunit delineates the binding site of ubiquinone (Pätsi et al. 2008). The mt T14319C mutation changes an asparagine in aspartic acid at position 119 of the ND6 subunit. Enzyme kinetic analysis of the NADH-ubiquinone oxidoreductase activity of complex I in normal and patient's fibroblasts showed an almost fivefold decrease of the apparent Km for both ubiquinone and NADH in the patient's sample (Piccoli et al. 2008b). The high affinity for the substrates in the patient's NADH: ubiquinone oxidoreductase, without compromising the overall electron transfer in the mitochondrial respiratory chain, may be, nevertheless, responsible for the enhanced production of ROS (see also Refs. Gonzalo et al. 2005; Ishikawa et al. 2008).

17.3.2 *Parkin Familial Parkinson*

Many different *Parkin* mutations have been reported (Abbas et al. 1999; Lücking et al. 2000; Hedrich et al. 2004). All types of mutations, including missense mutations leading to amino acid changes, nonsense mutations resulting in premature termination of translation, and exonic rearrangements (deletions, duplications and triplications) were identified (Lücking et al. 2001). Mutations have been found in several different ethnic populations (Hedrich et al. 2004). It is difficult to evaluate prevalence rates in these studies, as the frequency of *Parkin* mutations identified in a given cohort, depends on the age at onset of disease (Periquet et al. 2003). The various combinations of exon deletions, exon multiplications, and newly identified point mutations increase the already wide variety of disease-related mutations identified in *Parkin* gene (Lücking et al. 2000).

Parkin is made up of 465 amino acids, has a molecular weight of 52 kDa (Kitada et al. 1998) and has amino acid sequence homology with ubiquitin at the N-terminal end and two RING finger motifs at the C-terminal end, which could be responsible for adding ubiquitin to proteins. Because of these structural features, Parkin functions as an E3-ubiquitin ligase targeting misfolded proteins to the ubiquitin proteasome pathway for degradation (Tanaka et al. 2001). The position of the mutations indicates the functional importance of the protein regions such as the UBIQUITIN and RING–IBR–RING domains (Fig. 17.3).

Recently, there has been growing evidence indicating impaired mitochondrial function and morphology in Parkin deficiency in different model systems (Abou-Sleiman et al. 2006b). Mitochondrial respiratory defects and morphological abnormalities have been noted in brains of corsivo Parkin-knockout and corsivo Parkin-mutant transgenic mice (Palacino et al. 2004; Stichel et al. 2007) as well as in leukocytes from PD patients with *Parkin* mutations (Muftuoglu et al. 2004). Primary fibroblasts from patients carrying mutations in *Parkin*, or control fibroblasts treated with siRNA against *Parkin*, exhibited lower mitochondrial membrane potential and complex I activity, lower ATP level, decreased complex I-dependent ATP production, and increased susceptibility to rotenone toxicity (Mortiboys et al. 2008). The fibroblasts also exhibited mitochondrial morphological abnormalities, revealing mitochondria that were longer and more highly branched (Mortiboys et al. 2008). Investigations in the author's laboratory have detected a marked decrease in the activity of complex I and IV, in the fibroblasts of two patients with familial Parkinson, one with homozygous deletions of exons 3–4 (depression higher than 50%), the other with compound heterozygous for deletions of exon 5 and point mutation in the

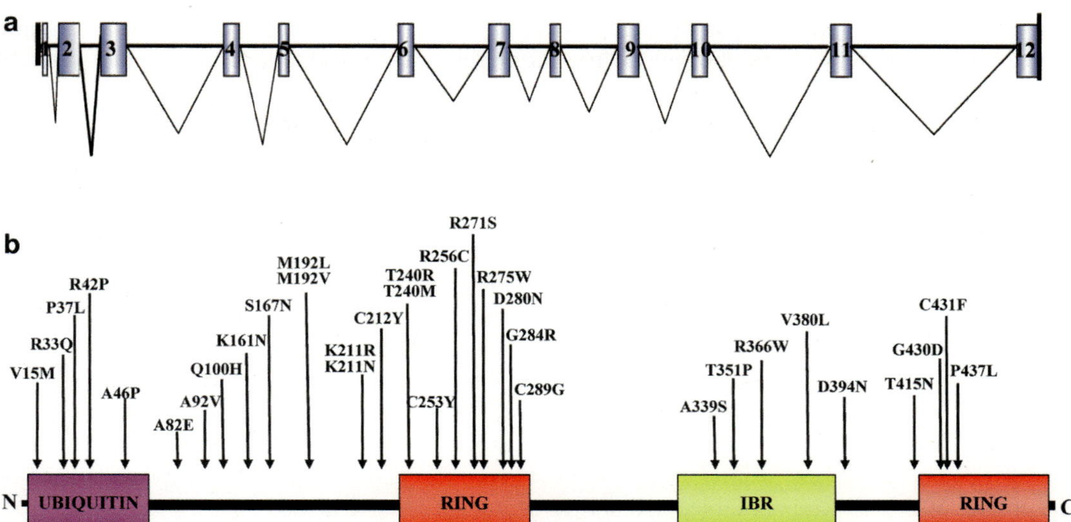

Fig.17.3 Structure of the gene (*PARK2*) (**a**) coding for the Parkin protein (**b**). In (**b**), the domains of the Parkin protein (http://www.uniprot.org) and the mutations found in patients with familial Parkinson are shown. The Parkin protein is made up of 465 amino acids, it has amino acid sequence homology with ubiquitin at the N-terminal end and two RING finger motifs at the C-terminal end, which could be responsible for binding of ubiquitin to proteins. Parkin IBR domain (in between RINGs) is also denominated as DRIL domain (double ring finger link)

exon 7 leading to substitution Cys253Tyr (30% depression). In the first case there was also a 50% decrease in the cellular level of ATP. How these Parkin mutations can impair the activity of respiratory chain complexes is under investigation. As already pointed out Parkin can be phosphorylated by PINK1 (Keeney et al. 2006). Phosphorylated Parkin appears to migrate into mitochondria where it stimulates autophagy (Narendra et al. 2008; Matsuda et al. 2010).

Recent works show that PINK1 kinase activity and its mitochondrial localization are prerequisites to induce translocation of the E3 ligase Parkin in depolarized mitochondria (Geisler et al. 2010; Matsuda et al. 2010). Once Parkin is recruited to the mitochondria, damaged mitochondria are delivered to the perinuclear area, where they are degraded by autophagy (Vives-Bauza et al. 2010). This mechanism can explain the functional interplay between ubiquitylation promoted by Parkin and mitochondrial quality control by PINK1. Mutations in either Parkin or PINK1 may alter mitochondrial turnover with accumulation of defective mitochondria.

17.4 Remarks and Perspectives

The genetic and biochemical observations reported in the present chapter highlight different mechanisms by which genetic defects of complex I may alter mitochondrial bioenergetics. Mutations in the *NDUFS4* and *NDUFS1* nuclear genes are associated with various forms of encephalopathies. The *NDUFS4* mutations have more unfavourable cell consequences—disappearance of the protein, block of the last step of complex I assembly, loss of the enzymatic activity and its response to cAMP-activation, accumulation of unproductive alternative transcripts—leading to a fatal outcome of the disease. The *NDUFS1* mutation resulting at cellular level, in an incomplete depression of complex I content and activity, enhancement of ROS production, both effects reversible by cAMP, is associated with a less severe encephalopathy. In this case, treatment with β-adrenergic agonists and antioxidants could exert a beneficial effect on the clinical course of the disease. The case of familial chronic epilepsy and progressive encephalopathy is paradigmatic of cases of complex I deficit not associated to mutations in structural genes. In this case an enhanced proteolytic degradation of the complex by a mitochondrial protease is observed but the genetic determinants and the biochemical mechanisms remain to be elucidated.

Genetic and functional analysis of mitochondria in familial PD associated with *PINK1* mutation revealed that co-segregation of mutations in the mitochondrial genes of complex I are determinant in developing the clinical course of the disease. This finding underscores the importance of mutational analysis of mitochondrial DNA in patients with hetero or homozygous familial forms of Parkinsonism as well as in sporadic PD. This would help not only in better understanding the pathogenesis of this devastating neurodegenerative disease but also in preventing its progress by earlier diagnosis.

The involvement of mitochondria in human diseases may be currently underestimated. In "primary" defects of respiratory chain, a phenotypic variability can exist both in the cases of mtDNA and nDNA mutations: thus mitochondriopathies fall outside the model of "one gene-one disease". In addition, it emerges that defects of the respiratory chain can be "secondary" and almost invariably at the basis of the progressive dysfunction observed in common neurodegenerative disorders.

A deeper understanding of cellular and clinical consequences associated to complex I deficiency is fundamental to develop therapeutic strategies. Treatment regimens of complex I deficient patients are so far purely empirical and unsuccessful. Although important links between clinical features and cellular dysfunction are still missing, any therapeutic strategy must combine clinical, genetic and cell physiology investigations to provide useful approaches to open new perspectives for treatments that could implement current strategies.

Acknowledgements This work was supported by: National Project, "Progetto FIRB Rete Nazionale per lo Studio della Proteomica Umana (Italian Human ProteomeNet)", 2009, Ministero dell'Istruzione, dell'Università e della Ricerca (MIUR) and University of Bari Research grant, 2009.

References

Abbas N, Lücking CB, Ricard S, Dürr A, Bonifati V, De Michele G, Bouley S, Vaughan JR, Gasser T, Marconi R, Broussolle E, Brefel-Courbon C, Harhangi BS, Oostra BA, Fabrizio E, Böhme GA, Pradier L, Wood NW, Filla A, Meco G, Denefle P, Agid Y, Brice A (1999) A wide variety of mutations in the parkin gene are responsible for autosomal recessive parkinsonism in Europe. Hum Mol Genet 8:567–574

Abou-Sleiman PM, Muqit MM, McDonald NQ, Yang YX, Gandhi S, Healy DG, Harvey K, Harvey RJ, Deas E, Bhatia K, Quinn N, Lees A, Latchman DS, Wood NW (2006a) A heterozygous effect for PINK1 mutations in Parkinson's disease? Ann Neurol 60:414–419

Abou-Sleiman PM, Muqit MM, Wood NW (2006b) Expanding insights of mitochondrial dysfunction in Parkinson's disease. Nat Rev Neurosci 7:207–219

Antonicka H, Ogilvie I, Taivassalo T, Anitori RP, Haller RG, Vissing J, Kennaway NG, Shoubridge EA (2003) Identification and characterization of a common set of complex I assembly intermediates in mitochondria from patients with complex I deficiency. J Biol Chem 278:43081–43088

Atorino L, Silvestri L, Koppen M, Cassina L, Ballabio A, Marconi R, Langer T, Casari G (2003) Loss of m-AAA protease in mitochondria causes complex I deficiency and increased sensitivity to oxidative stress in hereditary spastic paraplegia. J Cell Biol 163:777–787

Bénit P, Chretien D, Kadhom N, de Lonlay-Debeney P, Cormier-Daire V, Cabral A, Peudenier S, Rustin P, Munnich A, Rötig A (2001) Large-scale deletion and point mutations of the nuclear NDUFV1 and NDUFS1 genes in mitochondrial complex I deficiency. Am J Hum Genet 68:1344–1352

Bénit P, Beugnot R, Chretien D, Giurgea I, De Lonlay-Debeney P, Issartel JP, Corral-Debrinski M, Kerscher S, Rustin P, Rötig A, Munnich A (2003) Mutant NDUFV2 subunit of mitochondrial complex I causes early onset hypertrophic cardiomyopathy and encephalopathy. Hum Mutat 21:582–586

Bénit P, Slama A, Cartault F, Giurgea I, Chretien D, Lebon S, Marsac C, Munnich A, Rötig A, Rustin P (2004) Mutant NDUFS3 subunit of mitochondrial complex I causes Leigh syndrome. J Med Genet 41:14–17

Berger I, Hershkovitz E, Shaag A, Edvardson S, Saada A, Elpeleg O (2008) Mitochondrial complex I deficiency caused by a deleterious NDUFA11 mutation. Ann Neurol 63:405–408

Bonifati V, Rohé CF, Breedveld GJ, Fabrizio E, De Mari M, Tassorelli C, Tavella A, Marconi R, Nicholl DJ, Chien HF, Fincati E, Abbruzzese G, Marini P, De Gaetano A, Horstink MW, Maat-Kievit JA, Sampaio C, Antonini A, Stocchi F, Montagna P, Toni V, Guidi M, Dalla Libera A, Tinazzi M, De Pandis F, Fabbrini G, Goldwurm S, de Klein A, Barbosa E, Lopiano L, Martignoni E, Lamberti P, Vanacore N, Meco G, Oostra BA, Network Italian Parkinson Genetics (2005) Early-onset parkinsonism associated with PINK1 mutations: frequency, genotypes, and phenotypes. Neurology 65:87–95

Brandt U (2006) Energy converting NADH: quinone oxidoreductase (complex I). Annu Rev Biochem 75:69–92

Budde SM, van den Heuvel LP, Janssen AJ, Smeets RJ, Buskens CA, DeMeirleir L, Van Coster R, Baethmann M, Voit T, Trijbels JM, Smeitink JA (2000) Combined enzymatic complex I and III deficiency associated with mutations in the nuclear encoded NDUFS4 gene. Biochem Biophys Res Commun 275:63–68

Büeler H (2009) Impaired mitochondrial dynamics and function in the pathogenesis of Parkinson's disease. Exp Neurol 218:235–246

Bugiani M, Invernizzi F, Alberio S, Briem E, Lamantea E, Carrara F, Moroni I, Farina L, Spada M, Donati MA, Uziel G, Zeviani M (2004) Clinical and molecular findings in children with complex I deficiency. Biochim Biophys Acta 1659:136–147

Carelli V, Ghelli A, Bucchi L, Montagna P, De Negri A, Leuzzi V, Carducci C, Lenaz G, Lugaresi E, Degli Esposti M (1999) Biochemical features of mtDNA 14484 (ND6/M64V) point mutation associated with Leber's hereditary optic neuropathy. Ann Neurol 45:320–328

Chinnery PF, Brown DT, Andrews RM, Singh-Kler R, Riordan-Eva P, Lindley J, Applegarth DA, Turnbull DM, Howell N (2001) The mitochondrial ND6 gene is a hot spot for mutations that cause Leber's hereditary optic neuropathy. Brain 124:209–218

Chinta SJ, Andersen JK (2008) Redox imbalance in Parkinson's disease. Biochim Biophys Acta 1780:1362–1367

Civitarese AE, Ravussin E (2008) Mitochondrial energetics and insulin resistance. Endocrinology 149:950–954

Clark IE, Dodson MW, Jiang C, Cao JH, Huh JR, Seol JH, Yoo SJ, Hay BA, Guo M (2006) Drosophila pink1 is required for mitochondrial function and interacts genetically with parkin. Nature 441:1163–1166

Criscuolo C, Volpe G, De Rosa A, Varrone A, Marongiu R, Mancini P, Salvatore E, Dallapiccola B, Filla A, Valente EM, De Michele G (2006) PINK1 homozygous W437X mutation in a patient with apparent dominant transmission of parkinsonism. Mov Disord 21:1265–1267

Duchen MR (2004) Mitochondria in health and disease: perspectives on a new mitochondrial biology. Mol Aspects Med 25:365–451

Dunning CJ, McKenzie M, Sugiana C, Lazarou M, Silke J, Connelly A, Fletcher JM, Kirby DM, Thorburn DR, Ryan MT (2007) Human CIA30 is involved in the early assembly of mitochondrial complex I and mutations in its gene cause disease. EMBO J 26:3227–3237

Elliott HR, Samuels DC, Eden JA, Relton CL, Chinnery PF (2008) Pathogenic mitochondrial DNA mutations are common in the general population. Am J Hum Genet 83:254–260

Farrer MJ (2006) Genetics of Parkinson disease: paradigm shifts and future prospects. Nat Rev Genet 7:306–318

Fernandez-Moreira D, Ugalde C, Smeets R, Rodenburg RJ, Lopez-Laso E, Ruiz-Falco ML, Briones P, Martin MA, Smeitink JA, Arenas J (2007) X-linked NDUFA1 gene mutations associated with mitochondrial encephalomyopathy. Ann Neurol 61:73–83

Fitzgerald JC, Plun-Favreau H (2008) Emerging pathways in genetic Parkinson's disease: autosomal-recessive genes in Parkinson's disease—a common pathway? FEBS J 275:5758–5766

Friedrich T, Böttcher B (2004) The gross structure of the respiratory complex I: a Lego System. Biochim Biophys Acta 1657:71–83

Gandhi S, Muqit MM, Stanyer L, Healy DG, Abou-Sleiman PM, Hargreaves I, Heales S, Ganguly M, Parsons L, Lees AJ, Latchman DS, Holton JL, Wood NW, Revesz T (2006) PINK1 protein in normal human brain and Parkinson's disease. Brain 129:1720–1731

Geisler S, Holmström KM, Skujat D, Fiesel FC, Rothfuss OC, Kahle PJ, Springer W (2010) PINK1/Parkin-mediated mitophagy is dependent on VDAC1 and p62/SQSTM1. Nat Cell Biol 12:119–131

Gonzalo R, Garcia-Arumi E, Llige D, Marti R, Solano A, Montoya J, Arenas J, Andreu AL (2005) Free radicals-mediated damage in transmitochondrial cells harbouring the T14487C mutation in the ND6 gene of mtDNA. FEBS Lett 579:6909–6913

Hedrich K, Eskelson C, Wilmot B, Marder K, Harris J, Garrels J, Meija-Santana H, Vieregge P, Jacobs H, Bressman SB, Lang AE, Kann M, Abbruzzese G, Martinelli P, Schwinger E, Ozelius LJ, Pramstaller PP, Klein C, Kramer P (2004) Distribution, type, and origin of Parkin mutations: review and case studies. Mov Disord 19:1146–1157

Hirst J, Carroll J, Fearnley IM, Shannon RJ, Walker JE (2003) The nuclear encoded subunits of complex I from bovine heart mitochondria. Biochim Biophys Acta 1604:135–150

Hoefs SJ, Dieteren CE, Distelmaier F, Janssen RJ, Epplen A, Swarts HG, Forkink M, Rodenburg RJ, Nijtmans LG, Willems PH, Smeitink JA, van den Heuvel LP (2008) NDUFA2 complex I mutation leads to Leigh disease. Am J Hum Genet 82:1306–1315

Ishikawa K, Takenaga K, Akimoto M, Koshikawa N, Yamaguchi A, Imanishi H, Nakada K, Honma Y, Hayashi J (2008) ROS-generating mitochondrial DNA mutations can regulate tumor cell metastasis. Science 320:661–664

Isken O, Maquat LE (2007) Quality control of eukaryotic mRNA: safeguarding cells from abnormal mRNA function. Genes Dev 21:1833–1856

Iuso A, Scacco S, Piccoli C, Bellomo F, Petruzzella V, Trentadue R, Minuto M, Ripoli M, Capitanio N, Zeviani M, Papa S (2006) Dysfunctions of cellular oxidative metabolism in patients with mutations in the NDUFS1 and NDUFS4 genes of complex I. J Biol Chem 281:10374–10380

Janssen RJ, van den Heuvel LP, Smeitink JA (2004) Genetic defects in the oxidative phosphorylation (OXPHOS) system. Expert Rev Mol Diagn 4:143–156

Keeney PM, Xie J, Capaldi RA, Bennett JP Jr (2006) Parkinson's disease brain mitochondrial complex I has oxidatively damaged subunits and is functionally impaired and misassembled. J Neurosci 26(19):5256–5264

Kim Y, Park J, Kim S, Song S, Kwon SK, Lee SH, Kitada T, Kim JM, Chung J (2008) PINK1 controls mitochondrial localization of Parkin through direct phosphorylation. Biochem Biophys Res Commun 377:975–980

Kirby DM, Crawford M, Cleary MA, Dahl HH, Dennett X, Thorburn DR (1999) Respiratory chain complex I deficiency: an underdiagnosed energy generation disorder. Neurology 52:1255–1264

Kirby DM, Salemi R, Sugiana C, Ohtake A, Parry L, Bell KM, Kirk EP, Boneh A, Taylor RW, Dahl HH, Ryan MT, Thorburn DR (2004) NDUFS6 mutations are a novel cause of lethal neonatal mitochondrial complex I deficiency. J Clin Invest 114:837–845

Kitada T, Asakawa S, Hattori N, Matsumine H, Yamamura Y, Minoshima S, Yokochi M, Mizuno Y, Shimizu N (1998) Mutations in the Parkin gene cause autosomal recessive juvenile parkinsonism. Nature 392:605–608

Lang AE, Lozano AM (1998) Parkinson's disease. First of two parts. N Engl J Med 339:1044–1053

Leigh D (1951) Subacute necrotizing encephalomyelopathy in an infant. J Neurol Neurosurg Psychiatry 14:216–221

Lin MT, Beal MF (2006) Mitochondrial dysfunction and oxidative stress in neurodegenerative diseases. Nature 443:787–795

Loeffen J, Smeitink J, Triepels R, Smeets R, Schuelke M, Sengers R, Trijbels F, Hamel B, Mullaart R, van den Heuvel L (1998) The first nuclear-encoded complex I mutation in a patient with Leigh syndrome. Am J Hum Genet 63:1598–1608

Loeffen JL, Smeitink JA, Trijbels JM, Janssen AJ, Triepels RH, Sengers RC, van den Heuvel LP (2000) Isolated complex I deficiency in children: clinical, biochemical and genetic aspects. Hum Mutat 15:123–134

Loeffen J, Elpeleg O, Smeitink J, Smeets R, Stöckler-Ipsiroglu S, Mandel H, Sengers R, Trijbels F, van den Heuvel L (2001) Mutations in the complex I NDUFS2 gene of patients with cardiomyopathy and encephalomyopathy. Ann Neurol 49:195–201

Lücking CB, Dürr A, Bonifati V, Vaughan J, De Michele G, Gasser T, Harhangi BS, Meco G, Denèfle P, Wood NW, Agid Y, Brice A, French Parkinson's Disease Genetics Study Group, European Consortium on Genetic Susceptibility in Parkinson's Disease (2000) Association between early-onset Parkinson's disease and mutations in the Parkin gene. N Engl J Med 342:1560–1567

Lücking CB, Bonifati V, Periquet M, Vanacore N, Brice A, Meco G (2001) Pseudo-dominant inheritance and exon 2 triplication in a family with parkin gene mutations. Neurology 57:924–927

Luft R, Ikkos D, Palmieri G, Ernster L, Afzelius B (1962) A case of severe hypermetabolism of nonthyroid origin with a defect in the maintenance of mitochondrial respiratory control: a correlated clinical, biochemical, and morphological study. J Clin Invest 41:1776–1804

Majander A, Finel M, Wikstrom M (1994) Diphenyleneiodonium inhibits reduction of iron–sulfur clusters in the mitochondrial NADH-ubiquinone oxidoreductase (Complex I). J Biol Chem 269:21037–21042

Matsuda N, Sato S, Shiba K, Okatsu K, Saisho K, Gautier CA, Sou Y, Saiki S, Kawajiri S, Sato F, Kimura M, Komatsu M, Hattori N, Tanaka K (2010) PINK1 stabilized by mitochondrial depolarization recruits Parkin to damaged mitochondria and activates latent Parkin for mitophagy. J Cell Biol 189:211–221

McBride HM (2008) Parkin mitochondria in the autophagosome. J Cell Biol 183:757–759

Mortiboys H, Thomas KJ, Koopman WJ, Klaffke S, Abou-Sleiman P, Olpin S, Wood NW, Willems PH, Smeitink JA, Cookson MR, Bandmann O (2008) Mitochondrial function and morphology are impaired in parkin-mutant fibroblasts. Ann Neurol 64:555–565

Muftuoglu M, Elibol B, Dalmizrak O, Ercan A, Kulaksiz G, Ogus H, Dalkara T, Ozer N (2004) Mitochondrial complex I and IV activities in leukocytes from patients with parkin mutations. Mov Disord 19:544–548

Narendra D, Tanaka A, Suen DF, Youle RJ (2008) Parkin is recruited selectively to impaired mitochondria and promotes their autophagy. J Cell Biol 183:795–803

Ogilvie I, Kennaway NG, Shoubridge EA (2005) A molecular chaperone for mitochondrial complex I assembly is mutated in a progressive encephalopathy. J Clin Invest 115:2784–2792

Ohnishi T (1998) Iron-sulfur clusters/semiquinones in complex I. Biochim Biophys Acta 1364:186–206

Ohnishi T, Salerno JC (2005) Conformation-driven and semiquinone-gated proton-pump mechanism in the NADH-ubiquinone oxidoreductase (complex I). FEBS Lett 579:4555–4561

Orth M, Schapira AHV (2001) Mitochondria and degenerative disorders. Am J Med Genet 106:27–36

Pagliarini DJ, Calvo SE, Chang B, Sheth SA, Vafai SB, Ong SE, Walford GA, Sugiana C, Boneh A, Chen WK, Hill DE, Vidal M, Evans JG, Thorburn DR, Carr SA, Mootha VK (2008) A mitochondrial protein compendium elucidates complex I disease biology. Cell 134:112–123

Palacino JJ, Sagi D, Goldberg MS, Krauss S, Motz C, Wacker M, Klose J, Shen J (2004) Mitochondrial dysfunction and oxidative damage in parkin-deficient mice. J Biol Chem 279:18614–18622

Panelli D, Petruzzella V, Vitale R, De Rasmo D, Munnich A, Rötig A, Papa S (2008) The regulation of PTC containing transcripts of the human NDUFS4 gene of complex I of respiratory chain and the impact of pathological mutations. Biochimie 90:1452–1460

Papa S (1996) Mitochondrial oxidative phosphorylation changes in the life span. Molecular aspects and physiopathological implications. Biochim Biophys Acta 1276:87–105

Papa S, Capitanio N, Villani G (1999) Proton pumps of respiratory chain enzymes. In: Papa S, Guerrieri F, Tager JM (eds) Frontiers of cellular bioenenergetics: molecular biology, biochemistry and physiopathology. Plenum Press, London/New York, pp 49–88

Papa S, Scacco S, Sardanelli AM, Vergari R, Papa F, Budde S, van den Heuvel L, Smeitink J (2001) Mutation in the NDUFS4 gene of complex I abolishes cAMP-dependent activation of the complex in a child with fatal neurological syndrome. FEBS Lett 489:259–262

Papa S, Petruzzella V, Scacco S (2007) Structure, redox-coupled protonmotive activity and pathological disorders of respiratory chain complexes. In: Gibson G, Dienel GA (eds) Handbook of neurochemistry and molecular neurobiology, vol 5, 3rd edn. Springer, Berlin/Heidelberg, pp 94–118

Papa S, Sardanelli AM, Capitanio N, Piccoli C (2009a) Mitochondrial respiratory dysfunction and mutations in mitochondrial DNA in PINK1 familial parkinsonism. J Bioenerg Biomembr 41:509–516

Papa S, Petruzzella V, Scacco S, Sardanelli AM, Iuso A, Panelli D, Vitale R, Trentadue R, De Rasmo D, Capitanio N, Piccoli C, Papa F, Scivetti M, Bertini E, Rizza T, De Michele G (2009b) Pathogenetic mechanisms in hereditary dysfunctions of complex I of the respiratory chain in neurological diseases. Biochim Biophys Acta 1787:502–517

Parker WD Jr, Parks JK, Swerdlow RH (2008) Complex I deficiency in Parkinson's disease frontal cortex. Brain Res 1189:215–218

Pätsi J, Kervinen M, Finel M, Hassinen IE (2008) Leber hereditary optic neuropathy mutations in the ND6 subunit of mitochondrial complex I affect ubiquinone reduction kinetics in a bacterial model of the enzyme. Biochem J 409:129–137

Periquet M, Latouche M, Lohmann E, Rawal N, De Michele G, Ricard S, Teive H, Fraix V, Vidailhet M, Nicholl D, Barone P, Wood NW, Raskin S, Deleuze JF, Agid Y, Dürr A, Brice A, French Parkinson's Disease Genetics Study Group, European Consortium on Genetic Susceptibility in Parkinson's Disease (2003) Parkin mutations are frequent in patients with isolated early-onset parkinsonism. Brain 126:1271–1278

Petruzzella V, Vergari R, Puzziferri I, Boffoli D, Lamantea E, Zeviani M, Papa S (2001) A nonsense mutation in the NDUFS4 gene encoding the 18 kDa (AQDQ) subunit of complex I abolishes assembly and activity of the complex in a patient with Leigh-like syndrome. Hum Mol Genet 10:529–535

Petruzzella V, Di Giacinto G, Scacco S, Piemonte F, Torraco A, Carrozzo R, Vergari R, Dionisi-Vici C, Longo D, Tessa A, Papa S, Bertini E (2003) Atypical Leigh syndrome associated with the D393N mutation in the mitochondrial ND5 subunit. Neurology 61:1017–1018

Petruzzella V, Panelli D, Torraco A, Stella A, Papa S (2005) Mutations in the NDUFS4 gene of mitochondrial complex I alter stability of the splice variants. FEBS Lett 579:3770–3776

Piccoli C, Sardanelli AM, Scrima R, Ripoli M, Quarato G, D'Aprile A, Bellomo F, Scacco S, De Michele G, Filla A, Iuso A, Boffoli D, Capitanio N, Papa S (2008a) Mitochondrial respiratory dysfunction in familiar Parkinsonism associated with PINK1 mutation. Neurochem Res 33:2565–2574

Piccoli C, Ripoli M, Quarato G, Scrima R, D'Aprile A, Boffoli D, Margaglione M, Criscuolo C, De Michele G, Sardanelli AM, Papa S, Capitanio N (2008b) Coexistence of mutations in PINK1 and mitochondrial DNA in early onset parkinsonism. J Med Genet 45:596–602

Pitkanen S, Feigenbaum A, Laframboise R, Robinson BH (1996) NADH-coenzyme Q reductase (complex I) deficiency: heterogeneity in phenotype and biochemical findings. J Inherit Metab Dis 19:675–686

Plun-Favreau H, Klupsch K, Moisoi N, Gandhi S, Kjaer S, Frith D, Harvey K, Deas E, Harvey RJ, McDonald N, Wood NW, Martins LM, Downward J (2007) The mitochondrial protease HtrA2 is regulated by Parkinson's disease-associated kinase PINK1. Nat Cell Biol 9:1243–1252

Pridgeon JW, Olzmann JA, Chin LS, Li L (2007) PINK1 protects against oxidative stress by phosphorylating mitochondrial chaperone TRAP1. PLoS Biol 5:e172

Rahman S, Blok RB, Dahl HH, Danks DM, Kirby DM, Chow CW, Christodoulou J, Thorburn DR (1996) Leigh syndrome: clinical features and biochemical and DNA abnormalities. Ann Neurol 39:343–351

Robinson BH (1998) Human complex I deficiency: clinical spectrum and involvement of oxygen free radicals in the pathogenicity of the defect. Biochim Biophys Acta 1364:271–286

Saada A, Edvardson S, Rapoport M, Shaag A, Amry K, Miller C, Lorberboum-Galski H, Elpeleg O (2008) C6ORF66 is an assembly factor of mitochondrial complex I. Am J Hum Genet 82:32–38

Sazanov LA, Hinchliffe P (2006) Structure of the hydrophilic domain of respiratory complex I from *Thermus thermophilus*. Science 311:1430–1436

Scacco S, Petruzzella V, Budde S, Vergari R, Tamborra R, Panelli D, van den Heuvel LP, Smeitink JA, Papa S (2003) Pathological mutations of the human NDUFS4 gene of the 18-kDa (AQDQ) subunit of complex I affect the expression of the protein and the assembly and function of the complex. J Biol Chem 278:44161–44167

Schapira AH (2008) Mitochondria in the aetiology and pathogenesis of Parkinson's disease. Lancet Neurol 7:97–109

Scheffler IE, Yadava N, Potluri P (2004) Molecular genetics of complex I-deficient Chinese hamster cell lines. Biochim Biophys Acta 1659:160–171

Schuelke M, Smeitink J, Mariman E, Loeffen J, Plecko B, Trijbels F, Stöckler-Ipsiroglu S, van den Heuvel L (1999) Mutant NDUFV1 subunit of mitochondrial complex I causes leukodystrophy and myoclonic epilepsy. Nat Genet 21:260–261

Silvestri L, Caputo V, Bellacchio E, Atorino L, Dallapiccola B, Valente EM, Casari G (2005) Mitochondrial import and enzymatic activity of PINK1 mutants associated to recessive parkinsonism. Hum Mol Genet 14:3477–3492

Sim CH, Lio DS, Mok SS, Masters CL, Hill AF, Culvenor JG, Cheng HC (2006) C-terminal truncation and Parkinson's disease associated mutations down-regulate the protein serine/threonine kinase activity of PTEN-induced kinase-1. Hum Mol Genet 15:3251–3262

Smeitink JAM, van den Heuvel LP, DiMauro S (2001) The genetics and pathology of oxidative phosphorylation. Nat Rev Genet 2:342–352

Stichel CC, Zhu XR, Bader V, Linnartz B, Schmidt S, Lubbert H (2007) Mono- and double-mutant mouse models of Parkinson's disease display severe mitochondrial damage. Hum Mol Genet 16:2377–2393

Sugiana C, Pagliarini DJ, McKenzie M, Kirby DM, Salemi R, Abu-Amero KK, Dahl HH, Hutchison WM, Vascotto KA, Smith SM, Newbold RF, Christodoulou J, Calvo S, Mootha VK, Ryan MT, Thorburn DR (2008) Mutation of C20orf7 disrupts complex I assembly and causes lethal neonatal mitochondrial disease. Am J Hum Genet 83:468–478

Tanaka K, Suzuki T, Chiba T, Shimura H, Hattori N, Mizuno Y (2001) Parkin is linked to the ubiquitin pathway. J Mol Med 79:482–494

Thomas B, Beal MF (2007) Parkinson's disease. Hum Mol Genet 16(2):183–194

Triepels RH, van den Heuvel LP, Loeffen JL, Buskens CA, Smeets RJ, Rubio Gozalbo ME, Budde SM, Mariman EC, Wijburg FA, Barth PG, Trijbels JM, Smeitink JA (1999) Leigh syndrome associated with a mutation in the NDUFS7 (PSST) nuclear encoded subunit of complex I. Ann Neurol 45:787–790

Valente EM, Abou-Sleiman PM, Caputo V, Muqit MM, Harvey K, Gispert S, Ali Z, Del Turco D, Bentivoglio AR, Healy DG, Albanese A, Nussbaum R, González-Maldonado R, Deller T, Salvi S, Cortelli P, Gilks WP, Latchman DS, Harvey RJ, Dallapiccola B, Auburger G, Wood NW (2004) Hereditary early-onset Parkinson's disease caused by mutations in PINK1. Science 304:1158–1160

van den Heuvel L, Ruitenbeek W, Smeets R, Gelman-Kohan Z, Elpeleg O, Loeffen J, Trijbels F, Mariman E, de Bruijn D, Smeitink J (1998) Demonstration of a new pathogenic mutation in human complex I deficiency: a 5-bp duplication in the nuclear gene encoding the 18-kD (AQDQ) subunit. Am J Hum Genet 62:262–268

Ventura B, Genova ML, Bovina C, Formiggini G, Lenaz G (2002) Control of oxidative phosphorylation by Complex I in rat liver mitochondria: implications for aging. Biochim Biophys Acta 1553:249–260

Vives-Bauza C, Zhou C, Huang Y, Cui M, de Vries RL, Kim J, May J, Tocilescu MA, Liu W, Ko HS, Magrané J, Moore DJ, Dawson VL, Grailhe R, Dawson TM, Li C, Tieu K, Przedborski S (2010) PINK1-dependent recruitment of Parkin to mitochondria in mitophagy. Proc Natl Acad Sci USA 107(1):378–383

Vogel RO, Smeitink JA, Nijtmans LG (2007) Human mitochondrial complex I assembly: a dynamic and versatile process. Biochim Biophys Acta 1767:1215–1227

Walker JE (1992) The NADH: ubiquinone oxidoreductase (complex I) of respiratory chains. Q Rev Biophys 25:232–253

Yagi T, Matsuno-Yagi A (2003) The proton-translocating NADH-quinone oxidoreductase in the respiratory chain: the secret unlocked. Biochemistry 42:2266–2274

Yang Y, Ouyang Y, Yang L, Beal MF, McQuibban A, Vogel H, Lu B (2008) Pink1 regulates mitochondrial dynamics through interaction with the fission/fusion machinery. Proc Natl Acad Sci USA 10(5):7070–7073

Zadikoff C, Rogaeva E, Djarmati A, Sato C, Salehi-Rad S, St George-Hyslop P, Klein C, Lang AE (2006) Homozygous and heterozygous PINK1 mutations: considerations for diagnosis and care of Parkinson's disease patients. Mov Disord 21:875–879

Zhou C, Huang Y, Shao Y, May J, Prou D, Perier C, Dauer W, Schon EA, Przedborski S (2008) The kinase domain of mitochondrial PINK1 faces the cytoplasm. Proc Natl Acad Sci USA 105:2022–2027

Chapter 18
Anthracyclines and Mitochondria

Alvaro Mordente, Elisabetta Meucci, Andrea Silvestrini, Giuseppe Ettore Martorana, and Bruno Giardina

Abstract Anthracyclines remain the cornerstone in the treatment of many malignancies including lymphomas, leukaemias, and sarcomas. Unfortunately, the clinical use of these potent chemotherapeutics is severely limited by the development of a progressive dose-dependent cardiomyopathy that irreversibly evolves toward congestive heart failure. The molecular mechanisms responsible for anthracycline anticancer activity as well as those underlying anthracycline-induced cardiotoxicity are incompletely understood and remain a matter of remarkable controversy. Anthracyclines have long been considered to induce cardiotoxicity by mechanisms different from those mediating their anticancer activity. In particular, anthracycline antitumor efficacy is associated with nuclear DNA intercalation, topoisomerase II inhibition and drug-DNA adducts formation, whereas the cardiotoxicity is prevalently ascribed to oxidative stress and mitochondrial dysfunction. At present, however, the view that distinct mechanisms are implied in anticancer and cardiotoxic responses to anthracycline therapy does not seem fully convincing since beneficial (anticancer) and detrimental (cardiotoxic) effects are to some extent overlapping, share the subcellular organelle targets, the molecular effectors and the pathophysiological processes (i.e. DNA strand breaks, oxidative stress, signalling pathways, mitochondrial dysfunctions, apoptosis etc.).

Here, we review the potential role of mitochondria in the molecular mechanisms underlying anthracyclines anticancer activity as well as in the pathogenesis of anthracycline-induced cardiotoxicity

Keywords Anthracycline • Cardiotoxicity • Mitochondria

18.1 Anthracyclines: Anticancer Activity Versus Cardiotoxicity

Anthracyclines remain among the most potent anticancer drugs ever developed and, despite their extensive and long-standing (about half a century) clinical use, they continue to play, alone or in combination with other chemotherapeutics, an undisputed role in the treatment of a variety of solid tumours like carcinomas and sarcomas and haematological malignancies as leukemias and lymphomas (Minotti et al. 2004; Ewer and Ewer 2010; van Dalen et al. 2011). Unfortunately, the therapeutic potential of

A. Mordente (✉) • E. Meucci • A. Silvestrini • G.E. Martorana • B. Giardina
Institute of Biochemistry and Clinical Biochemistry, Catholic University School
of Medicine, Largo F. Vito 1, 00168 Rome, Italy
e-mail: alvaro.mordente@rm.unicatt.it

R. Scatena et al. (eds.), *Advances in Mitochondrial Medicine*, Advances in Experimental
Medicine and Biology 942, DOI 10.1007/978-94-007-2869-1_18,
© Springer Science+Business Media B.V. 2012

anthracyclines and, consequently, their clinical utility are severely limited by their selective toxicity for myocardial tissue which may lead to a progressive cardiomyopathy that can be neither predicted nor prevented and that irreversibly evolves to congestive heart failure (CHF) (Gianni et al. 2008; Ewer and Ewer 2010; Lipshultz and Adams 2010; Peng et al. 2010; Chen et al. 2011; Menna et al. 2011). Despite recent medical progress, current therapies for CHF are still limited and the prognosis for heart failure is disappointing (Eschenhagen et al. 2011; Larsen et al. 2011).

The molecular mechanisms responsible for anthracycline anticancer activity as well as those underlying anthracycline-induced cardiotoxicity remain not yet completely understood, thus constituting a matter of considerable controversy (Gewirtz 1999; Minotti et al. 2004; Chen et al. 2007a; Mordente et al. 2009; Peng et al. 2010; Menna et al. 2011). Anthracyclines have long been considered to induce cardiotoxicity by mechanisms different from those mediating their anticancer activity, a concept that has raised hopes to design new strategies for protecting the heart without diminishing the drug's antitumor efficiency (Gewirtz 1999; Minotti et al. 2004; Tokarska-Schlattner et al. 2006; Mordente et al. 2009; Sawyer et al. 2010). In particular, the antitumor activity of anthracyclines is commonly attributed to their ability to rapidly diffuse to the nucleus and interact with DNA by intercalation of their planar rings between nucleotide base pairs thus poisoning topoisomerases IIα (Nitiss 2009; Pommier et al. 2010) and/or by formation of anthracycline-DNA covalent adducts (Cutts et al. 2005; Swift et al. 2006). Anthracycline-DNA interactions result in inhibition of DNA, RNA, and protein synthesis, leading ultimately to cell death (Gewirtz 1999; Swift et al. 2006; Chen et al. 2007a). Conversely, the prevailing pathogenetic mechanism underlying anthracycline-induced cardiotoxicity provides a harmful cycle constituted by reactive oxygen species (ROS) overproduction, mitochondrial dysfunction, impairment of energy metabolism, and cardiomyocytes apoptosis (Gewirtz 1999; Minotti et al. 2004; Tokarska-Schlattner et al. 2006; Menna et al. 2011). At present, however, the view that anticancer and cardiotoxic effects rely on distinct molecular mechanisms in response to anthracycline therapy can be however questioned (Tokarska-Schlattner et al. 2006).

Here, we review: (*a*) chemistry, subcellular distribution and metabolism of anthracyclines; (*b*) the molecular mechanisms of anthracyclines anticancer activity; (*c*) the pathogenic mechanisms of anthracycline-induced cardiotoxicity; (*d*) the potential mechanistic role of mitochondria in anthracycline anticancer activity as well as in anthracycline-induced cardiotoxicity; (*d*) the role of different apoptotic pathways on the anthracycline antineoplastic and toxic activity.

18.2   Anthracyclines: Chemistry, Subcellular Distribution and Metabolism

The main anthracyclines approved by Food and Drug Administration for clinical use are doxorubicin (DOX; the best recognized and most frequently used agent in this group), daunorubicin (DNR), epirubicin (EPI) and idarubicin (IDA) (Fig. 18.1). DOX and DNR are natural compounds isolated for the first time in the early 1960s from the actinobacterium *Streptomyces peucetius* var. *caesius*. Conversely, EPI (4′-epidoxorubicin) and IDA (4-demethoxydaunorubicin) are synthetic analogues (second-generation anthracyclines) of DOX and DNR, respectively, from which the former two drugs differ by relatively small chemical modifications.

Structurally all the anthracyclines share aglyconic and sugar moieties. The aglycone consists of a planar tetracyclic ring (7,8,9,10-tetrahydrotetracene-5, 12-quinone) structure, with adjacent quinone-hydroquinone moieties in rings C-B, a methoxy substituent at C-4 in the ring D and a short side chain at C-9 with a carbonyl group at C-13. The sugar, daunosamine, is an amino-substituted trideoxyl fucosyl moiety attached to the C-7 of ring A by a glycosidic bond.

DOX differs from DNR only by a single hydroxyl group in the side chain (Fig. 18.1); DOX terminates with a primary alcohol at C-14, whereas DNR terminates with a methyl group. Despite the minor difference in structure, DOX and DNR present a different spectrum of anticancer activity.

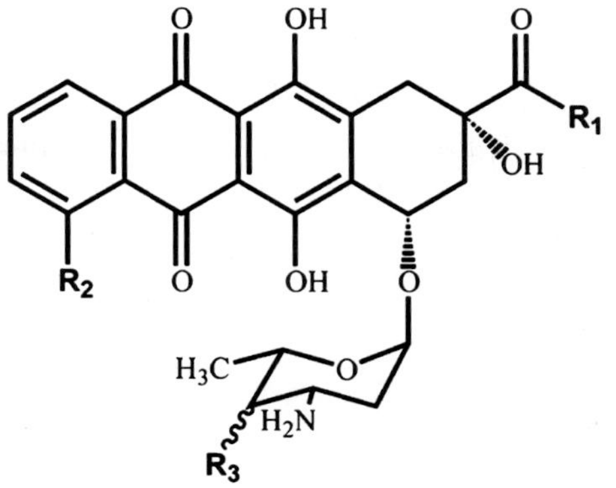

ANTHRACYCLINE	R_1	R_2	R_3	APPROVED INDICATIONS
DOX	CH₂OH	OCH₃	OH axial	Carcinomas, sarcomas
EPI	CH₂OH	OCH₃	OH equatorial	Lymphomas
DNR	CH₃	OCH₃	OH axial	Acute myeloblastic leukaemia
IDA	CH₃	H	OH axial	AIDS-related Kaposi's sarcoma

Fig. 18.1 Chemical structure of anthracyclines approved for clinical use and effects of substituents on the clinical spectrum of antitumor activity

While DOX is an essential component in the treatment of breast cancer, childhood solid tumours, soft tissue sarcomas, and aggressive lymphomas, DNR shows activity in acute lymphoblastic and myeloblastic leukemias.

EPI differs from DOX in an axial-to-equatorial epimerization of the hydroxyl group at C-4′ in daunosamine sugar. This positional change has little effect on the mode of action and spectrum of activity of EPI compared with DOX, but renders EPI a much better substrate than DOX for human liver UDP-glucuronosyltransferase 2B7 and consequently facilitates the formation of glucuronides that are excreted in bile and urine (Innocenti et al. 2001). Furthermore, such a limited modification favours EPI sequestration in cytoplasmic acidic organelles as recycling endosomes, lysosomes, and vesicles of the *trans*-Golgi network; hence, EPI fails to reach mitochondria and forms essentially no ROS compared with DOX (Salvatorelli et al. 2006). EPI also exhibits an impaired two-electron reduction of its side-chain carbonyl group in such a way that the levels of formation of its secondary alcohol metabolite always average ≤50% of those of DOX (Salvatorelli et al. 2006).

IDA differs from DNR in the absence of the 4-methoxy group in ring D, and it is widely used to treat acute myeloid leukemia (AML) and relapsed/refractory acute lymphoblastic leukaemia (ALL) because it is more effective in multi-drug-resistant cell lines and has a high penetration rate into the central nervous system compared to DNR or DOX. The broader spectrum of activity of IDA in respect to DNR is attributed to increased lipophilicity and cellular uptake and improved stabilization of a ternary drug-topoisomerase II-DNA complex (Binaschi et al. 2001).

Since most of the data regard DOX, this drug has been here assumed to represent all the anthracyclines unless otherwise specified whenever data regarding the other compounds are available.

Anthracyclines are cationic (the pK_a value of DOX, DNR, EPI and IDA is 8.34, 8.46, 8.08, and 8.5, respectively), lipophilic drugs. Consequently, a substantial fraction of the molecules is uncharged at

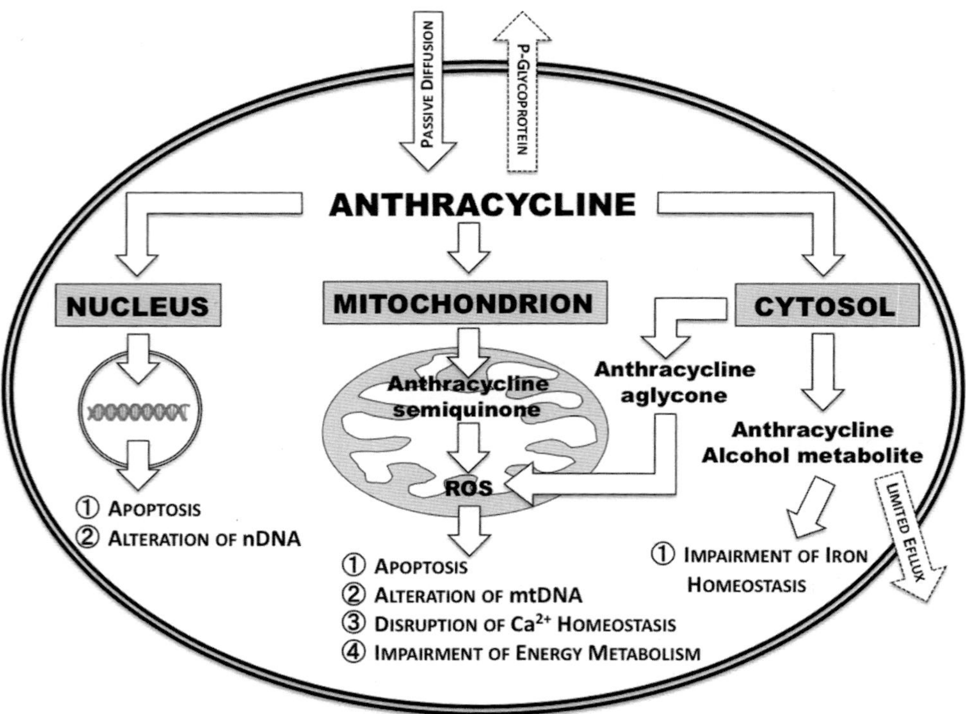

Fig. 18.2 Anthracyclines major cellular targets with their relative pathophysiological effects

normal intracellular pH, allowing them to freely penetrate the membranes of cytoplasmic organelles and vesicles. Anthracyclines have a relatively high volume of distribution (V_d) ranging from 700 to 1,100 l/m² and a plasma protein binding ranging from 50% to 85% (Morotti et al. 2011). They are rapidly cleared from plasma through liver metabolism (Danesi et al. 2002) and are excreted primarily through the hepatobiliary route (Wildiers et al. 2003). Approximately 50% DOX is eliminated from the body unchanged (Joerger et al. 2005). The pharmacokinetics of anthracyclines is most commonly described by a triphasic model, with half-life values for each phase of approximately 3–5 min, 1–3 and 24–48 h (Robert and Gianni 1993). Anthracycline pharmacokinetics exhibits large interpatient and intrapatient differences that may be important both for the individual antitumor response and for the anthracycline-related cardiotoxicity (Robert and Gianni 1993; Lal et al. 2010). The reasons for the interindividual variability are unknown but they may be due to functional polymorphisms in genes encoding proteins involved in anthracycline transport and metabolism (Lal et al. 2010).

Different tissues (Houba et al. 2001) and intracellular structures (Nicolay et al. 1986; Tokarska-Schlattner et al. 2005, 2006) accumulate the chemotherapic antibiotics at various degrees. The highest accumulation of anthracyclines among tissues is seen in the liver, heart, white blood cells and bone marrow (Lal et al. 2010).

The mechanisms underlying anthracyclines uptake by the cells are not completely understood. Anthracyclines are generally believed to be transported into the cells through passive diffusion (Frezard and Garnier-Suillerot 1991), but other studies indicate that specific transport proteins might be involved in cellular anthracycline uptake (Nagasawa et al. 2001). Furthermore, evidence for such transport mediated uptake were not found in normal mononuclear blood cells (Nagasawa et al. 2001) opening up the possibility of different uptake mechanisms in normal and malignant cells.

Intracellularly, anthracyclines accumulate primarily in two distinct sites (Fig. 18.2): nucleus and mitochondria (Nicolay et al. 1986; Jung and Reszka 2001; Wallace 2003; Tokarska-Schlattner et al.

2005, 2010), which therefore represent the major subcellular targets of anthracyclines cytotoxic activity. It should always be kept in mind that the nucleus and mitochondria selectively accumulate DOX up to concentrations much higher than plasma levels (Tokarska-Schlattner et al. 2006; Lal et al. 2010). Under clinically relevant plasma DOX concentrations of 0.5–1.0 μM, intramitochondrial concentrations can reach approximately 50–100 μM (Sokolove 1994; Tokarska-Schlattner et al. 2006). Analogously, nuclear concentrations of DOX are 50-fold higher than in the cytoplasm, reaching 340 μM at saturation, representing one molecule intercalated every five base pairs of DNA (Lal et al. 2010).

In cells, anthracyclines may undergo at least three major metabolic pathways (Licata et al. 2000; Mordente et al. 2001, 2009; Salvatorelli et al. 2006; Menna et al. 2011): (1) one-electron reduction to anthracycline semiquinone radicals; (2) two-electron reduction to secondary alcohol metabolites; (3) deglycosidation to anthracycline aglycones.

The quinone moiety in ring C of anthracyclines can be reduced by several mono-electronic oxidoreductases producing a semiquinone radical that quickly regenerates its parent quinone by reducing oxygen to reactive oxygen species (ROS) that are still considered the main (or sole) responsible for anthracycline-induced cardiotoxicity (Doroshow and Davies 1986; Gewirtz 1999; Menna et al. 2011) (see Sect. 18.4.3.1).

Alternatively, anthracyclines may undergo two-electron reduction of the C-13 carbonyl group in the side chain yielding anthracycline secondary alcohol metabolites, which are strongly implied in anthracycline-induced cardiotoxicity (Minotti et al. 1999, 2004; Licata et al. 2000; Mordente et al. 2003, 2009; Menna et al. 2007, 2011) (see Sect. 18.4.3.2). The C-13 hydroxy metabolites of DOX, DNR, EPI or IDA are known as doxorubicinol (DOXol), daunorubicinol (DNRol), epirubicinol (EPIol) and idarubicinol (IDAol), respectively. This reductive pathway is catalyzed by cytoplasmic oxidoreductases that exhibit a variable expression pattern in different human tissues (Penning and Drury 2007; Bains et al. 2009, 2010a, b).

Lastly, anthracyclines can be metabolized by deglycosidation reactions catalyzed by poorly characterized NADPH-dependent reductase- and hydrolase-type glycosidases into hydroxyaglycones (hydrolytic deglycosidation) or deoxyaglycones (reductive deglycosidation), respectively (Licata et al. 2000; Mordente et al. 2009; Menna et al. 2011). It is noteworthy, however, that in human myocardium DOX hydroxyaglycone is quickly reduced to DOXol hydroxyaglycone whereas DOX 7-deoxyaglycone is scarcely (or not at all) converted to DOXol 7-deoxyaglycone, thus representing a poor substrate for myocardial carbonyl reductases (Licata et al. 2000). Moreover, anthracycline 7-deoxyaglycone can also be produced by the oxidation of the glycosidic bond between ring A and the sugar daunosamine by anthracycline semiquinone radical (Minotti et al. 2004). Unlike C-13 hydroxy metabolites, anthracycline aglycones may cause cell damage in virtue of their prominent oxidizing properties (Sokolove 1994; Licata et al. 2000; Minotti et al. 2004; Salvatorelli et al. 2006) (see Sect. 18.4.3.1).

18.3 Anthracyclines as Antitumor Agents

The potential mechanisms of cytotoxicity of anthracyclines towards cancer cells are diverse (critically reviewed in Gewirtz 1999) including: (1) inhibition of both DNA replication and RNA transcription, leading to inhibition of macromolecules biosynthesis; (2) generation of reactive oxygen species (ROS), leading to DNA damage and/or lipid peroxidation; (3) DNA adduct formation; (4) DNA cross-linking; (5) interference with DNA unwinding or DNA strand separation and helicase activity; (6) direct membrane damages; (7) inhibition of topoisomerase II. In response to some or all of these effects, tumor cell growth is inhibited, and cells are likely prone to die by one (or more than one) mechanism (apoptosis or necrosis or autophagy?) (Sawyer et al. 2010).

Although the precise mechanisms by which anthracyclines kill tumor cells still remain poorly understood, compelling evidence (consistent with the high DNA affinity and nuclear localization of anthracyclines) suggest that anthracyclines anticancer activities (particularly at clinically relevant drug concentrations) are mainly due to their abilities to intercalate between nuclear DNA base pairs thus poisoning topoisomerase activity and/or to form toxic anthracycline-DNA adducts, which trigger the death of rapidly dividing cancer cells (Cutts et al. 2005; Swift et al. 2006; Coldwell et al. 2008; Nitiss 2009; Pommier et al. 2010).

18.3.1 Anthracyclines as Topoisomerase Poisons

The anthracyclines are normally classified as "topoisomerase II poisons". DNA topoisomerases are ubiquitous, highly conserved enzymes involved in maintaining genomic integrity of the cell. Mechanistically, topoisomerases regulate the topology of cellular DNA by modulating the degree of DNA supercoiling through DNA strand cleavage, strand passage and religation without altering its structure and sequence (Nitiss 2009; Pommier et al. 2010). Therefore, topoisomerases supervise numerous nuclear processes such as replication, transcription, chromatin remodeling, chromosome condensation/decondensation, recombination, and repair. Topoisomerases, moreover, are also implicated in apoptotic DNA degradation. In accordance with their reaction mechanism, topoisomerases are broadly divided into two distinct families: type I (Top1) and type II (Top2) topoisomerases. Type I topoisomerases cleave a single strand of DNA and relax a supercoil either by passing the other strand through an enzyme-DNA linked intermediate (type IA) or by a strand-swivel mechanism (type IB). Type II topoisomerases cleave duplex DNA and then relax the supercoil by passing a second duplex DNA through the transient enzyme-DNA linked intermediate (Koster et al. 2010). The two families are further divided into subfamilies, which can be distinguished on the basis of protein architecture (monomer versus oligomer), DNA substrate preference (duplex versus single-strand), reaction outcomes (net loss or gain of supercoils; complete or partial supercoil removal), and requirements for metals and ATP (Koster et al. 2010). Human cells contain six different topoisomerases: two type IA (Top3α and Top3β), two type IB (Top1 and Top1mt), and two type IIA topoisomerases (Top2α and Top2β), each enzyme being coded by a different gene (Pommier et al. 2010). It is noteworthy, that five different human enzymes (Top1, Top2α, Top2β, Top3α and Top3β) provide topoisomerase activity for the nucleus and one (Top1mt) for mitochondria. Actually, two (i.e. Top3α and Top2β) of the five topoisomerases are also targeted to the mitochondria via posttranscriptional mechanisms: mitochondrial Top3α is created by alternative translation initiation of the same mRNA that encodes nuclear Top3α (Wang et al. 2002); mitochondrial Top2β seems derived directly from the nuclear enzyme Top2β by proteolysis (Low et al. 2003). Up to date, the pathophysiological role of mitochondrial topoisomerases and their putative involvement in anthracycline anticancer activity are completely unknown and warrant further studies.

Among topoisomerases, Top2α is widely considered the primary molecular target for anthracycline antibiotics, which inhibit the enzymes by stabilizing a normally transient intermediate (termed the "cleavable or cleavage complex") in the enzyme's catalytic cycle where the topoisomerase remains covalently attached to DNA after strand cleavage. Through the stabilization of the topoisomerase cleavable complex, anthracyclines convert Top2α into a potent toxin and cause the accumulation of DNA double-stranded breaks (DSBs), which, if not repaired, lead to cell death. Moreover, anthracyclines as well as other topoisomerase-directed anticancer drugs (i.e. etoposide, amsacrine, and mitoxantrone) target both Top2α and Top2β isozymes (Toyoda et al. 2008). Despite similar structural features (~70% homology at the amino acid level) and biological properties, the two human enzyme isoforms are differently regulated and play distinct roles in living cells. Top2α is a nuclear isozyme highly expressed in rapidly growing tissues (i.e. tumor cells) and its expression is cell cycle-regulated, peaking in G$_2$/M phase. Top2α has been shown to be essential for embryonic development and cell proliferation (Akimitsu et al. 2003; Carpenter and Porter 2004) and the high efficacy of anthracyclines chemotherapy is thought to be due to the highly elevated expression of Top2α in cancer cells (Mukherjee et al. 2010; Desmedt et al. 2011). By contrast, Top2β is expressed throughout the cell cycle in virtually all tissues, including postmitotic cells, where it seems to play a key role in transcription and differentiation (Lyu et al. 2007). It is unclear, however, whether these two isozymes play different roles in tumor-cell killing and/or in the development of secondary malignancies during the course of Top2-based chemotherapy (Azarova et al. 2007; Lyu et al. 2007). Interestingly, Top2β, but not Top2α, is highly expressed in adult heart (Capranico et al. 1992) suggesting a possible involvement of Top2β in anthracyclines cardiotoxicity. To date, however, the role of Top2β in anthracyclines cardiotoxicity can be only presumed. Nevertheless, the idea that Top2β targeting may be involved in anthracyclines cardiotoxicity has significant clinical implications. It provides the rationale for developing Top2α-specific anticancer drugs to prevent tissue toxicities (i.e. cardiotoxicity) in patients receiving Top2-based chemotherapy (Lyu et al. 2007).

18.3.2 *Anthracycline-DNA Adducts*

In addition to the primary anticancer role as Top2α poisons, anthracyclines are also capable of forming covalent adducts with DNA that result more cytotoxic than the lesions (i.e. DSBs) induced by topoisomerase IIα inhibition (Swift et al. 2006), thereby contributing to the anticancer activity of anthracyclines. Anthracycline-DNA adducts were first reported in 1979 by Sinha and Chignell (1979), but adducts were difficult to isolate and characterize (unless at supraclinical levels of anthracyclines, typically ≥10 µM) due to the limited sensitivity of pre-existing assays. Recently, however, the use of accelerator mass spectrometry (which exhibits over five orders of magnitude higher sensitivity for detection of radio-carbon labelled anthracycline than other routinely-used assays) has provided the first direct evidence of anthracycline-DNA adducts formation in cells at clinically relevant anthracycline concentrations (10–500 nM) (Coldwell et al. 2008). These results confirm that anthracycline-DNA adducts formation is a realistic mechanism of action of anthracyclines that may be active during the clinical use of these anticancer drugs.

The anthracycline-induced adducts are formed predominantly at 5′-GC-3′ sites in DNA (Cullinane and Phillips 1990) where daunosamine, the sugar group of anthracyclines, is covalently linked to the N-2 amino group of guanine via an aminal (N–C–N) bond (Wang et al. 1991; Zeman et al. 1998; Ugarenko et al. 2010). The central carbon atom in the aminal bond is derived from formaldehyde (i.e. formaldehyde supplies a methylene group which links the 3′-amino group of DOX to the 2-amino group of deoxyguanosine residues of DNA via Schiff base chemistry) (Wang et al. 1991), that is, hence, absolutely essential for anthracycline-DNA adduct formation. These DNA lesions are in fact mono-adducts attached covalently to one strand of DNA, but they are stabilized through intercalation and hydrogen bonding with the second strand of DNA (Zeman et al. 1998; Ugarenko et al. 2010). The term "virtual crosslink" has been also used to describe this mode of DNA binding (Taatjes et al. 1997). All four clinically important anthracyclines can be activated by formaldehyde to form drug-DNA adducts, although EPI forms only low levels of adducts (Cutts et al. 2007). Notably, anthracycline-DNA adducts occur in both nuclear and mitochondrial DNA at similar rates (Cullinane et al. 2000; Swift et al. 2008).

Apoptosis resulting from anthracycline-DNA adducts formation does not depend on topoisomerase status, reflecting an independent mechanism of cell killing and highlighting that formaldehyde availability switches the mechanism of anthracyclines action from topoisomerase impairment to the formation of more cytotoxic DNA adducts (Swift et al. 2006).

Seminal works by Taatjes, Koch, and associates (Taatjes et al. 1997; Taatjes and Koch 2001) have already shown that formaldehyde can be produced from carbon cellular sources (e.g. lipid and spermine) under oxidative stress conditions induced by anthracycline iron-catalyzed free radical reactions. Formaldehyde levels are often higher in tumor cells (1.5–4.0 μM) than in normal cells or in anthracycline-resistant cancer cells equipped with higher levels of ROS-detoxifying enzymes (Kato et al. 2000).

The finding that formaldehyde is an absolute requirement for adduct formation prompted the synthesis of new anthracycline derivatives conjugated to formaldehyde (named doxoform, daunoform, and epiform, for DOX, DNR, and EPI, respectively) (Taatjes and Koch 2001) or the use of formaldehyde-releasing prodrugs in combination with the classical anthracyclines (Cutts et al. 2007). Compared to the parent drugs plus formaldehyde, new anthracycline derivatives conjugated to formaldehyde form the same adducts with DNA oligomers but at a greatly enhanced rate. Although these new anthracyclines exhibit greater growth inhibitory effects than their parent drugs, further development of these compounds as chemotherapeutics is impaired because of poor solubility characteristics, short lifetime in the vascular system, hydrolytic instability and non-specific toxicity (Burke and Koch 2004).

18.4 Anthracycline-Induced Cardiotoxicity: An Old, Evergreen Problem

The clinical efficacy of anthracyclines is seriously hampered by the development of a progressive, dose-dependent, dilated (a restrictive cardiomyopathy is occasionally observed in children) cardiomyopathy, which may become evident even years after completion of therapy and that leads to an irreversible and life threatening congestive heart failure.

Endomyocardial biopsies from anthracycline-treated patients show: vacuolar degeneration, cell loss (apoptosis and/or necrosis), compensatory hypertrophy, and interstitial fibrosis even at a low dose of anthracyclines, suggesting that all doses of anthracycline cause cardiac damage on a cellular level (Bernaba et al. 2010). Electron microscopy studies evidence: myofibrillar disarray and dropout, dilation of the sarcoplasmic reticulum, cytoplasmic vacuolization, mitochondrial swelling, disordered nuclear chromatin, increased lysosomal number (Peng et al. 2005; Chen et al. 2007a; Gianni et al. 2008). This morphologic pattern is seen almost universally in patients and laboratory animals, indicating a non species-specific mechanism of toxicity (Robert 2007), although the underlying molecular mechanisms and/or chemical mediators may be species-specific.

18.4.1 Dimension of the Problem

Formal estimates of the worldwide prevalence of anthracycline-induced cardiotoxicity are still lacking. In addition, differences between paediatric, adult, and elderly patients and the lack of uniformity in detecting and reporting cardiac events make such estimates even more difficult to carry out (Gianni et al. 2008). However, anthracycline-induced cardiotoxicity remains a serious and remarkable problem whose incidence will continue to grow because more than 50% of long-term cancer survivors (the term "cancer survivor" refers to an individual who has been diagnosed with cancer, starting from the time of diagnosis throughout his or her life) has received at least one treatment with anthracycline during their chemotherapy.

The advent of anthracyclines in chemotherapy regimens has greatly contributed to markedly improve cancer survival, particularly among childhood cancers, with an increase in the 5-year survival rates from 30% in the 1960s to about 80% today (Jemal et al. 2010; Lipshultz and Adams 2010; Trachtenberg et al. 2011). In the United States, the overall number of cancer survivors has been estimated to 11.7 million in 2007 (3.9% of the U.S. population) with a marked increase compared to 3.0

million in 1971 (1.5%) and to 9.8 million in 2001 (3.5%) (Cancer survivors–United States 2007 (2011)). Among them, there are currently an estimated 328,000 long-term childhood cancer survivors (Mariotto et al. 2009), namely 1 in 640 young adults between the ages of 20 and 39 is a survivor of childhood cancer (Armstrong et al. 2009). This ever-increasing population of cancer survivors is actually considered "a testament to the enormous progress made by modern anticancer therapeutics and medical care" (Chen et al. 2011).

Nevertheless, childhood or adulthood cancer survivors are at a substantial risk for anthracycline-induced complications that can markedly affect their mortality, morbidity and quality of life. Childhood Cancer Survivor Study (CCSS) reveals that 30 years after the cancer diagnosis, 73% of long term survivors has a chronic illness, 42% of which has a severe disabling, life threatening or fatal illness such as cardiovascular disease, stroke, pulmonary fibrosis, kidney failure or a second malignancy (Oeffinger et al. 2006). Cardiac complications are the leading noncancerous cause of severe complications in this group (Trachtenberg et al. 2011). When compared with their contemporaries who do not suffer from cancer, survivors have 8.2-fold higher rates of cardiac death (Mertens et al. 2001), 15-fold higher rates of CHF, 10-fold higher rates of cardiovascular disease, and 9-fold higher rates of kidney failure or stroke (Oeffinger et al. 2006). Similar findings have been reported in long-term survivors of childhood cancer from the Nordic countries (Moller et al. 2001).

18.4.2 Types, Clinical Presentations and Risk Factors of Anthracycline-Induced Cardiotoxicity

Anthracycline-induced cardiotoxicity has been termed type I chemotherapy related cardiac dysfunction (type I CRCD) (Ewer and Lippman 2005), which, in contrast to type II CRCD, is characterized by defined, although unspecific, ultra-structural changes of cell morphology and has a greater tendency to become irreversible.

Clinically, the cardiotoxic effects of anthracyclines manifest in distinct forms that are commonly classified by the time of onset as: (a) acute, (b) early-onset and (c) late-onset chronic progressive cardiotoxicity (Franco et al. 2011). Acute anthracycline-induced cardiotoxicity occurs within the first week of the anthracycline treatment and often manifests itself as disturbances in intracardiac conduction and/or transient arrhythmias (Franco et al. 2011). Acute cardiotoxicity is rarely observed with the current therapeutic schemes, it is usually reversible, not dose-dependent and does not preclude further anthracycline use. However, single cases of acute dilated cardiomyopathy and sudden cardiac death were also reported (Floyd et al. 2005). Early-onset chronic progressive cardiomyopathy refers to heart damage that develops during anthracycline therapy or in the first year after it is completed while late-onset chronic progressive cardiomyopathy refers to heart damage that occurs when more than 1 year has elapsed after the completion of anthracycline therapy (Franco et al. 2011). Both early- and late-onset cardiotoxicity are characterized by a dose-dependent, symptomatic or asymptomatic, progressive decrease in left ventricular function often resulting in CHF (Swain et al. 2003; van Dalen et al. 2006; Pinder et al. 2007). It is noteworthy that adults typically develop a dilated cardiomyopathy whereas children at the end of anthracycline treatment have a dilated cardiomyopathy, which may then progress to a restrictive cardiomyopathy (Giantris et al. 1998). However, the true limit between early and late toxicity is actually arbitrarily set because, as it will be seen hereafter, myocardial damage may just start with the first dose of the drug and each administration constitutes additive or sequential damage since this cardiomyopathy is to be considered a progressive disease (Elliott 2006).

Early retrospective studies identified total cumulative dose as a major risk factor for anthracycline-related CHF (Lefrak et al. 1973; Von Hoff et al. 1979). In particular, Von Hoff and colleagues (Von Hoff et al. 1979) reported that the overall incidence of doxorubicin-induced CHF was rather low and the probability of developing CHF increased exponentially after doses of anthracycline of

450–550 mg/m^2 of body surface area. Therefore, an empirical dose limit of 500 mg/m^2 has been suggested as a strategy to minimize the risk of doxorubicin-induced cardiomyopathy (Lefrak et al. 1973; Von Hoff et al. 1979) and most treatment protocols for adults and childhood cancer still limit the maximum cumulative dose of doxorubicin to this value. However, several risk factors depending on patient and treatment characteristics may increase the incidence and severity of anthracycline-related cardiotoxicity (Carver et al. 2007). Age at treatment (children-adolescents and the elderly had long been considered to be more vulnerable to anthracyclines but recent studies have shown that late-onset cardiotoxicity could occur independently of age of first treatment) (Swerdlow et al. 2007), sex (female), race (black), pre-existing cardiovascular disease (coronary artery disease, left ventricular dysfunction, hypertension etc.), metabolic (diabetes) or genetic (trisomy 21) diseases, meanwhile higher administration rates, concomitant radiation therapy, and combination chemotherapy are known to increase the risk of developing anthracycline-induced cardiotoxicity at much lower cumulative doses.

However, a more recent retrospective analysis conducted by Swain and colleagues (2003) demonstrates that the doxorubicin-induced CHF occurs with greater frequency (5.1%) and at lower doses ($\leq$300 mg/m^2) than those previously reported by Von Hoff et al. (1979). Again, data obtained from longitudinal studies examining morbidity and mortality in anthracycline-treated survivors of childhood cancer reveal that asymptomatic cardiac abnormalities (i.e. reduction of left ventricular mass and dimension) are common, persistent and, for many patients, progressive even at low (45 mg/m^2) cumulative doses of doxorubicin (Lipshultz et al. 2005). These observations suggest that there is no completely "safe" dose of anthracyclines for cardiomyocytes (Lipshultz et al. 2005). Then, the final question is: when and why do these subclinical cardiac abnormalities become symptomatic?

As already suggested (Menna et al. 2008), anthracycline-induced cardiac abnormalities can became symptomatic when the subclinical myocardial damage overlaps with changes in lifestyle, comorbidities or environmental stressors that would be harmless to age-matched normal individuals.

18.4.3 Mechanisms of Anthracycline-Induced Cardiotoxicity

The pathophysiology of anthracycline cardiotoxicity is complex and, despite decades of research, incompletely defined. Over the years, different molecular mechanisms have been proposed to account for the cardiotoxicity of anthracyclines but, actually, no single mechanism seems to comprehend all the existing experimental and clinical data.

Anthracycline-induced cardiotoxicity is considered a complex multifactorial process (Minotti et al. 2004; Salvatorelli et al. 2006). The current thinking is that anthracyclines are toxic *per se* but gain further toxicity after intracellular reductive metabolism. One-electron reduction of the quinone moiety of anthracyclines and the subsequent semiquinone redox-cycling results in the formation of ROS (Davies and Doroshow 1986; Doroshow and Davies 1986) that cause oxidative stress and energy depletion (Minotti et al. 2004; Tokarska-Schlattner et al. 2006; Menna et al. 2011) in cardiomyocytes (see Sect. 18.4.3.1). Two-electron reduction of the side-chain C-13 carbonyl group converts anthracyclines to secondary alcohol metabolites (see Sect. 18.4.3.2) that are remarkably more potent than the parent compound at impairing calcium (Gambliel et al. 2002; Wallace 2007) and iron homeostasis (Minotti et al. 1998, 1999, 2004).

Oxidative stress (Minotti et al. 2004; Berthiaume and Wallace 2007; Chen et al. 2007b; Swift et al. 2007), mitochondrial dysfunction and energy depletion (Minotti et al. 2004; Tokarska-Schlattner et al. 2006), ion dysregulation (Minotti et al. 1998, 1999, 2004; Wallace 2007) and concomitant alterations of the cardiac-specific signalling pathways (Minotti et al. 2004; Sawyer et al. 2010; Spallarossa et al. 2010) may eventually combine at inducing cardiomyopathy.

18.4.3.1 Role of Oxidative/Nitrosative Stress in Anthracycline-Induced Cardiotoxicity

Anthracyclines can induce ROS generation through two major molecular pathways: an enzymatic mechanism catalyzed by several mono-electronic oxidoreductases and a non-enzymatic mechanism involving anthracycline–iron complexes.

In the enzymatic mechanism, one electron reduction of the quinone moiety in anthracycline C ring results in formation of a semiquinone radical that quickly regenerates its parent quinone by reducing molecular oxygen to superoxide anion ($O_2^{\cdot-}$) and its dismutation product hydrogen peroxide (H_2O_2), thus increasing ROS concentration above the physiologic levels generated during normal aerobic metabolism (Doroshow and Davies 1986; Minotti et al. 1999, 2004; Mordente et al. 2001). This futile cycle is catalyzed by a number of oxidoreductases located primarily in mitochondria (NADH-ubiquinone oxidoreductase; see also Sect. 18.5.1) (Davies and Doroshow 1986; Doroshow and Davies 1986), as well as in microsomes (NADPH-cytochrome P450 or NADPH-cytochrome b_5 reductases) (Cummings et al. 1992; Pawlowska et al. 2004), nucleus (NADPH-cytochrome b_5 reductases) and cytosol (xanthine dehydrogenase, nitric oxide synthase) (Vasquez-Vivar et al. 1997; Yee and Pritsos 1997; Garner et al. 1999; Neilan et al. 2007). Alternatively, ROS production may also occur via a non-enzymatic pathway triggered by anthracycline-iron complexes. Anthracyclines, indeed, bind avidly Fe^{3+}, forming a drug-metal complex that, in the presence of oxygen, can cycle between the Fe^{2+} and Fe^{3+} oxidation states forming $O_2^{\cdot-}$ and H_2O_2 (Minotti et al. 1999, 2004).

Anthracycline aglycones may generate ROS as well (Sokolove 1994). Due to their higher lipophilicity, aglycones can intercalate into mitochondrial membranes better than the parent anthracyclines and thus divert more electrons towards oxygen thereby generating ROS in the closest proximity to sensitive targets (Sokolove 1994). Although neither $O_2^{\cdot-}$ nor H_2O_2 are particularly toxic *per se*, cell damage occurs rapidly when they react with redox-active iron generating more damaging radical species like hydroxyl radicals ($^{\cdot}OH$) and/or iron-centered perferryl or perferryl radicals (Minotti et al. 1999). On the whole, one-electron redox cycling of anthracyclines increases the intracellular levels of both $O_2^{\cdot-}$, H_2O_2 and redox-active iron, setting the stage for the formation of more damaging radical species (Minotti et al. 1999, 2004).

Numerous evidence, furthermore, show that anthracycline treatment also increases nitric oxide (NO) production by up-regulating the expression of the inducible isoform of nitric oxide synthase (iNOS) (Aldieri et al. 2002). The concurrent overproduction of $O_2^{\cdot-}$ and NO yields, in its turn, peroxinitrite ($ONOO^-$) (Weinstein et al. 2000; Mihm et al. 2002; Fogli et al. 2004), a powerful oxidant which, like $^{\cdot}OH$ or species of equivalent reactivity, may directly damage every type of cellular macromolecules, resulting in lipid peroxidation, protein covalent modifications and DNA strand breaks. At this regard, anthracycline-related oxidative and nitrosative stress may interfere with many aspects of cardiac function, particularly by inducing mitochondrial dysfunction (Wallace 2003, 2007; Oliveira et al. 2006; Oliveira and Wallace 2006; Tao et al. 2006; Xiong et al. 2006), energy imbalance (Tao et al. 2006; Tokarska-Schlattner et al. 2006), disruption of the cardiac-specific gene expression program (Minotti et al. 2004), and apoptosis (Kalyanaraman et al. 2002; Clementi et al. 2003; Minotti et al. 2004).

In most cells, the chances to form $^{\cdot}OH$, iron-centered radicals and $ONOO^-$ are kept to a minimum by the presence of detoxifying enzymes, namely superoxide dismutase, catalase, and glutathione peroxidase, that concur in reducing $O_2^{\cdot-}$ and H_2O_2 to water. Unfortunately, cardiomyocytes are more susceptible than other tissues to ROS injury for several reasons, among which their high metabolic activity (Goffart et al. 2004), the high concentration of cardiolipin, and relatively weak defences against oxidative damage (Doroshow et al. 1980; Chen et al. 1994). In fact, cardiomyocytes contain low levels of catalase (Chen et al. 1994; Li et al. 1997) and glutathione peroxidase (Chen et al. 1994), whose activity, moreover, diminishes readily after DOX administration (Doroshow et al. 1980; Siveski-Iliskovic et al. 1995). In addition, DOX also decreases the protein levels and enzymatic activity of cytosolic superoxide dismutase, suggesting that inhibition of different antioxidant enzymes represents a common response to anthracycline treatment (Doroshow et al. 1980; Li and Singal 2000; Li et al. 2002).

In this view, a recent study (Tokarska-Schlattner et al. 2010), by applying a genome-wide transcriptome analysis, has shown that DOX reduces several transcripts related to antioxidant response as: heme oxygenase, glutamate-cysteine ligase (the rate-limiting enzyme in glutathione biosynthesis) and glutathione S-transferase (GST) M4. The last isoenzyme is a member of the large, multifunctional GST family that catalyses the conjugation of reduced glutathione to electrophilic compounds, thereby detoxifying xenobiotics, including anthracyclines (L'Ecuyer et al. 2004), and protecting cells from oxidative stress.

Although ROS overproduction, and consequently oxidative stress, can probably explain several aspects of anthracycline-induced cardiotoxicity (i.e. acute cardiotoxicity), it is nonetheless unsatisfactory if applied uncritically to explain chronic progressive cardiomyopathy (Olson and Mushlin 1990; Minotti et al. 1999). In fact, it has been demonstrated that: (a) anthracycline cardiotoxicity can develop in the absence of biological indices of oxidative damage (Rajagopalan et al. 1988; Keizer et al. 1990), and DOX can even decrease the myocardial release of conjugated dienes and hydroperoxides (Minotti et al. 1996); and (b) ROS scavengers and/or antioxidants, that afford protection in small animals, fail in preventing or decreasing chronic cardiac dysfunction in large animals (e.g. dogs) (Van Vleet et al. 1980; Herman et al. 1985) or in patients treated with multiple doses of anthracycline (Legha et al. 1982; Myers et al. 1983). In particular, as far as vitamin E protection against anthracycline-induced cardiotoxicity is concerned, only one study out of four published trials has found that vitamin E could prevent a decrease in left ventricular ejection fraction (LVEF); however, the effect of vitamin E is moreover confounded by concomitant administration of the calcium antagonist, nifedipine, which likely contributes protective effects such as, for example, reduced cardiac afterload (Ladas et al. 2004).

18.4.3.2 Role of Secondary Alcohol Metabolites in Anthracycline-Induced Cardiotoxicity

Anthracyclines may gain cardiotoxicity also after a two-electron reduction of the side-chain carbonyl group at C-13 and formation of a secondary alcohol metabolite (Minotti et al. 1998, 2004; Forrest et al. 2000; Licata et al. 2000; Mordente et al. 2003; Menna et al. 2008). The production mechanisms (Mordente et al. 2001, 2009; Minotti et al. 2004), the different outcomes in single nucleotide polymorphisms of aldo-keto and carbonyl reductase superfamilies (Hoffmann and Maser 2007; Jin and Penning 2007; Penning and Drury 2007; Bains et al. 2009, 2010a, b), the involvement of secondary alcohol metabolites in the pathogenesis of anthracycline-induced cardiomyopathy (Forrest et al. 2000; Mordente et al. 2001, 2009; Minotti et al. 2004; Menna et al. 2011) are treated exhaustively in several reviews and/or articles to which the reader is strongly recommended to refer.

18.5 Anthracyclines and Mitochondria

"Mitochondria are truly the Dr. Jekyll and Mr. Hyde of the cell" (Halestrap and Pasdois 2009; Baines 2010). On the one hand, mitochondria are essential for the cell's survival providing the vast majority of energy required for cellular functions. On the other hand, they also possess the power to kill the cell. In response to a variety of stress, mitochondria can quickly shut off the energy supply, produce vast amounts of damaging ROS, and release an array of death-inducing proteins into the cellular milieu (Baines 2010). Mitochondrial dysfunctions have been observed in the heart and in tumours of animal treated with anthracyclines (Solem et al. 1996; Bellarosa et al. 2001; Zhou et al. 2001b; Childs et al. 2002). The main ultra-structural changes observed within mitochondria following treatment with anthracyclines include: mitochondrial swelling, membrane and mitochondrial cristae disruption and the presence of myelin figures (Yen et al. 1996; Chaiswing et al. 2004). Numerous evidence (Sokolove 1994; Ashley and Poulton 2009) demonstrate that anthracyclines rapidly penetrate into mitochondria and interact with several molecular targets including: (1) multienzyme complexes of the electron transport chain (ETC)/oxidative phosphorylation system (OXPHOS); (2) mitochondrial DNA (mtDNA); (3) mitochondrial permeability transition pore (MPTP). Anthracycline-mediated mitochondrial damage results in energy metabolism impairment and/or in apoptosis. Mitochondria, therefore, emerge as an intriguing (or primary?) cellular target for both anthracycline anticancer activity and anthracycline-induced cardiotoxicity.

18.5.1 Anthracyclines and Electron Transfer Chain/Oxidative Phosphorylation System

Numerous reports based on studies either with isolated mitochondria exposed to anthracycline or with mitochondria isolated from chemotherapeutic-treated animals demonstrate that anthracyclines can affect mitochondrial function by inhibiting/inactivating the different components of ETC (Muhammed et al. 1983; Bianchi et al. 1987; Ji and Mitchell 1994) with a particular vulnerability of NADH-ubiquinone oxidoreductase (complex I) and cytochrome c oxidase (complex IV)(Bianchi et al. 1987; Nicolay and de Kruijff 1987; Marcillat et al. 1989; Trapp et al. 1989; Tokarska-Schlattner et al. 2006; Berthiaume and Wallace 2007; Chandran et al. 2009; Lebrecht et al. 2010).

The impairment of mitochondrial ETC components, rather than a direct anthracycline-protein interaction actually demonstrated only in the case of cytochrome c oxidase (Chandran et al. 2009), is probably due to indirect damaging mechanisms (Goormaghtigh et al. 1990) as: (a) protein (and/or membrane phospholipid) oxidative damage induced by ROS overproduction and (b) membrane chaotropic effects caused by the formation of electrostatic complexes between anthracyclines and cardiolipin.

As suggested (Pointon et al. 2010), anthracyclines have redox potentials (DOX redox potential is −328 mV) that, while not ideal for redox activity (Land et al. 1983), do actually allow them to be reduced slowly by a number of oxidoreductases within the cell (Wallace 2003). Additionally, anthracyclines have a high affinity for cardiolipin (Goormaghtigh et al. 1986, 1990), an acidic phospholipid that is localized exclusively in the inner mitochondrial membrane and that facilitates the drugs accumulation in the inner mitochondrial membrane where they can be easily reduced by complex I of ETC, thereby triggering ROS overproduction and then ETC complexes oxidative damages. Alternatively, the interaction of anthracyclines with cardiolipin can provoke ETC dysfunctions, as cardiolipin is required for enzyme activity of mitochondrial complexes playing an important role in their allosteric regulation (Fry and Green 1980, 1981; Nicolay and de Kruijff 1987). Clustering of cardiolipin due to the presence of anthracyclines can therefore lead to the formation of local non-bilayer arrangements within the mitochondrial membranes and consequently to changes in fluidity and functionality of ETC complexes (Jung and Reszka 2001).

In the mammalian mitochondria, furthermore, each multienzyme complex helps to maintain the assembly and stabilization of the other complexes; therefore, damages to a single complex can easily spread to all the other ETC complexes (Li et al. 2007b; Hiraumi et al. 2009). Indeed, complex IV (Diaz et al. 2006) or complex III (Schagger et al. 2004) deficiency results in a marked decrease in the level of complex I. The reciprocal action of each ETC complex seems to be more pronounced in rapidly dividing than in post-mitotic cells (Li et al. 2007b; Hiraumi et al. 2009). Cardiomyocytes, that have almost completely lost the ability to divide, might be therefore "the exception that proves the rule" (Hiraumi et al. 2009).

18.5.2 Anthracyclines and Mitochondrial DNA

Human cells contain thousands copies of mitochondrial DNA (mtDNA), approximately 2–10 copies of mtDNA for mitochondrion (Santos et al. 2008). The human mitochondrial genome consists of a double-stranded circular DNA molecule of 16,569 nucleotide pairs, containing 37 genes encoding for 13 essential ETC/OXPHOS polypeptide subunits, plus 2 ribosomal RNAs and 22 transfer RNAs, required for mitochondrial protein synthesis (Calvo and Mootha 2010).

In cells, mtDNA is arranged in discrete, punctate structures termed "nucleoids" (Ashley and Poulton 2009) constituted by several copies of mtDNA bound to nucleoid proteins. Although the functional significance of nucleoids remains obscure, in yeast these structures seem to protect mtDNA from damage occurring in response to metabolic stress (Kucej et al. 2008).

Mitochondria are the primary sites of ROS generation (Schagger et al. 2004; Selivanov et al. 2011) and human mtDNA is exquisitely sensitive to oxidative damage induced by ROS and this sensitivity is related to: (a) the close proximity of mtDNA (located in the mitochondrial matrix close to the inner mitochondrial membrane) to the electron transport chain (the major source of ROS); (b) the lack of introns and protective histone proteins; and (c) the limited DNA repair capacity of mitochondria, partially compensated by the increased number of mtDNA copies (Rohan et al. 2010; Wallace et al. 2010).

As a consequence, mtDNA has a high mutation rate (10–200 times higher than that of nuclear genomic DNA) and defects in mtDNA (together with mitochondrial decline) have been involved in the pathogenesis of numerous degenerative and metabolic diseases (Medikayala et al. 2011) as well as in cancer and aging (Wallace et al. 2010). In particular, increased frequencies of mtDNA mutations characterize the aging heart and are also found in idiopathic dilated cardiomyopathy and end-stage heart failure (Zaragoza et al. 2011).

A recent study (Ashley and Poulton 2009), by exploiting the fluorescent DNA intercalating dye PicoGreen that selectively labels both nDNA and mtDNA within living cells, has evidenced for the first time that anthracyclines, at clinically relevant concentrations, rapidly penetrate into the mito-chondrial matrix where they directly interact with mtDNA. Quantitative (copy number depletion) and/ or qualitative (mutations and/or deletions) mtDNA damages have been identified in cancer cells (Cullinane et al. 2000; Sharples et al. 2000; Kluza et al. 2004) as well as in animal (Palmeira et al. 1997; Serrano et al. 1999) and in human cardiomyocytes treated with anthracyclines (Lebrecht et al. 2003, 2005, 2010; Lebrecht and Walker 2007).

The anthracycline-mediated mitochondrial heart toxicity results strictly tissue specific, as no detectable mtDNA lesions have been reported in the skeletal muscle (Lebrecht et al. 2003, 2005). Furthermore, mtDNA injuries are not secondary to apoptosis because they largely precede anthracy-cline-induced cell death and can be mimicked by nontoxic doses of DNA intercalating probe ethidium bromide, but not induced by the apoptosis inducer staurosporine.

Anthracyclines can damage mtDNA through a variety of mechanisms (Lebrecht and Walker 2007). First of all, anthracyclines can directly intercalate into mtDNA causing large-scale deletions within the molecule (Adachi et al. 1993), or can form a covalent bond with mtDNA after metabolic transfor-mation of anthracycline quinone ring into quinone methide (Abdella and Fisher 1985). Conversely, anthracyclines can also damage the mitochondrial genome indirectly by increasing ROS production (Lebrecht et al. 2005; Lebrecht and Walker 2007).

Mitochondrial DNA damages initiate, although in an unapparent form, early during short-term anthracyclines exposure and accumulate with time and ultimately impinge on the bioenergetics capac-ity of the organelles even when the initial anthracycline insult is no longer present, thus representing an important factor in the delayed onset of the anthracycline-induced cardiomyopathy (Lebrecht and Walker 2007). This mechanism hinges on the fact that the ETC dysfunction, associated with the mtDNA-damage, can subsequently lead to ROS overproduction, which, in turn, may either attack the multienzyme complexes itself or damage the mitochondrial genome. ROS therefore close a "vicious circle" (Fig. 18.3) composed of interconnected mtDNA and reverberating respiratory chain insults (i.e., ROS production, mtDNA mutations, ETC dysfunction, further stimulation of ROS production, etc.). This vicious circle explains the observation that oxidative stress can persist and even accumulate for weeks after acute anthracycline exposure (Zhou et al. 2001a). The clinical onset of anthracycline

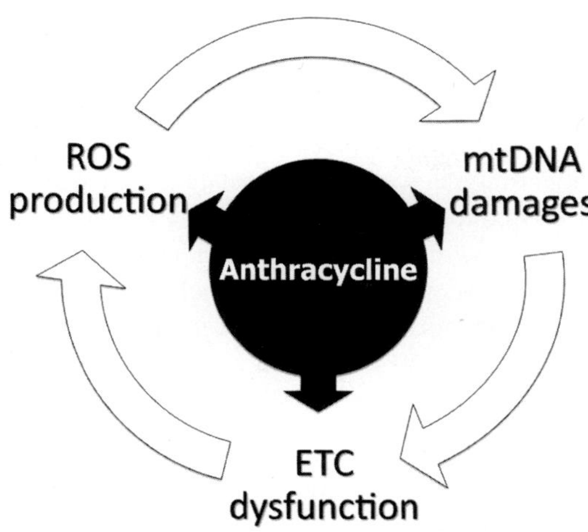

Fig. 18.3 Anthracycline-induced mitochondrial dysfunction. The "vicious circle" linking ROS overproduction, mtDNA damages, and ETC dysfunction

cardiomyopathy may occur when the mtDNA-damages and/or ETC dysfunctions exceed a threshold. Ultimately, mtDNA lesions appear to be pivotally associated with the fixation and temporal propagation of the anthracycline-induced lesions and thus are likely to represent the molecular mechanism of dose memory (Lebrecht and Walker 2007).

18.5.3 *Anthracyclines and Mitochondrial Permeability Transition Pore*

The mitochondrial permeability transition pore (MPTP) is a non-selective (permeable to any molecule of less than 1.5 kDa), high conductance channel that spans the inner and outer mitochondrial membranes (Halestrap and Pasdois 2009; Baines 2010). The precise structural identity of the MPTP is still controversial but recent data provide the strongest evidence for an involvement of at least three proteins in the molecular composition of this channel: a matrix protein, cyclophilin-D (CYPD), and two inner membrane proteins, the adenine nucleotide translocase (ANT) and the phosphate carrier (PIC) (Halestrap and Pasdois 2009; Baines 2010).

The opening of MPTP can be induced by a myriad of effectors among which, in particular, mitochondrial de-energization, high mitochondrial levels of Ca^{2+} or P_i (Varanyuwatana and Halestrap 2011) and, most important, ROS overproduction (Halestrap and Pasdois 2009; Baines 2010). The opening of MPTP leads to mitochondrial swelling with release of proapoptotic proteins and uncoupling of mitochondrial oxidative phosphorylation because of the increased permeability to protons. The resulting ATP deprivation causes disruption of ionic homeostasis, ROS overproduction, and ultimately ruptures of cell membrane and necrosis (Halestrap and Pasdois 2009; Kinnally et al. 2011). The opening of the MPTP is now recognized as a major cause of necrotic cell death (Halestrap and Pasdois 2009; Kinnally et al. 2011).

There is now considerable biochemical, pharmacological, and genetic evidence that the MPTP plays an essential role in the pathogenesis of multiple cardiac diseases, including cardiomyopathies (Halestrap and Pasdois 2009; Halestrap 2010) and, accordingly, the inhibition of the MPTP appears to be protective against numerous heart pathologies. On the other hand, an increasing number of studies on a variety of animal tumor models and cancer cell lines demonstrate that induction of MPTP opening by pharmacological interventions initiates cell death and prevents cell differentiation in tumorigenesis (Fulda et al. 2010).

A growing body of evidence demonstrates that MPTP is one of the primary molecular targets of anthracyclines (Montaigne et al. 2011), involved in mitochondrial dysfunction that characterizes anthracycline-induced cardiotoxicity as well as drug-related anticancer activity (Kluza et al. 2004). Studies with mitochondria exposed to the drug *in vitro* and with mitochondria isolated from animals treated with the drug *in vivo* do show that anthracyclines induce MPTP opening (Zhou et al. 2001b; De Oliveira et al. 2006). Accordingly, cyclosporine A, which blocks the MPTP opening by binding to matrix CYPD, prevents the mitochondrial failure and cell killing caused by anthracyclines (Zhou et al. 2001b). Moreover, deletion of CYPD protects the mouse myocardium against doxorubicin induced myocyte death, fibrosis, and contractile dysfunction.

18.6 Anthracyclines and Apoptosis

Apoptosis is a highly regulated genetic program of cell death that, in multi-cellular organisms, plays a pivotal role in the removal of transformed, damaged or infected cells as well as in a variety of biological processes including morphogenesis, tissue homeostasis, and aging (Tait and Green 2010). Accordingly, dysregulation of apoptotic signalling pathways contributes not only to the pathogenesis of diverse human diseases (e.g. cardiovascular, immune and neurodegenerative diseases) but also to the development of cancer and to the resistance to anti-cancer therapies (Tait and Green 2010; Kepp et al. 2011).

In mammals, two distinct, but interconnected, molecular signalling pathways mediate apoptosis: the intrinsic and extrinsic pathways both of which converge on activating the executioner caspases (i.e. caspases 3, 6 and 7).

The intrinsic or mitochondrial apoptotic pathway is activated by various developmental cues or cytotoxic insults such as viral infection, DNA damage and growth factor or cytokine deprivation and is strictly regulated by the B cell lymphoma-2 (BCL-2) family proteins. The crucial event in triggering the intrinsic pathway is mitochondrial outer membrane permeabilization (MOMP), which leads to the release of cytochrome *c* and other pro-apoptotic proteins, such as second mitochondrial activator of caspase (SMAC; also known as DIABLO) and a serine protease named high temperature requirement A2 (HTRA2; also known as OMI), from the mitochondrial intermembrane space into the cytosol. Following its release from mitochondria, cytochrome *c* binds apoptotic protease-activating factor-1 (APAF-1) inducing its oligomerization and leading to the formation of a caspase activation platform termed the apoptosome. The apoptosome recruits, dimerizes and activates an initiator caspase, caspase 9, which, in turn, cleaves and activates the executioner caspases 3, 6 and 7. Concurrently, mitochondrial release of SMAC/DIABLO and HTRA2/OMI block cytosolic inhibitor of apoptosis proteins (IAP) and thus relieves the IAP-mediated inhibition of caspase 3 and caspase 9 activity (Wang and Youle 2009).

Although the molecular events controlling the execution phase of this pathway are well characterized, those prior to the mitochondrial dysfunction and, in particular, the mechanisms underlying MOMP remain both elusive and controversial (Baines 2010; Lopez-Royuela et al. 2010). Nevertheless, MOMP results in a highly regulated process, primarily controlled through interactions between pro- and anti-apoptotic members of the BCL-2 family proteins.

Conversely, the extrinsic apoptotic pathway is triggered upon binding of proapoptotic "death ligands" to their respective "death receptors" on the surface of a target cell (Gonzalvez and Ashkenazi 2010; Wiezorek et al. 2010).

Death receptors are members of the tumor necrosis factor (TNF) receptor superfamily, and are characterized by cysteine-rich extracellular domains. The best-described death ligands belong to the

TNF family of cytokines. These TNF family death ligands comprise: FS-7-associated surface antigen ligand (FASL), TNFα, and TNF related apoptosis inducing ligand (TRAIL), which are predominantly produced by cells of the immune system.

Once activated, death receptors undergo clusterization and oligomerization thereby facilitating the recruitment of the adapter protein, FAS-associated protein with death domain (FADD) or TNF receptor type 1-associated death domain (TRADD), the binding of which further promotes the recruitment and the activation of initiator procaspases 8 and 10 within a death inducing signalling complex (DISC). If activation of these initiator caspases is sufficiently robust, they directly activate effector caspases 3, 6, and 7, which in turn result in cellular demise by the so-called Type I death receptor pathway of apoptosis (Johnstone et al. 2008; Kurita et al. 2011). However, if the magnitude of caspases 8 and 10 activation is not sufficient to directly activate effector caspases, they may still induce apoptosis through cleavage of the proapoptotic BCL-2 homology 3 (BH3)-interacting domain death agonist (BID) to generate truncated BID (tBID). tBID protein triggers MOMP by promoting oligomerization of either BCL-2-associated X protein (BAX) or BCL-2 antagonist or killer (BAK) within this membrane. The dependence on mitochondrial dysfunction for cell death is referred as the Type II death receptor pathway of apoptosis (Johnstone et al. 2008; Kurita et al. 2011).

Until a few years ago, apoptosis was disregarded as a possible mechanism underlying anthracycline-induced cardiomyopathy (Minotti et al. 2004). This picture is now changed dramatically and numerous evidence demonstrate that anthracyclines are able to activate both intrinsic (see Sect. 18.6.1) and extrinsic (see Sect. 18.6.2) pathways of apoptosis.

18.6.1   Effects of Anthracyclines on Intrinsic Apoptotic Pathway

The mechanisms whereby anthracyclines promote intrinsic, mitochondrial apoptosis are still incompletely understood. Nevertheless, anthracyclines, their metabolic derivatives (alcohol metabolites and aglycones) and/or by-products (ROS and RNS) may trigger intrinsic apoptosis pathway by regulating (activating or inhibiting) the activity of several components of the apoptotic machinery and in particular: (*a*) p53 tumor suppressor protein, (*b*) mitogen-activated protein kinases (MAPKs) superfamily and (*c*) BCL-2 family proteins.

The p53 tumor suppressor protein (referred as a "cellular gatekeeper" or "the guardian of the genome") is a pivotal transcription factor that plays a crucial role in maintaining genomic stability and preventing tumor formation by integrating and coordinating the cellular responses to a variety of intrinsic and extrinsic stress signals. Depending upon the cell type, the transformed state of a cell and the type or degree of stress placed upon a cell, activated p53 induces cell cycle arrest, DNA repair, apoptosis or senescence to prevent the propagation of damaged or mutant cells that could potentially become cancerous (Feng and Levine 2010).

Normally, p53 has a short half-life and it is maintained at low concentrations and in an inactive state in unstressed mammalian cells through a negative feedback loop with murine double minute 2 (MDM2). MDM2 is an E3 ubiquitin ligase that binds to and polyubiquitinates p53 thereby promoting its rapid proteolysis by proteasome. The expression of MDM2 is in its turn regulated by p53 at the transcription level so closing a negative feedback loop to maintain p53 protein at low levels under normal conditions. Moreover, p300 protein, acting as specific ubiquitin E4 ligase for p53 (Shi et al. 2009), cooperates with MDM2 in catalyzing p53 polyubiquitination, thus facilitating p53 degradation and inhibiting p53-mediated apoptosis.

The stability of p53 and consequently its functional role strictly depends on an array of protein post-translational modifications (e.g. phosphorylation, methylation, acetylation, glycosylation etc.) effective both during normal homeostasis and in stress-induced responses. Phosphorylation of p53 is classically regarded as the first crucial step of p53 stabilization. p53 can be phosphorylated by a broad range of kinases (Chua et al. 2006) mainly of the MAPKs superfamily (Wu 2004). p53 protein phosphorylation, diminishing p53/MDM2 interactions, decreases p53 ubiquitination and leads to the stabilization and accumulation of p53 protein in the cytoplasm and/or in mitochondria (Liu et al. 2008).

p53 may control intrinsic mitochondria-mediated pathway of apoptosis in two ways: by transactivating nuclear genes involved in apoptosis (*transcription-dependent actions*) and/or by physically and functionally interacting with mitochondrial proteins that carry out apoptosis (*transcription-independent actions*). As a nuclear transcription factor, p53 stimulates the expression of several pro-apoptotic BCL-2 family genes including BAX, p53 up-regulated modulator of apoptosis (PUMA), NOXA, and BID and represses the transcription of certain anti-apoptotic BCL-2 genes including BCL-2, BCL-2-like protein 1 (BCL-XL). Moreover, p53 upregulates the MAPK superfamily genes and APAF-1, a scaffolding protein for caspase-9 activation, whereas it downregulates MnSOD expression thereby increasing ROS production from mitochondria. Finally, p53 accumulation induces the expression of FAS receptor gene so affecting the extrinsic apoptotic pathway, too.

In addition to its complex function as a nuclear transcription factor, p53 can also act in the cytosol and, prevalently, in mitochondria promoting apoptosis through transcription-independent mechanisms. This alternative pro-apoptotic function of p53 relies on its capabilities of physically interacting with several members of the BCL-2 family proteins that regulate mitochondrial cell death by controlling MOMP.

Numerous studies prove that anthracyclines increase the expression and/or promote the activation of p53 tumor suppressor protein in cardiomyocytes (Chua et al. 2006; Liu et al. 2008; Sardao et al. 2009; Venkatesan et al. 2010) as well as in cancer cell lines (Panaretakis et al. 2002; Zantl et al. 2007; Lopez-Royuela et al. 2010; Misra and Pizzo 2010). Moreover, anthracycline treatment is also capable of increasing p53 levels in mitochondria (Nithipongvanitch et al. 2007a, b), an event that occurs early and may participate in mtDNA repair as a rapid adaptive response to oxidative stress (Nithipongvanitch et al. 2007b). Accordingly, pharmacological inhibition (by treatment with pifithrin-α, a chemical inhibitor of p53 activity) (Liu et al. 2004; Misra and Pizzo 2010) or genetic deletion of p53 (Shizukuda et al. 2005) abrogates anthracycline-induced cell death, thus confirming the crucial role of p53 in anthracycline-mediated apoptosis.

Preclinical and clinical studies seem to support this suggestion (Penault-Llorca et al. 2003; Ruiz-Ruiz et al. 2003; Stearns et al. 2003), but reports expressing opposite considerations have been also published (Inoue et al. 2000; Perego et al. 2001; Bertheau et al. 2002; Gariboldi et al. 2003; Manna et al. 2011). Uncertainties about the role of p53 in anthracycline-induced apoptosis may be attributed to a variety of factors as heterogeneity of the tumours examined or the methods used for assessing p53 status and tumor response (Bertheau et al. 2002; Minotti et al. 2004).

The molecular mechanisms whereby anthracyclines promote p53 activation, its translocation to mitochondria as well as the pathways underlying p53-mediated mitochondrial apoptosis are not clearly defined. However, the involvement of MAPK signalling transduction pathways in p53-mediated anthracycline-induced apoptosis has been widely suggested (Lou et al. 2005; Chua et al. 2006; Venkatakrishnan et al. 2006; Nithipongvanitch et al. 2007b; Venkatesan et al. 2010), although conflicting data actually exist in literature (Spallarossa et al. 2006; Tokarska-Schlattner et al. 2010).

MAPKs are highly conserved serine/threonine kinases that are activated in response to a wide variety of stimuli and that, therefore, play important roles in cell growth, proliferation, differentiation and death (Rose et al. 2010). MAPK signaling pathways, moreover, are the primary intermediators for the induction of apoptotic program by oxidative stress (Lou et al. 2005). There are three major MAPK family members: extracellular signal-regulated kinases (ERKs), p38 MAPKs, and c-Jun N-terminal kinases (JNKs). In the cardiomyocytes, ERKs are potently and rapidly activated by growth factors and hypertrophic agents thereby mediating cell survival and cytoprotection (Lou et al. 2005). In contrast, JNKs and p38 MAPKs are activated by cellular stresses, including oxidative stress, correlating with the cardiac pathophysiology and the cardiomyocyte apoptosis (Lou et al. 2005).

Anthracyclines activate MAPKs in cardiomyocytes (Zhu et al. 1999; Lou et al. 2005, 2006; Tokarska-Schlattner et al. 2010; Venkatesan et al. 2010) as well as in different human cancer cell lines, including: epidermoid carcinoma (Osborn and Chambers 1996), T leukemia (Yu et al. 1996), lung adenocarcinoma (Zhao et al. 2004), breast carcinoma (Small et al. 2003, 2007), and neuroblastoma (Guise et al. 2001).

All the three major MAPK families are activated by phosphorylation following DOX treatment although different activation patterns are described for the three kinase members (Lou et al. 2005, 2006). ERKs, indeed, are upregulated early (this activation is considered an adaptive and/or protective response), but transiently and downregulated during the heart failure stage. Conversely, phosphorylation of p38 MAPKs and JNKs increases early and persists until the heart failure stage, suggesting that these kinases may play a dominant role in the progression of anthracycline-induced cardiomyopathy and heart failure (Lou et al. 2005, 2006).

In contrast to previous findings, a more recent study on H9c2 cells and neonatal rat cardiomyocytes shows that, at clinically relevant DOX concentrations (i.e. 1 μM), anthracycline-induced cytotoxic effects are strictly associated with the increased activation and nuclear translocation of ERKs and p53, while no effect is observed on the phosphorylation levels of p38 MAPKs and JNKs (Liu et al. 2008). However, when the dose of DOX is increased fivefold (5 μM), significant increases also in p38 MAPKs and JNKs phosphorylation are reported in H9c2 cells (Chua et al. 2006). Ultimately, this study indicates that the cardiotoxic effects of DOX seem mediated by ERKs/p53 signal transduction pathway rather than by p38 MAPKs or JNKs cascades and the discrepancies found in the involvement of the three major MAPKs family members may be related, at least in part, to the differences in the doses of anthracyclines and experimental conditions. However, evidences for a predominant or exclusive role of p38 MAPKs and/or JNKs signal transduction pathways in anthracycline-induced apoptosis in cardiomyocytes (Thandavarayan et al. 2010; Chang et al. 2011; Das et al. 2011; Ghosh et al. 2011; Velez et al. 2011), in endothelial progenitor cells (Spallarossa et al. 2010) and in cancer cells (Nelyudova et al. 2007; Lagadinou et al. 2008; Aroui et al. 2010; El Btaouri et al. 2011; Feng et al. 2011) have been recently reported.

Anyway, whatever the MAPKs (i.e. ERKs, p38 MAPKs and/or JNK) signal transduction pathway is involved in anthracycline-induced apoptosis, p53 activation is often associated with the upregulation of pro-apoptotic BCL-2 proteins and/or downregulation of anti-apoptotic BCL-2 members (Lou et al. 2005; Chua et al. 2006; Liu et al. 2008) as well as with the disruption of mitochondrial potential and caspase activation.

The BCL-2 family proteins consist of more than 20 members characterized by the presence of one or more of four BCL-2 homology (BH) domains. The BCL-2 family proteins are divided into three subfamilies based on their structure and function: (*a*) pro-apoptotic BCL-2 proteins (BAX, BAK) contain three BH domains and promote apoptosis by inducing MOMP through the formation of the proteolipid pores on outer mitochondrial membrane; (*b*) anti-apoptotic members (chiefly BCL-2, BCL-XL, BCL-W, and MCL-1) contain BH1-4 domains and suppress apoptosis by antagonizing MOMP through the sequestration of their pro-apoptotic counterparts in an inactive state; (*c*) a third subfamily of BCL-2 proteins, the so-called BH3-only-domain proteins (chiefly BAD, BIK, BID, NOXA and PUMA), contains a single conserved BH3 domain that binds and regulates both the pro- and the anti-apoptotic BCL-2 family members. The BH3-only proteins are largely responsible for sensing the apoptotic signals and then transmitting them to other BCL-2 family members. Functionally, BH3-only proteins fall into two subgroups: "activators" and "derepressors", according to how they trigger apoptosis. Activators (BID and BIM) trigger MOMP by direct activation of BAX and BAK, while derepressors such as PUMA, NOXA and BAD inhibit the antiapoptotic BCL-2 family members to release pro-apoptotic members from their inhibition (e.g. BAX from BCL-XL and BAK from MCL1) (reviewed in Kroemer et al. 2007).

In this view, the activation of BAX and/or BAK is the 'point of no return' in the intrinsic apoptotic pathway; cells from BAX and BAK double knockout mice are highly resistant to drug-induced apoptosis. Upon activation, BAK (located within OMM) and BAX (translocating from the cytosol to OMM) oligomerize so forming dynamic proteolipid pores that promote MOMP and trigger apoptotic cascade. Nevertheless, the biochemical nature of such pores and how anti-apoptotic BCL-2 family proteins regulate them remains a key and controversial issue in the field of cell death (Youle and Strasser 2008).

Consistent with the scenario outlined above, treatment with anthracyclines induces upregulation/activation of BAX (Liu et al. 2004; Tikoo et al. 2011), BAK (Lopez-Royuela et al. 2010) or both BAK and BAX (Lopez-Royuela et al. 2010) in cardiomyocytes and in leukemia cells (Lopez-Royuela et al. 2010) as well as inhibits BCL-2 and BCL-XL in cardiomyocytes (Venkatesan et al. 2010). Accordingly, the ratio of BAX to BCL-XL increases with the progress of apoptotic death. In these cells lines, BAX/BAK upregulation is caspase-independent, suggesting that caspase activation occurs exclusively downstream mitochondria and that the caspase amplification loop is not involved in BAX/BAK activation (Lopez-Royuela et al. 2010). Finally, in cells exposed to anthracyclines, PUMA and/or NOXA are upregulated, too (Kurata et al. 2008; Wang et al. 2009; Lopez-Royuela et al. 2010).

18.6.2 Effects of Anthracyclines on Extrinsic Apoptosis Pathway

Standard chemotherapy and radiotherapy for cancer predominantly initiate apoptosis via the intrinsic mitochondrial pathway. However, it has been suggested that death receptor signalling also contributes to the overall anti-tumor response to diverse chemotherapeutic drugs, including anthracyclines (Sayers 2011).

The extrinsic apoptosis pathway transmits signals from extracellular death ligands through the appropriate death receptors to the cells' apoptotic machinery (Gonzalvez and Ashkenazi 2010). The most extensively studied receptor-ligand signalling systems are (a) FAS (also called CD95, APO-1)-FASL; (b) TNF receptor 1 (TNFR1)-TNFα; (c) TRAIL receptor 1 (TRAILR1)-TRAIL, and TRAIL receptor 2 (TRAILR2)-TRAIL (Guicciardi and Gores 2009; Gonzalvez and Ashkenazi 2010).

Anthracyclines promote extrinsic apoptosis pathway by altering the expression of death receptors and/or potentiating the activity of death receptors ligands.

The FAS/FASL system is one of the key regulators of the apoptotic pathway in many cell types, particularly in cells related to the immune system. The FAS/FASL system has been implicated in chemotherapy-induced tumor cell death and FAS/FASL down-regulation seems to be involved in cancer drug resistance (Gonzalvez and Ashkenazi 2010). Moreover, FAS/FASL is abundantly expressed in the heart (Setsuta et al. 2004), playing an important role in the development and progression of anthracycline-induced cardiomyopathy (Miyata et al. 2010). In experimental models, myocardial FAS expression and cardiomyocyte apoptosis are concomitantly increased in response to DOX administration (Nakamura et al. 2000; Lien et al. 2006a, b). Accordingly, blocking of the FAS/FASL interaction with FASL-neutralizing antibody inhibits both FAS overexpression and DOX-induced cardiotoxicity (Nakamura et al. 2000; Wu et al. 2002a). In addition, FAS/FAS ligand interaction increases the susceptibility of cultured neonatal cardiomyocytes to DOX-induced apoptosis (Yamaoka et al. 2000). Furthermore, DOX upregulates FAS expression in cancer cell lines and in solid tumor (Massart et al. 2004; Yoshimoto et al. 2005; Kim et al. 2009). In addition, in MCF-7 breast cancer cell line, DOX enhances FAS oligomerization (i.e. activation) without increasing the level of FAS, in a FAS/FASL-independent manner (Li et al. 2007a). Again, the apoptotic levels of hepatocellular carcinoma (HCC) cells treated with FASL plus DOX are significantly higher than those treated with FASL or DOX alone, suggesting that a combined treatment of FASL with anthracyclines may be an useful approach to improve the efficacy of chemotherapy for HCC (Liu et al. 2009).

In contrast to the previous data, other reports show that DOX-induced apoptosis in cardiomyocytes (Jeremias et al. 2005; Malugin et al. 2006) or in several different cancer cell lines (Eischen et al. 1997;

Gamen et al. 1997; Bellarosa et al. 2001; Wieder et al. 2001; Malugin et al. 2006) is independent from FAS signal pathway. Therefore, the role of FAS/FASL-dependent apoptosis in the mechanisms of anthracycline citotoxicity remains controversial. Recent studies indicate that FAS signalling also exerts biological effects unrelated to apoptosis, such as induction of inflammation and fibrosis, ROS generation, acceleration of proliferation/differentiation, and induction of hypertrophy (Miyata et al. 2010). Indeed, its proinflammatory and hypertrophic effects have been noted in both heart and cardiomyocytes. It has been therefore hypothesized that FAS signalling might contribute to the pathogenesis of anthracycline-induced cardiotoxicity through mechanisms unrelated to induction of cardiomyocyte apoptosis (Miyata et al. 2010).

TNF-α is a potent proinflammatory cytokine locally produced by many cell types including cardiomyocytes where it elicits a variety of responses ranging from cardioprotective to pathological ones (Wang et al. 2007; Kleinbongard et al. 2010, 2011). Chronically elevated levels of TNF-α have been identified as a risk factor for coronary heart disease and congestive heart failure (Wang et al. 2007; Kleinbongard et al. 2010, 2011). In particular, TNF-α seems to play an important role in the development of heart failure by contributing to depression of myocardial contractile function, induction of cardiomyocyte apoptosis, as well as induction of proinflammatory signalling (Wang et al. 2007; Kleinbongard et al. 2010, 2011). TNF-α transduces its signal through two distinct surface receptors, TNFR1 and TNFR2, which are both expressed in cardiac myocytes (Wang et al. 2007; Kleinbongard et al. 2010, 2011). It has been reported that through TNFR1, TNFα exerts negative inotropic effects on the myocardial contractile function and induces cardiac myocyte apoptosis.

DOX stimulates TNF-α expression by immune cells (Ujhazy et al. 2003) and cardiomyocytes (Mukherjee et al. 2003) and increases serum TNF-α levels in patients undergoing chemotherapy (Morsi et al. 2006) and in rodent models of chemotherapy (Tangpong et al. 2006; Gilliam et al. 2009). A recent study (Gilliam et al. 2011) demonstrates that TNF-α/TNFR1 system mediates diaphragm weakness induced by DOX. Etanercept, a soluble TNF-α receptor, prevented the depression in force caused by DOX. No change in circulating or muscle-derived TNF-α is detected but DOX, rather, appears to stimulate expression and sarcolemmal localization of TNFR1 (Gilliam et al. 2011). Genetic TNFR1 deficiency protects the diaphragm against DOX-induced weakness, confirming an essential role for TNF-α/TNFR1 signalling (Gilliam et al. 2011).

TRAIL is another member of the TNF superfamily that selectively triggers apoptotic cell death in a wide variety of human and mouse tumor cell lines by interacting with its proapoptotic receptors, TRAILR1 (also termed as DR4) and TRAILR2 (or DR5), while exhibiting low toxicity towards most of normal cells or tissues (Humphreys and Halpern 2008; Johnstone et al. 2008; Yang et al. 2010). Accordingly, TRAIL is considered a promising anticancer agent, currently tested in phase I clinical trials (Johnstone et al. 2008; Abdulghani and El-Deiry 2010). In addition to TRAIL, agonistic antibodies against TRAILR1 and/or TRAILR2 have been also developed (Wiezorek et al. 2010). These antibodies mimic TRAIL's function by activating death receptor-mediated apoptosis with potential as cancer therapeutic agents and have progressed to phase I (Ashkenazi and Herbst 2008; Herbst et al. 2010; Wiezorek et al. 2010) or phase II (Ashkenazi and Herbst 2008; Herbst et al. 2010; Trarbach et al. 2010) trials in treatment of multiple types of cancers.

Nonetheless, growing evidence suggest that many primary tumors are resistant to TRAIL-induced apoptosis despite the expression of the death-inducing TRAIL receptors on the surface of the tumor cells (Dyer et al. 2007). The cause of TRAIL resistance is under investigation and several mechanisms underlying TRAIL sensitivity/resistance have been proposed (Dyer et al. 2007). This has prompted intense interest in the identification of compounds that can sensitize cancer cells to TRAIL.

Among cytotoxic agents tested, anthracyclines have proved to be really efficient in sensitizing various human cancer cell lines to TRAIL or to agonistic antibodies to TRAIL death receptors, potentiating their proapoptotic activity and thereby overcoming tumor cell resistance towards these agents. In particular, DOX pre-treatment significantly enhances TRAIL-induced citotoxicity in various cancer cell lines including: breast (Singh et al. 2003; Aroui et al. 2009a, b; Malin et al. 2011), colon (Xu et al.

2003, 2011), gastric (Xu et al. 2011), hepatocellular (Koehler et al. 2009), ovarian (Cuello et al. 2001), prostate (Kelly et al. 2002; Voelkel-Johnson et al. 2002; Wu et al. 2002b; Kang et al. 2005), renal (Wu et al. 2003), small cell lung carcinoma (Vaculova et al. 2010; Guo et al. 2011), glioblastoma multiforme (Guo et al. 2011), rhabdomyosarcoma (Komdeur et al. 2004), osteosarcoma and soft tissue sarcoma (Bouralexis et al. 2004; Wang et al. 2010), all of which, vice versa, result resistant to either one of the above said agents when used alone.

Analogously to TRAIL, DOX (but not 5-fluorouracil, vinblastine, paclitaxel, or docetaxel) enhances proapoptotic and cytotoxic activity of human agonistic TRAIL-receptors antibodies in various human solid cancer cells, including renal, prostate, bladder, and lung carcinoma (Voelkel-Johnson et al. 2002; Wu et al. 2007). The synergistic cytotoxicity of DOX and TRAIL-receptor antibody requires relatively low concentrations of both agents, thus minimizing drug toxicity and maximizing potential therapeutic applications in vivo.

The molecular mechanisms underlying these synergistic effects are not well defined. Although the sensitivity of cancer cells to TRAIL does not seem to be a simple function of TRAIL death receptor expression level, the augmentation of TRAIL-induced apoptosis by chemotherapeutic drugs has been suggested to be, at least in part, the result of anthracycline-induced upregulation of death receptors (Wang et al. 2010). Low concentrations of DOX (0.1 and 1 μg/mL), indeed, significantly upregulated TRAILR1 and/or TRAILR2 expression in several cancer cells at both the mRNA and protein levels in a dose- and time-dependent manner (Wu et al. 2007).

## 18.7	Conclusions

Anthracyclines perform a wide repertoire of biological activities in cancer cells as well as in the cardiomyocytes. The long-held assumption that anthracyclines exert their pharmacological/toxicological effects by distinct molecular mechanisms in cancer or in heart tissue does not seem fully convincing because beneficial (antitumoral/therapeutic) and detrimental (cardiotoxic) responses to drug treatment are to some extent overlapping, sharing the subcellular organelle targets (i.e. mitochondrion and/or nucleus), the molecular effectors (i.e. anthracycline by-products and/or metabolites) and the pathophysiological processes (i.e. DNA strand breaks, oxidative stress, signalling pathways, mitochondrial dysfunctions, apoptosis etc.) (Tokarska-Schlattner et al. 2006). The speculation that anthracyclines may damage cancer and myocardial cells by impairing the same molecular pathways still leaves unresolved some important questions, namely: why cancer and heart are more vulnerable than other tissues to anthracyclines treatment or, in other words, what do tumor cells and cardiomyocytes have in common that render them the preferential targets of anthracyclines?

In 2002 Hoshijima and Chien drew, for the first time, an intriguing theoretical parallel between the dysregulation of the signalling pathways driving cancer and those driving cardiac hypertrophy.

Lessons from cardiotoxicity associated with modern anticancer therapies with new "targeted therapeutics" which target specific protein kinases that are dysregulated (mutated and/or overexpressed) in cancer, confirm that there are really numerous parallels between signalling pathways that drive tumor growth and survival and signalling pathways that regulate functional homeostasis and hypertrophic responses in cardiomyocytes (Cheng and Force 2010a, b). Hence, inhibition of the "key" kinases that drive cancerogenesis could potentially compromise the survival of cardiomyocytes.

Recently, moreover, in reviewing emerging anticancer therapeutic targets (i.e. c-Met receptor tyrosine kinase, Notch and Hedgehog signalling, insulin-like growth factor receptor pathway, phosphoinositide-specific phospholipase C isozyme, epigenetic modulators, transcription factor, and microRNAs, and so on) Peng et al. (2010) have highlighted that many of these pathways, in addition to being involved in the proliferation, angiogenesis and differentiation of neoplasm, are also expressed in the cardiovascular system. Hence, heart cells share signalling pathways and biological processes with cancer cells. Therefore, understanding the molecular mechanisms and function of those targets in the cardiovascular system and other vital tissues becomes an important step in the development of newer anticancer therapies (Peng et al. 2010).

May be ultimately assumed that novel targeted therapeutics and anthracyclines share similar cellular targets?

In a recent study, aimed at a global characterization of the cardiac transcriptomic response to a low DOX dose, Tokarska-Schlattner et al. (2010), have evidenced that many of the genes sensitive to DOX not only respond similarly in heart and cancer, but they also encode proteins that are putative targets of new anticancer therapies: heat shock proteins (Peng et al. 2010; Subjeck and Repasky 2011), MAPK (Pratilas and Solit 2010), certain G proteins (Tang et al. 2008), IGF (Clemmons 2007), HIF (Welsh et al. 2006), VEGF (Kerbel 2008), and TGF-β, the latter playing a dual role as tumor suppressor and prooncogenic factor (Jakowlew 2006). Moreover, as further suggested by Tokarska-Schlattner et al. (2010), DOX exhibits certain mechanistic details in common with the tyrosine kinase inhibitors (i.e. imatinib and gefitinib), a novel class of anticancer drugs. DOX, indeed, represses transcripts of pathways targeted by imatinib and, like gefitinib, induces expression of quiescin Q6, a gene that may play a role in tissue growth by affecting repartition between cells in the proliferative cycle, in quiescence, and in apoptosis (Yano et al. 2006). It is also worthy to note that targeting these genes, which is supposed to be beneficial for cytotoxic action in cancer, may be rather detrimental to the heart.

Finally, mitochondria are emerging as one the major cellular targets for both anthracycline anticancer activity and drug-induced cardiotoxicity for their pivotal role in oxidative stress, bioenergetics impairment, disruption of Ca^{2+} homeostasis, and apoptotic pathways.

References

Abdella BR, Fisher J (1985) A chemical perspective on the anthracycline antitumor antibiotics. Environ Health Perspect 64:4–18

Abdulghani J, El-Deiry WS (2010) TRAIL receptor signaling and therapeutics. Expert Opin Ther Targets 14(10): 1091–1108

Adachi K, Fujiura Y, Mayumi F, Nozuhara A, Sugiu Y, Sakanashi T, Hidaka T, Toshima H (1993) A deletion of mitochondrial DNA in murine doxorubicin-induced cardiotoxicity. Biochem Biophys Res Commun 195(2):945–951

Akimitsu N, Adachi N, Hirai H, Hossain MS, Hamamoto H, Kobayashi M, Aratani Y, Koyama H, Sekimizu K (2003) Enforced cytokinesis without complete nuclear division in embryonic cells depleting the activity of DNA topoisomerase IIalpha. Genes Cells 8(4):393–402

Aldieri E, Bergandi L, Riganti C, Costamagna C, Bosia A, Ghigo D (2002) Doxorubicin induces an increase of nitric oxide synthesis in rat cardiac cells that is inhibited by iron supplementation. Toxicol Appl Pharmacol 185(2):85–90

Armstrong GT, Liu Q, Yasui Y, Huang S, Ness KK, Leisenring W, Hudson MM, Donaldson SS, King AA, Stovall M, Krull KR, Robison LL, Packer RJ (2009) Long-term outcomes among adult survivors of childhood central nervous system malignancies in the Childhood Cancer Survivor Study. J Natl Cancer Inst 101(13):946–958

Aroui S, Brahim S, De Waard M, Breard J, Kenani A (2009a) Efficient induction of apoptosis by doxorubicin coupled to cell-penetrating peptides compared to unconjugated doxorubicin in the human breast cancer cell line MDA-MB 231. Cancer Lett 285(1):28–38

Aroui S, Brahim S, Hamelin J, De Waard M, Breard J, Kenani A (2009b) Conjugation of doxorubicin to cell penetrating peptides sensitizes human breast MDA-MB 231 cancer cells to endogenous TRAIL-induced apoptosis. Apoptosis 14(11):1352–1365

Aroui S, Mili D, Brahim S, De Waard M, Kenani A (2010) Doxorubicin coupled to penetratin promotes apoptosis in CHO cells by a mechanism involving c-Jun NH2-terminal kinase. Biochem Biophys Res Commun 396(4):908–914

Ashkenazi A, Herbst RS (2008) To kill a tumor cell: the potential of proapoptotic receptor agonists. J Clin Invest 118(6):1979–1990

Ashley N, Poulton J (2009) Mitochondrial DNA is a direct target of anti-cancer anthracycline drugs. Biochem Biophys Res Commun 378(3):450–455

Azarova AM, Lyu YL, Lin CP, Tsai YC, Lau JY, Wang JC, Liu LF (2007) Roles of DNA topoisomerase II isozymes in chemotherapy and secondary malignancies. Proc Natl Acad Sci USA 104(26):11014–11019

Baines CP (2010) The cardiac mitochondrion: nexus of stress. Annu Rev Physiol 72:61–80

Bains OS, Karkling MJ, Grigliatti TA, Reid RE, Riggs KW (2009) Two nonsynonymous single nucleotide polymorphisms of human carbonyl reductase 1 demonstrate reduced in vitro metabolism of daunorubicin and doxorubicin. Drug Metab Dispos 37(5):1107–1114

Bains OS, Grigliatti TA, Reid RE, Riggs KW (2010a) Naturally occurring variants of human aldo-keto reductases with reduced in vitro metabolism of daunorubicin and doxorubicin. J Pharmacol Exp Ther 335(3):533–545

Bains OS, Karkling MJ, Lubieniecka JM, Grigliatti TA, Reid RE, Riggs KW (2010b) Naturally occurring variants of human CBR3 alter anthracycline in vitro metabolism. J Pharmacol Exp Ther 332(3):755–763

Bellarosa D, Ciucci A, Bullo A, Nardelli F, Manzini S, Maggi CA, Goso C (2001) Apoptotic events in a human ovarian cancer cell line exposed to anthracyclines. J Pharmacol Exp Ther 296(2):276–283

Bernaba BN, Chan JB, Lai CK, Fishbein MC (2010) Pathology of late-onset anthracycline cardiomyopathy. Cardiovasc Pathol 19(5):308–311

Bertheau P, Plassa F, Espie M, Turpin E, de Roquancourt A, Marty M, Lerebours F, Beuzard Y, Janin A, de The H (2002) Effect of mutated TP53 on response of advanced breast cancers to high-dose chemotherapy. Lancet 360(9336):852–854

Berthiaume JM, Wallace KB (2007) Adriamycin-induced oxidative mitochondrial cardiotoxicity. Cell Biol Toxicol 23(1):15–25

Bianchi C, Bagnato A, Paggi MG, Floridi A (1987) Effect of adriamycin on electron transport in rat heart, liver, and tumor mitochondria. Exp Mol Pathol 46(1):123–135

Binaschi M, Bigioni M, Cipollone A, Rossi C, Goso C, Maggi CA, Capranico G, Animati F (2001) Anthracyclines: selected new developments. Curr Med Chem Anticancer Agents 1(2):113–130

Bouralexis S, Clayer M, Atkins GJ, Labrinidis A, Hay S, Graves S, Findlay DM, Evdokiou A (2004) Sensitivity of fresh isolates of soft tissue sarcoma, osteosarcoma and giant cell tumour cells to Apo2L/TRAIL and doxorubicin. Int J Oncol 24(5):1263–1270

Burke PJ, Koch TH (2004) Design, synthesis, and biological evaluation of doxorubicin-formaldehyde conjugates targeted to breast cancer cells. J Med Chem 47(5):1193–1206

Calvo SE, Mootha VK (2010) The mitochondrial proteome and human disease. Annu Rev Genomics Hum Genet 11:25–44

Cancer survivors–United States, 2007 (2011) MMWR Morb Mortal Wkly Rep 60(9):269–272

Capranico G, Tinelli S, Austin CA, Fisher ML, Zunino F (1992) Different patterns of gene expression of topoisomerase II isoforms in differentiated tissues during murine development. Biochim Biophys Acta 1132(1):43–48

Carpenter AJ, Porter AC (2004) Construction, characterization, and complementation of a conditional-lethal DNA topoisomerase IIalpha mutant human cell line. Mol Biol Cell 15(12):5700–5711

Carver JR, Shapiro CL, Ng A, Jacobs L, Schwartz C, Virgo KS, Hagerty KL, Somerfield MR, Vaughn DJ (2007) American Society of Clinical Oncology clinical evidence review on the ongoing care of adult cancer survivors: cardiac and pulmonary late effects. J Clin Oncol 25(25):3991–4008

Chaiswing L, Cole MP, St Clair DK, Ittarat W, Szweda LI, Oberley TD (2004) Oxidative damage precedes nitrative damage in adriamycin-induced cardiac mitochondrial injury. Toxicol Pathol 32(5):536–547

Chandran K, Aggarwal D, Migrino RQ, Joseph J, McAllister D, Konorev EA, Antholine WE, Zielonka J, Srinivasan S, Avadhani NG, Kalyanaraman B (2009) Doxorubicin inactivates myocardial cytochrome c oxidase in rats: cardioprotection by Mito-Q. Biophys J 96(4):1388–1398

Chang WT, Li J, Huang HH, Liu H, Han M, Ramachandran S, Li CQ, Sharp WW, Hamann KJ, Yuan CS, Hoek TL, Shao ZH (2011) Baicalein protects against doxorubicin-induced cardiotoxicity by attenuation of mitochondrial oxidant injury and JNK activation. J Cell Biochem 112(10):2873–2881

Chen Y, Saari JT, Kang YJ (1994) Weak antioxidant defenses make the heart a target for damage in copper-deficient rats. Free Radic Biol Med 17(6):529–536

Chen B, Peng X, Pentassuglia L, Lim CC, Sawyer DB (2007a) Molecular and cellular mechanisms of anthracycline cardiotoxicity. Cardiovasc Toxicol 7(2):114–121

Chen Y, Jungsuwadee P, Vore M, Butterfield DA, St Clair DK (2007b) Collateral damage in cancer chemotherapy: oxidative stress in nontargeted tissues. Mol Interv 7(3):147–156

Chen MH, Colan SD, Diller L (2011) Cardiovascular disease: cause of morbidity and mortality in adult survivors of childhood cancers. Circ Res 108(5):619–628

Cheng H, Force T (2010a) Molecular mechanisms of cardiovascular toxicity of targeted cancer therapeutics. Circ Res 106(1):21–34

Cheng H, Force T (2010b) Why do kinase inhibitors cause cardiotoxicity and what can be done about it? Prog Cardiovasc Dis 53(2):114–120

Childs AC, Phaneuf SL, Dirks AJ, Phillips T, Leeuwenburgh C (2002) Doxorubicin treatment in vivo causes cytochrome C release and cardiomyocyte apoptosis, as well as increased mitochondrial efficiency, superoxide dismutase activity, and Bcl-2:Bax ratio. Cancer Res 62(16):4592–4598

Chua CC, Liu X, Gao J, Hamdy RC, Chua BH (2006) Multiple actions of pifithrin-alpha on doxorubicin-induced apoptosis in rat myoblastic H9c2 cells. Am J Physiol Heart Circ Physiol 290(6):H2606–H2613

Clementi ME, Giardina B, Di Stasio E, Mordente A, Misiti F (2003) Doxorubicin-derived metabolites induce release of cytochrome C and inhibition of respiration on cardiac isolated mitochondria. Anticancer Res 23(3B):2445–2450

Clemmons DR (2007) Modifying IGF1 activity: an approach to treat endocrine disorders, atherosclerosis and cancer. Nat Rev Drug Discov 6(10):821–833

Coldwell KE, Cutts SM, Ognibene TJ, Henderson PT, Phillips DR (2008) Detection of Adriamycin-DNA adducts by accelerator mass spectrometry at clinically relevant Adriamycin concentrations. Nucleic Acids Res 36(16):e100

Cuello M, Ettenberg SA, Nau MM, Lipkowitz S (2001) Synergistic induction of apoptosis by the combination of trail and chemotherapy in chemoresistant ovarian cancer cells. Gynecol Oncol 81(3):380–390

Cullinane C, Phillips DR (1990) Induction of stable transcriptional blockage sites by adriamycin: GpC specificity of apparent adriamycin-DNA adducts and dependence on iron(III) ions. Biochemistry 29(23):5638–5646

Cullinane C, Cutts SM, Panousis C, Phillips DR (2000) Interstrand cross-linking by adriamycin in nuclear and mitochondrial DNA of MCF-7 cells. Nucleic Acids Res 28(4):1019–1025

Cummings J, Allan L, Willmott N, Riley R, Workman P, Smyth JF (1992) The enzymology of doxorubicin quinone reduction in tumour tissue. Biochem Pharmacol 44(11):2175–2183

Cutts SM, Nudelman A, Rephaeli A, Phillips DR (2005) The power and potential of doxorubicin-DNA adducts. IUBMB Life 57(2):73–81

Cutts SM, Swift LP, Pillay V, Forrest RA, Nudelman A, Rephaeli A, Phillips DR (2007) Activation of clinically used anthracyclines by the formaldehyde-releasing prodrug pivaloyloxymethyl butyrate. Mol Cancer Ther 6(4):1450–1459

Danesi R, Fogli S, Gennari A, Conte P, Del Tacca M (2002) Pharmacokinetic-pharmacodynamic relationships of the anthracycline anticancer drugs. Clin Pharmacokinet 41(6):431–444

Das J, Ghosh J, Manna P, Sil PC (2011) Taurine suppresses doxorubicin-triggered oxidative stress and cardiac apoptosis in rat via up-regulation of PI3-K/Akt and inhibition of p53, p38-JNK. Biochem Pharmacol 81(7):891–909

Davies KJ, Doroshow JH (1986) Redox cycling of anthracyclines by cardiac mitochondria. I. Anthracycline radical formation by NADH dehydrogenase. J Biol Chem 261(7):3060–3067

De Oliveira F, Chauvin C, Ronot X, Mousseau M, Leverve X, Fontaine E (2006) Effects of permeability transition inhibition and decrease in cytochrome c content on doxorubicin toxicity in K562 cells. Oncogene 25(18):2646–2655

Desmedt C, Di Leo A, de Azambuja E, Larsimont D, Haibe-Kains B, Selleslags J, Delaloge S, Duhem C, Kains JP, Carly B, Maerevoet M, Vindevoghel A, Rouas G, Lallemand F, Durbecq V, Cardoso F, Salgado R, Rovere R, Bontempi G, Michiels S, Buyse M, Nogaret JM, Qi Y, Symmans F, Pusztai L, D'Hondt V, Piccart-Gebhart M, Sotiriou C (2011) Multifactorial approach to predicting resistance to anthracyclines. J Clin Oncol 29(12):1578–1586

Diaz F, Fukui H, Garcia S, Moraes CT (2006) Cytochrome c oxidase is required for the assembly/stability of respiratory complex I in mouse fibroblasts. Mol Cell Biol 26(13):4872–4881

Doroshow JH, Davies KJ (1986) Redox cycling of anthracyclines by cardiac mitochondria. II. Formation of superoxide anion, hydrogen peroxide, and hydroxyl radical. J Biol Chem 261(7):3068–3074

Doroshow JH, Locker GY, Myers CE (1980) Enzymatic defenses of the mouse heart against reactive oxygen metabolites: alterations produced by doxorubicin. J Clin Invest 65(1):128–135

Dyer MJ, MacFarlane M, Cohen GM (2007) Barriers to effective TRAIL-targeted therapy of malignancy. J Clin Oncol 25(28):4505–4506

Eischen CM, Kottke TJ, Martins LM, Basi GS, Tung JS, Earnshaw WC, Leibson PJ, Kaufmann SH (1997) Comparison of apoptosis in wild-type and Fas-resistant cells: chemotherapy-induced apoptosis is not dependent on Fas/Fas ligand interactions. Blood 90(3):935–943

El Btaouri H, Morjani H, Greffe Y, Charpentier E, Martiny L (2011) Role of JNK/ATF-2 pathway in inhibition of thrombospondin-1 (TSP-1) expression and apoptosis mediated by doxorubicin and camptothecin in FTC-133 cells. Biochim Biophys Acta 1813(5):695–703

Elliott P (2006) Pathogenesis of cardiotoxicity induced by anthracyclines. Semin Oncol 33(3 suppl 8):S2-7

Eschenhagen T, Force T, Ewer MS, de Keulenaer GW, Suter TM, Anker SD, Avkiran M, de Azambuja E, Balligand JL, Brutsaert DL, Condorelli G, Hansen A, Heymans S, Hill JA, Hirsch E, Hilfiker-Kleiner D, Janssens S, de Jong S, Neubauer G, Pieske B, Ponikowski P, Pirmohamed M, Rauchhaus M, Sawyer D, Sugden PH, Wojta J, Zannad F, Shah AM (2011) Cardiovascular side effects of cancer therapies: a position statement from the Heart Failure Association of the European Society of Cardiology. Eur J Heart Fail 13(1):1–10

Ewer MS, Ewer SM (2010) Cardiotoxicity of anticancer treatments: what the cardiologist needs to know. Nat Rev Cardiol 7(10):564–575

Ewer MS, Lippman SM (2005) Type II chemotherapy-related cardiac dysfunction: time to recognize a new entity. J Clin Oncol 23(13):2900–2902

Feng Z, Levine AJ (2010) The regulation of energy metabolism and the IGF-1/mTOR pathways by the p53 protein. Trends Cell Biol 20(7):427–434

Feng R, Zhai WL, Yang HY, Jin H, Zhang QX (2011) Induction of ER stress protects gastric cancer cells against apoptosis induced by cisplatin and doxorubicin through activation of p38 MAPK. Biochem Biophys Res Commun 406(2):299–304

Floyd JD, Nguyen DT, Lobins RL, Bashir Q, Doll DC, Perry MC (2005) Cardiotoxicity of cancer therapy. J Clin Oncol 23(30):7685–7696

Fogli S, Nieri P, Breschi MC (2004) The role of nitric oxide in anthracycline toxicity and prospects for pharmacologic prevention of cardiac damage. FASEB J 18(6):664–675

Forrest GL, Gonzalez B, Tseng W, Li X, Mann J (2000) Human carbonyl reductase overexpression in the heart advances the development of doxorubicin-induced cardiotoxicity in transgenic mice. Cancer Res 60(18):5158–5164

Franco VI, Henkel JM, Miller TL, Lipshultz SE (2011) Cardiovascular effects in childhood cancer survivors treated with anthracyclines. Cardiol Res Pract 2011:134679

Frezard F, Garnier-Suillerot A (1991) Comparison of the membrane transport of anthracycline derivatives in drug-resistant and drug-sensitive K562 cells. Eur J Biochem 196(2):483–491

Fry M, Green DE (1980) Cardiolipin requirement by cytochrome oxidase and the catalytic role of phospholipid. Biochem Biophys Res Commun 93(4):1238–1246

Fry M, Green DE (1981) Cardiolipin requirement for electron transfer in complex I and III of the mitochondrial respiratory chain. J Biol Chem 256(4):1874–1880

Fulda S, Galluzzi L, Kroemer G (2010) Targeting mitochondria for cancer therapy. Nat Rev Drug Discov 9(6):447–464

Gambliel HA, Burke BE, Cusack BJ, Walsh GM, Zhang YL, Mushlin PS, Olson RD (2002) Doxorubicin and C-13 deoxydoxorubicin effects on ryanodine receptor gene expression. Biochem Biophys Res Commun 291(3):433–438

Gamen S, Anel A, Lasierra P, Alava MA, Martinez-Lorenzo MJ, Pineiro A, Naval J (1997) Doxorubicin-induced apoptosis in human T-cell leukemia is mediated by caspase-3 activation in a Fas-independent way. FEBS Lett 417(3):360–364

Gariboldi MB, Ravizza R, Riganti L, Meschini S, Calcabrini A, Marra M, Arancia G, Dolfini E, Monti E (2003) Molecular determinants of intrinsic resistance to doxorubicin in human cancer cell lines. Int J Oncol 22(5):1057–1064

Garner AP, Paine MJ, Rodriguez-Crespo I, Chinje EC, Ortiz De Montellano P, Stratford IJ, Tew DG, Wolf CR (1999) Nitric oxide synthases catalyze the activation of redox cycling and bioreductive anticancer agents. Cancer Res 59(8):1929–1934

Gewirtz DA (1999) A critical evaluation of the mechanisms of action proposed for the antitumor effects of the anthracycline antibiotics adriamycin and daunorubicin. Biochem Pharmacol 57(7):727–741

Ghosh J, Das J, Manna P, Sil PC (2011) The protective role of arjunolic acid against doxorubicin induced intracellular ROS dependent JNK-p38 and p53-mediated cardiac apoptosis. Biomaterials 32(21):4857–4866

Gianni L, Herman EH, Lipshultz SE, Minotti G, Sarvazyan N, Sawyer DB (2008) Anthracycline cardiotoxicity: from bench to bedside. J Clin Oncol 26(22):3777–3784

Giantris A, Abdurrahman L, Hinkle A, Asselin B, Lipshultz SE (1998) Anthracycline-induced cardiotoxicity in children and young adults. Crit Rev Oncol Hematol 27(1):53–68

Gilliam LA, Ferreira LF, Bruton JD, Moylan JS, Westerblad H, St Clair DK, Reid MB (2009) Doxorubicin acts through tumor necrosis factor receptor subtype 1 to cause dysfunction of murine skeletal muscle. J Appl Physiol 107(6):1935–1942

Gilliam LA, Moylan JS, Ferreira LF, Reid MB (2011) TNF/TNFR1 signaling mediates doxorubicin-induced diaphragm weakness. Am J Physiol Lung Cell Mol Physiol 300(2):L225–L231

Goffart S, von Kleist-Retzow JC, Wiesner RJ (2004) Regulation of mitochondrial proliferation in the heart: power-plant failure contributes to cardiac failure in hypertrophy. Cardiovasc Res 64(2):198–207

Gonzalvez F, Ashkenazi A (2010) New insights into apoptosis signaling by Apo2L/TRAIL. Oncogene 29(34):4752–4765

Goormaghtigh E, Huart P, Brasseur R, Ruysschaert JM (1986) Mechanism of inhibition of mitochondrial enzymatic complex I-III by adriamycin derivatives. Biochim Biophys Acta 861(1):83–94

Goormaghtigh E, Huart P, Praet M, Brasseur R, Ruysschaert JM (1990) Structure of the adriamycin-cardiolipin complex. Role in mitochondrial toxicity. Biophys Chem 35(2–3):247–257

Guicciardi ME, Gores GJ (2009) Life and death by death receptors. FASEB J 23(6):1625–1637

Guise S, Braguer D, Carles G, Delacourte A, Briand C (2001) Hyperphosphorylation of tau is mediated by ERK activation during anticancer drug-induced apoptosis in neuroblastoma cells. J Neurosci Res 63(3):257–267

Guo L, Fan L, Pang Z, Ren J, Ren Y, Li J, Chen J, Wen Z, Jiang X (2011) TRAIL and doxorubicin combination enhances anti-glioblastoma effect based on passive tumor targeting of liposomes. J Control Release 154(1):93–102

Halestrap AP (2010) A pore way to die: the role of mitochondria in reperfusion injury and cardioprotection. Biochem Soc Trans 38(4):841–860

Halestrap AP, Pasdois P (2009) The role of the mitochondrial permeability transition pore in heart disease. Biochim Biophys Acta 1787(11):1402–1415

Herbst RS, Eckhardt SG, Kurzrock R, Ebbinghaus S, O'Dwyer PJ, Gordon MS, Novotny W, Goldwasser MA, Tohnya TM, Lum BL, Ashkenazi A, Jubb AM, Mendelson DS (2010) Phase I dose-escalation study of recombinant human Apo2L/TRAIL, a dual proapoptotic receptor agonist, in patients with advanced cancer. J Clin Oncol 28(17):2839–2846

Herman EH, Ferrans VJ, Myers CE, Van Vleet JF (1985) Comparison of the effectiveness of (+/-)-1,2-bis(3,5-dioxopiperazinyl-1-yl)propane (ICRF-187) and N-acetylcysteine in preventing chronic doxorubicin cardiotoxicity in beagles. Cancer Res 45(1):276–281

Hiraumi Y, Iwai-Kanai E, Baba S, Yui Y, Kamitsuji Y, Mizushima Y, Matsubara H, Watanabe M, Watanabe K, Toyokuni S, Nakahata T, Adachi S (2009) Granulocyte colony-stimulating factor protects cardiac mitochondria in the early phase of cardiac injury. Am J Physiol Heart Circ Physiol 296(3):H823–H832

Hoffmann F, Maser E (2007) Carbonyl reductases and pluripotent hydroxysteroid dehydrogenases of the short-chain dehydrogenase/reductase superfamily. Drug Metab Rev 39(1):87–144

Hoshijima M, Chien KR (2002) Mixed signals in heart failure: cancer rules. J Clin Invest 109(7):849–855

Houba PH, Boven E, van der Meulen-Muileman IH, Leenders RG, Scheeren JW, Pinedo HM, Haisma HJ (2001) A novel doxorubicin-glucuronide prodrug DOX-GA3 for tumour-selective chemotherapy: distribution and efficacy in experimental human ovarian cancer. Br J Cancer 84(4):550–557

Humphreys RC, Halpern W (2008) Trail receptors: targets for cancer therapy. Adv Exp Med Biol 615:127–158

Innocenti F, Iyer L, Ramirez J, Green MD, Ratain MJ (2001) Epirubicin glucuronidation is catalyzed by human UDP-glucuronosyltransferase 2B7. Drug Metab Dispos 29(5):686–692

Inoue A, Narumi K, Matsubara N, Sugawara S, Saijo Y, Satoh K, Nukiwa T (2000) Administration of wild-type p53 adenoviral vector synergistically enhances the cytotoxicity of anti-cancer drugs in human lung cancer cells irrespective of the status of p53 gene. Cancer Lett 157(1):105–112

Jakowlew SB (2006) Transforming growth factor-beta in cancer and metastasis. Cancer Metastasis Rev 25(3):435–457

Jemal A, Siegel R, Xu J, Ward E (2010) Cancer statistics, 2010. CA Cancer J Clin 60(5):277–300

Jeremias I, Stahnke K, Debatin KM (2005) CD95/Apo-1/Fas: independent cell death induced by doxorubicin in normal cultured cardiomyocytes. Cancer Immunol Immunother 54(7):655–662

Ji LL, Mitchell EW (1994) Effects of Adriamycin on heart mitochondrial function in rested and exercised rats. Biochem Pharmacol 47(5):877–885

Jin Y, Penning TM (2007) Aldo-keto reductases and bioactivation/detoxication. Annu Rev Pharmacol Toxicol 47:263–292

Joerger M, Huitema AD, Meenhorst PL, Schellens JH, Beijnen JH (2005) Pharmacokinetics of low-dose doxorubicin and metabolites in patients with AIDS-related Kaposi sarcoma. Cancer Chemother Pharmacol 55(5):488–496

Johnstone RW, Frew AJ, Smyth MJ (2008) The TRAIL apoptotic pathway in cancer onset, progression and therapy. Nat Rev Cancer 8(10):782–798

Jung K, Reszka R (2001) Mitochondria as subcellular targets for clinically useful anthracyclines. Adv Drug Deliv Rev 49(1–2):87–105

Kalyanaraman B, Joseph J, Kalivendi S, Wang S, Konorev E, Kotamraju S (2002) Doxorubicin-induced apoptosis: implications in cardiotoxicity. Mol Cell Biochem 234–235(1–2):119–124

Kang J, Bu J, Hao Y, Chen F (2005) Subtoxic concentration of doxorubicin enhances TRAIL-induced apoptosis in human prostate cancer cell line LNCaP. Prostate Cancer Prostatic Dis 8(3):274–279

Kato S, Burke PJ, Fenick DJ, Taatjes DJ, Bierbaum VM, Koch TH (2000) Mass spectrometric measurement of formaldehyde generated in breast cancer cells upon treatment with anthracycline antitumor drugs. Chem Res Toxicol 13(6):509–516

Keizer HG, Pinedo HM, Schuurhuis GJ, Joenje H (1990) Doxorubicin (adriamycin): a critical review of free radical-dependent mechanisms of cytotoxicity. Pharmacol Ther 47(2):219–231

Kelly MM, Hoel BD, Voelkel-Johnson C (2002) Doxorubicin pretreatment sensitizes prostate cancer cell lines to TRAIL induced apoptosis which correlates with the loss of c-FLIP expression. Cancer Biol Ther 1(5):520–527

Kepp O, Galluzzi L, Lipinski M, Yuan J, Kroemer G (2011) Cell death assays for drug discovery. Nat Rev Drug Discov 10(3):221–237

Kerbel RS (2008) Tumor angiogenesis. N Engl J Med 358(19):2039–2049

Kim HS, Lee YS, Kim DK (2009) Doxorubicin exerts cytotoxic effects through cell cycle arrest and Fas-mediated cell death. Pharmacology 84(5):300–309

Kinnally KW, Peixoto PM, Ryu SY, Dejean LM (2011) Is mPTP the gatekeeper for necrosis, apoptosis, or both? Biochim Biophys Acta 1813(4):616–622

Kleinbongard P, Heusch G, Schulz R (2010) TNFalpha in atherosclerosis, myocardial ischemia/reperfusion and heart failure. Pharmacol Ther 127(3):295–314

Kleinbongard P, Schulz R, Heusch G (2011) TNFalpha in myocardial ischemia/reperfusion, remodeling and heart failure. Heart Fail Rev 16(1):49–69

Kluza J, Marchetti P, Gallego MA, Lancel S, Fournier C, Loyens A, Beauvillain JC, Bailly C (2004) Mitochondrial proliferation during apoptosis induced by anticancer agents: effects of doxorubicin and mitoxantrone on cancer and cardiac cells. Oncogene 23(42):7018–7030

Koehler BC, Urbanik T, Vick B, Boger RJ, Heeger S, Galle PR, Schuchmann M, Schulze-Bergkamen H (2009) TRAIL-induced apoptosis of hepatocellular carcinoma cells is augmented by targeted therapies. World J Gastroenterol 15(47):5924–5935

Komdeur R, Meijer C, Van Zweeden M, De Jong S, Wesseling J, Hoekstra HJ, van der Graaf WT (2004) Doxorubicin potentiates TRAIL cytotoxicity and apoptosis and can overcome TRAIL-resistance in rhabdomyosarcoma cells. Int J Oncol 25(3):677–684

Koster DA, Crut A, Shuman S, Bjornsti MA, Dekker NH (2010) Cellular strategies for regulating DNA supercoiling: a single-molecule perspective. Cell 142(4):519–530

Kroemer G, Galluzzi L, Brenner C (2007) Mitochondrial membrane permeabilization in cell death. Physiol Rev 87(1):99–163

Kucej M, Kucejova B, Subramanian R, Chen XJ, Butow RA (2008) Mitochondrial nucleoids undergo remodeling in response to metabolic cues. J Cell Sci 121(Pt 11):1861–1868

Kurata K, Yanagisawa R, Ohira M, Kitagawa M, Nakagawara A, Kamijo T (2008) Stress via p53 pathway causes apoptosis by mitochondrial Noxa upregulation in doxorubicin-treated neuroblastoma cells. Oncogene 27(6):741–754

Kurita S, Mott JL, Cazanave SC, Fingas CD, Guicciardi ME, Bronk SF, Roberts LR, Fernandez-Zapico ME, Gores GJ (2011) Hedgehog inhibition promotes a switch from Type II to Type I cell death receptor signaling in cancer cells. PLoS One 6(3):e18330

L'Ecuyer T, Allebban Z, Thomas R, Vander Heide R (2004) Glutathione S-transferase overexpression protects against anthracycline-induced H9C2 cell death. Am J Physiol Heart Circ Physiol 286(6):H2057–H2064

Ladas EJ, Jacobson JS, Kennedy DD, Teel K, Fleischauer A, Kelly KM (2004) Antioxidants and cancer therapy: a systematic review. J Clin Oncol 22(3):517–528

Lagadinou ED, Ziros PG, Tsopra OA, Dimas K, Kokkinou D, Thanopoulou E, Karakantza M, Pantazis P, Spyridonidis A, Zoumbos NC (2008) c-Jun N-terminal kinase activation failure is a new mechanism of anthracycline resistance in acute myeloid leukemia. Leukemia 22(10):1899–1908

Lal S, Mahajan A, Chen WN, Chowbay B (2010) Pharmacogenetics of target genes across doxorubicin disposition pathway: a review. Curr Drug Metab 11(1):115–128

Land EJ, Mukherjee T, Swallow AJ, Bruce JM (1983) One-electron reduction of adriamycin: properties of the semiquinone. Arch Biochem Biophys 225(1):116–121

Larsen RL, Canter CE, Naftel DC, Tressler M, Rosenthal DN, Blume ED, Mahle WT, Yung D, Morrow WR, Orav EJ, Wilkinson JD, Towbin JA, Lipshultz SE (2011) The impact of heart failure severity at time of listing for cardiac transplantation on survival in pediatric cardiomyopathy. J Heart Lung Transplant 30(7):755–760

Lebrecht D, Walker UA (2007) Role of mtDNA lesions in anthracycline cardiotoxicity. Cardiovasc Toxicol 7(2):108–113

Lebrecht D, Setzer B, Ketelsen UP, Haberstroh J, Walker UA (2003) Time-dependent and tissue-specific accumulation of mtDNA and respiratory chain defects in chronic doxorubicin cardiomyopathy. Circulation 108(19):2423–2429

Lebrecht D, Kokkori A, Ketelsen UP, Setzer B, Walker UA (2005) Tissue-specific mtDNA lesions and radical-associated mitochondrial dysfunction in human hearts exposed to doxorubicin. J Pathol 207(4):436–444

Lebrecht D, Kirschner J, Geist A, Haberstroh J, Walker UA (2010) Respiratory chain deficiency precedes the disrupted calcium homeostasis in chronic doxorubicin cardiomyopathy. Cardiovasc Pathol 19(5):e167–e174

Lefrak EA, Pitha J, Rosenheim S, Gottlieb JA (1973) A clinicopathologic analysis of adriamycin cardiotoxicity. Cancer 32(2):302–314

Legha SS, Wang YM, Mackay B, Ewer M, Hortobagyi GN, Benjamin RS, Ali MK (1982) Clinical and pharmacologic investigation of the effects of alpha-tocopherol on adriamycin cardiotoxicity. Ann N Y Acad Sci 393:411–418

Li T, Singal PK (2000) Adriamycin-induced early changes in myocardial antioxidant enzymes and their modulation by probucol. Circulation 102(17):2105–2110

Li G, Chen Y, Saari JT, Kang YJ (1997) Catalase-overexpressing transgenic mouse heart is resistant to ischemia-reperfusion injury. Am J Physiol 273(3 Pt 2):H1090–H1095

Li T, Danelisen I, Singal PK (2002) Early changes in myocardial antioxidant enzymes in rats treated with adriamycin. Mol Cell Biochem 232(1–2):19–26

Li S, Zhou Y, Dong Y, Ip C (2007a) Doxorubicin and selenium cooperatively induce fas signaling in the absence of Fas/Fas ligand interaction. Anticancer Res 27(5A):3075–3082

Li Y, D'Aurelio M, Deng JH, Park JS, Manfredi G, Hu P, Lu J, Bai Y (2007b) An assembled complex IV maintains the stability and activity of complex I in mammalian mitochondria. J Biol Chem 282(24):17557–17562

Licata S, Saponiero A, Mordente A, Minotti G (2000) Doxorubicin metabolism and toxicity in human myocardium: role of cytoplasmic deglycosidation and carbonyl reduction. Chem Res Toxicol 13(5):414–420

Lien YC, Daosukho C, St Clair DK (2006a) TNF receptor deficiency reveals a translational control mechanism for adriamycin-induced Fas expression in cardiac tissues. Cytokine 33(4):226–230

Lien YC, Lin SM, Nithipongvanitch R, Oberley TD, Noel T, Zhao Q, Daosukho C, St Clair DK (2006b) Tumor necrosis factor receptor deficiency exacerbated Adriamycin-induced cardiomyocytes apoptosis: an insight into the Fas connection. Mol Cancer Ther 5(2):261–269

Lipshultz SE, Adams MJ (2010) Cardiotoxicity after childhood cancer: beginning with the end in mind. J Clin Oncol 28(8):1276–1281

Lipshultz SE, Lipsitz SR, Sallan SE, Dalton VM, Mone SM, Gelber RD, Colan SD (2005) Chronic progressive cardiac dysfunction years after doxorubicin therapy for childhood acute lymphoblastic leukemia. J Clin Oncol 23(12):2629–2636

Liu X, Chua CC, Gao J, Chen Z, Landy CL, Hamdy R, Chua BH (2004) Pifithrin-alpha protects against doxorubicin-induced apoptosis and acute cardiotoxicity in mice. Am J Physiol Heart Circ Physiol 286(3):H933–H939

Liu J, Mao W, Ding B, Liang CS (2008) ERKs/p53 signal transduction pathway is involved in doxorubicin-induced apoptosis in H9c2 cells and cardiomyocytes. Am J Physiol Heart Circ Physiol 295(5):H1956–H1965

Liu Z, Liu R, Qiu J, Yin P, Luo F, Su J, Li W, Chen C, Fan X, Zhang J, Zhuang G (2009) Combination of human Fas (CD95/Apo-1) ligand with adriamycin significantly enhances the efficacy of antitumor response. Cell Mol Immunol 6(3):167–174

Lopez-Royuela N, Perez-Galan P, Galan-Malo P, Yuste VJ, Anel A, Susin SA, Naval J, Marzo I (2010) Different contribution of BH3-only proteins and caspases to doxorubicin-induced apoptosis in p53-deficient leukemia cells. Biochem Pharmacol 79(12):1746–1758

Lou H, Danelisen I, Singal PK (2005) Involvement of mitogen-activated protein kinases in adriamycin-induced cardiomyopathy. Am J Physiol Heart Circ Physiol 288(4):H1925–H1930

Lou H, Kaur K, Sharma AK, Singal PK (2006) Adriamycin-induced oxidative stress, activation of MAP kinases and apoptosis in isolated cardiomyocytes. Pathophysiology 13(2):103–109

Low RL, Orton S, Friedman DB (2003) A truncated form of DNA topoisomerase IIbeta associates with the mtDNA genome in mammalian mitochondria. Eur J Biochem 270(20):4173–4186

Lyu YL, Kerrigan JE, Lin CP, Azarova AM, Tsai YC, Ban Y, Liu LF (2007) Topoisomerase IIbeta mediated DNA double-strand breaks: implications in doxorubicin cardiotoxicity and prevention by dexrazoxane. Cancer Res 67(18):8839–8846

Malin D, Chen F, Schiller C, Koblinski JE, Cryns VL (2011) Enhanced metastasis suppression by targeting TRAIL receptor 2 in a murine model of triple-negative breast cancer. Clin Cancer Res 17(15):5005–5015

Malugin A, Kopeckova P, Kopecek J (2006) HPMA copolymer-bound doxorubicin induces apoptosis in ovarian carcinoma cells by the disruption of mitochondrial function. Mol Pharm 3(3):351–361

Manna SK, Gangadharan C, Edupalli D, Raviprakash N, Navneetha T, Mahali S, Thoh M (2011) Ras puts the brake on doxorubicin-mediated cell death in p53-expressing cells. J Biol Chem 286(9):7339–7347

Marcillat O, Zhang Y, Davies KJ (1989) Oxidative and non-oxidative mechanisms in the inactivation of cardiac mitochondrial electron transport chain components by doxorubicin. Biochem J 259(1):181–189

Mariotto AB, Rowland JH, Yabroff KR, Scoppa S, Hachey M, Ries L, Feuer EJ (2009) Long-term survivors of childhood cancers in the United States. Cancer Epidemiol Biomarkers Prev 18(4):1033–1040

Massart C, Barbet R, Genetet N, Gibassier J (2004) Doxorubicin induces Fas-mediated apoptosis in human thyroid carcinoma cells. Thyroid 14(4):263–270

Medikayala S, Piteo B, Zhao X, Edwards JG (2011) Chronically elevated glucose compromises myocardial mitochondrial DNA integrity by alteration of mitochondrial topoisomerase function. Am J Physiol Cell Physiol 300(2):C338–C348

Menna P, Recalcati S, Cairo G, Minotti G (2007) An introduction to the metabolic determinants of anthracycline cardiotoxicity. Cardiovasc Toxicol 7(2):80–85

Menna P, Salvatorelli E, Minotti G (2008) Cardiotoxicity of antitumor drugs. Chem Res Toxicol 21(5):978–989

Menna P, Gonzalez Paz O, Chello M, Covino E, Salvatorelli E, Minotti G (2011) Anthracycline cardiotoxicity. Expert Opin Drug Saf (in press)

Mertens AC, Yasui Y, Neglia JP, Potter JD, Nesbit ME Jr, Ruccione K, Smithson WA, Robison LL (2001) Late mortality experience in five-year survivors of childhood and adolescent cancer: the Childhood Cancer Survivor Study. J Clin Oncol 19(13):3163–3172

Mihm MJ, Yu F, Weinstein DM, Reiser PJ, Bauer JA (2002) Intracellular distribution of peroxynitrite during doxorubicin cardiomyopathy: evidence for selective impairment of myofibrillar creatine kinase. Br J Pharmacol 135(3):581–588

Minotti G, Mancuso C, Frustaci A, Mordente A, Santini SA, Calafiore AM, Liberi G, Gentiloni N (1996) Paradoxical inhibition of cardiac lipid peroxidation in cancer patients treated with doxorubicin. Pharmacologic and molecular reappraisal of anthracycline cardiotoxicity. J Clin Invest 98(3):650–661

Minotti G, Recalcati S, Mordente A, Liberi G, Calafiore AM, Mancuso C, Preziosi P, Cairo G (1998) The secondary alcohol metabolite of doxorubicin irreversibly inactivates aconitase/iron regulatory protein-1 in cytosolic fractions from human myocardium. FASEB J 12(7):541–552

Minotti G, Cairo G, Monti E (1999) Role of iron in anthracycline cardiotoxicity: new tunes for an old song? FASEB J 13(2):199–212

Minotti G, Menna P, Salvatorelli E, Cairo G, Gianni L (2004) Anthracyclines: molecular advances and pharmacologic developments in antitumor activity and cardiotoxicity. Pharmacol Rev 56(2):185–229

Misra UK, Pizzo SV (2010) PFT-alpha inhibits antibody-induced activation of p53 and pro-apoptotic signaling in 1-LN prostate cancer cells. Biochem Biophys Res Commun 391(1):272–276

Miyata S, Takemura G, Kosai K, Takahashi T, Esaki M, Li L, Kanamori H, Maruyama R, Goto K, Tsujimoto A, Takeyama T, Kawaguchi T, Ohno T, Nishigaki K, Fujiwara T, Fujiwara H, Minatoguchi S (2010) Anti-Fas gene therapy prevents doxorubicin-induced acute cardiotoxicity through mechanisms independent of apoptosis. Am J Pathol 176(2):687–698

Moller TR, Garwicz S, Barlow L, Falck Winther J, Glattre E, Olafsdottir G, Olsen JH, Perfekt R, Ritvanen A, Sankila R, Tulinius H (2001) Decreasing late mortality among five-year survivors of cancer in childhood and adolescence: a population-based study in the Nordic countries. J Clin Oncol 19(13):3173–3181

Montaigne D, Marechal X, Preau S, Baccouch R, Modine T, Fayad G, Lancel S, Neviere R (2011) Doxorubicin induces mitochondrial permeability transition and contractile dysfunction in the human myocardium. Mitochondrion 11(1):22–26

Mordente A, Meucci E, Martorana GE, Giardina B, Minotti G (2001) Human heart cytosolic reductases and anthracycline cardiotoxicity. IUBMB Life 52(1–2):83–88

Mordente A, Minotti G, Martorana GE, Silvestrini A, Giardina B, Meucci E (2003) Anthracycline secondary alcohol metabolite formation in human or rabbit heart: biochemical aspects and pharmacologic implications. Biochem Pharmacol 66(6):989–998

Mordente A, Meucci E, Silvestrini A, Martorana GE, Giardina B (2009) New developments in anthracycline-induced cardiotoxicity. Curr Med Chem 16(13):1656–1672

Morotti M, Valenzano Menada M, Venturini PL, Ferrero S (2011) Pharmacokinetic and toxicity considerations for the use of anthracyclines in ovarian cancer treatment. Expert Opin Drug Metab Toxicol 7(6):707–720

Morsi MI, Hussein AE, Mostafa M, El-Abd E, El-Moneim NA (2006) Evaluation of tumour necrosis factor-alpha, soluble P-selectin, gamma-glutamyl transferase, glutathione S-transferase-pi and alpha-fetoprotein in patients with hepatocellular carcinoma before and during chemotherapy. Br J Biomed Sci 63(2):74–78

Muhammed H, Ramasarma T, Kurup CK (1983) Inhibition of mitochondrial oxidative phosphorylation by adriamycin. Biochim Biophys Acta 722(1):43–50

Mukherjee S, Banerjee SK, Maulik M, Dinda AK, Talwar KK, Maulik SK (2003) Protection against acute adriamycin-induced cardiotoxicity by garlic: role of endogenous antioxidants and inhibition of TNF-alpha expression. BMC Pharmacol 3:16

Mukherjee A, Shehata M, Moseley P, Rakha E, Ellis I, Chan S (2010) Topo2alpha protein expression predicts response to anthracycline combination neo-adjuvant chemotherapy in locally advanced primary breast cancer. Br J Cancer 103(12):1794–1800

Myers C, Bonow R, Palmeri S, Jenkins J, Corden B, Locker G, Doroshow J, Epstein S (1983) A randomized controlled trial assessing the prevention of doxorubicin cardiomyopathy by N-acetylcysteine. Semin Oncol 10(1 suppl 1):53–55

Nagasawa K, Nagai K, Ohnishi N, Yokoyama T, Fujimoto S (2001) Contribution of specific transport systems to anthracycline transport in tumor and normal cells. Curr Drug Metab 2(4):355–366

Nakamura T, Ueda Y, Juan Y, Katsuda S, Takahashi H, Koh E (2000) Fas-mediated apoptosis in adriamycin-induced cardiomyopathy in rats: In vivo study. Circulation 102(5):572–578

Neilan TG, Blake SL, Ichinose F, Raher MJ, Buys ES, Jassal DS, Furutani E, Perez-Sanz TM, Graveline A, Janssens SP, Picard MH, Scherrer-Crosbie M, Bloch KD (2007) Disruption of nitric oxide synthase 3 protects against the cardiac injury, dysfunction, and mortality induced by doxorubicin. Circulation 116(5):506–514

Nelyudova A, Aksenov N, Pospelov V, Pospelova T (2007) By blocking apoptosis, Bcl-2 in p38-dependent manner promotes cell cycle arrest and accelerated senescence after DNA damage and serum withdrawal. Cell Cycle 6(17):2171–2177

Nicolay K, de Kruijff B (1987) Effects of adriamycin on respiratory chain activities in mitochondria from rat liver, rat heart and bovine heart. Evidence for a preferential inhibition of complex III and IV. Biochim Biophys Acta 892(3):320–330

Nicolay K, Fok JJ, Voorhout W, Post JA, de Kruijff B (1986) Cytofluorescence detection of adriamycin-mitochondria interactions in isolated, perfused rat heart. Biochim Biophys Acta 887(1):35–41

Nithipongvanitch R, Ittarat W, Cole MP, Tangpong J, Clair DK, Oberley TD (2007a) Mitochondrial and nuclear p53 localization in cardiomyocytes: redox modulation by doxorubicin (Adriamycin)? Antioxid Redox Signal 9(7):1001–1008

Nithipongvanitch R, Ittarat W, Velez JM, Zhao R, St Clair DK, Oberley TD (2007b) Evidence for p53 as guardian of the cardiomyocyte mitochondrial genome following acute adriamycin treatment. J Histochem Cytochem 55(6):629–639

Nitiss JL (2009) Targeting DNA topoisomerase II in cancer chemotherapy. Nat Rev Cancer 9(5):338–350

Oeffinger KC, Mertens AC, Sklar CA, Kawashima T, Hudson MM, Meadows AT, Friedman DL, Marina N, Hobbie W, Kadan-Lottick NS, Schwartz CL, Leisenring W, Robison LL (2006) Chronic health conditions in adult survivors of childhood cancer. N Engl J Med 355(15):1572–1582

Oliveira PJ, Wallace KB (2006) Depletion of adenine nucleotide translocator protein in heart mitochondria from doxorubicin-treated rats–relevance for mitochondrial dysfunction. Toxicology 220(2–3):160–168

Oliveira PJ, Santos MS, Wallace KB (2006) Doxorubicin-induced thiol-dependent alteration of cardiac mitochondrial permeability transition and respiration. Biochemistry (Moscow) 71(2):194–199

Olson RD, Mushlin PS (1990) Doxorubicin cardiotoxicity: analysis of prevailing hypotheses. FASEB J 4(13):3076–3086

Osborn MT, Chambers TC (1996) Role of the stress-activated/c-Jun NH2-terminal protein kinase pathway in the cellular response to adriamycin and other chemotherapeutic drugs. J Biol Chem 271(48):30950–30955

Palmeira CM, Serrano J, Kuehl DW, Wallace KB (1997) Preferential oxidation of cardiac mitochondrial DNA following acute intoxication with doxorubicin. Biochim Biophys Acta 1321(2):101–106

Panaretakis T, Pokrovskaja K, Shoshan MC, Grander D (2002) Activation of Bak, Bax, and BH3-only proteins in the apoptotic response to doxorubicin. J Biol Chem 277(46):44317–44326

Pawlowska J, Priebe W, Paine MJ, Wolf CR, Borowski E, Tarasiuk J (2004) The ability of new sugar-modified derivatives of antitumor anthracycline, daunorubicin, to stimulate NAD(P)H oxidation in different cellular oxidoreductase systems: NADH dehydrogenase, NADPH cytochrome P450 reductase, and xanthine oxidase. Oncol Res 14(10):469–474

Penault-Llorca F, Cayre A, Bouchet Mishellany F, Amat S, Feillel V, Le Bouedec G, Ferriere JP, De Latour M, Chollet P (2003) Induction chemotherapy for breast carcinoma: predictive markers and relation with outcome. Int J Oncol 22(6):1319–1325

Peng X, Chen B, Lim CC, Sawyer DB (2005) The cardiotoxicology of anthracycline chemotherapeutics: translating molecular mechanism into preventative medicine. Mol Interv 5(3):163–171

Peng X, Pentassuglia L, Sawyer DB (2010) Emerging anticancer therapeutic targets and the cardiovascular system: is there cause for concern? Circ Res 106(6):1022–1034

Penning TM, Drury JE (2007) Human aldo-keto reductases: function, gene regulation, and single nucleotide polymorphisms. Arch Biochem Biophys 464(2):241–250

Perego P, Corna E, De Cesare M, Gatti L, Polizzi D, Pratesi G, Supino R, Zunino F (2001) Role of apoptosis and apoptosis-related genes in cellular response and antitumor efficacy of anthracyclines. Curr Med Chem 8(1):31–37

Pinder MC, Duan Z, Goodwin JS, Hortobagyi GN, Giordano SH (2007) Congestive heart failure in older women treated with adjuvant anthracycline chemotherapy for breast cancer. J Clin Oncol 25(25):3808–3815

Pointon AV, Walker TM, Phillips KM, Luo J, Riley J, Zhang SD, Parry JD, Lyon JJ, Marczylo EL, Gant TW (2010) Doxorubicin in vivo rapidly alters expression and translation of myocardial electron transport chain genes, leads to ATP loss and caspase 3 activation. PLoS One 5(9):e12733

Pommier Y, Leo E, Zhang H, Marchand C (2010) DNA topoisomerases and their poisoning by anticancer and antibacterial drugs. Chem Biol 17(5):421–433

Pratilas CA, Solit DB (2010) Targeting the mitogen-activated protein kinase pathway: physiological feedback and drug response. Clin Cancer Res 16(13):3329–3334

Rajagopalan S, Politi PM, Sinha BK, Myers CE (1988) Adriamycin-induced free radical formation in the perfused rat heart: implications for cardiotoxicity. Cancer Res 48(17):4766–4769

Robert J (2007) Long-term and short-term models for studying anthracycline cardiotoxicity and protectors. Cardiovasc Toxicol 7(2):135–139

Robert J, Gianni L (1993) Pharmacokinetics and metabolism of anthracyclines. Cancer Surv 17:219–252

Rohan TE, Wong LJ, Wang T, Haines J, Kabat GC (2010) Do alterations in mitochondrial DNA play a role in breast carcinogenesis? J Oncol 2010:604304

Rose BA, Force T, Wang Y (2010) Mitogen-activated protein kinase signaling in the heart: angels versus demons in a heart-breaking tale. Physiol Rev 90(4):1507–1546

Ruiz-Ruiz C, Robledo G, Cano E, Redondo JM, Lopez-Rivas A (2003) Characterization of p53-mediated up-regulation of CD95 gene expression upon genotoxic treatment in human breast tumor cells. J Biol Chem 278(34):31667–31675

Salvatorelli E, Guarnieri S, Menna P, Liberi G, Calafiore AM, Mariggio MA, Mordente A, Gianni L, Minotti G (2006) Defective one- or two-electron reduction of the anticancer anthracycline epirubicin in human heart. Relative importance of vesicular sequestration and impaired efficiency of electron addition. J Biol Chem 281(16):10990–11001

Santos C, Martinez M, Lima M, Hao YJ, Simoes N, Montiel R (2008) Mitochondrial DNA mutations in cancer: a review. Curr Top Med Chem 8(15):1351–1366

Sardao VA, Oliveira PJ, Holy J, Oliveira CR, Wallace KB (2009) Doxorubicin-induced mitochondrial dysfunction is secondary to nuclear p53 activation in H9c2 cardiomyoblasts. Cancer Chemother Pharmacol 64(4):811–827

Sawyer DB, Peng X, Chen B, Pentassuglia L, Lim CC (2010) Mechanisms of anthracycline cardiac injury: can we identify strategies for cardioprotection? Prog Cardiovasc Dis 53(2):105–113

Sayers TJ (2011) Targeting the extrinsic apoptosis signaling pathway for cancer therapy. Cancer Immunol Immunother 60(8):1173–1180

Schagger H, de Coo R, Bauer MF, Hofmann S, Godinot C, Brandt U (2004) Significance of respirasomes for the assembly/stability of human respiratory chain complex I. J Biol Chem 279(35):36349–36353

Selivanov VA, Votyakova TV, Pivtoraiko VN, Zeak J, Sukhomlin T, Trucco M, Roca J, Cascante M (2011) Reactive oxygen species production by forward and reverse electron fluxes in the mitochondrial respiratory chain. PLoS Comput Biol 7(3):e1001115

Serrano J, Palmeira CM, Kuehl DW, Wallace KB (1999) Cardioselective and cumulative oxidation of mitochondrial DNA following subchronic doxorubicin administration. Biochim Biophys Acta 1411(1):201–205

Setsuta K, Seino Y, Ogawa T, Ohtsuka T, Seimiya K, Takano T (2004) Ongoing myocardial damage in chronic heart failure is related to activated tumor necrosis factor and Fas/Fas ligand system. Circ J 68(8):747–750

Sharples RA, Cullinane C, Phillips DR (2000) Adriamycin-induced inhibition of mitochondrial-encoded polypeptides as a model system for the identification of hotspots for DNA-damaging agents. Anticancer Drug Des 15(3):183–190

Shi D, Pop MS, Kulikov R, Love IM, Kung AL, Grossman SR (2009) CBP and p300 are cytoplasmic E4 polyubiquitin ligases for p53. Proc Natl Acad Sci USA 106(38):16275–16280

Shizukuda Y, Matoba S, Mian OY, Nguyen T, Hwang PM (2005) Targeted disruption of p53 attenuates doxorubicin-induced cardiac toxicity in mice. Mol Cell Biochem 273(1–2):25–32

Singh TR, Shankar S, Chen X, Asim M, Srivastava RK (2003) Synergistic interactions of chemotherapeutic drugs and tumor necrosis factor-related apoptosis-inducing ligand/Apo-2 ligand on apoptosis and on regression of breast carcinoma in vivo. Cancer Res 63(17):5390–5400

Sinha BK, Chignell CF (1979) Binding mode of chemically activated semiquinone free radicals from quinone anticancer agents to DNA. Chem Biol Interact 28(2–3):301–308

Siveski-Iliskovic N, Hill M, Chow DA, Singal PK (1995) Probucol protects against adriamycin cardiomyopathy without interfering with its antitumor effect. Circulation 91(1):10–15

Small GW, Somasundaram S, Moore DT, Shi YY, Orlowski RZ (2003) Repression of mitogen-activated protein kinase (MAPK) phosphatase-1 by anthracyclines contributes to their antiapoptotic activation of p44/42-MAPK. J Pharmacol Exp Ther 307(3):861–869

Small GW, Shi YY, Higgins LS, Orlowski RZ (2007) Mitogen-activated protein kinase phosphatase-1 is a mediator of breast cancer chemoresistance. Cancer Res 67(9):4459–4466

Sokolove PM (1994) Interactions of adriamycin aglycones with mitochondria may mediate adriamycin cardiotoxicity. Int J Biochem 26(12):1341–1350

Solem LE, Heller LJ, Wallace KB (1996) Dose-dependent increase in sensitivity to calcium-induced mitochondrial dysfunction and cardiomyocyte cell injury by doxorubicin. J Mol Cell Cardiol 28(5):1023–1032

Spallarossa P, Altieri P, Garibaldi S, Ghigliotti G, Barisione C, Manca V, Fabbi P, Ballestrero A, Brunelli C, Barsotti A (2006) Matrix metalloproteinase-2 and -9 are induced differently by doxorubicin in H9c2 cells: the role of MAP kinases and NAD(P)H oxidase. Cardiovasc Res 69(3):736–745

Spallarossa P, Altieri P, Barisione C, Passalacqua M, Aloi C, Fugazza G, Frassoni F, Podesta M, Canepa M, Ghigliotti G, Brunelli C (2010) p38 MAPK and JNK antagonistically control senescence and cytoplasmic p16INK4A expression in doxorubicin-treated endothelial progenitor cells. PLoS One 5(12):e15583

Stearns V, Singh B, Tsangaris T, Crawford JG, Novielli A, Ellis MJ, Isaacs C, Pennanen M, Tibery C, Farhad A, Slack R, Hayes DF (2003) A prospective randomized pilot study to evaluate predictors of response in serial core biopsies to single agent neoadjuvant doxorubicin or paclitaxel for patients with locally advanced breast cancer. Clin Cancer Res 9(1):124–133

Subjeck JR, Repasky EA (2011) Heat shock proteins and cancer therapy: the trail grows hotter! Oncotarget 2(6):433–434

Swain SM, Whaley FS, Ewer MS (2003) Congestive heart failure in patients treated with doxorubicin: a retrospective analysis of three trials. Cancer 97(11):2869–2879

Swerdlow AJ, Higgins CD, Smith P, Cunningham D, Hancock BW, Horwich A, Hoskin PJ, Lister A, Radford JA, Rohatiner AZ, Linch DC (2007) Myocardial infarction mortality risk after treatment for Hodgkin disease: a collaborative British cohort study. J Natl Cancer Inst 99(3):206–214

Swift LP, Rephaeli A, Nudelman A, Phillips DR, Cutts SM (2006) Doxorubicin-DNA adducts induce a non-topoisomerase II-mediated form of cell death. Cancer Res 66(9):4863–4871

Swift L, McHowat J, Sarvazyan N (2007) Anthracycline-induced phospholipase A2 inhibition. Cardiovasc Toxicol 7(2):86–91

Swift LP, Cutts SM, Nudelman A, Levovich I, Rephaeli A, Phillips DR (2008) The cardio-protecting agent and topoisomerase II catalytic inhibitor sobuzoxane enhances doxorubicin-DNA adduct mediated cytotoxicity. Cancer Chemother Pharmacol 61(5):739–749

Taatjes DJ, Koch TH (2001) Nuclear targeting and retention of anthracycline antitumor drugs in sensitive and resistant tumor cells. Curr Med Chem 8(1):15–29

Taatjes DJ, Gaudiano G, Koch TH (1997) Production of formaldehyde and DNA-adriamycin or DNA-daunomycin adducts, initiated through redox chemistry of dithiothreitol/iron, xanthine oxidase/NADH/iron, or glutathione/iron. Chem Res Toxicol 10(9):953–961

Tait SW, Green DR (2010) Mitochondria and cell death: outer membrane permeabilization and beyond. Nat Rev Mol Cell Biol 11(9):621–632

Tang Y, Olufemi L, Wang MT, Nie D (2008) Role of Rho GTPases in breast cancer. Front Biosci 13:759–776

Tangpong J, Cole MP, Sultana R, Joshi G, Estus S, Vore M, St Clair W, Ratanachaiyavong S, St Clair DK, Butterfield DA (2006) Adriamycin-induced, TNF-alpha-mediated central nervous system toxicity. Neurobiol Dis 23(1):127–139

Tao Z, Withers HG, Penefsky HS, Goodisman J, Souid AK (2006) Inhibition of cellular respiration by doxorubicin. Chem Res Toxicol 19(8):1051–1058

Thandavarayan RA, Watanabe K, Sari FR, Ma M, Lakshmanan AP, Giridharan VV, Gurusamy N, Nishida H, Konishi T, Zhang S, Muslin AJ, Kodama M, Aizawa Y (2010) Modulation of doxorubicin-induced cardiac dysfunction in dominant-negative p38alpha mitogen-activated protein kinase mice. Free Radic Biol Med 49(9):1422–1431

Tikoo K, Sane MS, Gupta C (2011) Tannic acid ameliorates doxorubicin-induced cardiotoxicity and potentiates its anticancer activity: potential role of tannins in cancer chemotherapy. Toxicol Appl Pharmacol 251(3):191–200

Tokarska-Schlattner M, Zaugg M, da Silva R, Lucchinetti E, Schaub MC, Wallimann T, Schlattner U (2005) Acute toxicity of doxorubicin on isolated perfused heart: response of kinases regulating energy supply. Am J Physiol Heart Circ Physiol 289(1):H37–H47

Tokarska-Schlattner M, Zaugg M, Zuppinger C, Wallimann T, Schlattner U (2006) New insights into doxorubicin-induced cardiotoxicity: the critical role of cellular energetics. J Mol Cell Cardiol 41(3):389–405

Tokarska-Schlattner M, Lucchinetti E, Zaugg M, Kay L, Gratia S, Guzun R, Saks V, Schlattner U (2010) Early effects of doxorubicin in perfused heart: transcriptional profiling reveals inhibition of cellular stress response genes. Am J Physiol Regul Integr Comp Physiol 298(4):R1075–R1088

Toyoda E, Kagaya S, Cowell IG, Kurosawa A, Kamoshita K, Nishikawa K, Iiizumi S, Koyama H, Austin CA, Adachi N (2008) NK314, a topoisomerase II inhibitor that specifically targets the alpha isoform. J Biol Chem 283(35):23711–23720

Trachtenberg BH, Landy DC, Franco VI, Henkel JM, Pearson EJ, Miller TL, Lipshultz SE (2011) Anthracycline-associated cardiotoxicity in survivors of childhood cancer. Pediatr Cardiol 32(3):342–353

Trapp BD, Andrews SB, Wong A, O'Connell M, Griffin JW (1989) Co-localization of the myelin-associated glycoprotein and the microfilament components, F-actin and spectrin, in Schwann cells of myelinated nerve fibres. J Neurocytol 18(1):47–60

Trarbach T, Moehler M, Heinemann V, Kohne CH, Przyborek M, Schulz C, Sneller V, Gallant G, Kanzler S (2010) Phase II trial of mapatumumab, a fully human agonistic monoclonal antibody that targets and activates the tumour necrosis factor apoptosis-inducing ligand receptor-1 (TRAIL-R1), in patients with refractory colorectal cancer. Br J Cancer 102(3):506–512

Ugarenko M, Nudelman A, Rephaeli A, Kimura K, Phillips DR, Cutts SM (2010) ABT-737 overcomes Bcl-2 mediated resistance to doxorubicin-DNA adducts. Biochem Pharmacol 79(3):339–349

Ujhazy P, Zaleskis G, Mihich E, Ehrke MJ, Berleth ES (2003) Doxorubicin induces specific immune functions and cytokine expression in peritoneal cells. Cancer Immunol Immunother 52(7):463–472

Vaculova A, Kaminskyy V, Jalalvand E, Surova O, Zhivotovsky B (2010) Doxorubicin and etoposide sensitize small cell lung carcinoma cells expressing caspase-8 to TRAIL. Mol Cancer 9:87

van Dalen EC, van der Pal HJ, Kok WE, Caron HN, Kremer LC (2006) Clinical heart failure in a cohort of children treated with anthracyclines: a long-term follow-up study. Eur J Cancer 42(18):3191–3198

van Dalen EC, Raphael MF, Caron HN, Kremer LC (2011) Treatment including anthracyclines versus treatment not including anthracyclines for childhood cancer. Cochrane Database Syst Rev (1):CD006647

Van Vleet JF, Ferrans VJ, Weirich WE (1980) Cardiac disease induced by chronic adriamycin administration in dogs and an evaluation of vitamin E and selenium as cardioprotectants. Am J Pathol 99(1):13–42

Varanyuwatana P, Halestrap AP (2011) The roles of phosphate and the phosphate carrier in the mitochondrial permeability transition pore. Mitochondrion (in press)

Vasquez-Vivar J, Martasek P, Hogg N, Masters BS, Pritchard KA Jr, Kalyanaraman B (1997) Endothelial nitric oxide synthase-dependent superoxide generation from adriamycin. Biochemistry 36(38):11293–11297

Velez JM, Miriyala S, Nithipongvanitch R, Noel T, Plabplueng CD, Oberley T, Jungsuwadee P, Van Remmen H, Vore M, St Clair DK (2011) p53 Regulates oxidative stress-mediated retrograde signaling: a novel mechanism for che-motherapy-induced cardiac injury. PLoS One 6(3):e18005

Venkatakrishnan CD, Tewari AK, Moldovan L, Cardounel AJ, Zweier JL, Kuppusamy P, Ilangovan G (2006) Heat shock protects cardiac cells from doxorubicin-induced toxicity by activating p38 MAPK and phosphorylation of small heat shock protein 27. Am J Physiol Heart Circ Physiol 291(6):H2680–H2691

Venkatesan B, Prabhu SD, Venkatachalam K, Mummidi S, Valente AJ, Clark RA, Delafontaine P, Chandrasekar B (2010) WNT1-inducible signaling pathway protein-1 activates diverse cell survival pathways and blocks doxorubicin-induced cardiomyocyte death. Cell Signal 22(5):809–820

Voelkel-Johnson C, King DL, Norris JS (2002) Resistance of prostate cancer cells to soluble TNF-related apoptosis-inducing ligand (TRAIL/Apo2L) can be overcome by doxorubicin or adenoviral delivery of full-length TRAIL. Cancer Gene Ther 9(2):164–172

Von Hoff DD, Layard MW, Basa P, Davis HL Jr, Von Hoff AL, Rozencweig M, Muggia FM (1979) Risk factors for doxorubicin-induced congestive heart failure. Ann Intern Med 91(5):710–717

Wallace KB (2003) Doxorubicin-induced cardiac mitochondrionopathy. Pharmacol Toxicol 93(3):105–115

Wallace KB (2007) Adriamycin-induced interference with cardiac mitochondrial calcium homeostasis. Cardiovasc Toxicol 7(2):101–107

Wallace DC, Fan W, Procaccio V (2010) Mitochondrial energetics and therapeutics. Annu Rev Pathol 5:297–348

Wang C, Youle RJ (2009) The role of mitochondria in apoptosis*. Annu Rev Genet 43:95–118

Wang AH, Gao YG, Liaw YC, Li YK (1991) Formaldehyde cross-links daunorubicin and DNA efficiently: HPLC and X-ray diffraction studies. Biochemistry 30(16):3812–3815

Wang Y, Lyu YL, Wang JC (2002) Dual localization of human DNA topoisomerase IIIalpha to mitochondria and nucleus. Proc Natl Acad Sci USA 99(19):12114–12119

Wang M, Markel T, Crisostomo P, Herring C, Meldrum KK, Lillemoe KD, Meldrum DR (2007) Deficiency of TNFR1 protects myocardium through SOCS3 and IL-6 but not p38 MAPK or IL-1beta. Am J Physiol Heart Circ Physiol 292(4):H1694–H1699

Wang JX, Li Q, Li PF (2009) Apoptosis repressor with caspase recruitment domain contributes to chemotherapy resistance by abolishing mitochondrial fission mediated by dynamin-related protein-1. Cancer Res 69(2):492–500

Wang S, Ren W, Liu J, Lahat G, Torres K, Lopez G, Lazar AJ, Hayes-Jordan A, Liu K, Bankson J, Hazle JD, Lev D (2010) TRAIL and doxorubicin combination induces proapoptotic and antiangiogenic effects in soft tissue sarcoma in vivo. Clin Cancer Res 16(9):2591–2604

Weinstein DM, Mihm MJ, Bauer JA (2000) Cardiac peroxynitrite formation and left ventricular dysfunction following doxorubicin treatment in mice. J Pharmacol Exp Ther 294(1):396–401

Welsh SJ, Koh MY, Powis G (2006) The hypoxic inducible stress response as a target for cancer drug discovery. Semin Oncol 33(4):486–497

Wieder T, Essmann F, Prokop A, Schmelz K, Schulze-Osthoff K, Beyaert R, Dorken B, Daniel PT (2001) Activation of caspase-8 in drug-induced apoptosis of B-lymphoid cells is independent of CD95/Fas receptor-ligand interaction and occurs downstream of caspase-3. Blood 97(5):1378–1387

Wiezorek J, Holland P, Graves J (2010) Death receptor agonists as a targeted therapy for cancer. Clin Cancer Res 16(6):1701–1708

Wildiers H, Highley MS, de Bruijn EA, van Oosterom AT (2003) Pharmacology of anticancer drugs in the elderly population. Clin Pharmacokinet 42(14):1213–1242

Wu GS (2004) The functional interactions between the p53 and MAPK signaling pathways. Cancer Biol Ther 3(2):156–161

Wu S, Ko YS, Teng MS, Ko YL, Hsu LA, Hsueh C, Chou YY, Liew CC, Lee YS (2002a) Adriamycin-induced cardiomyocyte and endothelial cell apoptosis: in vitro and in vivo studies. J Mol Cell Cardiol 34(12):1595–1607

Wu XX, Kakehi Y, Mizutani Y, Kamoto T, Kinoshita H, Isogawa Y, Terachi T, Ogawa O (2002b) Doxorubicin enhances TRAIL-induced apoptosis in prostate cancer. Int J Oncol 20(5):949–954

Wu XX, Kakehi Y, Mizutani Y, Nishiyama H, Kamoto T, Megumi Y, Ito N, Ogawa O (2003) Enhancement of TRAIL/Apo2L-mediated apoptosis by adriamycin through inducing DR4 and DR5 in renal cell carcinoma cells. Int J Cancer 104(4):409–417

Wu XX, Jin XH, Zeng Y, El Hamed AM, Kakehi Y (2007) Low concentrations of doxorubicin sensitizes human solid cancer cells to tumor necrosis factor-related apoptosis-inducing ligand (TRAIL)-receptor (R) 2-mediated apoptosis by inducing TRAIL-R2 expression. Cancer Sci 98(12):1969–1976

Xiong Y, Liu X, Lee CP, Chua BH, Ho YS (2006) Attenuation of doxorubicin-induced contractile and mitochondrial dysfunction in mouse heart by cellular glutathione peroxidase. Free Radic Biol Med 41(1):46–55

Xu LH, Deng CS, Zhu YQ, Liu SQ, Liu DZ (2003) Synergistic antitumor effect of TRAIL and doxorubicin on colon cancer cell line SW480. World J Gastroenterol 9(6):1241–1245

Xu L, Qu X, Luo Y, Zhang Y, Liu J, Qu J, Zhang L, Liu Y (2011) Epirubicin enhances TRAIL-induced apoptosis in gastric cancer cells by promoting death receptor clustering in lipid rafts. Mol Med Rep 4(3):407–411

Yamaoka M, Yamaguchi S, Suzuki T, Okuyama M, Nitobe J, Nakamura N, Mitsui Y, Tomoike H (2000) Apoptosis in rat cardiac myocytes induced by Fas ligand: priming for Fas-mediated apoptosis with doxorubicin. J Mol Cell Cardiol 32(6):881–889

Yang A, Wilson NS, Ashkenazi A (2010) Proapoptotic DR4 and DR5 signaling in cancer cells: toward clinical translation. Curr Opin Cell Biol 22(6):837–844

Yano S, Matsuyama H, Hirata H, Inoue R, Matsumoto H, Ohmi C, Miura K, Shirai M, Iizuka N, Naito K (2006) Identification of genes linked to gefitinib treatment in prostate cancer cell lines with or without resistance to androgen: a clue to application of gefitinib to hormone-resistant prostate cancer. Oncol Rep 15(6):1453–1460

Yee SB, Pritsos CA (1997) Comparison of oxygen radical generation from the reductive activation of doxorubicin, streptonigrin, and menadione by xanthine oxidase and xanthine dehydrogenase. Arch Biochem Biophys 347(2):235–241

Yen HC, Oberley TD, Vichitbandha S, Ho YS, St Clair DK (1996) The protective role of manganese superoxide dismutase against adriamycin-induced acute cardiac toxicity in transgenic mice. J Clin Invest 98(5):1253–1260

Yoshimoto Y, Kawada M, Ikeda D, Ishizuka M (2005) Involvement of doxorubicin-induced Fas expression in the antitumor effect of doxorubicin on Lewis lung carcinoma in vivo. Int Immunopharmacol 5(2):281–288

Youle RJ, Strasser A (2008) The BCL-2 protein family: opposing activities that mediate cell death. Nat Rev Mol Cell Biol 9(1):47–59

Yu R, Shtil AA, Tan TH, Roninson IB, Kong AN (1996) Adriamycin activates c-jun N-terminal kinase in human leukemia cells: a relevance to apoptosis. Cancer Lett 107(1):73–81

Zantl N, Weirich G, Zall H, Seiffert BM, Fischer SF, Kirschnek S, Hartmann C, Fritsch RM, Gillissen B, Daniel PT, Hacker G (2007) Frequent loss of expression of the pro-apoptotic protein Bim in renal cell carcinoma: evidence for contribution to apoptosis resistance. Oncogene 26(49):7038–7048

Zaragoza MV, Brandon MC, Diegoli M, Arbustini E, Wallace DC (2011) Mitochondrial cardiomyopathies: how to identify candidate pathogenic mutations by mitochondrial DNA sequencing, MITOMASTER and phylogeny. Eur J Hum Genet 19(2):200–207

Zeman SM, Phillips DR, Crothers DM (1998) Characterization of covalent adriamycin-DNA adducts. Proc Natl Acad Sci USA 95(20):11561–11565

Zhao Y, You H, Yang Y, Wei L, Zhang X, Yao L, Fan D, Yu Q (2004) Distinctive regulation and function of PI 3 K/Akt and MAPKs in doxorubicin-induced apoptosis of human lung adenocarcinoma cells. J Cell Biochem 91(3):621–632

Zhou S, Palmeira CM, Wallace KB (2001a) Doxorubicin-induced persistent oxidative stress to cardiac myocytes. Toxicol Lett 121(3):151–157

Zhou S, Starkov A, Froberg MK, Leino RL, Wallace KB (2001b) Cumulative and irreversible cardiac mitochondrial dysfunction induced by doxorubicin. Cancer Res 61(2):771–777

Zhu W, Zou Y, Aikawa R, Harada K, Kudoh S, Uozumi H, Hayashi D, Gu Y, Yamazaki T, Nagai R, Yazaki Y, Komuro I (1999) MAPK superfamily plays an important role in daunomycin-induced apoptosis of cardiac myocytes. Circulation 100(20):2100–2107

Part IV
Applications of Mitochondrial Science

Chapter 19
Mitochondrial Proteomic Approaches for New Potential Diagnostic and Prognostic Biomarkers in Cancer

Patrizia Bottoni, Bruno Giardina, Alessandro Pontoglio, Salvatore Scarà, and Roberto Scatena

Abstract Mitochondrial dysfunction and mutations in mitochondrial DNA have been implicated in a wide variety of human diseases, including cancer. In recent years, considerable advances in genomic, proteomic and bioinformatic technologies have made it possible the analysis of mitochondrial proteome, leading to the identification of over 1,000 proteins which have been assigned unambiguously to mitochondria. Defining the mitochondrial proteome is a fundamental step for fully understanding the organelle functions as well as mechanisms underlying mitochondrial pathology. In fact, besides giving information on mitochondrial physiology, by characterizing all the components of this subcellular organelle, the application of proteomic technologies permitted now to study the proteins involved in many crucial properties in cell signaling, cell differentiation and cell death and, in particular, to identify mitochondrial proteins that are aberrantly expressed in cancer cells. An improved understanding of the mitochondrial proteome could be essential to shed light on the connection between mitochondrial dysfunction, deregulation of apoptosis and tumorigenesis and to discovery new therapeutic targets for mitochondria-related diseases.

Keywords Biomarkers • Cancer • Mitochondria • Mitochondrial proteome • Oncoproteomics

19.1 Introduction

Mitochondria represent the main intracellular source of energy, playing a key role in cellular bioenergetics, ion omeostasis, carbohydrate and fatty acid metabolism. Most of cellular energy is producted by the mitochondrial complexes in the oxidative phosphorylation system (OXPHOS). During beta oxidation of lipids and Krebs cycle, reducing equivalent derived from oxidation of substrates are transferred to NAD^+ and FAD (forming NADH and $FADH_2$) which are oxidized by a system of electron carriers located in the inner membrane, the electron transport chain. This process generate a proton gradient between the mitochondrial matrix and the intermembrane space, that is used to produce ATP. The oxidative phosphorylation is not the sole metabolic pathway located in mitochondria.

P. Bottoni (✉) • B. Giardina • A. Pontoglio • S. Scarà • R. Scatena
Institute of Biochemistry and Clinical Biochemistry, Catholic University,
School of Medicine, Largo F. Vito 1, 00168 Rome, Italy
e-mail: patrizia.bottoni@rm.unicatt.it

R. Scatena et al. (eds.), *Advances in Mitochondrial Medicine*, Advances in Experimental
Medicine and Biology 942, DOI 10.1007/978-94-007-2869-1_19,
© Springer Science+Business Media B.V. 2012

These subcellular organelles host other metabolic processes, including the tricarboxylic acid cycle (TCA cycle), β-oxidation of fatty acid, steroid synthesis, heme biosynthesis. In addition, two of the five reactions of urea cycle are located within mitochondria, as well as several reactions of ketogenesis and gluconeogenesis (Michal 1999). Mitochondria play a crucial role not only for energy production (obtained by breaking down carbohydrates and lipids), but also in controlling intracellular Ca⁺⁺ homeostasis and in regulating apoptosis by releasing cytochrome c, procaspases and other proapoptotic factors. Moreover, the majority of reactive oxygen species (ROS) are by-products of oxidative metabolism. Physiological levels of ROS are involved in the regulation of numerous cellular processes, acting as intracellular signaling transducers and even as oncosuppressors (Takahashi et al. 2006). If produced excessively, ROS can be noxious to the cell, leading to the activation of the intrinsic apoptotic pathway.

One of the major targets of ROS is mitochondrial DNA (mtDNA), a circular 16.5 Kb genome, of which each human cell may contain several hundred of copies. The mitochondrial genome contains 13 protein-coding genes and encodes several proteins essential for the function of mitochondrial respiratory chain, such as 13 Krebs cycle and respiratory-chain subunits, 22 transfer RNAs and 2 ribosomal RNAs (rRNAs)-12S and 16S (Fliss et al. 2000). Owing to its closeness to the mitochondrial electron transfer chain and a lack of protective histones, mtDNA is extremely sensitive to oxidative damage induced by ROS which is probably a major source of mitochondrial genomic instability causing respiratory dysfunction.

19.2 Role of Mitochondria in Cancer

Considering the essential involvement of mitochondria in cellular bioenergetic and in various important cellular processes such as apoptosis and cellular oxidative stress responses, it is not surprising that mitochondria dysfunction could contribute to the development of numerous human diseases including the genesis and/or progression of cancer. The first hypothesis of the possible existence of tight connection between mitochondrial bioenergetics and tumourigenesis was advanced several decades ago by Otto Warburg (1956) who demonstrated that cancer cells, contrary to normal cells, use glycolysis to generate energy even when oxygen is available. He assumed that this particular metabolic shift characterized by high glucose uptake and elevated lactate production was caused by mitochondrial impairment and was the origin of malignant transformation. Warburg's brilliant observation has had a great impact, profoundly stimulating the investigation of mitochondrial function in tumor cells and has nowadays important clinical applications in the visualization of tumors by positron emission tomography (PET) imaging technique. However, in light of recent findings, there must be at present a significant re-evaluation of the role of mitochondria in cancer cell metabolism. Recent studies, in showing that mutations in the nuclear genes encoding succinate dehydrogenase (SDH) and fumarate hydratase (FH), both enzymes of the TCA cycle, predispose to development of hereditary paraganglioma or leiomyoma and papillary renal cell cancer (Baysal et al. 2000; Tomlinson et al. 2002), revealed the existence of an important link between mitochondrial malfunctioning and tumourigenesis. Consequent changes in the expression and activity of enzymes that determine the rate of metabolic fluxes can promote metabolic reprogramming which confers replicative advantages to rapidly proliferating cancer cells (De Berardinis et al. 2008a). In reality, it is becoming evident that "aerobic glycolysis" typical of cancer cell is only an aspect of a more complex metabolic shift aimed to provide not only energy by increasing ATP production in an oxygen independent manner, but also to convert extracellular nutrients into biosynthetic precursors required for synthesize nucleotides, proteins and lipids necessary for the rapidly growing cells (Hammerman et al. 2004; Garber 2006; Moreno-Sanchez et al. 2007; Kim and Dang 2007). Increasing evidences have implicated mitochondria in the pathogenesis of cancer, showing the presence of somatic mutations in the mitochondrial genome (mtDNA) that has been observed in a wide variety of tumors (Brandon et al. 2006), with a frequency that was reported to be ten times higher than that of nuclear DNA mutations (Verma et al. 2003). The six hallmark that characterize the malignant transformations (limitless proliferative potential, self-sufficient in growth signals, insensitivity to anti-proliferative signals, disabled apoptosis, sustained angiogenesis and invasiveness/metastatic potential) that have been described in a milestone article by Hanahan and Weinberg (2000) may be directly or indirectly related to mitochondrial dysfunction (Galluzzi et al. 2010). Notwithstanding a growing number of evidences suggesting a more active role for mitochondrial physiology in cancer cell metabolism, it is complex issue to define how the different mitochondrial activities and functions could be associated to cancer and to identify the mechanisms by which mitochondria can contribute to malignant transformation and tumor progression.

19.3 Proteomic Strategies for Studying Mitochondrial Proteome

The important role that mitochondria dysfunction seems to play in several diseases, including cancer, has aroused great interest in studying mitochondrial proteome, in an attempt to identify new potential diagnostic markers and therapeutic targets (Gaucher et al. 2004). Several tools exist to study mitochondria and, among them, proteomics technologies are becoming to play an ever more active role in investigating mitochondrial physiology in cancer cell metabolism. The most direct approach to obtain the complete mitochondrial proteome is to isolate highly purified mitochondria and determine the subset of mitochondrial proteins by mass spectrometry. Once isolated these organelles by classical differential centrifugation, gradient ultracentrifugation or free-flow electrophoresis, mitochondria can be solubilized and the proteins can be separated in various ways (Pflieger et al. 2002; Mootha et al. 2003; Sickmann et al. 2003; Taylor et al. 2003). As recently reviewed by Mathy and Sluse (2008), the techniques available to carry out valid comparative proteomics are fundamentally based on two different approaches: two-dimensional electrophoresis (2-DE electrophoresis) and peptide mass fingerprinting (PMF) or shotgun proteomics. These methods differ by the means utilized to separate and identify proteins and involve a series of advantages and disadvantages intrinsically related to the method of choice and to the type of sample to analyze. A classical proteomic approach frequently applied by researchers working in proteomic field is conducted by using 2-DE as powerful separation method and mass spectrometry (MS spectrometry) as efficacious identification method. In short, 2-DE, the most popular proteomic technology that separates proteins based on their isoelectric point and molecular weight, is a method that offers several advantages, giving the best resolution in terms of separation and permitting also to identify post-translationally modified forms of proteins, such as phosphorylation that are responsible for the appearance of trains of spot in 2-DE map (Mathy and Sluse 2008). Therefore, at least theoretically, it should be able to resolve the estimated 1,500 mitochondrial proteins on a single gel. However, this technique presents several limits in its ability to analyze the mitochondrial proteome for various reasons. A large percentage of mitochondrial proteins (such as the complexes of the respiratory chain) are integral or peripheral membrane proteins which, due to their extremely hydrophobic character, tends to precipitate during electrophoresis. In addition, mitochondria contain many low molecular weight proteins (<10 kDa), and very basic proteins ($pI > 9$), which are difficult to resolve by standard 2-DE (Wilkins et al. 1998). Some of these problems was recently solved with the introduction of labelling methodologies like DIGE that has enhanced notably the versatility of 2-DE, allowing not only the identification of low abundant proteins but also suppressing the inter-gel variability and considerably improving the reproducibility of the quantitative proteomic analysis (Unlu et al. 1997). All protein spots of interest can be excised from the gel, digested by a specific protease and identified by MS spectrometry.

In another type of proteomic approach, commonly named shotgun proteomics, the protein separation is not carried out by the traditional 2-DE electrophoresis but by liquid chromatography. Peptides resulting from specific protease's digestion are separated and then identified by injecting them into a mass spectrometer via electrospray ionization (ESI) or by spotting them onto a MALDI (matrix-assisted laser desorption ionization-mass spectrometry) plate. Besides having the advantage of the extreme rapidity of execution, the shotgun strategy permits to overcome some important limits of the traditional approach with 2-DE, such as the identification of proteins with extreme hydrophobicity, mass, or isoelectric point. However, in same cases of particular complexity of the sample, it could be appropriate to carried out a cellular fractionation to obtain a better separation and consequently an undoubted identification of a major number of proteins. Several methods of comparative proteomics have been introduced for shotgun proteomics. In one of the first technique used, the ICATs (Isotope-coded affinity tags), proteins or peptides derived from two different samples are labeled with heavy and light stable isotopic probes. Both samples are then mixed, digested with a protease and subjected to avidin affinity chromatography to isolate peptides labeled with isotope-coded tagging reagents. The ICAT peptides are then analyzed by liquid chromatography-mass spectrometry (LC-MS) to calculate the relative abundance levels by comparing signal intensities of the labeled peptides (Gygi et al. 1999). The method, however, is applicable only to cysteine-containing proteins, which make up about 30% of the total proteome. Differently from ICAT, SILAC (stable isotope labeling by amino acids in cell culture) technique avoids any chemical modification of proteins in the process of encoding quantitative information. Protein labeling is not carried out after protein extraction, but directly in cell culture, by metabolic incorporation of the heavy and light amino acids into the proteins that results in a mass shift of the corresponding peptides which can be detected by a mass spectrometer. This technique, that obviously presents all the advantages of shotgun proteomics, allows comparison samples from different conditions or treatments which are combined and treated as a single sample throughout subsequent purification and analyses (Ong and Mann 2006). This approach has been applied to study cell signaling, post translational modifications such as phosphorylation (Ibarrola et al. 2004; Harsha et al. 2008), protein-protein interaction and regulation of gene expression. Moreover, some tags used in this type of approach offer the possibility of simultaneously analyzing relative protein levels from multiple complex samples, such as the iTRAQ (isobaric tag for relative and absolute quantitation) and the ExacTag reagent, that permit to compare up to eight and up to ten samples respectively (Griffin et al. 2007; Parman et al. 2007). More recently, SELDI-TOF, an extension of MALDI-TOF has been introduced as powerful tool for rapid identification of cancer-specific biomarkers and proteomic signatures. This technology has been applied to a wide variety of cancers, but needing raw samples it is not very suitable for the application on isolated mitochondria.

As discussed previously, each of these methods suffers from intrinsic technical limitations and can be suitable for some type of samples rather than others. Undoubtedly the advent of new techniques of comparative proteomics offers new possibility for investigating mitochondrial proteome. However at present there is no single proteomic technology that has the analytical capacity to permit the complete coverage of proteome of a whole cell or organelle, including mitochondria. Generally, each strategy has been found to successfully resolve a particular type of cellular components, then, depending on the aim of the study that is undertaken, one technique can be better performing for the analysis rather than others. Therefore to minimize the biases and problems associated with the individual methods it is often appropriate to combine various proteomic technologies in an attempt to obtain the maximum of proteome coverage. That is the approach carried out by McDonald et al. (2006), who compared the ability of three protein separation methods (two dimensional liquid chromatography with ProteomeLabTM PF 2D Protein Fractionation System, one-dimensional reversed phase high performance liquid chromatography, and 2-DE) to determine the relative overlap in protein separation for these technologies. In particular, isolating mitochondria and using the inner mitochondrial membrane (IMM) subproteome as model of proteome, the authors obtained a little overlap (7%) between the proteins observed by the three different separation technologies and less than 24% of proteins common between any two methods, highlighting how an integrative approach can allow a major coverage of the IMM proteome.

19.4   Mitochondrial Proteome

Although the mitochondria possess their own independent genome, the majority of the recently estimate 1,500 human mitochondrial proteins (Meisinger et al. 2008) are transcribed from the nuclear genome, translated in the cytoplasm and imported into the mitochondria, where they carry out their specific function. The proteins encoded by the mtDNA include a subset of OXPHOS components, ribosomal RNAs and transfer RNAs. Therefore the mitochondrial proteome is a dynamic program (Balaban 2010) defined both by the nuclear and the mtDNA, that can vary significantly depending on specific cellular requirements and consequently can be reprogrammed in many different pathologic conditions, such as numerous genetic defects (Pagliarini et al. 2008), metabolic diseases such as diabetes (Johnson et al. 2009) and, not least, the cancer (Krieg et al. 2004). Really, the important role that mitochondria play in a wide spectrum of human diseases is well known, typically reported in metabolic and neuromuscular diseases. By matching the 1,100 proteins from MitoCarta, a collection of nuclear and mtDNA genes encoding proteins, against genetic disorders using the Online Mendelian Inheritance in Man database (OMIM), an online catalog of human genes and genetic disorders, it has been esteemed that approximately 170 mitochondrial proteins in OMIM are involved in about 160 diseases (Huynen et al. 2009). The important association of mitochondria with various pathologies profoundly stimulated the proteomic research, leading to an increasing interest in investigating the mitochondrial proteome. During the last decade, considerable advances in genomics, proteomics and bioinformatics have made it possible to characterize the mitochondrial proteome and to systematically identify a list of over 1,000 proteins that constitute them. In particular, the human mitochondrial proteome has been extensively studied in highly purified heart mitochondria.

One of the first study on the mammalian mitochondrial proteome has been published by Taylor et al. (2003), who by analyzing highly purified mitochondria from human heart by one-dimensional SDS-PAGE and LC MS/MS, identified a set of 615 distinct proteins and estimated the total human mitochondrial proteome to be about 1,500 proteins. One year later, the same group published another study where multidimensional liquid chromatography MS/MS was investigated as an alternative means for characterizing the same sample (Gaucher et al. 2004). Taken together, the gel- and non gel-based methods applied to human heart mitochondrial proteome permitted to identified 680 proteins likely to be present in or closely associated with the mitochondria. Interestingly, a good coverage of the OXPHOS machinery was obtained. Considering that all the OXPHOS complexes were reported to be involved in one or more diseases states, these results are of particular interest and could be useful as a basis for differential expression studies of these subunits in various disease states.

This paper was followed by other interesting studies, investigating mitochondrial proteome in rat tissues by using both 2D-DIGE and quantitative mass approaches (Forner et al. 2006; Johnson et al. 2007). More recently, Pagliarini and coworkers (2008) performed a MS-based proteomics study on both highly purified mitochondrial preparations to discover genuine mitochondrial proteins and distinguish them from cytosolic contaminants. By integrating MS data with other genome-scale datasets of mitochondrial localization, they created a mitochondrial compendium of 1,098 genes and their protein expression across 14 mouse tissues. Additionally, by analyzing MS data together with a study of the evolutionary aspects of the respiratory chain formation, the authors are able to predict 19 proteins to be important for the normal function of Complex I of the electron transport chain and whose defects can cause diseases. This database represents an accurate and comprehensive molecular characterization of the organelle.

With the wealth of data arriving from wide-genomic and large-scale proteomics approaches, numerous databases have been created, that combine information on genetic, functional and pathogenetic aspects of nuclear-encoded mitochondrial proteins (MitoP2, Mitomap, MitoProteome, Human Mitochondrial Protein Database, and so on). Among these, MitoP2 (Andreoli et al. 2004) is one of the most comprehensive database, providing all relevant data on mitochondrial proteomic studies and making them readily accessible via search tools and links (http://www.mitop2.de). This database, released in 2004 in replace of an earlier version called MITOP (Scharfe et al. 2000) and regularly updated, collects results from proteome mapping, mutant screening, expression profiling, protein-protein interaction and cellular sublocalization studies, with the aim to provide a comprehensive list of mitochondrial proteins of various species, including human, also giving information about putative mitochondrial proteins identified by homology search tools.

Recently, the increasing number of identified mitochondrial protein sequences and completed mitochondrial genomes together with the need of gain an in-depth understanding of the molecular functions and processes of mitochondria has lead to the creation of the MitoInteractome, a comprehensive multi-species database containing a wealth of information on predicted protein-protein interactions, physico-chemical properties, polymorphism and diseases related to the mitochondrial proteome (Reja et al. 2009). MitoInteractome database contains 6,549 protein sequences which were extracted from the SwissProt, MitoP, MitoProteome, HPRD and Gene Ontology databases, and aims to offer aid in understanding of the molecular functions and interaction networks of mitochondrial proteins and help in identifying biomarkers for diagnosis and new molecular targets for drug development related to mitochondria. Another more recent freely accessible database, the InterMitoDatabase (Gu et al. 2011) integrates information from a wide range of resources including PubMed, KEGG, BioGRID, HPRD, DIP and IntAct.

Taken together, these databases are valuable tools for all researchers who are investigating mitochondrial physiology and dysfunction, notwithstanding they comprise only part of the estimated 697–4,532 total mitochondrial proteins (Calvo et al. 2006). It is evident that the completion of the mitochondrial proteome and the in-depth knowledge of its functions is essential not only for the possible discovery of new mitochondrial disease proteins, but also for study how the mitochondrial functional capacity could adapt to the different needs of the cell in disease state.

19.5 Proteomic Approach to Study Mitochondria and Cancer

Generally, the two major lines of research currently under investigations in mitochondrial proteomic field are: (i) a structural proteomics, which aims to identify a complete list of components of subcellular proteomes and is supported by the development of subproteome databases and (ii) a comparative proteomics, which describes proteome variations induced under various conditions (Douette and Sluse 2006).

Comparative proteomic analysis has frequently reported extensive protein alterations between normal and transformed cells, including qualitative and/or quantitative differences in several mitochondrial proteins, confirming that multiple cellular pathways were involved in the complex process of tumorigenesis. For example, in the article published by Chen and co-workers (2004), a number of proteins were found to be significantly over-expressed in squamous cell carcinoma of the oral mucosa, such as glycolytic enzymes, heat-shock proteins, tumor antigens, cytoskeleton proteins, enzymes involved in detoxification and anti-oxidation systems, and proteins involved in mitochondrial and intracellular signaling pathways.

19.6 Mitochondria, Warburg Effect and Proteomics

The proteomic approach to cancer cell metabolism seems to confirm the Warburg's original hypothesis, regarding a characteristic hyperactivation of glycolysis. In fact, a number of studies have been published describing a great heterogeneity of alterations in protein expression patterns that confirm a particular metabolic state in different neoplasias.

As recently reviewed by Scatena et al. (2010), these studies showed an altered expression of glycolytic enzymes in cancer (HK, LDH-A, aldolase – ALD-A and C, pyruvate kinase – PK-M2), even if in some case there are evident contradictory data in term of up- or down-regulation of some of them. In addition to induction of glycolytic enzymes, it is observed also an enzymes elevation of the pentose phosphate pathway, a significant reduction in the levels of components of the Krebs cycle and oxidative phosphorylation, and an increase in glucose transporter (GLUT) levels (i.e. GLUT-1). Moreover, various studies have shown induction of the HIF-1a, HIF-2a and phosphatidyl inositol 3-kinase (PI3K)/Akt. All these altered protein expression patterns, even if confirm the Warburg effect, suggest that it could be only an aspect of a more complex functional adaptation of which the cancer cell needs to fulfill the new metabolic requests.

Of particular relevance in the study of the metabolic alterations occurring in cancer cells is the role of hexokinase II (HKII), an enzyme that is physically associated to the outer surface of the external membrane of mitochondria through specific binding to a porin (voltage-dependent anion channel). This association confers HK direct access to mitochondrially generated ATP, which is one of the two substrates of HK. Importantly, mitochondrial HK is strongly elevated in rapidly growing tumour cells, being its gene promoter sensitive to typical tumour markers such as HIF-1 and P53. (Mathupala et al. 2010). These findings indicate hexokinase II as an important tool used by cancer cells to survive and proliferate under even adverse conditions, including hypoxia, being able to inhibit programmed death in cancer cells by modulating the interplay, directly and indirectly via Akt, between pro- and anti-apoptotic factors related to the Bcl-2 family (Kim and Dang 2005; Robey and Hay 2006). These observations render HK in general and mitochondrial HK in particular an interesting target for the investigation of cellular and molecular basis for the association of mitochondrial bioenergetics with tumours and could have important implications for glycolysis inhibition in cancer treatment, as demonstrated by the introduction of multiple HK inhibitors in preclinical and clinical Phase trials (for review: Scatena et al. 2008).

A number of oncoproteomic studies reported overexpression of HK in cancer cells, but few of these have correlated this induction to a specific pathogenetic mechanism involving mitochondrial physiology. For example, Danial et al. (2003) used proteomic analysis to show that BAD, a pro-apoptotic BCL-2 family member, resides in mitochondria in a functional holoenzyme complex together with the catalytic subunits of protein kinase A and protein phosphatase 1, Wiskott-Aldrich family member WAVE-1 (an A kinase-anchoring protein) and glucokinase (HK IV). This complex is fundamental for regulating the activity of this HK isoform in response to glucose, and it links the molecular mechanisms which modulate glycolysis to those which regulate apoptosis. Interestingly, in a following proteomic study, Miller et al. (2007) hypothesised that the high levels of HK present in rapidly growing tumours may serve not only to sustain elevated glycolytic rates, but also to minimize protein oxidative damage that might result in a decline in cellular activity, thereby compromising energy metabolism.

Similarly, in renal cancer, a proteomic approach based on 2-DE and MS confirmed the overexpression of proteins involved in the majority of steps in the glycolytic pathway and decreases in gluconeogenic reactions and in the levels of several mitochondrial enzymes (Unwin et al. 2003). In particular, among the various alterations reported, this study showed a tumor-specific elevation of pyruvate kinase M2. Interestingly, the dimeric form of M2-PK is predominant in cancer cells and seems to be caused by direct interaction of M2-PK with several oncoproteins (Du et al. 2007). The M2 isoform of this glycolytic protein has been studied by Christofk et al. (2008), who, by using a novel proteomic screening approach to identify phosphotyrosine-binding proteins, observed that the activity of M2-PK can be regulated by tyrosine kinase signalling pathways. In particular, binding of phosphotyrosine peptides to M2-PK results in release of the allosteric activator fructose-1,6-bisphosphate, which in turn leads to inhibition of M2-PK enzymatic activity. The authors suggest that cancer cells, by reexpressing M2-PK, acquire the ability to use glucose for anabolic processes. In addition to already cited protein modifications, the study by Unwin et al. (2003) reported an increased expression of LDH-A in renal cancer compared to normal kidney cortex. This finding is in accordance with results from other studies demonstrating that LDH-A is strongly up-regulated in neoplasia in response to intratumoural hypoxia (Fantin et al. 2006), being controlled by HIF, which binds DNA, thereby influencing transcription (Pelicano et al. 2006). It is recently demonstrated in cancer cells a shift from A/B isoenzyme pattern to the LDH-A form, that better support the conversion of pyruvate into lactate particularly under hypoxic conditions, thereby conferring a metabolic advantage to tumour cell. Conversely, a lack of LDH-B expression has been identified by MS/MS in human prostate metastatic cancer (Leiblich et al. 2006) and confirmed by an iTRAQ facilitated proteomic analysis in human prostate cancer cells with different metastatic potential (Glen et al. 2008). This a loss of LDH-B expression seems to involve promoter hypermethylation, an event frequently associated with development of prostate cancer (Leiblich et al. 2006). Interestingly, an involvement of LDH-B in tumour progression and metastasis is demonstrated also in a differential proteome analysis of hepatocellular carcinoma cells showing a downregulation of this subunit in the clone with high metastatic potential (Ding et al. 2004). Although the silencing of LDH-B has been demonstrated in a variety of tumours (Balinsky et al. 1983; Kawamoto 1994; Koukourakis et al. 2005, 2006), the underlying molecular mechanism has not been elucidated in detail. Further investigations are needed to clarify how loss of LDH-B contributes to tumour progression.

19.7 Mitochondrial Oxidative Metabolism and Oncoproteomics

After the Warburg's observation on the changes of energetic metabolism of cancer cells, an enormous amount of studies have been carried out to focus on the metabolic and structural alterations of mitochondria in many different tumours. These data have typically shown a characteristic derangement of mitochondrial metabolism in the genesis and progression of cancer (Gottschalk et al. 2004; Shaw 2006; Moreno-Sanchez et al. 2007; De Berardinis et al. 2008b).

From an oncoproteomic point of view, it is interesting to note that several mitochondrial proteins have been observed to be altered in a variety of tumour types.

In analyzing the protein expression profiles of poorly or moderately differentiated gastric carcinoma as well as those of adjacent normal tissues from 14 surgical patients, Nishigaki et al. (2005) reported several mitochondrial proteins that are differentially expressed in the tumors. Among them, three proteins, namely CLPP, COX5A, and mitochondrial enoyl coenzyme-A hydratase (ECH1), are known to play a role in mitochondrial metabolism, including redox regulation, suggesting a possible novel link between changes in mitochondrial metabolism and gastric carcinogenesis. In particular an altered expression of ECH1, that is localized to the mitochondrial matrix and functions in the second step of the mitochondrial fatty acid beta-oxidation pathway, has been reported in hepatocellular carcinoma and in prostate cancer (Wozny et al. 2007).

Similarly, a proteomic approach involving two-dimensional electrophoresis and mass spectrometry revealed that a notable group of enzymes involved in cellular redox balance results significantly altered by Ras-mediated oncogenic transformation of ovarian epithelial cell lines (Young et al. 2004). This up-regulation of the overall antioxidant capacity of transformed cells may constitute a common mechanism for tumor cells to evade apoptosis induced by high levels of ROS.

One year later, a more systematic approach to characterize mitochondrial proteome from human T leukemia cells was carried out by Rezaul et al. (2005) who identified 227 known mitochondrial proteins (membrane and soluble) and 453 additional proteins likely to be associated with mitochondria. Most of these proteins are known to functionally participate in various processes such as respiration, TCA cycle, amino acid and nucleotide metabolism, glycolysis, protection against oxidative stress, mitochondrial assembly, molecular transport, protein biosynthesis, cell cycle control, and other known cellular processes.

An altered energy metabolism in cancer cells is observed also in a study of Kim et al. (2007). Interestingly, two-dimensional electrophoresis proteomics on the mitochondria-enriched fraction in the human gastric cancer cell line AGS revealed high expression of four mitochondrial proteins: ubiquinol-cytochrome c reductase, mitochondrial short-chain ECH1, heat shock protein 60, and mitochondria elongation factor Tu. The increased levels of stress-related and chaperoning proteins (i.e. HSP70, HSP60, and mitochondrial translation elongation factor Tu protein) provide evidence of translational machinery remodelling in the gastric cancer cells, that requires not only an alternative source of energy but also an adequate support of chaperone systems. Interestingly, the mitochondrial elongation factor Tu was reported to be up-regulated also in a more recent proteomic analysis of tumorigenic and metastatic breast cancer cells (Chen et al. 2011).

Another metabolic adaptation frequently observed in cancer cells is the accelerated rate of fatty acid degradation, showed by the overexpression ECH1, which catalyzes the second step of the β-oxidation pathway. This emphasizes how the cancer cell exploit also this energy source for its altered metabolism and represent only an aspect of a more complex metabolic rearrangement that the cancer cell puts into practice to respond to the new primary requests of its uncontrolled proliferation.

Consistent with previous studies reporting a decrease of cytochrome oxidase in different neoplasias, Krieg et al. (2004) demonstrated a specific association between altered cytochrome c oxidase subunit levels and tumor-altered metabolism in normal and tumor prostate-derived cell lines.

Oncoproteomic studies have shown a downregulation of mitochondrial proteins in hepatocellular carcinoma tissues (Sun et al. 2007) and of two mitochondrial ATPase subunits (ATP5a1 and ATP5b) (Chafey et al. 2009) in mice with liver-specific deletion of Apc resulting in acute activation of beta-catenin signaling. Mitochondrial isocitrate dehydrogenase subunit α was reported overexpressed more strongly in cancer tissues than normal ones in oral squamous cell carcinoma (Hayashi et al. 2009).

The comparison of membrane fraction proteomic profiles of normal and cancerous human colorectal tissues performed with a gel-assisted digestion method and iTRAQ labeling mass spectrometry highlights various changes of protein profiles associated with the process of colorectal tumorigenesis. Among the differentially expressed proteins is SLC25A4, a member of mitochondrial solute carrier family 25A4, which consists of a number of proteins transporters of a large variety of molecules, that is significantly increased in colorectal cancer tissues compared with matched normal tissues. This protein is suggested to be one of the potential biomarkers for monitoring colorectal carcinoma (Chen et al. 2010).

In order to thoroughly understand the molecular mechanisms associated with tumorigenesis and metastasis, a subcellular proteomic strategy has been applied by Chen et al. (2011) to identify specific tumor-related markers in mitochondria. To this aim, mitochondrial proteins has been purified from three breast cells, MCF10A, MCF7, and MDA-MB-231, respectively corresponding to the normal luminal epithelial cells, the non-invasive breast cancer cells derived from luminal duct, and the invasive breast cancer cells derived from the same tissues, and subjected to 2D-DIGE and MALDI-TOF mass spectrometry. Among the numerous differentially expressed spots identified by their peptide fingerprint, 33 proteins belonged to mitochondrial proteins, most of which are involved in electron transport, metabolism and protein folding. These include cytochrome c oxidase subunit 5B, malate dehydrogenase and elongation factor Tu which are highly expressed in both low invasive and aggressive breast cancer cells. Interestingly, several of the identified proteins such as calcium-binding mitochondrial carrier protein SCaMC-1 is overexpressed in common non-invasive and invasive breast cancer cells.

19.8 Mitochondria, Oncoproteomics and HIFs

It is well known that the cancer cells are frequently exposed to reduced availability of nutrient and inadequate O_2 concentrations, which decline as the distance from the vessel increases (Harris 2002; Brahimi-Horn et al. 2007). This may lead to epigenetic and genetic adaptation of clones that, escaping this oxygen deficient microenvironment, acquire increased invasiveness and metastasis.

A major mechanism mediating adaptive responses to reduced O_2 availability is the regulation of transcription by hypoxia-inducible factor 1 (HIF-1) (Semenza 2009). The levels of HIF-1a itself can be regulated by hypoxia transcriptionally and posttranslationally through ubiquitination. In addition, adaptive response mediated by HIF-1 complex involves the regulation of genes that respond to changes in available oxygen in the cellular environment, specifically to decreases in oxygen concentration. The hundreds of genes that are induced by hypoxia in an HIF-1-dependent manner encode proteins that have key roles in every critical aspect of cancer biology. Among these functions, the most fundamental may be angiogenesis (Liao and Johnson 2007), which has been a major focus of cancer biology and therapy over the past decade, and glucose/energy metabolism (Swietach et al. 2007; Chiche et al. 2009; Semenza 2009), which is already being studied and probably will be more extensively investigated in the next decade.

In response to hypoxia, HIF-1 is up-regulated, which enhances expression of glycolytic enzymes and concurrently it down regulates mitochondrial respiration through up-regulation of pyruvate dehydrogenase kinase 1 (PDK1) (see recent reviews Semenza 2009; Solaini et al. 2010). Specifically, HIF-1 induces expression of PDK1, PDK1 phosphorylates and inactivates PDH, the mitochondrial enzyme that converts pyruvate into acetyl-CoA. Thereby, in combination with the hypoxia-induced expression of LDH-A, which converts pyruvate into lactate, PDK1 reduces the delivery of acetyl-CoA to the tricarboxylic acid cycle. Moreover, the subunit composition of cytochrome oxidase (COX) is altered in hypoxic cells by increased expression of the COX4-2 subunit, which optimises COX activity under hypoxic conditions, and increased degradation of the COX4-1 subunit, which optimises COX activity under aerobic conditions (Semenza 2007).

Proteomic studies have confirmed the fundamental role for HIF-1a in breast and prostate cancer biology, specifically in the early stages of mammary and prostate carcinogenesis (Kimbro and Simons 2006). Moreover, its expression is correlated with diagnostic and prognostic indicators for early relapse and metastatic disease. For these reasons, HIF-1a is considered a potential prognostic biomarker in proteomic assessments of breast, prostate, lung and gastric cancers (Vaupel 2004; Kimbro and Simons 2006; Semenza 2007; Denko 2008; Vander Heiden et al. 2009).

Interestingly, Liu et al. showed in gastric cancer a novel thyroid hormone-mediated tumourigenic signaling pathway in which T(3)-induced overexpression of HIF1-a was mediated by fumarate accumulation (Liu et al. 2009). It could be interesting to evaluate the potential role of succinate accumulation in stabilizing HIF-1a (due to mutations in the succinate dehydrogenase B or succinate dehydrogenase D genes that inhibit HIF prolylhydroxylase) via a proteomic approach to clarify the complex protein modulation mediating this important phenomenon (Frezza and Gottlieb 2009).

Taken together, these experimental and clinical data delineate an important role for HIF-1 in mediating radiation resistance and provide a therapeutic rationale for clinical trials that combine radiation therapy with HIF-1 inhibitors (Semenza 2010).

One aspect that has been partially disregarded in the analysis of cancer cell metabolism in general and in that of the Warburg effect in particular is the pentose phosphate pathway. Interestingly, oncoproteomic studies have already detected the enzymes induction of this metabolic in liver cancers, breast cancer metastases and in different prostate cancer cell lines (Vaupel 2004; Lee et al. 2005; Shaw 2006; Bottoni et al. 2009). As previously noted, some proteomic studies showed an impaired tricarboxylic acid cycle in certain types of cancers, while it was variable in others. However, the meaning of this impairment should be carefully evaluated. In fact, the Krebs cycle, such as mitochondrial oxidative metabolism in general, could be reduced simply due to the shifting of some substrates towards anabolic pathways (Moreno-Sanchez et al. 2007; De Berardinis et al. 2008a; Scatena et al. 2008).

19.9 Mitochondrial HSP-70 and Oncoproteomics

Another interesting mitochondrial protein over-expressed in cancer is mortalin, also known as mitochondrial heat-shock protein 70, to which have been ascribed numerous cellular functions, such as the control of cell proliferation, cellular senescence and immortalisation. Different proteomic approaches have confirmed the correlation between HSP70 overexpression and the differentiation level and/or aggressiveness of various types of cancer. As examples, we cite proteomic studies of gastric adenocarcinoma (He et al. 2004), hepatocarcinoma (Bottoni et al. 2009) and oesophageal cancer (Jazii et al. 2006). Interestingly, in colorectal adenocarcinoma mortalin overexpression was found to correlate with a poor prognosis (Dundas et al. 2005). More interestingly from a therapeutic point of view for potential clinical applications, various oncoproteomics studies correlate elevated levels of HSP70 with therapeutic resistance (Voss et al. 2001; Castagna et al. 2004; Allal et al. 2004; Smith et al. 2007; Short et al. 2007). A useful example is the study of Pocaly et al. (2008), which utilised a proteomic approach to analyse the molecular basis of resistance to imatinib, a tyrosine kinase inhibitor that is used as a front-line therapy in chronic myeloid leukaemia. Among the identified proteins, the authors observed a differential expression of HSP70 suggesting a role for these proteins in the development of imatinib resistance. Of note, elevated levels of mortalin have also been observed in many in vitro-immortalized and tumor-derived cells, and tumor tissues and has been evidenced to significantly contribute to cancerogenesis. Interestingly, this protein is mainly found in mitochondria, but also in cytosol. Depending on its intracellular distribution and on its interactions with other proteins, numerous different effects have been ascribed to mortalin. In cytosol this protein is able to sequester the tumor suppressor protein p53 (Wadhwa et al. 2002), as well as to activate the oncogenic Ras-Raf signaling pathway (Wadhwa et al. 2003), which controls cell proliferation and is often deregulated in tumors.

19.10 Mitochondria, Oncoproteomics and Resistance

Another important consequence of malignant transformation of the cells is their acquired resistance to apoptotic cell death. As well known, two are the major apoptotic pathways. The extrinsic one (receptor-mediated) involves formation of a death-inducing signal complex (DISC) consisting of Fas, Fas-associated death domain (FADD), and procaspase 8, which subsequently activates procaspase 3 and other effector caspases. By contrast, the permeabilization of the outer mitochondrial membrane followed by release of cytochrome c is considered a key event during the early phase of the mitochondria-mediated apoptotic process. The resulting cascade of events, involving the activation of procaspase 9 and other effector caspases, determine the cleavage of a variety of cellular proteins, leading to cell death via intrinsic apoptosis. In addition, mitochondrial production of ROS also seems to play a role in cell death, in regulating the process involved in the initiation of apoptotic signaling. Most chemotherapeutic agents induce apoptosis through at least one of these pathways. Several functional proteomic studies were undertaken in an attempt to investigate the mechanisms by which chemotherapeutic agents perform their antineoplastic action. For example, by applying 2-DE approach on human nasopharyngeal carcinoma cell lines exposed to gold(III) porphyrin 1a, Wang et al. (2005) identified a number of altered proteins, including enzymes participating in energy production and proteins involved in cellular redox balance. These alteration suggest that gold(III) porphyrin 1a induced apoptosis by mitochondrial death pathways related to ROS.

In evaluating the variation of proteomic profile in the mitochondrial fraction of adrenocortical carcinoma cell line after exposure to mitotane, Stigliano et al. (2008) observed an alteration of proteins involved in energetic metabolism, stress response, cytoskeleton structure, and tumorigenesis. In particular, owing to drug-treatment, aldolase A, peroxiredoxin I, heterogenous nuclear ribonucleoprotein A2/B1, tubulin-beta isoform II, heat shock cognate 71 kDa protein, and D, and heat shock 70 kDa protein 1A were up regulated.

In addition to analyze the modulation of protein expression profiles in cancer cells induced by antineoplastic drugs, the knowledge of signaling pathways and proteins that contributes to the resistance against apoptosis-inducing therapeutic regimens is fundamental for establish new therapeutic protocols aimed to selectively target rapidly proliferating cancer cells. To this aim, various researchers deemed advantageous to use a proteomic approach. In fact, from an oncoproteomic point of view, it is reasonable to expect that drug radioresistance reveals a global changes in expression levels of proteins involved in various intracellular pathways. Various proteomic studies have been recently published investigating molecular mechanisms by which cancer cells overcome the cytotoxic effects of radiation and showing alterations in protein expression levels associated with anticancer drug-resistances.

Changes in mitochondrial protein abundances were found in MCF-7 human breast cancer cells selected for resistance to adriamycin accompanied by verapamil (Strong et al. 2006). Specifically, the increased abundance detected for two key enzymes involved in fatty acid oxidation, 3,2 trans-enoyl CoA isomerase and the trifunctional enzyme α-subunit, suggests that this metabolic alteration could favor drug-resistant cancer cells in supporting ATP synthesis. Moreover increased levels of proteins involved in ATP production, such as adenylate kinase 2 and three truncated α-ATP synthase isoforms were reported in this study, whereas decreased levels of cytochrome c oxidase subunit Vb were also detected.

Another study investigating the alterations of mitochondrial proteome induced in non-Hodgkin lymphoma by adriamycin reported increased levels of HSP70, ATP-binding cassette transporter isoform B6 (ABCB6) and prohibitin (PHB), that seem to be closely related to chemoresistance (Jiang et al. 2009).

By shotgun analysis, alterations in the abundances of proteins in soluble mitochondrial fractions of a mitoxantrone-resistant MCF-7 cell line and its parental drug susceptible cell line were investigated by Wang et al. (2007) to provide enhanced understanding of drug resistance. Of particular interest are several proteins shown to have altered abundances in the drug-resistant cell line, such as apoptosis inhibitor 5 and PHB, that are reported to be potent suppressors of the E2F-dependent apoptotic pathway. Also galectin-3 binding protein, which is involved in regulation of tumor proliferation, angiogenesis and apoptosis, was found increased in MX cells, thereby contributing to evasion of apoptosis and cell survival.

Consistent with previous results reporting a bioenergetic dysfunction of mitochondria in many types of cancers, Shin et al. (2005), to screen for proteins possibly responsible for 5-fluorouacil (5-FU) resistance, showed a down-regulation of the alpha subunit of mitochondrial F(1)F(0)-ATP synthase (ATP-α) that results in decreased ATP synthase activity in drug-resistant cells compared with parent cells. They also established a positive correlation between ATP synthase expression and 5-FU sensitivity in human colorectal cancer cell lines. Other findings supporting a link between chemoresistance and ATP synthase down-regulation, probably imputable to reduced oxidative phosphorylation capability that hampers the apoptotic potential of the cancer cell (Dey and Moraes 2000), were provided by Dai et al. (2010). In mitochondrial comparative proteomics of human ovarian cancer cells and their platinum-resistant sublines, they identified a list of differentially expressed spots, among which five mitochondrial proteins involved energy metabolism and electron transfer respiratory chain, including such as ATP-α, thioredoxin-dependent peroxide reductase, mitochondrial precursor (PRDX), PHB, ETF (electron transfer flavoprotein), and ALDH (aldehyde dehydrogenase) that were all downregulated platinum-resistant cell lines. In particular, the differential expression in tumor cells of one of them, the PHB, has been examined in several studies, many of which reported elevated levels in transformed cells in respect to normal. The precise molecular function of the PHB complex is not clear, but a growing body of evidence suggests for PHB a role in apoptosis, by modulation of transcription (Fusaro et al. 2003) or by inhibition of the intrinsic apoptotic pathway (Gregory-Bass et al. 2008), in addition to its action as chaperone for respiration chain proteins. It is recently showed by a proteomic approach that PHB1 levels are significantly elevated in membrane fractions isolated from paclitaxel-resistant sublines compared to their normal drug-sensitive sublines, but whole cell levels of protein were unchanged (Patel et al. 2010). Also a comparative analysis of the proteome of ribosomal proteins of human colon cancer cell line and its 5-FU-resistant subline showed a significative upregulation of PHB, whose modulation may be related to 5-FU resistance (Kimura et al. 2010). In the already cited study, Chen et al. (2011) reported that PHB was is downregulated in mitochondrial fractions of non-invasive and invasive breast cancer cells, but appears confined in their nucleous. Moreover it has been demonstrated that PHB may accumulate on the cell membrane where it can interact with peptides and endogenous ligands. Then, these apparently contrasting results could be explain with a differential distribution of the PHB not only between normal and tumor cells, but also between various intracellular compartments. Intriguingly, this protein has been shown to migrate from an intracellular compartment to one on the cell surface that mediates the drug-resistant phenotype (Fusaro et al. 2003). This suggests that the cellular localization of the PHB rather than the total amount of this protein in the cell, may be relevant to drug-resistance phenotype (Patel et al. 2010).

From a therapeutic point of view, considering that mitochondria are the cellular powerhouse and the primary source of energy for the cell, there is an increasing interest in developing compounds selectively targeting mitochondria for the treatment of neoplasia. Proteomic methods and bioinformatics tools are currently utilized also for preclinical evaluation of a series of novel, small molecule compounds with presumed anti-cancer activities, to assess their anti-proliferative efficacy in a panel of cancer cell lines as well as in a mouse model of human breast cancer (Millard et al. 2010). The mechanism of action of these compounds containing a triphenylphosphine, that are able to significantly affected signaling pathways relevant to growth and proliferation, includes mitochondrial localization that causes decreased oxygen consumption, with concomitant increase in superoxide production and attenuation of growth factor signaling.

19.11 Mitochondrial Phosphoproteome and Cancer

Protein phosphorylation is the posttranslational modification commonly more investigated by proteomic analysis. As well know reversible phosphorylation of proteins is an important regulatory mechanism which plays a significant role in a wide range of cellular processes, including in the signaling process targeting proteins to the mitochondria. One of the first examples of systematic documentation of mitochondrial phosphoproteome in cancer was provided by the research of Guo et al. (2011). The integration of LC-MS/MS-based and protein antibody array-based proteomics with genomics approaches permitted to investigate the phosphoproteome and transcriptome of gastric cancer cell lines and endoscopic gastric biopsies from normal subjects and patients suffering from benign gastritis or gastric cancer (Guo et al. 2011). Of note, a percentage of overexpressed phosphoproteins were associated with mitochondria, including proteins of the electron transfer chain, mitochondrial permeability transition pore, mitochondrial ribosomal proteins, as well as various enzymes involved in apoptosis and metabolism. These results support the role of the poorly understood regulation of the posttranslational signaling network within the mitochondria, further confirming (providing additional evidence of) as critical is their role in oncogenic process in general and in cancer oncogenesis in particular. It could be advantageous to explore also this interesting area of mitochondrial posttranslational modifications to have an expansive view of key regulatory mechanisms that control oncogenesis and to better understand the role and function of the mitochondria in health and disease.

19.12 Concluding Remarks

In last years, it is becoming clear the importance of the proteomic approach as a useful tool to gain valuable information on mitochondrial physiology. Advances in proteomic technologies have made possible not only to carry out a structural proteomic analysis on complete set of proteins which composes the mitochondrial proteome, but also to perform a quantitative analysis of protein expression in mitochondria cancer cells, in an attempt to obtain differential mitochondrial protein profiles in normal and cancer cells. In addition, the recent creation of mitochondrial proteomic databases permits to integrate information on genetic, functional and pathogenetic aspects of nuclear-encoded mitochondrial proteins. We believe that, besides providing data on up- or down-regulation of one or a number of proteins that result altered in carcinogenesis process, the mitochondrial proteomics, if compared to data obtained from the cell proteome, can give more interesting information on the true mitochondrial status in the cell. Undoubtedly these integrative studies can lead to the identification of markers for clinical detection of cancer, and contribute to an better understanding of how differential protein expression might influence the development of the disease. Additionally, integrative analysis of the phosphoproteome and transcriptome could provide a more complete picture of molecular signaling pathways and of key regulatory mechanisms that control oncogenesis. At present, the proteomic approach to cancer cell metabolism seems to confirm the Warburg's subtle observation regarding an hyperactivation of glycolysis. However, continuing to consider glycolysis as the sole energetic metabolic pathway that neoplastic cell uses for its remarkable metabolic request will never permit to fully understand the mechanisms regulating the environmental adaptation of cancer. In fact, it is becoming ever more evident that the aerobic glycolytic state of cancer cells is only an aspect of a more complex metabolic rearrangement that occurs into neoplastic cell. Also oncoproteomic field, in demonstrating all the complexity of cancer cell metabolism, confirmed the results of other studies in suggesting a more active role of mitochondria in cancer and requiring a revision of so-called Warburg effect. Importantly, accumulating evidence of a strict correlation among glycolysis, oxidative phosphorylation and cancer cell phenotype underlines that cancer cell adopts, by a strong selective program, a particular metabolic profile that tends to utilize every available metabolic pathway to fulfill its only purpose, (i.e. uncontrolled proliferation). Finally, a more systematic approach to the definition of the mitochondrial proteomic profile of normal and neoplastic cell could have important biological and clinical implications, not only for evaluating new and more effective anticancer therapies, but also for biomarker identification and monitoring of disease progression.

References

Allal AS, Kahne T, Reverdin AK et al (2004) Radioresistance-related proteins in rectal cancer. Proteomics 4:2261–2269

Andreoli C, Prokisch H, Hortnagel K et al (2004) MitoP2, an integrated database on mitochondrial proteins in yeast and man. Nucleic Acids Res 32:D459–D462

Balaban RS (2010) The mitochondrial proteome: a dynamic functional program in tissues and disease states. Environ Mol Mutagen 51:352–359

Balinsky D, Platz CE, Lewis JW (1983) Isozyme patterns of normal, benign, and malignant human breast tissues. Cancer Res 43:5895–5901

Baysal BE, Ferrell RE, Willett-Brozick JE et al (2000) Mutations in SDHD, a mitochondrial complex II gene, in hereditary paraganglioma. Science 287:848–851

Bottoni P, Giardina B, Vitali A et al (2009) A proteomic approach to characterizing ciglitazone-induced cancer cell differentiation in Hep-G2 cell line. Biochim Biophys Acta 1794:615–626

Brahimi-Horn MC, Chiche J, Pouysségur J (2007) Hypoxia and cancer. J Mol Med 85:1301–1307

Brandon M, Baldi P, Wallace DC (2006) Mitochondrial mutations in cancer. Oncogene 25:4647–4662

Calvo S, Mohit J, Xie X et al (2006) Systematic identification of human mitochondrial disease genes through integrated genomics. Nat Genet 38:576–582

Castagna A, Antonioli P, Astner H et al (2004) A proteomic approach to cisplatin resistance in the cervix squamous cell carcinoma cell line A431. Proteomics 4:3246–3267

Chafey P, Finzi L, Boisgard R et al (2009) Proteomic analysis of beta-catenin activation in mouse liver by DIGE analysis identifies glucose metabolism as a new target of the Wnt pathway. Proteomics 9:3889–3900

Chen J, He QY, Yuen AP, Chiu JF (2004) Proteomics of buccal squamous cell carcinoma: the involvement of multiple pathways in tumorigenesis. Proteomics 4:2465–2475

Chen JS, Chen KT, Fan CW et al (2010) Comparison of membrane fraction proteomic profiles of normal and cancerous human colorectal tissues with gel-assisted digestion and iTRAQ labeling mass spectrometry. FEBS J 277: 3028–3038

Chen YW, Chou HC, Lyu PC et al (2011) Mitochondrial proteomics analysis of tumorigenic and metastatic breast cancer markers. Funct Integr Genomics 11:225–239

Chiche J, Ilc K, Laferrière J et al (2009) Hypoxia-inducible carbonic anhydrase IX and XII promote tumor cell growth by counteracting acidosis through the regulation of the intracellular pH. Cancer Res 69:358–368

Christofk HR, Vander Heiden MG, Wu N (2008) Pyruvate kinase M2 is a phosphotyrosinebinding protein. Nature 452: 181–186

Dai Z, Yin J, He H et al (2010) Mitochondrial comparative proteomics of human ovarian cancer cells and their platinum-resistant sublines. Proteomics 10:3789–3799

Danial NN, Gramm CF, Scorrano L et al (2003) BAD and glucokinase reside in a mitochondrial complex that integrates glycolysis and apoptosis. Nature 424:896–897

De Berardinis RJ, Lum JJ, Hatzivassiliou G, Thompson CB (2008a) The biology of cancer: metabolic reprogramming fuels cell growth and proliferation. Cell Metab 7:11–20

De Berardinis RJ, Sayed N, Ditsworth D, Thompson CB (2008b) Brick by brick: metabolism and tumor cell growth. Curr Opin Genet Dev 18:54–61

Denko NC (2008) Hypoxia, HIF1 and glucose metabolism in the solid tumour. Nat Rev Cancer 8:705–713

Dey R, Moraes CT (2000) Lack of oxidative phosphorylation and low mitochondrial membrane potential decrease susceptibility to apoptosis and do not modulate the protective effect of Bcl-x(L) in osteosarcoma cells. J Biol Chem 275:7087–7094

Ding SJ, Li Y, Shao XX et al (2004) Proteome analysis of hepatocellular carcinoma cell strains, MHCC97- H and MHCC97-L, with different metastasis potentials. Proteomics 4:982–994

Douette P, Sluse FE (2006) Mitochondrial uncoupling proteins: new insights from functional and proteomic studies. Free Radic Biol Med 40:1097–1107

Du XL, Hu H, Lin DC et al (2007) Proteomic profiling of proteins dysregulated in Chinese esophageal squamous cell carcinoma. J Mol Med 85:863–875

Dundas SR, Lawrie LC, Rooney PH, Murray GI (2005) Mortalin is over-expressed by colorectal adenocarcinomas and correlates with poor survival. J Pathol 205:74–81

Fantin VR, St-Pierre J, Leder P (2006) Attenuation of LDH-A expression uncovers a link between glycolysis, mitochondrial physiology, and tumor maintenance. Cancer Cell 9:425–434

Fliss MS, Usadel H, Caballero OL et al (2000) Facile detection of mitochondrial DNA mutations in tumors and bodily fluids. Science 287:2017–2019

Forner F, Foster LJ, Campanaro S et al (2006) Quantitative proteomic comparison of rat mitochondria from muscle, heart, and liver. Mol Cell Proteomics 5:608–619

Frezza C, Gottlieb E (2009) Mitochondria in cancer: not just innocent bystanders. Semin Cancer Biol 19:4–11

Fusaro G, Dasgupta P, Rastogi S et al (2003) Prohibitin induces the transcriptional activity of p53 and is exported from the nucleus upon apoptotic signaling. J Biol Chem 278:47853–47861

Galluzzi L, Morselli E, Kepp O et al (2010) Mitochondrial gateways to cancer. Mol Aspects Med 31:1–20

Garber K (2006) Energy deregulation: licensing tumor to grow. Science 312:1158–1159

Gaucher SP, Taylor SW, Fahy E et al (2004) Expanded coverage of the human heart mitochondrial proteome using multidimensional liquid chromatography coupled with tandem mass spectrometry. J Proteome Res 3:495–505

Glen A, Gan CS, Hamdy FC et al (2008) iTRAQfacilitated proteomic analysis of human prostate cancer cells identifies proteins associated with progression. J Proteome Res 7:897–907

Gottschalk S, Anderson N, Hainz C et al (2004) Imatinib (STI571) – mediated changes in glucose metabolism in human leukaemia BCR-ABL-positive cells. Clin Cancer Res 10:6661–6668

Gregory-Bass RC, Olatinwo M, Xu W et al (2008) Prohibitin silencing reverses stabilization of mitochondrial integrity and chemoresistance in ovarian cancer cells by increasing their sensitivity to apoptosis. Int J Cancer 122:1923–1930

Griffin TJ, Xie H, Brandhakavi S et al (2007) iTRAQ reagent-based quantitative proteomic analysis on a linear ion trap mass spectrometer. J Proteome Res 6:4200–4209

Gu Z, Li J, Gao S et al (2011) InterMitoBase: an annotated database and analysis platform of protein-protein interactions for human mitochondria. BMC Genomics 12:335

Guo T, Lee SS, Ng WH et al (2011) Global molecular dysfunctions in gastric cancer revealed by an integrated analysis of the phosphoproteome and transcriptome. Cell Mol Life Sci 68:1983–2002

Gygi SP, Rist B, Gerber SA et al (1999) Quantitative analysis of complex protein mixtures using isotope-coded affinity tags. Nat Biotechnol 17:994–999

Hammerman PS, Fox CJ, Thompson CB (2004) Beginnings of a signal-transduction pathway for bioenergetic control of cell survival. Trends Biochem Sci 29:586–592

Hanahan D, Weinberg RA (2000) The hallmarks of cancer. Cell 100:57–70

Harris AL (2002) Hypoxia-a key regulatory factor in tumor growth. Nat Rev Cancer 2:38–47

Harsha HC, Jimeno A, Molina H et al (2008) Activated epidermal growth factor receptor as a novel target in pancreatic cancer therapy. J Proteome Res 7:4651–4658

Hayashi E, Kuramitsu Y, Fujimoto M et al (2009) Proteomic profiling of differential display analysis for human oral squamous cell carcinoma: 14-3-3 σ Protein is upregulated in human oral squamous cell carcinoma and dependent on the differentiation level. Proteomics Clin Appl 3:1338–1347

He QY, Cheung YH, Leung SY et al (2004) Diverse proteomic alterations in gastric adenocarcinoma. Proteomics 4:3276–3287

Huynen MA, de Hollander M, Szklarczyk R (2009) Mitochondrial proteome evolution and genetic disease. Biochim Biophys Acta 1792:1122–1129

Ibarrola N, Molina H, Iwahori A, Pandey A (2004) A novel proteomic approach for specific identification of tyrosine kinase substrates using 13C tyrosine. J Biol Chem 279:15805–15813

Jazii FR, Najafi Z, Malekzadeh R et al (2006) Identification of squamous cell carcinoma associated proteins by proteomics and loss of beta tropomyosin expression in esophageal cancer. World J Gastroenterol 12:7104–7112

Jiang YJ, Sun Q, Fang XS, Wang X (2009) Comparative mitochondrial proteomic analysis of Rji cells exposed to adriamycin. Mol Med 15:173–182

Johnson DT, Harris RA, French S et al (2007) Tissue heterogeneity of the mammalian mitochondrial proteome. Am J Physiol Cell Physiol 292:C689–C697

Johnson DT, Harris RA, French S et al (2009) Proteomic changes associated with diabetes in the BB-DP rat. Am J Physiol Endocrinol Metab 293:E422–E432

Kawamoto M (1994) Breast cancer diagnosis by lactate dehydrogenase isozymes in nipple discharge. Cancer 73:1836–1841

Kim JW, Dang CV (2005) Multifaceted roles of glycolytic enzymes. Trends Biochem Sci 30:142–150

Kim JW, Dang CV (2007) Cancer's molecular sweet tooth and the Warburg effect. Cancer Res 66:8927–8930

Kim HK, Park WS, Kang SH et al (2007) Mitochondrial alterations in human gastric carcinoma cell line. Am J Physiol Cell Physiol 293:C761–C771

Kimbro KS, Simons JW (2006) Hypoxia-inducible factor-1 in human breast and prostate cancer. Endocr Relat Cancer 13:739–749

Kimura K, Wada A, Ueta M et al (2010) Comparative proteomic analysis of the ribosomes in 5-fluorouracil resistance of a human colon cancer cell line using the radical-free and highly reducing method of two-dimensional polyacrylamide gel electrophoresis. Int J Oncol 37:1271–1278

Koukourakis MI, Giatromanolaki A, Simopoulos C et al (2005) Lactate dehydrogenase 5 (LDH5) relates to up-regulated hypoxia inducible factor pathway and metastasis in colorectal cancer. Clin Exp Metastasis 22:25–30

Koukourakis MI, Giatromanolaki A, Polychronidis A et al (2006) Endogenous markers of hypoxia/ anaerobic metabolism and anemia in primary colorectal cancer. Cancer Sci 97:582–588

Krieg RC, Knuechel R, Schiffmann E et al (2004) Mitochondrial proteome: cancer-altered metabolism associated with cytochrome c oxidase subunit level variation. Proteomics 4:2789–2795

Lee JD, Yang WI, Park YN et al (2005) Different glucose uptake and glycolytic mechanisms between hepatocellular carcinoma and intrahepatic mass-forming cholangiocarcinoma with increased (18)F-FDG uptake. J Nucl Med 46:1753–1759

Leiblich A, Cross SS, Catto JW et al (2006) Lactate dehydrogenase-B is silenced by promoter hypermethylation in human prostate cancer. Oncogene 25:2953–2960

Liao D, Johnson RS (2007) Hypoxia: a key regulator of angiogenesis in cancer. Cancer Metastasis Rev 26:281–290

Liu R, Li Z, Bai S et al (2009) Mechanism of cancer cell adaptation to metabolic stress: proteomics identification of a novel thyroid hormone-mediated gastric carcinogenic signaling pathway. Mol Cell Proteomics 8:70–85

Mathupala SP, Ko YH, Pedersen PL (2010) The pivotal roles of mitochondria in cancer: Warburg and beyond and encouraging prospects for effective therapies. Biochim Biophys Acta 1797:1225–1230

Mathy G, Sluse FE (2008) Mitochondrial comparative proteomics: strengths and pitfalls. Biochim Biophys Acta 1777:1072–1077

McDonald T, Sheng S, Stanley B et al (2006) Expanding the subproteome of the inner mitochondria using protein separation technologies: one- and two-dimensional liquid chromatography and two-dimensional gel electrophoresis. Mol Cell Proteomics 5:2392–2411

Meisinger C, Sickmann A, Pfanner N (2008) The mitochondrial proteome: from inventory to function. Cell 134:22–24

Michal G (1999) Biochemical pathways: an atlas of biochemistry and molecular biology. Wiley, New York

Millard M, Pathania D, Shabaik Y et al (2010) Preclinical evaluation of novel triphenylphosphonium salts with broad-spectrum activity. PLoS One 5(10):e13131

Miller S, Ross-Inta C, Giulivi C (2007) Kinetic and proteomic analyses of S-nitrosoglutathione-treated hexokinase A: consequences for cancer energy metabolism. Amino Acids 32:593–602

Mootha VK, Bunkenborg J, Olsen JV et al (2003) Integrated analysis of protein composition, tissue diversity, and gene regulation in mouse mitochondria. Cell 115:629–640

Moreno-Sanchez R, Rodriguez-Enriquez S, Marin-Hernandez A, Saavedra E (2007) Energy metabolism in tumor cells. FEBS J 274:1393–1418

Nishigaki R, Osaki M, Hiratsuka M et al (2005) Proteomic identification of differentially-expressed genes in human gastric carcinomas. Proteomics 5:3205–3213

Ong SE, Mann M (2006) A practical recipe for stable isotope labeling by amino acids in cell culture (SILAC). Nat Protoc 1:2650–2660

Pagliarini DJ, Calvo SE, Chang B et al (2008) A mitochondrial protein compendium elucidates complex I disease biology. Cell 134:112–123

Parman CE, Javali H, Wood D et al (2007) P207-T protein identification and quantitative analysis of complex mixtures using a peptide-based isobaric mass tagging technology. J Biomol Technol 18:72

Patel N, Chatterjee SK, Vrbanac V et al (2010) Rescue of paclitaxel sensitivity by repression of Prohibitin1 in drug-resistant cancer cells. Proc Natl Acad Sci USA 107:2503–2508

Pelicano H, Martin DS, Xu RH, Huang P (2006) Glycolysis inhibition for anticancer treatment. Oncogene 25:4633–4646

Pflieger D, Le Caer JP, Lemaire C et al (2002) Systematic identification of mitochondrial proteins by LC-MS/MS. Anal Chem 74:2400–2406

Pocaly M, Lagarde V, Etienne G et al (2008) Proteomic analysis of an imatinib-resistant K562 cell line highlights opposing roles of heat shock cognate 70 and heat shock 70 proteins in resistance. Proteomics 8:2394–2406

Reja R, Venkatakrishnan AJ, Lee J et al (2009) MitoInteractome: mitochondrial protein interactome database, and its application in 'aging network' analysis. BMC Genomics 10(Suppl 3):S20

Rezaul K, Wu L, Mayya V et al (2005) A systematic characterization of mitochondrial proteome from human T leukemia cells. Mol Cell Proteomics 4:169–181

Robey RB, Hay N (2006) Mitochondrial hexokinases, novel mediators of the antiapoptotic effects of growth factors and Akt. Oncogene 25:4683–4696

Scatena R, Bottoni P, Pontoglio A et al (2008) Glycolytic enzyme inhibitors in cancer treatment. Expert Opin Investig Drugs 17:1533–1545

Scatena R, Bottoni P, Pontoglio A, Giardina B (2010) Revisiting the Warburg effect in cancer cells with proteomics. The emergence of new approaches to diagnosis, prognosis and therapy. Proteomics Clin Appl 4:143–158

Scharfe C, Zaccaria P, Hoertnagel K et al (2000) MITOP, the mitochondrial proteome database: 2000 update. Nucleic Acids Res 28:155–158

Semenza GL (2007) Oxygen-dependent regulation of mitochondrial respiration by hypoxia-inducible factor 1. Biochem J 405:1–9

Semenza GL (2009) Regulation of cancer cell metabolism by hypoxia-inducible factor 1. Semin Cancer Biol 19:12–16

Semenza GL (2010) Defining the role of hypoxia-inducible factor 1 in cancer biology and therapeutics. Oncogene 29:625–634

Shaw RJ (2006) Glucose metabolism and cancer. Curr Opin Cell Biol 18:598–608

Shin YK, Yoo BC, Chang HJ et al (2005) Down-regulation of mitochondrial F1F0-ATP synthase in human colon cancer cells with induced 5-fluorouracil resistance. Cancer Res 65:3162–3170

Short DM, Heron ID, Birse-Archbold JL et al (2007) Apoptosis induced by staurosporine alters chaperone and endoplasmic reticulum proteins: identification by quantitative proteomics. Proteomics 7:3085–3096

Sickmann A, Reinders J, Wagner Y et al (2003) The proteome of Saccharomyces cerevisiae mitochondria. Proc Natl Acad Sci USA 100:13207–13212

Smith L, Welham KJ, Watson MB et al (2007) The proteomic analysis of cisplatin resistance in breast cancer cells. Oncol Res 16:497–506

Solaini G, Baracca A, Lenaz G, Sgarbi G (2010) Hypoxia and mitochondrial oxidative metabolism. Biochim Biophys Acta 1797:1171–1177

Stigliano A, Cerquetti L, Borro M et al (2008) Modulation of proteomic profile in H295R adrenocortical cell line induced by mitotane. Endocr Relat Cancer 15:1–10

Strong R, Nakanishi T, Ross D, Fenselau C (2006) Alterations in the mitochondrial proteome of adriamycin resistant MCF-7 breast cancer cells. J Proteome Res 5:2389–2395

Sun W, Xing B, Sun Y et al (2007) Proteome analysis of hepatocellular carcinoma by two-dimensional difference gel electrophoresis: novel protein markers in hepatocellular carcinoma tissues. Mol Cell Proteomics 6:1798–1808

Swietach P, Vaughan-Jones RD, Harris AL (2007) Regulation of tumor pH and the role of carbonic anhydrase 9. Cancer Metastasis Rev 26:299–310

Takahashi A, Ohtani N, Yamakoshi K et al (2006) Mitogenic signalling and the p16INK4a-Rb pathway cooperate to enforce irreversible cellular senescence. Nat Cell Biol 8:1291–1297

Taylor SW, Fahy E, Zhang B et al (2003) Characterization of the human heart mitochondrial proteome. Nat Biotechnol 21:281–286

Tomlinson IP, Alam NA, Rowan AJ et al (2002) Germline mutations in FH predispose to dominantly inherited uterine fibroids, skin leiomyomata and papillary renal cell cancer. Nat Genet 30:406–410

Unlu M, Morgan ME, Minden JS (1997) Difference gel electrophoresis: a single gel method for detecting changes in protein extracts. Electrophoresis 18:2071–2077

Unwin RD, Craven RA, Harnden P et al (2003) Proteomic changes in renal cancer and co-ordinate demonstration of both the glycolytic and mitochondrial aspects of the Warburg effect. Proteomics 3:1620–1632

Vander Heiden MG, Cantley LC, Thompson CB (2009) Understanding the Warburg effect: the metabolic requirements of cell proliferation. Science 324:1029–1033

Vaupel P (2004) The role of hypoxia-induced factors in tumor progression. Oncologist 9:10–17

Verma M, Kagan J, Sidransky D, Srivastava S (2003) Proteomic analysis of cancer-cell mitochondria. Nat Rev Cancer 3:789–795

Voss T, Ahorn H, Haberl P et al (2001) Correlation of clinical data with proteomics profiles in 24 patients with B-cell chronic lymphocytic leukemia. Int J Cancer 91:180–186

Wadhwa R, Yaguchi T, Hasan MK et al (2002) Hsp70 family member, mot-2/mthsp70/GRP75, binds to the cytoplasmic sequestration domain of the p53 protein. Exp Cell Res 274:246–253

Wadhwa R, Yaguchi T, Hasan MK et al (2003) Mortalin-MPD (mevalonate pyrophosphate decarboxylase) interactions and their role in control of cellular proliferation. Biochem Biophys Res Commun 302:735–742

Wang Y, He QY, Sun RW et al (2005) GoldIII porphyrin 1a induced apoptosis by mitochondrial death pathways related to reactive oxygen species. Cancer Res 65:11553–11564

Wang J, Gutierrez P, Edwards N, Fenselau C (2007) Integration of 18O labeling and solution isoelectric focusing in a shotgun analysis of mitochondrial proteins. J Proteome Res 6:4601–4607

Warburg O (1956) On the origin of cancer cells. Science 123:309–314

Wilkins MR, Gasteiger E, Sanchez JC et al (1998) Two-dimensional gel electrophoresis for proteome projects: the effects of protein hydrophobicity and copy number. Electrophoresis 19:1501–1505

Wozny W, Schroer K, Schwall GP et al (2007) Differential radioactive quantification of protein abundance ratios between benign and malignant prostate tissues: cancer association of annexin A3. Proteomics 7:313–322

Young TW, Mei FC, Yang G et al (2004) Activation of antioxidant pathways in ras-mediated oncogenic transformation of human surface ovarian epithelial cells revealed by functional proteomics and mass spectrometry. Cancer Res 64:4577–4584

Chapter 20
Mitochondria in Anthropology and Forensic Medicine

Tomasz Grzybowski and Urszula Rogalla

Abstract Mitochondria's role in crucial metabolic pathways is probably the first answer which comes to our minds for the question: what do these tiny organelles serve for? However, specific features of their DNA made them extremely useful also in the field of anthropology and forensics. MtDNA analyses became a milestone in the complex task of unraveling earliest human migrations. Evidence provided by these experiments left no doubts on modern humans origins pointing to Africa being our cradle. It also contributed to interpretation of putative ways of our dispersal around Asia and Americas thousands years ago. On the other hand, analysis of mtDNA is well established and valuable tool in forensic genetics. When other definitely more popular markers give no answer on identity, it is the time to employ information carried by mitochondria. This chapter summarizes not only current reports on the role of mitochondria in forensics and reconstruction of modern humans phylogeny, but also calls one's attention to a broad range of difficulties and constraints associated with mtDNA analyses.

Keywords Anthropology • Forensic genetics • mtDNA analysis • Phylogenetics

20.1 Mitochondrial DNA Polymorphism in Anthropology

Soon after deciphering the entire sequence of mitochondrial DNA (Anderson et al. 1981) this tiny molecule let us reveal more and more of its potential. Alas, it has one "drawback" among plenty of indisputable advantages – sometimes it cannot replicate itself perfectly. Though, this relatively high rate of mutation changes makes mtDNA a good source of knowledge about recent history of *Homo sapiens* spanning 150,000 years back or even more. The only marker that played almost as important role as mtDNA in unraveling our species phylogeny is Y chromosome.

Obviously it is not possible to fully reconstruct phylogeny of any species using a single DNA marker, yet realizing that today's variation reflects past events – although seemed a challenge at first – allowed drawing reasonable conclusions concerning genetic history of *Homo sapiens*.

T. Grzybowski (✉) • U. Rogalla
Ludwik Rydygier Collegium Medicum, Department of Molecular and Forensic Genetics,
The Nicolaus Copernicus University, M. Curie-Skłodowskiej Str. 9, 85-094 Bydgoszcz, Poland
e-mail: tgrzyb@cm.umk.pl

R. Scatena et al. (eds.), *Advances in Mitochondrial Medicine*, Advances in Experimental Medicine and Biology 942, DOI 10.1007/978-94-007-2869-1_20,
© Springer Science+Business Media B.V. 2012

20.1.1 Introduction

While for most geneticists mtDNA sequence is fairly enough for subsequent inferences, phylogeneticist seeks for special features of the polynucleotide chain to firstly assign molecule under study to specific group, called haplogroup. Haplogroup is a cluster of closely related haplotypes that share mutations inherited from common ancestor. Term "haplotype", in turn, embraces all molecules that are characterized by the same order of nucleotides and fell into definite haplogroup. It is worth noting that mutations in mtDNA sequence are usually reported as deviations from the revised Cambridge Reference Sequence (rCRS, Andrews et al. 1999).

Skeleton of the world mtDNA phylogeny has been quite well reconstructed and most of the major haplogroups have been characterized quite deeply (Fig. 20.1). Nevertheless, any new haplogroup has to be named according to specific rules. Nomenclature of haplogroups is fixed and imposes using letters and numbers by turns beginning with a letter, for example U5a1b (Macaulay et al. 1999).

Mutual relationships of haplotypes can be depicted as trees – kind of graphs (as seen by mathematics) in which each pair of vertices is connected by exactly one straight path. Each path represents at least one mutation event. According to this theorem, haplotype can be found in almost every vertex and in every leaf (in case it has no offspring). Sometimes, when sequence under study has extremely high mutation rate, i.e. mtDNA control region, it is reasonable to present phylogeny in a form of cyclic graphs which are called networks by phylogeneticists. Their major attribute, which serves as a key factor for discriminating them from trees, is possibility of presenting various plausible simultaneous ways of evolution, including specific events like parallel and back-mutations.

Given a tree, one is able to estimate evolutionary age of each lineage and sometimes also its dispersal time. What has to be utilized is so called human mitochondrial molecular clock, which for general purposes might be treated as a direct assumption of mutation rate in certain mtDNA regions. There are several molecular clocks available, although no uniform calibration has been proposed, that would take both coding and non-coding regions into account. On the basis of human-chimp divergence time of 6.5 MYBP Mishmar et al. (2003) calculated mutation rate of 1 nucleotide change per 5,138 years that was probably most widely used so far. Its major drawback, however, is exclusion of influence of selection on shaping mtDNA diversity. Other authors (e.g. Kivisild et al. 2006) pointed out significant excess of non-synonymous mutations in younger mtDNA clades and therefore suggested counting only synonymous mutations for the calculations. According to their estimations one mutation event takes place in mtDNA coding region every 6,764 years, on average. Although the clock took effects of selection into account, it still didn't seem to be accurate enough since it excluded a significant portion of mtDNA genome from calculations. Problem of evident time-dependency of mutation rate was solved partially by Soares et al. (2009). Their calibration also utilizes human-chimp splitting time, yet is based on most recent fossil evidence. According to Soares et al. (2009), substitution rate in the whole molecule accounts to 1 per 3,624 years, while in coding region itself 1 mutation arises every 3,533 years.

20.1.2 MtDNA and the Origins of Modern Humans

It is widely accepted now that all modern humans derive from African populations. The most convincing proof was given by Alan Wilson's group (Cann et al. 1987) of the University of California, who used 12 restriction enzymes in their study to digest mtDNA taken from as little as 147 donors representing various contemporary populations – Americans (both of European and African origins), East Asia and New Guinea inhabitants and Australian Aborigines. Restriction mapping results allowed construction of a maximum parsimony phylogenetic tree (MP) depicting evolutionary relationships

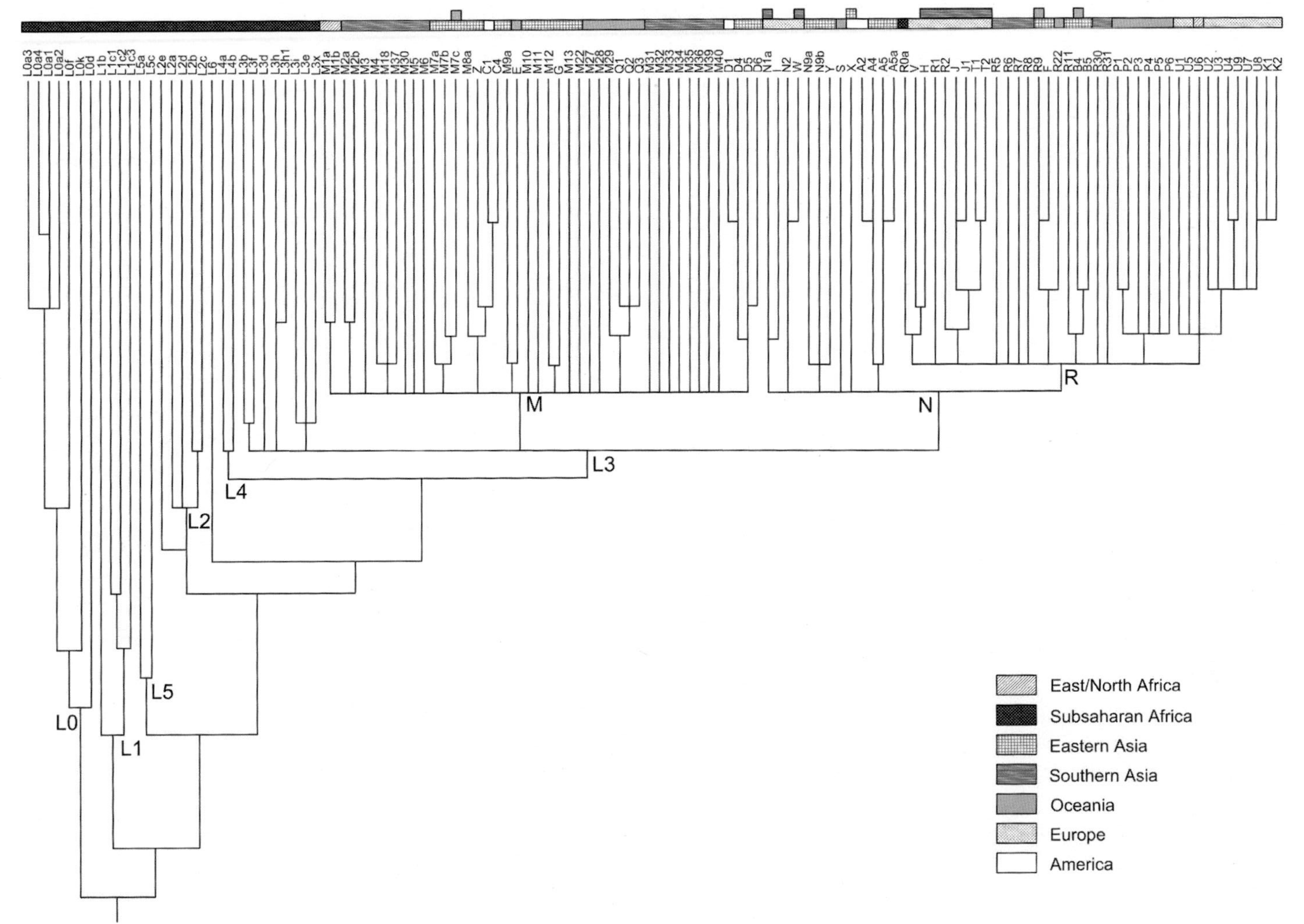

Fig. 20.1 Global mitochondrial DNA phylogenetic tree, with a basic branching pattern according to the updated tree of van Oven and Kayser (2009)

between all haplotypes. Two deepest roots in this tree were representing mtDNA of exclusively African origin and a mixture of African and non-African lineages. Surprisingly, most significant diversity was noted among purely African lineages. These observations were interpreted as a strong evidence supporting so called "out of Africa" hypothesis suggesting that *H. sapiens* is of African origin. Performing molecular dating of the tree has shown, that the last common ancestor of the all mtDNA sequences under study (so called "mitochondrial Eve") must have lived in Africa about 140,000–200,000 years ago. Many subsequent mtDNA analyses confirmed Wilson's conclusions (Vigilant et al. 1991; Mishmar et al. 2003; Macaulay et al. 2005). Global mtDNA tree can be divided into two daughter branches, L0 and L1'5 (Behar et al. 2008). The L1'5 branch encompasses sub-Saharan L3 that is dated 50,000–84,000 years back (Macaulay et al. 2005; Kivisild et al. 2006). Two macrohaplogroups, M and N, deriving directly from L3 cover all mtDNA molecules noted in all populations beyond Africa. Part of N haplogroup evolved into another numerous and also very divergent haplogroup – R.

Phylogenetic tree reconstructed on the basis of single nucleotide polymorphisms (SNPs) found on non-recombining part of Y chromosome (NRY) has a topology that highly resembles the one created for mtDNA. They both support the 'out of Africa' hypothesis, which assumes gene pool of *Homo sapiens* was dramatically reduced as a result of founder effect.

20.1.3   Earliest Human Migrations from Africa to Eurasia

The time and routes of earliest migrations of our ancestors from Africa to Eurasia were most widely reconstructed on the basis of mtDNA analyses. All non-African mtDNA lineages are classified as belonging to one out of two major macrohaplogroups M and N – both deriving from sub-Saharan L3 haplogroup. West Eurasian mitochondrial genomes fall almost exclusively into macrohaplogroup N. On the contrary, mtDNAs of inhabitants of East Eurasia belong both to M and N macrohaplogroups, which originate most probably from East Africa (Quintana-Murci et al. 1999; Kivisild et al. 2003; Metspalu et al. 2004). They reached Asia via so called southern route, during earliest waves of migration of *Homo sapiens sapiens* taking place ca. 70,000 years ago. Existence of the southern route, conducted from East Africa through Bab-el-Mandeb and southern part of Arabian Peninsula (Yemen), through tropical coasts of the Indian Ocean to Southeastern Asia and Oceania, is supported mostly by the M macrohaplogroup phylogeny. It's important to notice that its highest diversity and frequencies are noticed in India, while in the Near East and Southwest Asia it is very scarce (Kivisild et al. 2003; Metspalu et al. 2004; Sun et al. 2006; Chandrasekar et al. 2009). Distribution of frequencies and diversity of macrohaplogroup M indicates that existence of the ca. 45,000 years ago so called northern route of Eurasian colonization, presumed to lead along the Nile river, through Sinai to the Near East, is less plausible. Evolutionary ages of M and N haplogroups are similar – 50,000–70,000 years, respectively (Soares et al. 2009). Since all mtDNA lineages descending from African L3 haplogroup in India belong to M and N haplogroups that are of similar age, one may expect all founder lineages of both macrohaplogroups reached Eurasia via southern route during first migrations of *Homo sapiens* from Africa. First division into west- and east-Eurasian took place in the region between the Indus Plain and territories encompassing southwestern Asia (Metspalu et al. 2004). Haplogroup R arose from macrohaplogroup N relatively early (Kivisild et al. 2003). In eastern Eurasia it was divided into B and R9 and in western Eurasia – into HV, TJ and U clades. This scenario is reflected by the results of entire mtDNA genomes sequencing experiments encompassing some populations inhabiting regions adjacent to the southern route. For example, results of entire mtDNA genomes sequencing from indigenous peopling of Malaysia, named *Orang Asli,* showed existence of two haplogroups M21 and M22 of advanced age (ca. 57,000 years ago). Its appearance is limited almost exclusively to *Orang Asli* and a few Thailand inhabitants (Macaulay et al. 2005). Similar geographical specificity of some mtDNA clades, derived directly from M, N and R haplogroups, was spotted during full mtDNA sequencing experiments among

Australian Aborigines and Papua New Guinea inhabitants (Ingman and Gyllensten 2003). Age and geographical specificity of the abovementioned haplogroups indicate that they are regional relicts of earliest migrations of modern humans. According to these facts it seems obvious that no matter if first colonizers chose northern or southern route, they must have reached the Indian Ocean coasts soon after leaving Africa. Some authors assume that there was one wave of migration leading through the southern route which made all three M, N and R haplogroups reach Eurasia. On the basis of molecular dating of these clades (TMRCA) in the region between India and Australia it is assessed that first colonizers got to India, Eastern Asia (China) and Australia $66,100 \pm 5,700$, $64,500 \pm 3,800$ and $63,400 \pm 5,200$ years ago, respectively. Assuming that route of migration adjacent to the Indian Ocean coasts numbered ca. 12,000 km it can be estimated that the speed of dispersal of modern humans came to 0.7–4 km per year. Population which left Africa about 60,000 years ago probably wasn't numerous and consisted of as little as 500–2,000 women (Macaulay et al. 2005).

It seems that the results concerning scenario of colonization of Eurasia, as revealed by entire mtDNA sequencing, are consistent with the data obtained from population analyses based on the nonrecombining part of chromosome Y (NRY). Vital for the inference is the observation of C, D and F haplogroups of Y chromosome in populations of South Asia. It is probable that founders of these three clades reached Eurasia as a result of single migration event via the southern route. However, some authors suggest that beside the earliest wave of migration along southern route, which brought C and D clades to Europe, second wave also existed – one that led north, across the Near East, which took haplogroup F to West and East Eurasia (Richards et al. 2006).

One should be aware, however, that these discrepancies in opinions concerning Eurasia colonization events may be only apparent. Colonizing of west Eurasia, which according to soma anthropologists, archeologists and geneticist was carried out along northern route from Africa, across Sinai and the Near East, could be the result of early modification of the chosen direction of migration by some group of founders, who finally took the southern route. This hypothesis is supported by similar age of N and R mtDNA haplogroups in India and Europe ($66,100 \pm 5,700$ and $66,300 \pm 5,600$ years, respectively) (Macaulay et al. 2005). In compliance with this scenario, ancestors of contemporary Europeans would be this group of colonizers, which after having left Africa changed the route and sidetracked into north-western direction. Wanderers were restrained from further conquests by the harsh weather conditions, yet finally entered Near East and Europe 45–50 k years ago. There is also an evidence of back-migrations from the Near East into North Africa, based on the presence of haplogroups U6 and M1 in North and East Africa (Olivieri et al. 2006).

20.1.4 Time and Routes of the Americas Colonization in the Light of mtDNA Testing

Perfect climatic and topological conditions for conquering America by the modern humans were noticed in a period of time between 30,000 and 13,000 years ago due to existence of mainland between Siberia and Alaska. If first colonizers took a chance of migrating across the Bering Strait, they would run into unexpected obstacle, which blocked the main route into the continent for the vast part of Pleistocene. This barrier was an ice-cap lingering huge part of the North America. In the times between 55 and 30,000 years ago and about 13,500 y.a. the abovementioned obstacle was probably cut with the ice-free corridor between today's Yukon River, through Canada reaching Montana state. This piece of human-friendly ground could serve the colonizers as the promenade into America (Jobling et al. 2004).

Last decade was abound with intense genetic analyses which aimed in searching for Asian territories, which were associated with entering the New World. So far, most advanced research concerning mtDNA is currently made with maximum resolution – on the entire mitochondrial genome sequencing level.

After migration through Bering Strait was visualized, may scientists naturally paid their attention to Central Siberia populations, scarcely studied so far. In fact in the 1990s it was stated that the variety of mtDNA pool of Native Americans constitutes some part of diversity seen in Central-Asian and Siberian populations – in all three linguistic groups of American Indians (Amerindian, Na-Dene and Eskimo-Aleut) only four main founder mtDNA haplogroups were noted – A, B, C and D – and all that are also seen in Asia (Wallace 1995). Undoubtedly, these sought-after "founder territories" for the New World must be located somewhere in Central Asia and/or Siberia. The fifth founder clade seen among Native Americans is X – one that is spotted almost exclusively among some north Amerindian groups (i.e. Ojibwa speaking Algonquin language) and Navajo belonging to Na-Dene linguistic group (Brown et al. 1998). What characterizes the X haplogroup, and particularly its subclade X2 is its wide range of occurrence in Europe (Reidla et al. 2003). On the contrary, not much is known about its existence in Asian populations. Therefore, quite interesting was the discovery of its occurrence in southern Siberian populations – among Altaians and Buryats. On this basis it has been suggested that Siberian haplogroup X could have been one of the Asian founders for Paleoindian mtDNA pool (Derenko et al. 2001). Subsequent analyses of coding region sequence of mtDNA using PCR-RFLP technique and entire genome sequencing have shown that Altai, who were assigned to X haplogroup, belong to its subclade X2e, which seems much different from X2a typical for Native Americans (Reidla et al. 2003; Derenko et al. 2007). The latter hasn't been found in any Eurasian population so far.

Number and time periods of the first *Homo sapiens* migrations from Asia to the New World are still a matter of heated discussion. First hypothesis assumed existence of three waves corresponding to three main linguistic groups of Native Americans. Yet, it hasn't been proven to be true according to data obtained from various genetic markers analyses. Arguments against existence of these three waves come i.a. from mtDNA analyses, which demonstrate no correlation between genetic structure of Native Americans and their affinity to linguistic groups. More light has been shed on this issue by the mtDNA experiments held just 2–3 years ago.

Thanks to entire mtDNA genomes sequencing, phylogeny of Native American (A-D) haplogroups could be resolved in detail, distributions of frequencies of certain haplogroups were analyzed and their evolutionary age was assessed. It turned out that indigenously American origin characterizes only subclades A2, B2, C1 and D1 and their evolutionary age is very close (about 20,000 years), what suggests that they reached deeper American lands in just one wave of migration from Beringia (Tamm et al. 2007; Achilli et al. 2008). Until now, it is not clearly explained what was the number of founder haplotypes for these haplogroups that took part in colonizing the America. Each of the haplogroups could have been represented by single haplotype (its founder node) or multiple haplotypes – as suggested for C1 haplogroup, which is said to have three founder haplotypes among the New World colonizers (Achilli et al. 2008).

Irrespective of the number of founder haplotypes, molecular dating results (TMRCA) for A2, B2, C1 and D1 indicate that these haplogroups were brought to the North American continent about 19,000 years ago, right after the last glacial maximum (LGM). The data gathered so far support the hypothesis of an early settlement of modern humans in America, preceding Clovis culture. mtDNA sequencing results are absolutely consistent here with archeological data which points to arrival of modern humans to the South America (Monte Verde, Chile) at least 12,500 years ago.

20.1.5 Colonization of Europe as Revealed by mtDNA Analysis

After having left Africa, modern humans manned all the remaining continents and genetic drift in populations inhabiting geographically distant areas led to development of a kind of subdivision (structure) of the global population. It is reflected by the results of molecular variance analyses (AMOVA) performed for data coming from various genetic markers. For example, for autosomal biallelic loci (single nucleotide polymorphisms, SNPs), about 91% of diversity is observed within population, whereas as little as 9% is seen between main continental groups of populations (Li et al. 2008). For non-recombinant markers (mtDNA, NRY) part of diversity that is observed between continents is considerably higher (12–52%), what is a result of smaller effective population size (1/4 as compared to autosomal loci) and related increased impact of genetic drift favoring formation of stratification in global population (reviewed by Jobling et al. 2004). It is worth to notice that this structure is more evident in the case of Y chromosome than in mtDNA (about 12–22% and 16–52% between continents, respectively). To some extent, this difference follows patrilocality that is responsible for higher genetic distances between populations as inferred from Y chromosome analyses than mtDNA.

While intercontinental differences are easily noticed in a variety of markers, differences between populations inhabiting the same continent are definitely harder to be spotted. One of the existing exceptions is a clear structure of African populations (Tishkoff et al. 2009). The autosomal gene pool in Europe is homogeneous but at the same time small genetic differentiation that is present between subpopulations (an average of 0.17% of the total genetic variance) is characterized by a significant correlation between genetic and geographic distance (Lao et al. 2008).

Mitochondrial DNA pool of Europeans is even more homogenous (Simoni et al. 2000; McEvoy et al. 2004). As a result of early founder analyses of mtDNA in the Near East in Europe is was shown that the majority of mtDNA haplogroups in Europe shared a common regional ancestry from the Upper Paleolithic and Neolithic (Richards et al. 2000). The pioneer colonization of the Upper Paloolithic might have been marked by the most ancient haplogroups in Europe, U8 and U5, dated back to ca. 50,000 and 30,000 years, respectively (Soares et al. 2010; Malyarchuk et al. 2010). During the Last Glacial Maximum (LGM, between 19,000 and 22,000 YBP) human populations became concentrated in refugial areas in the western Caucasus and southern European peninsulas. Thus, re-colonisation of the continent from southern refugia in the wake of the major warming phase after 15 kya appears to be a major concept to explain the mtDNA diversity of the present-day Europeans. Recent analyses of the complete mitochondrial genomes point to the postglacial expansion times for most of the lineages spreading from south-west Europe. This re-expansion time frame is reflected mainly in the age of haplogroups V, H1 and H3 which all appear to have originated in south-west Europe and date to 11–11.5 kya—the end of the Younger Dryas glacial relapse (Soares et al. 2010). Near Eastern Neolithic contribution to the mtDNA pool of Europeans is probably minor and includes selected subclusters of haplogroups J and K, namely, J2a1a and K2a, both dating to 8–9 kya within Europe (Soares et al. 2010). One may predict that future analyses of complete mitochondrial genomes accompanied by dating with improved mtDNA clock will shed more light on the archeogenetics of Europe.

20.2 Mitochondrial DNA as a Tool in Forensic Investigations

20.2.1 Introduction

Solving many criminal cases is dependent on determining the origin of material evidence by the means of molecular biology techniques. Individual identification is a multidisciplinary field, gathering most exciting achievements of molecular biology, genetics, informatics, genomics and many more under just one name. The techniques that are currently in use in forensics, are mostly based on DNA analyses, so it is not surprising why so much emphasis is put on development of these.

The real breakthrough in forensic genetics took place when in vitro amplification of DNA was proposed. PCR technique revolutionized virtually all fields of experimental biology, but it is not an exaggeration to say that for forensics the new era began. It finally turned possible to draw DNA profiles from tiny amounts of biological stains and individual DNA identification, thanks to its improved (in order of several magnitudes) sensitivity, became first-line method in solving criminal cases where any biological trace is involved. Nevertheless, scientific aspects of individual identification are still evolving.

One may expect that the commonly used autosomal microsatellite (STR) profiles obtained from DNA analysis would be sufficient for individual identification in all cases, yet quite surprisingly it is not true. In certain cases, i.e. when it comes to maternity testing or the collected material is degraded or available from hair shaft only, the only hope for forensics expert is utilizing mtDNA analyses.

20.2.2 *Mitochondrial DNA Analyses in Forensics*

Although autosomal miniSTRs and single nucleotide polymorphism (SNP) loci are very effective tools in identification of most types of specimens, they face some restrictions when analyzed material spent some time in unfavorable conditions making nuclear DNA degrade. However, degraded DNA is not a deadlock anymore, as mitochondrial DNA testing works quite efficiently even if material underwent major damage.

Mitochondrial genome has some specific features making it more resistant than nuclear DNA. First of all, it is of circular shape, which ensures its small vulnerability to exonucleases that usually quite easily degrade DNA chains. Secondly, it is present in each somatic cell in high numbers – each mitochondrion contains up to 11 mtDNA particles (Cavalier et al. 2000), while there are 1,000–100,000 mitochondria in each cell (depending on its type) (Lightowlers et al. 1997). Therefore, it is more likely to survive under unfavorable conditions than nuclear DNA. Human mtDNA is inherited along maternal lineage and undergoes no recombination. Therefore, when used in identification, it doesn't allow pointing to a single person, but rather a group of relatives, descending from a single woman. Nevertheless, even if it is not as discriminating as set of microsatellite autosomal loci, it has other interesting yet unique attribute – it is quite clearly distinguishable between populations representing various continents and even specific regions. Therefore, in many cases mtDNA analysis results may serve as an important information concerning biogeographic ancestry of the donor.

Lack of recombination in mtDNA causes certain haplotypes to get fixed in population and mutations are the main source of diversity. Quite luckily, mutations occur there ten times more frequently, on average, that in nuclear genome (Brown et al. 1979, 1982). High rate of mutation is the main cause of high mtDNA diversity, that is noticed in human population, which in turn makes mtDNA highly useful tool in forensic genetics. Clear-cut differences are spotted when examining evolution rate in various mitochondrial DNA regions. They occur most frequently per unit of time in so called hypervariable regions of the D-loop – HVSI in region 16,024–16,400, HVSII between 44 and 340 nucleotide and HVSIII from 438 to 576 nucleotide. The highest mutation rate is seen in HVSI region (Brandstätter et al. 2004; Lutz et al. 1998).

In forensic genetics mtDNA analyses are performed usually when other methods are expected to or already failed, for example to identify human remains especially when they are old, skeletal remains or when the only available material is a hair deprived of bulb. It seems useful also in Disater Victims Identification (DVI) teams work, where it serves as a mean of determination of maternal kinship.

How it works? Specific fragments of mtDNA (usually hypervariable regions HVSI and HVSII) are amplified in PCR reaction followed by sequence analysis on automatic analyzers. Sequences obtained are tagged with haplotypes variants as a result of comparison with Anderson's reference sequence (rCRS) (Anderson et al. 1981; Andrews et al. 1999). If the expert observes conformity of the haplotype extracted from material evidence and from the suspect, he or she performs statistical analyses on the basis of population databases consisting of thousands of records representing haplotypes from persons unrelated in maternal lineage. The more seldom in the database the haplotype from evidence is seen, the more likely it actually belongs to the suspect. However, the strength of mtDNA haplotype frequency estimations is still limited by the size of the current forensic databases, especially for rare mtDNA sequences that have not been observed in databases. For rare types, the apparent frequency in the database will underestimate the true population frequency (Holland and Parsons 1999). Therefore, the painstaking efforts are currently being made to increase the size of control region population datasets and their geographical coverage (Pereira et al. 2004; Behar et al. 2007).

It is worth noting that forensic mtDNA analysis has recently been expanded by development of minisequencing strategies enabling haplogroup assignment of casework and reference samples. These could be extremely helpful in the preselection of samples deriving from suspects and crime scenes in high-volume cases (Brandstätter et al. 2006). Several systems of this kind, based on typing of haplogroup-specific SNPs have been proposed – e.g. the one allowing dissection of the most frequent in Europe haplogroup H into its subclades (Brandstätter et al. 2006) or multiplex minisequencing reaction for genotyping 32 selected coding region SNPs representing main and derived branches of the East Asian and Native American mtDNA phylogeny (Alvarez-Iglesias et al. 2007). In the near future one may envisage the introduction of complete genome sequencing in forensics, accompanied by a development entire mtDNA genome reference population data suitable for forensic comparisons (Irwin et al. 2010).

It is widely known that not only human genetic material is found on crime scene. When species of the donor of DNA has to be determined, mtDNA testing can be a method of choice. The point is to get to know *cytb* sequence. Why this particular one? It has been shown that *cytb* gene is characterized by high level of diversity between species and remains quite uniform in animals belonging to the same species. Therefore, simple PCR followed by sequencing reaction and aligning to *cytb* gene sequence entries in nucleotide databases using the program BLAST let expert witnesses answer questions concerning donor species with high confidence (Parson et al. 2000).

20.2.3 *Quality Control*

One of the absolutely most important issues in forensic genetics is appropriate and strict quality control. Although it is not that obvious at a first glance, molecular phylogenetics has a lot to do when it comes to assessing value of the data obtained and in forensics in general.

Undoubtedly when an attorney provides forensics expert with material evidence, he or she is usually interested not in evolutionary history but the identity of the donor of DNA to be found. Nevertheless, getting to know haplogroup's affinity of the donor, makes it possible to check the correctness of the results of the DNA analyses – to some extent. It is particularly important if the biological material is old and degraded and the analyses have to be performed in several time-consuming steps – each providing only a subset of the total DNA sequence. Good Laboratory Practice (GLP) justifiably forces experts to work in two independent groups yet nobody has a right to assume, that it would be enough for assuring top class analyses.

Haplotype which is obtained during the analyses has to make some "phylogenetic sense" – in other words, it has to conform to some haplogroup. All the mutations that are found have to be interpreted with known evolutionary events in expert's mind. If there are some deviations like presence of diagnostic mutations typical for two or more haplogroups in one specimen, it should arouse suspicion. In most cases such result arises as a consequence of contamination of the sample. In fact, experienced geneticist should be able to predict almost entire mtDNA sequence on the basis of its small fragment. If his/her predictions are inconsistent with the actual results, analysis should be repeated.

Forensic genetics are usually familiar with phylogenetics and use this knowledge in verification of the data *a posteriori* (Bandelt et al. 2001; Salas et al. 2007). Nevertheless, many older mtDNA databases created in Europe and USA contained some data that in the light of subsequent phylogenetics analyses turned out to be partially incorrect and had to be wiped off (Yao et al. 2004; Bandelt et al. 2004).

20.2.4   Databases

Publicly accessible DNA databases are of great importance in forensic genetics. They allow making statistical inferences on the results generated by automated sequencers. Definitely, the most reliable and most widely used mtDNA haplotypes' database is EMPOP (www.empop.org) maintained by The European DNA Profiling Group (EDNAP). It is an initiative towards gathering control region haplotypes from various world's populations in just one place and making them as credible as possible by harsh quality control procedures (Parson et al. 2004).

The first release of EMPOP, that turned online in October 2006, contained 16121 (Dec 2011) haplotypes (Parson and Dür 2007). The second release (EMPOP2, available from May, 2010) includes more than 5,000 new mtDNA haplotypes from more than 30 populations and thus contains now 10,970 haplotypes. The database is divided into two separate parts – first, "forensic", containing data obtained by collaborating forensic laboratories and second, "literature", built up with reliable data from literature. All haplotypes included in forensic part were submitted in the form of raw database files subsequently assembled into consensus sequences. For each new haplotype sequence of the both strands had to be confirmed and further verified by three separate scientific teams also by the means of phylogenetics. Similar testing concerns literature data, that undergoes *a posteriori* check for correctness before being published.

EMPOP database, although managed by Institute of Legal Medicine (GMI), Innsbruck Medical University, fruits from partnership of several forensic laboratories, that are into mtDNA analyses and passed special verification procedures.

Yet, EMPOP is not only well-shaped collection of haplotypes but also bioinformatics tools allowing to check any population dataset. One of the available tools is Network – an algorithm created by mathematicians that allows clear, graphical presentation of numerical input data. In fact, it serves as a mean to verify correctness of the data (Bandelt and Dür 2007).

20.2.5   Casework Examples

It has already been mentioned here that mtDNA plays a crucial role in individual identification especially if the available evidence seems to be degraded, destroyed by fire or simply old. Geneticists that cooperate with DVI teams are often performing mtDNA analyses as this is the only hope for obtaining satisfactory results. Humankind history is full of mass disasters like terrorist attack on WTC, tsunami in Indonesia or earthquake on Haiti, to name only a few. Sometimes identification by recognition by family member is not possible – this in an open gate for DNA testing. Probably the most extensive mass identification was held by ICMP (International Commission on Missing Persons) in former Yugoslavia (Huffine et al. 2001). It was assessed that in Bosnia and Herzegovina there were over 30,000 missing persons. ICMP had to create a network of fully functional forensic laboratories that would cope together with this huge identification challenge. Considerable part of human remains were bare scattered bones – material unsuitable for testing on the basis of nuclear DNA. In this cases the only choice was to perform mtDNA analyses and compare the results with the before-created database of genetic profiles of families seeking their missing relatives.

MtDNA testing can be also a useful tool for identification of historical remains. In 2005 at Frombork Cathedral (Poland) remains of a man were exhumed from area proximal to the altar Nicolaus Copernicus was responsible for during his life (Bogdanowicz et al. 2009). All the remains – three molar teeth and femurs – had the same mtDNA haplotype. In case of Copernicus it was very hard to find descendants, whose DNA could serve for comparative purposes. Nevertheless, an attempt was made to search for other biological material that would help answer the question whether what have been found are the remains of famous astronomer. In collections of Museum Gustavianum in Uppsala (Sweden) there was a book, "Calendarium Romanum Magnum", which was presumed to belong to Copernicus for the vast part of his life. It was a subject of thorough examination that let scientists reveal several hairs caught between the pages. MtDNA analysis gave surprising results – the haplotype found was identical to the one from remains from cathedral! It is very likely that these remains belong to Nicolas Copernicus as the haplotype observed was noticed only four times in the EMPOP1 database – once in Denmark and three times in Germany (Bogdanowicz et al. 2009).

References

Achilli A, Perego UA, Bravi CM, Coble MD, Kong QP, Woodward SR, Salas A, Torroni A, Bandelt H-J (2008) The phylogeny of the four pan-American MtDNA haplogroups: implications for evolutionary and disease studies. PLoS One 3:e1764

Alvarez-Iglesias V, Jaime JC, Carracedo A, Salas A (2007) Coding region mitochondrial DNA SNPs: targeting East Asian and Native American haplogroups. Forensic Sci Int Genet 1:44–55

Anderson S, Bankier AT, Barell BG, de Bruijn MH, Coulson AR, Drouin J, Eperon IC, Nierlich DP, Roe BA, Sanger F, Schreier PH, Smith AJ, Staden R, Young IG (1981) Sequence and organization of the human mitochondrial genome. Nature 290:457–465

Andrews RM, Kubacka I, Chinnery PF, Lightowlers RN, Turnbull DM, Howell N (1999) Reanalysis and revision of the Cambridge reference sequence for human mitochondrial DNA. Nat Genet 23:147

Bandelt H-J, Dür A (2007) Translating DNA data tables into quasi-median networks for parsimony analysis and error detection. Mol Phylogenet Evol 42:256–271

Bandelt HJ, Lahermo P, Richards M, Macaulay V (2001) Detecting errors in mtDNA data by phylogenetic analysis. Int J Legal Med 115:64–69

Bandelt H-J, Salas A, Lutz-Bonengel S (2004) Artificial recombination in forensic mtDNA population databases. Int J Legal Med 118:267–273

Behar DM, Rosset S, Blue-Smith J, Balanovsky O, Tzur S, Comas D, Mitchell RJ, Quintana-Murci L, Tyler-Smith C, Wells RS, Consortium G (2007) The genographic project public participation mitochondrial DNA database. PLoS Genet 3:e104

Behar DM, Villems R, Soodyall H, Blue-Smith J, Pereira L, Metspalu E, Scozzari R, Makkan H, Tzur S, Comas D, Bertranpetit J, Quintana-Murci L, Tyler-Smith C, Wells RS, Rosset S, Genographic Consortium (2008) The dawn of human matrilineal diversity. Am J Hum Genet 82:1130–40

Bogdanowicz W, Allen M, Branicki W, Lembring M, Gajewska M, Kupiec T (2009) Genetic identification of putative remains of the famous astronomer Nicolas Copernicus. Proc Natl Acad Sci USA 30:12279–12282

Brandstätter A, Peterson CT, Irwin JA, Mpoke S, Koech DK, Parson W, Parsons TJ (2004) Mitochondrial DNA control region sequences from Nairobi (Kenya): inferring phylogenetic parameters for the establishment of a forensic database. Int J Legal Med 118:294–306

Brandstätter A, Salas A, Niederstätter H, Gassner C, Carracedo A, Parson W (2006) Dissection of mitochondrial superhaplogroup H using coding region SNPs. Electrophoresis 27:2541–2550

Brown WM, George M, Wilson AC (1979) Rapid evolution of animal mitochondrial DNA. Proc Natl Acad Sci USA 76:1967–1971

Brown WM, Prager EM, Wan A, Wilson AC (1982) Mitochondrial DNA sequences in primates: tempo and mode of evolution. J Mol Evol 18:225–239

Brown MD, Hosseini SH, Torroni A, Bandelt HJ, Allen JC, Schurr TG, Scozza CF, Wallace DC (1998) mtDNA haplogroup X: an ancient link between Europe/Western Asia and North America? Am J Hum Genet 63:1852–1861

Cann RL, Stoneking M, Wilson AC (1987) Mitochondrial DNA and human evolution. Nature 325:31–36

Cavalier L, Johannisson A, Gyllensten U (2000) Analysis of mtDNA copy number and composition of single mitochondrial particles using flow cytometry and PCR. Exp Cell Res 259:79–85

Chandrasekar A, Kumar S, Sreenath J, Sarkar BN, Urade BP, Mallick S, Bandopadhyay SS, Barua P, Barik SS, Basu D, Kiran U, Gangopadhyay P, Sahani R, Prasad BV, Gangopadhyay S, Lakshmi GR, Ravuri RR, Padmaja K, Venugopal PN, Sharma MB, Rao VR (2009) Updating phylogeny of mitochondrial DNA macrohaplogroup M in India: dispersal of modern human in South Asian corridor. PLoS One 4:e7447

Derenko MV, Grzybowski T, Malyarchuk BA, Czarny J, Mi cicka-Sliwka D, Zakharov IA (2001) The presence of mitochondrial haplogroup x in Altaians from South Siberia. Am J Hum Genet 69:237–241

Derenko M, Malyarchuk B, Grzybowski T, Denisova G, Dambueva I, Perkova M, Dorzhu C, Luzina F, Lee HK, Vanecek T, Villems R, Zakharov I (2007) Phylogeographic analysis of mitochondrial DNA in northern Asian populations. Am J Hum Genet 81:1025–1041

Holland MM, Parsons TJ (1999) Mitochondrial DNA sequence analysis – validation and use for forensic casework. Forensic Sci Rev 11:21

Huffine E, Crews J, Kennedy B, Bomberger K, Zinbo A (2001) Mass identification of persons missing from the break-up of the former Yugoslavia: structure, function and role of the International Commission on Missing Persons. Croat Med J 42:271–275

Ingman M, Gyllensten U (2003) Mitochondrial genome variation and evolutionary history of Australian and New Guinean aborigines. Genome Res 13:1600–1606

Irwin JA, Parson W, Coble MD, Just RS (2010) mtGenome reference population databases and the future of forensic mtDNA analysis. Forensic Sci Int Genet. doi:10.1016/j.fsigen.2010.02.008

Jobling MA, Hurles ME, Tyler-Smith C (2004) Human evolutionary genetics: origins, peoples and disease. Garland Science Publishing, London/New York

Kivisild T, Rootsi S, Metspalu M, Mastana S, Kaldma K, Parik J, Metspalu E, Adojaan M, Tolk HV, Stepanov V, Gölge M, Usanga E, Papiha SS, Cinnio lu C, King R, Cavalli-Sforza L, Underhill PA, Villems R (2003) The genetic heritage of the earliest settlers persists both in Indian tribal and caste populations. Am J Hum Genet 72:313–332

Kivisild T, Shen P, Wall DP, Do B, Sung R, Davis K, Passarino G, Underhill PA, Scharfe C, Torroni A, Scozzari R, Modiano D, Coppa A, de Knijff P, Feldman M, Cavalli-Sforza LL, Oefner PJ (2006) The role of selection in the evolution of human mitochondrial genomes. Genetics 172:373–387

Lao O, Lu TT, Nothnagel M, Junge O, Freitag-Wolf S, Caliebe A, Balascakova M, Bertranpetit J, Bindoff LA, Comas D, Holmlund G, Kouvatsi A, Macek M, Mollet I, Parson W, Palo J, Ploski R, Sajantila A, Tagliabracci A, Gether U, Werge T, Rivadeneira F, Hofman A, Uitterlinden AG, Gieger C, Wichmann HE, Rüther A, Schreiber S, Becker C, Nürnberg P, Nelson MR, Krawczak M, Kayser M (2008) Correlation between genetic and geographic structure in Europe. Curr Biol 18:1241–1248

Li JZ, Absher DM, Tang H, Southwick AM, Casto AM, Ramachandran S, Cann HM, Barsh GS, Feldman M, Cavalli-Sforza LL, Myers RM (2008) Worldwide human relationships inferred from genome-wide patterns of variation. Science 319:1100–1104

Lightowlers RN, Chinnery PF, Turnbull DM, Howell N (1997) Mammalian mitochondrial genetics: heredity, heteroplasmy and disease. Trends Genet 13:450–455

Lutz S, Weisser HJ, Heizmann J, Pollak S (1998) Location and frequency of polymorphic positions in the mtDNA control region of individuals from Germany. Int J Legal Med 111:67–77

Macaulay V, Richards M, Hickey E, Vega E, Cruciani F, Guida V, Scozzari R, Bonné-Tamir B, Sykes B, Torroni A (1999) The emerging tree of West Eurasian mtDNAs: a synthesis of control-region sequences and RFLPs. Am J Hum Genet 64:232–249

Macaulay V, Hill C, Achilli A, Rengo C, Clarke D, Meehan W, Blackburn J, Semino O, Scozzari R, Cruciani F, Taha A, Shaari NK, Raja JM, Ismail P, Zainuddin Z, Goodwin W, Bulbeck D, Bandelt HJ, Oppenheimer S, Torroni A, Richards M (2005) Single, rapid coastal settlement of Asia revealed by analysis of complete mitochondrial genomes. Science 308:1034–1036

Malyarchuk B, Derenko M, Grzybowski T, Perkova M, Rogalla U, Vanecek T, Tsybovsky I (2010) The peopling of Europe from the mitochondrial haplogroup U5 perspective. PLoS One 5:e10285

McEvoy B, Richards M, Forster P, Bradley DG (2004) The Longue Durée of genetic ancestry: multiple genetic marker systems and Celtic origins on the Atlantic facade of Europe. Am J Hum Genet 75:693–702

Metspalu M, Kivisild T, Metspalu E, Parik J, Hudjashov G, Kaldma K, Serk P, Karmin M, Behar DM, Gilbert MT, Endicott P, Mastana S, Papiha SS, Skorecki K, Torroni A, Villems R (2004) Most of the extant mtDNA boundaries in south and southwest Asia were likely shaped during the initial settlement of Eurasia by anatomically modern humans. BMC Genet 5:26

Mishmar D, Ruiz-Pesini E, Golik P, Macaulay V, Clark AG, Hosseini S, Brandon M, Easley K, Chen E, Brown MD, Sukernik RI, Olckers A, Wallace DC (2003) Natural selection shaped regional mtDNA variation in humans. Proc Natl Acad Sci USA 100:171–176

Olivieri A, Achilli A, Pala M, Battaglia V, Fornarino S, Al-Zahery N, Scozzari R, Cruciani F, Behar DM, Dugoujon JM, Coudray C, Santachiara-Benerecetti AS, Semino O, Bandelt HJ, Torroni A (2006) The mtDNA legacy of the Levantine early Upper Palaeolithic in Africa. Science 314:1767–1770

Parson W, Pegoraro K, Niederstätter H, Föger M, Steinlechner M (2000) Species identification by means of the cytochrome b gene. Int J Legal Med 114:23–28

Parson W, Brandstätter A, Alonso A, Brandt N, Brinkmann B, Carracedo A, Corach D, Froment O, Furac I, Grzybowski T, Hedberg K, Keyser-Tracqui C, Kupiec T, Lutz-Bonengel S, Mevag B, Ploski R, Schmitter H, Schneider P, Syndercombe-Court D, Sørensen E, Thew H, Tully G, Scheithauer R (2004) The EDNAP mitochondrial DNA population database (EMPOP) collaborative exercises: organisation, results and perspectives. Forensic Sci Int 139:215–226

Parson W, Dür A (2007) EMPOP-a forsenic mtDNA database. Forsenic Sci Int Genet 1:88–92

Pereira L, Cunha C, Amorim A (2004) Predicting sampling saturation of mtDNA haplotypes: an application to an enlarged Portuguese database. Int J Legal Med 118:132–136

Quintana-Murci L, Semino O, Bandelt H-J, Passarino G, McElreavey K, Santachiara-Benerecetti AS (1999) Genetic evidence of an early exit of Homo sapiens sapiens from Africa through eastern Africa. Nat Genet 23:437–441

Reidla M, Kivisild T, Metspalu E, Kaldma K, Tambets K, Tolk HV, Parik J, Loogväli EL, Derenko M, Malyarchuk B, Bermisheva M, Zhadanov S, Pennarun E, Gubina M, Golubenko M, Damba L, Fedorova S, Gusar V, Grechanina E, Mikerezi I, Moisan JP, Chaventré A, Khusnutdinova E, Osipova L, Stepanov V, Voevoda M, Achilli A, Rengo C, Rickards O, De Stefano GF, Papiha S, Beckman L, Janicijevic B, Rudan P, Anagnou N, Michalodimitrakis E, Koziel S, Usanga E, Geberhiwot T, Herrnstadt C, Howell N, Torroni A, Villems R (2003) Origin and diffusion of mtDNA haplogroup X. Am J Hum Genet 73:1178–1190

Richards M, Macaulay V, Hickey E, Vega E, Sykes B, Guida V, Rengo C, Sellitto D, Cruciani F, Kivisild T, Villems R, Thomas M, Rychkov S, Rychkov O, Rychkov Y, Gölge M, Dimitrov D, Hill E, Bradley D, Romano V, Calì F, Vona G, Demaine A, Papiha S, Triantaphyllidis C, Stefanescu G, Hatina J, Belledi M, Di Rienzo A, Novelletto A, Oppenheim A, Nørby S, Al-Zaheri N, Santachiara-Benerecetti S, Scozzari R, Torroni A, Bandelt HJ (2000) Tracing European founder lineages in the Near Eastern mtDNA pool. Am J Hum Genet 67:1251–1257

Richards M, Bandelt H-J, Kivisild T, Oppenheimer S (2006) A model for the dispersal of modern humans out of Africa. In: Bandelt H-J, Macaulay V, Richards M (eds) Human mitochondrial DNA and the evolution of homo sapiens. Springer, Berlin/Heidelberg

Salas A, Bandelt H-J, Macaulay V, Richards MB (2007) Phylogeographic investigations: the role of trees in forensic genetics. Forensic Sci Int 168:1–13

Simoni L, Calafell F, Pettener D, Bertranpetit J, Barbujani G (2000) Geographic patterns of mtDNA diversity in Europe. Am J Hum Genet 66:262–278

Soares P, Ermini L, Thomson N, Mormina M, Rito T, Röhl A, Salas A, Oppenheimer S, Macaulay V, Richards MB (2009) Correcting for purifying selection: an improved human mitochondrial molecular clock. Am J Hum Genet 84:740–759

Soares P, Achilli A, Semino O, Davies W, Macaulay V, Bandelt H-J, Torroni A, Richards MB (2010) The archaeogenetics of Europe. Curr Biol 20:R174–R183

Sun C, Kong QP, Palanichamy MG, Agrawal S, Bandelt H-J, Yao YG, Khan F, Zhu CL, Chaudhuri TK, Zhang YP (2006) The dazzling array of basal branches in the mtDNA macrohaplogroup M from India as inferred from complete genomes. Mol Biol Evol 23:683–690

Tamm E, Kivisild T, Reidla M, Metspalu M, Smith DG, Mulligan CJ, Bravi CM, Rickards O, Martinez-Labarga C, Khusnutdinova EK, Fedorova SA, Golubenko MV, Stepanov VA, Gubina MA, Zhadanov SI, Ossipova LP, Damba L, Voevoda MI, Dipierri JE, Villems R, Malhi RS (2007) Beringian standstill and spread of Native American founders. PLoS One 2:e829

Tishkoff SA, Reed FA, Friedlaender FR, Ehret C, Ranciaro A, Froment A, Hirbo JB, Awomoyi AA, Bodo JM, Doumbo O, Ibrahim M, Juma AT, Kotze MJ, Lema G, Moore JH, Mortensen H, Nyambo TB, Omar SA, Powell K, Pretorius GS, Smith MW, Thera MA, Wambebe C, Weber JL, Williams SM (2009) The genetic structure and history of Africans and African Americans. Science 324:1035–1044

van Oven M, Kayser M (2009) Updated comprehensive phylogenetic tree of global human mitochondrial DNA variation. Hum Mutat 30:E386–E394

Vigilant L, Stoneking M, Harpending H, Hawkes K, Wilson AC (1991) African populations and the evolution of human mitochondrial DNA. Science 253:1503–1507

Wallace DC (1995) 1994 William Allan award address. Mitochondrial DNA variation in human evolution, degenerative disease, and aging. Am J Hum Genet 57:201–223

Yao YG, Bravi CM, Bandelt H-J (2004) A call for mtDNA data quality control in forensic science. Forensic Sci Int 141:1–6

Index

A

Abacavir, 333, 348, 349, 351, 353, 359, 360
Acetyl-CoA, 216, 240, 241, 288, 359, 432
AD. *See* Alzheimer's disease (AD)
Adefovir, 348–351, 353
Adenine nucleotide translocase (ANT), 58, 161, 162, 217, 237, 255, 262, 295, 318, 339, 341, 399
Adenosine analogs, 351
ADOAD. *See* Autosomal dominant optic atrophy and deafness (ADOAD)
ADP/ATP ratio, 152, 237, 240, 251
Aging, 10, 41, 100, 152, 202, 236, 257, 270, 300, 311–322, 398
AHS. *See* Alpers-Huttenlocher disease (AHS)
Akt, 26, 113, 257, 289, 296, 429
Aldolase, 429, 433
Alpers-Huttenlocher disease (AHS), 188, 193, 195–199
ALS. *See* Amyotrophic lateral sclerosis (ALS)
Alzheimer's disease (AD), 41, 43, 45, 120, 172, 269–274, 276, 279, 334, 339, 340, 372
Aminoaciduria, 195
Aminoglycoside-induced deafness, 190–191
Amyloidosis, 272
Amyotrophic lateral sclerosis (ALS), 269, 276–277, 372
ANT. *See* Adenine nucleotide translocase (ANT)
Anthracycline, induced adducts, 391
Anthropology, 441–451
Anticancer therapy, 296, 341–342
Antineoplastic agents, 336
Antioxidants
 enzymatic antioxidants, 115–116
 non-enzymatic antioxidants, 116–117
Apoptosis
 anti-apoptotic proteins, 64, 65, 159, 162–164, 295, 302, 356
 inducing factor (AIF), 295
 and mitochondrial fission, 158, 170–171
 and mitochondrial fusion, 158, 170–174
 pro-apoptotic proteins, 64, 162, 163, 295, 302, 356
Apoptosome, 159–162, 295, 400

B

Bad protein, 403, 429
Bak protein, 64, 162, 163, 174, 401, 403
Barth syndrome, 123, 188, 201, 261
Bax protein, 64, 159, 162, 163, 165, 174, 295, 302, 401, 403
Bcl-2 family proteins, 114, 161–165, 167, 174, 400–404
BCL-W, 295, 403
Bcl-XL, 64, 160, 163, 167, 169, 294, 295, 302, 402–404
Bc_1, ubiquinone-cytochrome c oxidoreductase (Complex III), 10–13
Benzodiazepine
 inhibitors, 260
 receptors, 103, 339, 341
Beta amyloid (Aβ), 270
Beta-oxidation, 141, 188, 259, 289, 338, 341, 423, 430
Bezafibrate, 335
Bioenergetics, 67, 76, 84, 86, 88, 122, 125, 153, 188, 273, 278, 289–292, 312, 313, 315, 330, 334, 336, 339, 356, 373, 379, 398, 407, 423, 424, 434
Biomarkers, 42, 119, 121, 299, 319, 423–436
Breakage syndromes, 188, 193, 195

ATP production, 59–61, 152, 170, 172, 194, 202, 217, 218, 223, 224, 226, 228, 236, 238, 242, 243, 251–253, 260, 273, 275, 290, 315, 319, 353, 378, 424, 434
Autosomal dominant optic atrophy and deafness (ADOAD), 188, 202

C

Calcium (Ca^{2+})
 efflux, 56–58, 61, 63, 252, 260
 homeostasis, 54, 55, 57, 58, 64, 269, 407
 intracellular deposits, 54
 mediated apoptosis, 63–65
 receptor-operated channels (ROCs), 54
 regulated processes, 54, 62
 role, 54, 60, 252

R. Scatena et al. (eds.), *Advances in Mitochondrial Medicine*, Advances in Experimental Medicine and Biology 942, DOI 10.1007/978-94-007-2869-1,
© Springer Science+Business Media B.V. 2012

Calcium (Ca^{2+}) (*cont.*)
  second-messenger-operated channels (SMOCs), 54
  store-operated channels (SOCs), 54
  transport, 55–58, 60, 63, 250, 252–256, 262, 300
  transporters, 55
  uniporter (MCU), 56, 59, 252
  uptake, 54–58, 60–63, 68, 114, 252–256,
    259, 260
  voltage-operated channels (VOCs), 60
Caloric restriction, 122, 313, 314, 320–321
Cancer, 40, 63, 113, 166, 287–304, 321, 330, 387,
    423–436
  metabolism, 342
  stem cell, 288, 298, 304, 342
Carcinogenesis, 107, 117, 298, 300, 301, 304, 336, 430,
    432, 436
Cardiolipin, 82, 114, 119, 123, 125, 165, 201, 221, 261,
    262, 318, 331, 334, 340, 395, 397
Cardiomyocytes, 86, 251, 253, 313, 352, 386, 394, 395,
    397, 398, 402–406
Cardiomyopathy, 5, 43, 44, 189–191, 193, 194, 201, 204,
    205, 258–261, 318, 339, 348, 361, 373, 386,
    392–394, 396, 398, 399, 401, 403, 404
Cardioprotection, 86, 105, 255–257
Cardiotoxicity, 106, 355, 385–386, 388, 389, 391–397,
    400, 404–407
Caspase
  activators, 159, 160, 162
  adaptator, 162
  effector, 62, 160, 162, 401, 433
  inhibitor, 160, 162
  initiator, 159–162, 400, 401
Catalase, 6, 61, 63, 94, 116, 236, 238, 239, 258, 277,
    297, 314, 317, 319, 395
CED family, 162, 163
Cell
  cycle regulation, 165, 300
  death, 54, 58, 59, 62, 63, 65, 68, 88, 112, 114, 116,
    158–162, 167, 171, 173, 174, 239, 254, 255, 270,
    274, 277, 290, 294, 298, 300, 301, 314, 319, 330,
    339, 341, 354, 386, 390, 398–402, 404, 405, 433
  differentiation, 294, 301–304, 400
  lines, 47, 103, 125, 166, 167, 200, 271, 272, 275,
    290, 292, 303, 342, 387, 399, 402–405, 430–435
  proliferation, 112, 113, 170, 173, 239, 291, 292, 298,
    302, 304, 342, 391, 432, 433
  respiration, 83, 87, 88
  transformation, 302
Cellular senescence, 113, 122, 300, 320, 432
Chemotherapy, 168, 341, 391–394, 404, 405
Ciglitazone, 335
Citrate synthase (CS), 220, 221, 226, 237, 259, 276
Clofibric acid, 335
Clonazepam, 57, 254, 256, 260
CMT2A neuropathy, 202
C-MYC, 291, 292
Coenzyme Q (CoQ) deficiency, 200
Complex I (NADH-ubiquinone oxidoreductase), 8–10,
    77, 108, 303, 335, 372, 374, 375, 378, 395, 397
Complex II (succinate-Q reductase complex), 95

Complex III (bc$_1$, ubiquinone-cytochrome c
    oxidoreductase), 10–13
Complex IV (Cytochrome c oxidase), 13–17
Complex V (F$_1$F$_o$ ATP Synthase), 17–20
Congenital heart disease, 250
Copper-zinc superoxide dismutase (SOD1), 276, 277
CREB-binding protein, 25, 26, 278
CS. *See* Citrate synthase (CS)
CsA. *See* Cyclosporine-A (CsA)
Cybrid technique, 271, 275, 276
Cyclophilin D (CypD), 58, 161, 255–257, 339, 341,
    399, 400
Cyclosporine-A (CsA), 58, 150, 254–257, 262, 339,
    341, 400
Cytidine analogs, 350
Cytochrome c oxidase. *See* Complex IV (Cytochrome c
    oxidase)
Cytochrome, release of cytochrome c, 58, 64, 65,
    103, 161, 173, 174, 294, 339, 341, 356,
    400, 433
Cytokines, 239, 244, 356, 361, 400, 401, 405

D
Daunorubicin (DNR), 386, 387, 389, 392
Deafness dystonia syndrome (DSS), 201
Death effector domain (DED), 160
Degenerative disease, 123, 296, 312, 334, 341,
    348, 372
Diabetes
  and aging, 321
  type 2, 42, 152, 153, 215, 236, 239–244
Diabetes Insipidus, Diabetes Mellitus, Optic Atrophy,
    And Deafness (DIDMOAD), 188, 202
Didanosine, 333, 348–354, 357, 359
Diltiazem, 57, 256, 260
DJ-1 protein, 274
DNA depletion, 46, 196, 198, 199, 302, 352–355,
    360, 361
DNA Polymerase-g, 168, 314, 318, 319, 332, 334,
    352–355, 357, 358, 360, 361
DNR. *See* Daunorubicin (DNR)
Doxorubicin (DOX), 106, 336, 337, 386–389, 391–397,
    400, 403–407
Drug effects, 330–332, 338

E
ECM. *See* Extracellular matrix (ECM)
Electrochemical gradient, 22, 54, 56, 58, 138–142, 170,
    236, 237, 295, 303, 331, 336
Electro transport chain (ETC), 54, 63, 83, 103, 138, 217,
    219, 221, 222, 229, 236–238, 240, 241, 270–272,
    276, 278, 293, 316, 319, 321, 331, 334, 336, 353,
    359, 396–399, 423, 427
Emtricitabine, 348, 349, 351, 353, 359, 360
Encephalo-Myopathic MDD, 188, 198
Encephalomyopathy, 43–45, 188, 189, 193, 200, 203,
    205, 374
Entecavir, 348, 349, 351, 353, 354, 360

Epirubicin (EPI), 386, 387, 389, 391, 392
ETC. *See* Electro transport chain (ETC)
Extracellular matrix (ECM), 294, 335

F
FADH2, 137, 216, 290
FAS/FASL system, 404, 405
FFAs. *See* Free fatty acids (FFAs)
F_1F_0 ATP synthase. *See* Complex V (F_1F_0 ATP Synthase)
FH. *See* Fumarate hydratase (FH)
Fibrates, 303, 335, 336, 338
Forensic genetics, 447–450
Free fatty acids (FFAs), 56, 118, 130–148, 151, 216, 218, 219, 228, 238, 244, 359, 360
Free radicals, 5, 6, 58, 62, 63, 102, 103, 118–120, 151, 153, 228, 250, 253, 254, 256, 260, 270, 272, 273, 296, 312, 316, 317, 319, 333, 334, 336, 337, 340, 341, 375, 378, 392
Fumarate hydratase (FH), 293, 294, 335–337, 424

G
Gemfibrozil, 335
Glucose transporters
    GLUT1, 125, 291, 429
    GLUT3, 291
Glutamine (Gln), 278, 291–294
Glutathione (GSH), 6, 63, 94, 112, 113, 115–117, 120, 148, 236, 238, 292, 318, 337, 396
Glycolysis, 4, 84, 124, 125, 152, 166, 240, 287–291, 295, 297, 335, 341, 424, 428–430, 436
Golgi, 54, 64, 387
GRACILE syndrome, 188, 194
Guanosine analogs, 350

H
HD. *See* Huntington's disease (HD)
Heart failure, 123, 124, 189, 190, 194, 250, 257–261, 386, 392, 398, 403, 405
Heat shock proteins, mtHSP70 (mortalin), 22, 300, 432, 433
Hepatitis
    B, 349, 352, 353, 357
    C, 339, 357
Hepato-cerebral (encephalo-hepatic) MDDI, 198–199
Hexokinase (HK)
    HKI, 291
    HKII, 289, 291, 429
HIV disease, 334, 348, 349, 353, 356–361
HtrA2 protease, 65, 161, 162, 274, 375, 400
Huntington's disease (HD), 86, 269, 277–278, 372
Hypertrophy, 222, 257–259, 261, 392, 405, 406
Hypoxia, 76–78, 83, 84, 87, 104, 166, 253–255, 289–291, 429–432
Hypoxia-inducible factor (HIF), 87, 104, 113, 288–289, 293, 335, 407, 430, 432
Hypoxia/reoxygenation, 119, 256

I
ICDH. *See* Isocitrate dehydrogenase (ICDH)
Idarubicin (IDA), 386, 387, 389
IDH2. *See* Isocitrate dehydrogenase 2 (IDH2)
Infantile-onset spinocerebellar ataxia (IOSCA), 188, 199
Inherited mitochondrial disorders (MIDs), 187–206
    non syndromic, 188, 194, 203–206
    syndromic, 188–206
Insulin resistance, 152, 153, 215–230, 238–241, 243, 244
Intramitochondrial space, 375
IOSCA. *See* Infantile-onset spinocerebellar ataxia (IOSCA)
Ischemia (I), 76, 78, 84, 85, 104, 124, 125
Isocitrate dehydrogenase (ICDH), 59, 237, 251, 293, 431
Isocitrate dehydrogenase 2 (IDH2), 293, 294

J
JNK/SAPK, 238, 239, 334, 402, 403

K
Kearns-Sayre syndrome (KSS), 42, 188, 189, 192, 242, 261

L
Lactacidosis, 189, 190, 192, 194, 195, 197–200, 204, 205
Lactate dehydrogenase (LDH)
    A (LDH-A), 290, 291, 429, 430, 432
    B (LDH-B), 429
Lamivudine, 333, 348–354, 357, 359, 360
LBSL syndrome, 188, 199–200
Leber's hereditary optic neuropathy (LHON), 20, 41, 44–46, 188, 191, 202
Leigh syndrome (LS), 43–45, 188, 189, 193–194, 197, 200, 203, 205, 373
Leucine-rich repeat kinase 2 (LRRK2), 274
LHON. *See* Leber's hereditary optic neuropathy (LHON)
Lipid peroxidation, 97, 112, 115, 116, 118–120, 122, 124, 143, 228, 297, 318, 355, 389, 395
Lipotoxicity, 216, 218
LRRK2. *See* Leucine-rich repeat kinase 2 (LRRK2)

M
Magnetic resonance spectroscopy (^{31}P-MRS), 223–224, 275, 277
Manganese-superoxide dismutase (MnSOD), 5, 61, 63, 236, 238, 258, 317, 318, 336, 402
MAPKs. *See* Mitogen activated protein kinases (MAPKs)
Maternally inherited diabetes and deafness (MIDD), 189, 190
Mb. *See* Myoglobin (Mb)
MCHS disorder. *See* Myo-cerebro-hepatopathy-spectrum (MCHS) disorder
Mcl-1, 163, 165, 169, 294, 295, 403
MDDs. *See* Mitochondrial depletion disorders (MDDs)
MDM2. *See* Murine double minute 2 (MDM2)

MELAS. *See* Mitochondrial encephalomyopathy (MELAS)
Membrane potential ($\Delta\Psi_m$), 25, 56, 86, 97, 102, 103, 112, 114, 161, 172, 219, 258, 317, 342
Membranes
  inner mitochondrial (IMM), 4–8, 12, 17, 21, 24, 55–58, 61, 68, 95, 96, 100, 101, 103, 110, 139, 165, 170, 172, 173, 199, 217–219, 221, 236–238, 242, 256, 261, 289, 293, 295, 331, 335, 339, 340, 375, 376, 397, 398, 426
  intermembrane space (IMS), 12, 21, 22, 55, 56, 58, 60, 61, 68, 96, 98, 99, 101, 102, 104, 114, 161, 162, 166, 171–174, 216, 217, 220, 277, 317, 375, 423
  outer mitochondrial (OMM), 21, 22, 55, 56, 58, 60, 61, 64, 66–68, 95, 105, 114, 159, 161, 162, 166, 167, 170, 172, 202, 216, 274, 277, 289, 295, 339, 399, 400, 403, 404, 433
MEMSA. *See* Myoclonic epilepsy, myopathy, and sensory ataxia (MEMSA)
MERRF syndrome. *See* Myoclonus epilepsy with RRF (MERRF) syndrome
Metabolic disease, 41, 241, 243, 330, 342, 398, 427
MIDD. *See* Maternally inherited diabetes and deafness (MIDD)
MIDs. *See* Inherited mitochondrial disorders (MIDs)
MIRAS. *See* Mitochondrial autosomal recessive ataxia syndrome (MIRAS)
Mitochondria
  biogenesis, 168, 202–206
  density, 220–222, 226, 228, 230, 239, 240
  dynamics, 67, 170–174, 201, 202, 313, 375
  fission, 65–68, 170–171, 202–206, 220
  function, 40, 54, 86, 124, 215, 239, 252, 270, 290, 313, 330, 358, 372, 397, 424
  fusion, 65–68, 171–174, 202–206
  matrix, 6, 8, 17, 55–59, 96, 98, 104, 115, 121, 138, 221, 241, 252, 317, 318, 331–333, 337, 339, 355, 372, 377, 398, 423, 430
  morphology, 67, 170, 173, 174, 219–222, 313, 353
  protein import, 26, 277
  as therapeutic targets, 294, 425
  trafficking, 65–68, 139, 169
Mitochondrial autosomal recessive ataxia syndrome (MIRAS), 188, 195, 196
Mitochondrial depletion disorders (MDDs), 197–199
Mitochondrial DNA (mtDNA)
  alterations in human diseases, 40, 46
  analysis, 446–449, 451
  common deletion, 42, 275, 276
  copy number alterations, 46
  duplications, 315, 333
  haplogroup, 41, 445–447
  haplotypes' database, 449, 450
  heteroplasmy, 40, 44–46
  mutation, 40–48, 122, 168, 188–193, 203, 243, 270, 272, 275, 298–299, 312–316, 319–322, 352, 355, 358, 377, 398
  mutations in protein coding genes, 44
  mutations in the control region or D-loop, 39, 42, 299, 442
  mutations in translational machinery, 43–44
  polymorphism, 41, 47, 115, 242, 272
Mitochondrial dysfunction, 40, 46, 47, 63, 68, 116, 216, 217, 225–230, 236, 239, 240, 242–244, 252–256, 258, 259, 269–275, 277, 278, 297, 316, 318, 332, 334, 336, 340, 348, 352, 360, 361, 375, 386, 394–396, 399–401, 406, 425
Mitochondrial encephalomyopathy (MELAS), 43–46, 188–191
Mitochondrial genome, 8, 13, 20, 23, 25, 39, 40, 168, 220, 261, 298, 299, 316, 319, 331, 333, 342, 397, 398, 424, 428, 444, 445, 447, 448
Mitochondrial myopathy, 43, 45, 192, 197, 200
Mitochondrial neuro-gastrointestinal encephalopathy (MNGIE), 188, 193, 195–196
Mitochondrial outer membrane permeabilization (MOMP), 158, 161, 162, 166, 167, 169, 171, 174, 295, 296, 400–404
Mitochondrial permeability transition pore (MPTP), 55, 58, 61, 63–65, 76, 103, 107, 115, 249, 250, 252–257, 262, 273, 295, 331, 334, 339, 341, 397, 399–400, 435
Mitochondrial pharmacology, 330, 342
Mitochondrial phosphoproteome, 435
Mitochondrial proteome, 25, 120, 425–428, 430, 434, 435
Mitochondrial toxicity, 333, 334, 338, 341, 348, 349, 352–361
Mitochondrial transcription factor (TFAM)
Mitofusin 2 (Mfn2), 60, 66–68, 171–173, 202, 229, 231, 330
Mitogen activated protein kinases (MAPKs), 296, 401–403
MNGIE. *See* Mitochondrial neuro-gastrointestinal encephalopathy (MNGIE)
MnSOD. *See* Manganese-superoxide dismutase (MnSOD)
MOMP. *See* Mitochondrial outer membrane permeabilization (MOMP)
MPTP. *See* Mitochondrial permeability transition pore (MPTP)
^{31}P-MRS. *See* Magnetic resonance spectroscopy (^{31}P-MRS)
mtDNA. *See* Mitochondrial DNA (mtDNA)
Multisystem disease, 191, 194
Murine double minute 2 (MDM2), 168, 169, 401, 402
Myo-cerebro-hepatopathy-spectrum (MCHS) disorder, 188, 195, 197
Myoclonic epilepsy, myopathy, and sensory ataxia (MEMSA), 188, 195–197
Myoclonus epilepsy with RRF (MERRF) syndrome, 189–190
Myoglobin (Mb), 76, 82, 85, 200, 225
Myopathic MDD, 188, 198
Myopathy, lactacidosis, and sideroblastic anemia (MLASA), 188, 189, 200

Index
459

N

NADH. *See* Nicotinamide adenine dinucleotide (NADH)

NADH-ubiquinone oxidoreductase. *See* Complex I (NADH-ubiquinone oxidoreductase)

NADPH, 63, 95, 104, 105, 107, 116, 117, 121, 237–241, 258, 288, 292, 293, 295, 389, 395

Na^+/K^+-ATPase, 253

NARP disease. *See* Neurogenic weakness, ataxia, and retinitis pigmentosa (NARP) disease

ND5 gene, 9, 44, 46, 47, 189, 194, 372, 376–378

ND6 gene, 9, 44, 47, 189, 191, 194, 299, 372, 376–378

NDUFS1 gene, 9, 194, 373, 379

NDUFS4 gene, 9, 10, 21, 22, 194, 373, 374, 379

Neoplasias, 428, 430, 431, 435

Neoplasm metabolism, 297

Neurodegenerative disease, 41, 68, 158, 171, 269–270, 276, 278, 279, 313, 332, 337, 375, 380, 400

Neurogenic weakness, ataxia, and retinitis pigmentosa (NARP) disease, 20, 44, 45, 191–192, 194

NF-kB, 238, 239

Nicotinamide adenine dinucleotide (NADH), 4, 6, 7, 61, 77, 78, 95–98, 101, 102, 104, 111, 116, 137, 140, 145, 216, 219, 221, 236, 237, 240–242, 251, 259, 290, 293–295, 302–304, 317, 338, 340, 355, 378, 423

Nitric oxide (NO)

and Complex I, 77–83, 86

and Complex IV, 76–83, 86–88

mitochondrial chemistry, 75–88

and pathophysiological relevance, 75–88

Nitric oxide synthase (NOS), 5, 77, 87, 88, 105–106, 258, 395

Nitrite

metabolic role, 84–85

pathway, 81–83

Nitrosative stress, 78, 80, 86, 88, 296, 297, 395–396

Nitrosyl pathway, 79–80, 82, 83

NRTI-associated toxicity, 349, 361, 385

NRTIs. *See* Nucleoside/nucleotide reverse transcriptase inhibitors (NRTIs)

Nuclear DNA (nDNA), 20, 23, 42, 121–123, 187, 188, 193–206, 258, 261, 272, 312, 317, 318, 331, 332, 335, 347, 353, 357, 373, 380, 390, 398, 425, 448, 450

Nuclear magnetic resonance (NMR), 223, 224, 230, 277, 315

Nucleoside/nucleotide reverse transcriptase inhibitors (NRTIs), 333, 334, 348, 349, 352, 353, 355–361

O

Obesity, 149, 150, 152, 153, 215, 216, 226, 227, 230, 330, 342

Oct, 291

OMI/HTRA2, 65, 161, 162, 274, 400

Oncogenic mutations, 293, 294

Oncoproteomics, 429–434, 436

Oxidative damages, 10, 42, 106, 115, 118, 120–122, 150, 153, 218, 273, 297, 312, 313, 316–318, 321, 333, 336, 353, 375, 395–398, 424, 429

Oxidative phosphorylation (OXPHOS), 3–27, 39, 41, 44, 46, 56, 61, 76, 84–87, 95, 106, 109, 110, 120, 122, 124, 125, 139, 141–143, 150, 152, 170, 172, 188, 217, 218, 220, 223, 224, 227, 228, 236–238, 250, 254, 255, 258, 260, 288–291, 312–315, 318, 319, 321, 332, 334, 335, 337–341, 348, 353, 355, 359, 371, 372, 377, 396–399, 423, 427, 429, 434, 436

Oxidative stress, 62, 94, 100, 104–107, 112–115, 117, 119–121, 123–125, 152, 153, 238, 239, 244, 250, 252, 255–259, 272–274, 276, 278, 290–292, 296–298, 300, 302, 313, 314, 316, 319–321, 334, 335, 338, 355, 356, 359, 361, 392, 394, 396, 398, 402, 406, 407, 424, 430

Oxoglutarate dehydrogenase (OGDH), 251, 259

P

p53

functions on mitochondria, 166–170

mitochondrial localization, 166–168

mitochondrial targeting, 169–170

Pancreatic cells, 357

Parkin, 45, 171, 274, 375, 378–379

Parkinson's disease, 41, 42, 86, 107, 125, 171, 243, 269, 273–276, 279, 334, 335, 339, 372, 375–380

Pearson-syndrome, 188, 192–193, 242

PEO. *See* Progressive external ophthalmoplegia (PEO)

Peroxisome proliferator activated receptor (PPAR), 223, 303, 342

Peroxisome proliferator-activated receptor gamma coactivator 1-alpha (PGC-1α), 25, 26, 223, 226, 275, 278

Peroxynitrite ($ONOO^-$), 5, 63, 80, 84, 88, 95, 105, 118, 120, 236, 336, 355, 395

PGC-1α. *See* Peroxisome proliferator-activated receptor gamma coactivator 1-alpha (PGC-1α)

Pharmacological approach, 342

Pharmacotoxicology, 331–332, 335, 336

Phosphofructokinase (PFK), isoenzyme 3 (PFKFB3), 291

Phosphoglycerate kinase (PGK), 291

Phosphoglycerate mutase (PGM),

Phosphorylation signalling pathways, 296

Phylogenetics, 23, 47, 57, 298, 442–444, 449, 450

PINK 1. *See* PTEN induced kinase 1 (PINK 1)

p58 MAPK, 25, 26, 56, 238, 269, 402, 403

Polymerase chain reaction (PCR) analyses, 316, 358

Pontocerebellar Hypoplasia, 199

Porines, 56

PPAR-ligands, 342

Progressive external ophthalmoplegia (PEO), 42–45, 189, 190, 192, 193, 195, 199, 202

Prohibitin, 173, 300, 434

Proton electrochemical gradient, 5, 17, 58, 95, 98

Proton leakage, 172, 290, 314

Protonophores, 57, 337

PTEN induced kinase 1 (PINK 1), 171, 274, 375–380

PUMA, 162–166, 295, 402–404
Pyruvate dehydrogenase (PDH), 54, 59, 104, 194, 237,
       240, 251–254, 259, 270, 271, 359, 432
Pyruvate kinase (PK), M2-PK, 429

R
RAS, 291, 301
Reactive nitrogen species (RNS), 94, 112, 113, 117, 120,
       236, 244, 296–298, 330, 334, 340, 401
Reactive oxygen species (ROS)
    and advanced glycation end products (AGE),
         118, 121
    and cell signalling, 94, 112–114
    and DNA damage, 114, 276, 297, 312, 313, 317, 318,
         331, 334, 340, 398
    generating reactions, 103, 105, 147, 395
    homeostasis, 94, 112, 113, 115, 152, 166, 359, 372,
         399, 424
    and lipid peroxidation, 97, 112, 115, 118–120, 122,
         124, 228, 297, 318, 355
    modulation of ROS production, 102–103
    mtROS in pathology, 44, 46, 102, 103, 113, 114,
         123–126, 149, 150, 239, 258, 296, 298, 302, 314,
         316–321
    and protein oxidation, 115, 119–120,
         276, 395
    sources of, 95–108
Redox centers, 4–6, 10, 11, 13, 15, 79,
       138, 372
Reperfusion (R), 76, 124, 125, 250–258,
       262, 332
Respiratory capacity, 230, 242, 270, 321
Respiratory chain complexes (RCC)
    assembly, 24, 25, 188, 372, 379
    biogenesis, 24–25, 188
    structure, 103, 110, 172, 188, 340
    supercomplexes, 24, 96, 109–111, 123–125
    transcriptional factors controlling the biogenesis,
         24–25
Respiratory control ratio, 314
RNS. *See* Reactive nitrogen species (RNS)
ROS. *See* Reactive oxygen species (ROS)
rRNA mutations, 43, 190–191
Ruthenium red (RuR), 56, 249, 253–255

S
SANDO. *See* Sensory ataxia, neuropathy, dysarthria,
       and ophthalmoplegia (SANDO)
Sarco-endoplasmic reticulum (SR/ER), 54, 63
SDH. *See* Succinate dehydrogenase (SDH)
Second mitochondrial activator of caspases (SMAC),
       294, 400
Sensory ataxia, neuropathy, dysarthria, and
       ophthalmoplegia (SANDO), 188, 195, 196
Signalling pathways, 94, 113, 114, 238, 239, 257, 291,
       296, 297, 301, 302, 335, 394, 400, 406, 429
SMAC. *See* Second mitochondrial activator of caspases
       (SMAC)

Smac/DIABLO, 62, 65, 161, 162, 295, 296, 400
Small ubiquitin-like modifier (SUMO), 170, 171
SODI. *See* Copper-zinc superoxide dismutase (SOD1)
SR/ER. *See* Sarco-endoplasmic reticulum (SR/ER)
State 3, 124, 141–146, 150, 218, 219,
       314, 337
State 4, 99, 103, 104, 141, 142, 145–147,
       150, 218
Stavudine, 333, 348–354, 357, 360
Succinate dehydrogenase (SDH)
    assembly factor (SDHAF2), 293
    SDHA, 194, 293
    SDHB, 293
    SDHC, 100, 293
    SDHD, 100, 293
Succinate-Q reductase *See* Complex II (succinate-Q
       reductase complex)
SUMO. *See* Small ubiquitin-like modifier (SUMO)
α-Synuclein protein, 273

T
TCA. *See* Tricarboxycylic acid (TCA) cycle
Telbivudine, 348–351, 353, 357
Tenofovir, 349–351, 353, 359
Tetramethyl-p-phenylendiamine (TMPD), 76, 82, 83,
       87, 376
Thymidine analogs, 352
Thymidine kinase-2 (TK2), 197, 198,
       352, 354
TNF-α. *See* Tumor necrosis factor-α (TNF-α)
TNF related apoptosis inducing ligand (TRAIL),
       401, 404–406
Topoisomerases, directed anticancer drugs,
       390, 391
Toxic effects, 335, 339, 343
TRAIL. *See* TNF related apoptosis inducing
       ligand (TRAIL)
Translation defects, 188, 199–200
TRAP1, 375, 377
Tricarboxycylic acid (TCA) cycle, 216, 224,
       230, 235–237, 240, 241, 291–294,
       424, 430
Tumor markers, 302, 429, 431
Tumor necrosis factor-α (TNF-α), 165, 239, 244, 357,
       401, 404, 405

U
Uncoupling proteins (UCPs)
    activity, 56, 103, 137–153, 236, 237, 342
    mitochondrial anion carrier family (MACF),
         138, 139
    pathological implications, 153
    physiological roles, 56, 138, 149–153
    proton and electron leaks, 140
    uncoupling protein 1 (UCP1), 138–146,
         148–152
    uncoupling protein 2 (UCP2), 139, 144, 146,
         149–153, 242

V

Voltage dependent anion-selective channels (VDAC), 55, 56, 58, 60, 61, 67, 102, 158, 161, 162, 165, 255, 289, 295, 296, 317, 331, 429

W

Warburg effect, 288, 289, 291, 295, 300, 303, 330, 341, 342, 428–430, 432, 436

Wolfram syndrome (WFS), 202

X

X-Linked Sideroblastic Anemia with Ataxia (XLSA/A), 201

Z

Zalcitabine, 333, 348–354, 356, 357

Zidovudine, 333, 348–357, 359, 360

Printed by Printforce, the Netherlands